Mental
Retardation

Mental Retardation
Nature, Cause, and Management

Second Edition

GEORGE S. BAROFF
Developmental Disabilities Training Institute
and Department of Psychology
University of North Carolina at Chapel Hill

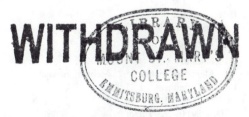

HEMISPHERE PUBLISHING CORPORATION, Washington
A subsidiary of Harper & Row, Publishers, Inc.

Cambridge New York Philadelphia San Francisco
London Mexico City São Paulo Singapore Sydney

MENTAL RETARDATION: Nature, Cause, and Management; Second Edition

1 2 3 4 5 6 7 8 9 0   E B E B   8 9 8 7 6

This book was set in Times Roman by Hemisphere Publishing Corporation. The editors were Christine Flint Lowry, Amy J. Whitmer, and Allison Brown; the designer was Sharon Martin DePass; the production supervisor was Peggy M. Rote; and the typesetter was Cynthia B. Mynhier.
Edwards Brothers, Inc., was printer and binder.

Library of Congress Cataloging-in-Publication Data

Baroff, George S.
  Mental retardation.

  Bibliography: p.
  Includes index.
    1. Mental retardation.   2. Mentally handicapped—
Care and treatment.   I. Title
RC570.B27   1985   616.85′88   85-8525
ISBN 0-89116-263-1 (cloth)
ISBN 0-89116-457-X (paper)

DEDICATION

To my wife Rishie—she has taught me the meaning of loyalty and courage.

To Bobbie Phillips, our Administrative Assistant, another personifier of loyalty.

To Ray Newnam, the long-time heart and conscience of the Institute. If I needed an "advocate," I'd choose Ray.

To recent and current colleagues in the Institute who have shown their commitment on behalf of handicapped persons:

Tony Dalton
Leslie Houston
Al Singer
Rudy Buckman
Suzi White
Mike Pickett
Meg Anderson
Toni James-Manus
Roger Manus

And to the staff that supports us:
Nancy Dotson
Judy Hall
Judy Jackson

Contents

10   Management of Behavior Problems Prominent in Severe
       and Profound Retardation   **415**

Preface

The content of this second edition, like that of its predecessor, reflects experiences in both undergraduate and graduate instruction and in the in-service training of workers in community and institutional mental retardation programs. The book offers the student a comprehensive treatment of mental retardation—what it is, what its causes are, and what you do about it. For the worker, professional or paraprofessional, there is the possibility of more selective use—dipping into chapters or sections that relate to the specific services with which one is involved.

The book retains its original organization. The first half presents what might be considered the "scientific" aspect of mental retardation—its nature and causation, while the latter half focuses on the service needs of retarded persons and their families and the programs provided to meet them.

The revision contains two new chapters—one on personality and mental retardation and including the related disorders of autism and learning disability, and the other on the management of behavior problems. The latter reflects the special concerns created by attempting to serve all segments of the retarded population in the community. The former presents a personality model through which the psychological problems of the retarded individual and family members can be understood. Its special focus is on our need for "self-esteem," the experiences that foster it, and how this need can be frustrated by mental retardation.

With regard to the book itself, the first chapter is devoted to the "nature" of mental retardation. There is an expanded treatment of intelligence as a way of introducing the disorder and calling attention to its essence. The nature of mental retardation is depicted in terms of the three components of the current definition of the American Association on Mental Deficiency: subaverage general intelligence, adaptive impairment, and onset during the "developmental" years. The chapter provides excerpts from the lives of two retarded individuals and concludes with "expectancy" tables for probable levels of functioning at maturity for each of the four degrees of retardation.

Chapter 2 is one of the two new chapters and, as noted, offers a "need" model of personality through which the psychological needs of all of us, normal and retarded, can be understood. Common personality characteristics and problem behaviors are described, and this is followed by descriptions of two other related disorders, autism and learning disability. Treatment procedures are introduced and then presented in depth in subsequent chapters.

Chapters 3 through 5 are concerned with the second major aspect of the condition, its causation. Chapters 3 and 4 are devoted to biological determinants, and Chapter 5 to psychological ones. Chapter 3 deals with chromosomal and gene-determined forms of retardation, while Chapter 4 describes the nongenetic biological conditions that can cause retardation during pregnancy, at birth, and postnatally. Chapter 4 contains a brand-new section on drug effects on the fetus and neonate and gives particular attention to chemical substances currently widely abused. Chapter 5 shifts the emphasis from the biological to the psychological. It describes the contribution of the psychological environment to the development of intelligence, the possibility of preventing "nonorganic" forms of retardation through early intervention, and the ingredients of "effective parenting."

The second half of the book is devoted to "services." These are introduced in Chapter 6 with sections on the "right" to services, the significance of normalization, and an overview of the full array of services from those of prevention and infancy to those for adults. Chapters 7 through 9 present the services within a developmental framework—from infancy to adulthood. Chapter 7 describes infant and preschool programs for retarded children. This chapter has been much expanded to reflect the proliferation of home-based and day center programs for these children and their families. And in light of the prominence of motor disorders in retarded children served in infancy and early childhood programs, a special section has been devoted to this topic.

Chapters 8 and 9 present both school-age and adult programs. Adult services commonly include educational activities and are therefore treated with school-age ones in the same chapters. Chapter 8 focuses on two topics, education and recreation. In education there is discussion of special education and mainstreaming, strategy training, and teaching methods for persons with profound retardation. The second part of the chapter describes the recreational needs of and services to retarded youth and adults, an oft-neglected area. Chapter 9 limits its focus to adolescent and adult services. Three topics are addressed—vocational, sexual, and residential. The vocational one describes the work potential of retarded youth and refers to evidence for some vocational capacity at even severe and profound levels of impairment. This chapter also includes a much-expanded treatment of sexuality in retarded youth and adults and the concerns of their parents and caregivers. It acknowledges retarded people as "sexual" and offers suggestions for assisting them in the management of their sexuality in socially appropriate ways. The third topic describes the growing array of residential options to the family home. It cites the research on the adaptive behavior benefits associated with community living and also characterizes the current status of our institutions and the population they increasingly serve.

The final chapter is devoted wholly to the management of the severe behavior problems seen in the most impaired segment of the population. Its focus is on the "behavioral" approach, and examples and procedures are offered for coping with aggression, stereotypic and self-injurious behavior, rumination, and pica. Though these problems are particularly prominent in those with profound retardation, they are found at all levels, and the treatment methods described have application to the full range of the retarded population.

Finally, in writing a new edition, the author has tried constantly to keep "readability" in the foreground. The first edition was considered readable; I hope that this one is also.

George S. Baroff

Preface
to the First Edition

The content of this book grew out of (1) classroom teaching of undergraduates and graduates, (2) supervising clinical psychology graduate students in the assessment of mentally retarded persons, and (3) training workers in community and institutional mental retardation programs. The author saw the need for a text that could deal adequately with *both* the scientific and practical aspects of mental retardation. Traditionally, books in this area have focused on the scientific side with relatively little attention to its practical dimension—the range of services which have been and are being developed at community and institutional levels. The present book seeks to balance the scientific with the practical as it presents both an in-depth treatment of the nature and causes of mental retardation and a description of the full array of services designed to assist retarded persons. With reference to "nature," the first chapter consists of an analysis of retardation as seen through the *1961 and 1973 "definitions"* of the American Association on Mental Deficiency and the offerings of *norms* of behavioral expectations based on mental age, chronological age, and degree of retardation. The second and third chapters deal, respectively, with *biological* and *psychological* factors; particular attention is paid to explaining *basic genetic principles* and to showing the *interrelationship* of genetic and environmental factors. The fourth and fifth chapters consist of an overview of mental retardation services—*prevention, identification, education, training, recreation, employment,* and *residential.* In the realm of "identification" (diagnosis), there is analysis of the diagnostic process from a multidisciplinary standpoint (medicine, psychology, social work, public health nursing) with particular emphasis on the role of the psychologist and on the assessment process itself. Much attention is also paid to the related diagnostic problems of childhood psychosis, autism, and organicity or brain damage. Chapter 6 begins the detailed presentation of service programs and it focuses on the *preschool* child.

It presents the objectives of preschool programs, describes the principles of behavior modification and their implementation in such programs, and offers a picture of the growth of the retarded child against a backdrop of normal child development. Chapter 7 addressed *school-age* programs. It includes a review of the so-called "efficacy" research, a presentation of curriculum objectives and appropriate organizational structures for their achievement, and treatment of special topics—work-study programs, sexuality in mental retardation, and direct efforts to alter mental functioning through cognitive training. Chapter 8 considers the *employability* of retarded persons in terms of competitive work, employment in sheltered workshops, and participation in activity centers. Chapter 9 looks at our large *residential institutions* and considers both their problems and possibilities while the last chapter offers *residential alternatives* at the community level (foster homes, group homes, and apartments).

Throughout the presentation of the "services" there is an interweaving of related scientific aspects so that one gains a sense of the theoretical basis on which they rest as well as the research that pertains to their effectiveness. For the *student* the book offers a comprehensive view of all aspects of mental retardation while *workers* in the field can dip into it selectively and find whole chapters or major portions thereof devoted to the particular programs in which they're engaged. My goal was to produce a book that could be useful at more than one level; I hope that I've succeeded.

George S. Baroff

September 1974

Mental
Retardation

The Nature of Mental Retardation

OVERVIEW

This is a book about *people* who have difficulty in coping with some of life's adjustive tasks because of *impaired general intelligence*. The extent of their coping or adaptive difficulty is primarily related to the degree of intellectual impairment, though it is also much affected by both society's general attitude toward persons with limited intelligence and the services provided to them. For individuals with relatively mild deficit, the impact may be largely confined to academic progress during the school years and to the level of job aspiration in adulthood. At more severe levels of deficit, virtually every aspect of living is involved, the paramount effect being to render the person incapable of assuming the degree of independence expected in our culture.

This book covers each of the three major dimensions of mental retardation— its nature, its cause, and its management. In the first two chapters, its *nature* is examined with the focus directed toward the intellectual, personality, and adaptive problems of the retarded individual and their effect on parents and siblings. In the next three chapters the *causation* of mental retardation is explored in terms of biological and psychological determinants. The remaining five chapters are devoted to the *management* of mental retardation—to the range of services developed for its prevention, detection, and habilitation from infancy to adulthood. The goal of habilitation services for retarded persons is not different from that for nonhandicapped ones—to enable each of us to achieve the highest level of competence of which we are capable.

In this initial chapter we consider (a) the nature of the intelligence; (b) issues related to the classification of individuals as mentally retarded; (c) the current definition of mental retardation as promulgated by the American Association on Mental Deficiency (AAMD); (d) a detailed elaboration of each of the three components of the AAMD definition—subaverage general intelligence, associated deficits in "adaptive behavior," and onset during the "development period"; and (e) expected levels of functioning at maturity as related to degree of mental retardation.

ON THE NATURE OF INTELLIGENCE

Historical and contemporary views have stressed several kinds of behaviors as reflective of "intelligence"—the ability to *learn* and *profit from experience* and to acquire knowledge in so doing, the ability to *reason,* and the ability to *adapt* to changing conditions (Sternberg, 1981). Each of these is "cognitive" in nature, but a fourth one, a motivational component, has also been posited (Sternberg, 1981). This is a kind of *will to succeed.*

Underlying "Factors" and "Processes"

Behaviors reflecting learning ability, knowledge, and adaptation can be re- garded as the outward manifestation or end product of more fundamental elements. There have been two approaches to the exploration of these underlying elements. One seeks to describe them in terms of *basic mental capacities,* whereas the other focuses on the *processes* actually used in problem solving. Of the two, the latter seems to offer a more fundamental understanding of intelligence and also includes elements that in recent years have been the subject of much research in mental retardation.

BASIC MENTAL CAPACITIES: THE "FACTORIAL" APPROACH

The factorial approach is the product of the statistical technique of factor analysis. The technique has been employed with various measures of intelligence for the purpose of seeking to isolate the fewest common factors that will explain the correlations between them. In the domain of intelligence we can distinguish two main factorial theories. One views intelligence as a relatively unitary phenom- enon, and the other sees it as composed of numerous independent abilities.

INTELLIGENCE AS RELATIVELY UNITARY

The creator of factor analysis, Spearman, regarded intelligence as depending on a single general factor (g) and on an indeterminate number of specific abilities (s) (Spearman, 1923, 1927). The general factor was found in all tests of intelli- gence as reflected in the positive correlation found among presumably different measures. Spearman's g continues to have a prominent role in theories of intelli- gence. Kaufman (1975), for example, considers that the Verbal Scale and Full Scale IQs on the Wechsler tests of intelligence are good measures of g. There has been little interest in $s,$ presumably because these "specific" abilities did not lend themselves to any form of reduction or grouping.

In 1923 Spearman characterized g as involving the apprehension of experi- ence, the educing of relations, and the educing of correlates (Spearman, 1923).

Sternberg (1980) illustrates Spearman's meaning in terms of a simple analogy; Lawyer:Client = Doctor: _____ . *Apprehension* refers to the mental *encoding* of each term in the analogy, recognizing its meaning. *Educing of relations* refers to the *inferring* of the relation between lawyer and client, and *educing of correlates* refers to the *application* of the "educed" relationship to "Doctor" so as to produce the missing term "Patient." To us, the task seems to reflect basic deductive reasoning. We shall again encounter encoding, inferring, and application as elements in the "process" approach to intelligence.

HIERARCHICAL MODELS OF *g*

Some more recent theorists, while accepting the primacy of *g,* consider that *g* alone does not offer a complete enough explanation of intelligence. They propose a hierarchical model with *g* at the highest level and subsuming at least two major ability subgroupings.

Cattell (1971) and Horn (1968) have identified core abilities called "crystallized" and "fluid." *Crystallized* ability represents the kind of capacity involved in answering questions on general information and word meaning and on understanding what one has read. It correlates closely with standard intelligence test scores and is distinguished from "fluid" ability in being much influenced by experience.

Fluid ability is represented by reasoning in nonverbal and visual-spatial contexts (see Fig. 1). In contrast with crystallized intelligence, tasks involving fluid intelligence are seen as relatively unpracticed in our culture. Cattell has been particularly interested in trying to develop "culture-fair" measures of intelligence.

Another two-stage hierarchical model is offered by Vernon (1971). Again, two major abilities are subsumed under *g*—"verbal-educational" and "practical-mechanical." The *verbal-education* factor is represented by tasks involving the use of language and appears to be very similar to crystallized ability in that it also incorporates a "verbal" and "educational" component. The *practical-mechanical* ability factor, like fluid intelligence, is also represented by nonverbal visual-spatial tasks, but the cognitive skills incorporated therein have more to do with understanding *spatial relationships* than with pure reasoning. Examples of practical-mechanical ability are matching block designs and assembling puzzles. This ability also incorporates some "mechanical" understanding.

INTELLIGENCE AS MULTIFACTORIAL

In contrast with theorists who regard *g* as underlying all mental functions, multifactorial ones have either deemphasized or rejected the role of *g* and have instead identified abilities that are regarded as independent of each other. Two of the best-known multifactor theories are those of the Thurstones (Thurstone, L. L., 1938; Thurstone, L. L., & Thurstone, T. G., 1941) and Guilford (1967).

The Thurstones' "Primary Mental Abilities"

The Thurstones identified a number of separate abilities, though they also found some evidence of *g*. The best known of their "primary mental abilities" are presented along with the kinds of intelligence test items that represent them. They

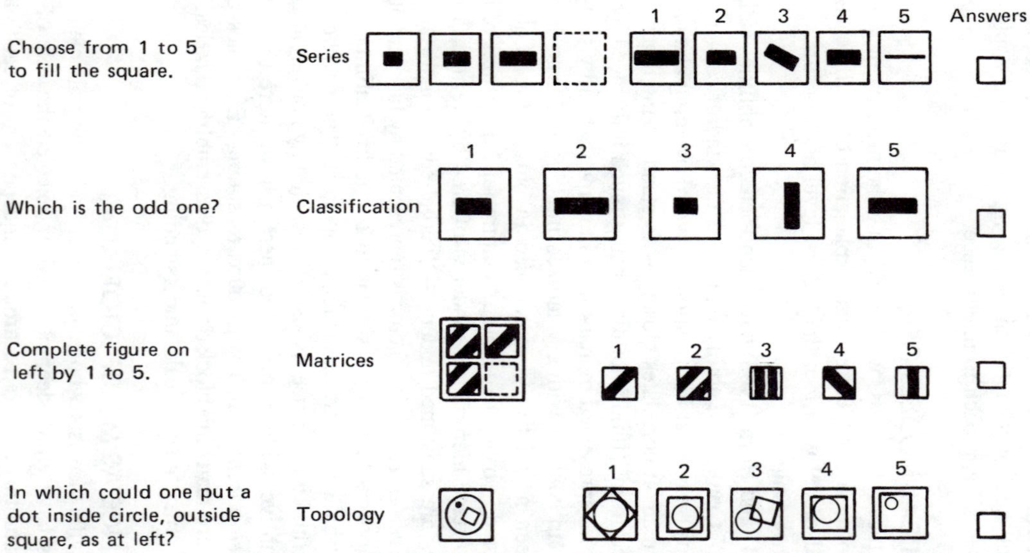

FIG. 1 Four forms of subtests of fluid intelligence (Excerpts from Culture-Fair Intelligence Scales 1, 2, and 3). From Cattell (1971b), by permission of Grune & Stratton.

are (a) *verbal comprehension* (reading comprehension, verbal analysis, disarranged sentences, verbal reasoning, and proverbs); (b) *number* (speed and accuracy of simple computations); (c) *space* (understanding spatial relationships); (d) *memory* (rote memory as in the immediate recall of a series of digits); and (e) *reasoning* (understanding syllogisms or finding a "rule").

Guilford's Three-Dimensional Model

By far the most complex of the factorial approaches, the Guilford model, conceptualizes intelligence in terms of three dimensions—operations, content, and products of information.

Operations are basic cognitive capacities and represent another way of depicting "primary" abilities. Five operations are postulated: *cognition* (knowing or grasping items of information); *memory* (recalling information); *divergent production* (generating alternatives); *convergent production* (identifying a best *single* choice among options); and *evaluation* (reaching judgments based on some standard).

Content refers to the "form" of the information the basic operations must process. Four types are represented—figural (pictorial), symbolic (numbers, letters, codes), semantic (words), and behavioral ("reading" the meaning of the behavior of others and ourselves). As will be seen, "content" has particular relevance for mental retardation. Though retarded individuals share the same operations as nonretarded persons (Guilford & Hoepfner, 1971), they certainly do better in the processing of figural (nonverbal) information than of semantic. This difference also is reflected in the Vernon model. Retarded persons tend to perform better on "practical-mechanical" tasks than on "verbal-educational" ones.

Products of information are the kinds of logical outcomes of the interactions between operations and content. Six kinds of products are proposed: *units* (relatively circumscribed ideas of information), *classes* (conceptions that underly items of information and permit their being grouped), *relations* (items of information with some specific connections), *systems* (organized aggregates of information), *transformations* (redefinition of items of information), and *implications* (expectancies growing from a piece of information). In Guilford's model, the interaction of five operations, four contents, and six products creates 120 possible different abilities (5 × 4 × 6)!

Of the three dimensions, "operations" has probably been of greatest interest to psychologists as they have sought to interpret items on intelligence tests according to these categories. With reference to the most widely used intelligence test for school-age children and adults, the Wechsler scales, subtest items have been grouped as (a) vocabulary (*cognition*), (b) comprehension (*evaluation*) (c) digit span (*memory*), and (d) picture arrangement (*convergent production* and *evaluation*). Items pertaining to *divergent production,* a measure of originality and creativity, are generally absent from current intelligence tests (Kaufman, 1979; Sattler, 1974).[1] Parenthetically, it should be acknowledged that the content of such univer-

---

[1]Meeker (1969) has been a major interpreter of the Guilford model in terms of the Wechsler tests and has also suggested its possible application in the classroom (Meeker, 1973).

sally used intelligence tests as the Wechsler scales and the Stanford-Binet have probably much more heavily influenced the conception of intelligence of their users than theories of intelligence per se.

INTELLIGENCE AS "PROCESS"

In distinguishing between the factorial and process approaches, the analogy of still and motion pictures seems appropriate. With the factorial approach represented by still pictures, "the process" one presumes to show us those same factors in action.

Piaget may be regarded as representing an intermediate position between factor and process theories. His theory still consists of a series of snapshots but ones taken fairly close together and over time. His major contribution has been the careful description of the *development* of thinking from infancy to maturity. He has identified four major stages in the development of intelligence: sensorimotor, preoperational, concrete operations, and formal operations (Flavell, 1963; Piaget, 1952). These stages are also presumed to represent the kinds of thinking seen in mentally retarded individuals, persons whose mental development at maturity will not have progressed to the stage of formal operations (Inhelder, 1968; Woodward, 1963, 1962).

Sensorimotor Intelligence

From birth to age 2 years, the infant moves through a series of developmental changes in cognition that involve a growing awareness of self and the external world, an ability to act on that world so as to produce an effect, an awareness of the existence of the world apart from the infant's perception of it ("object permanence"), and culminates with the appearance of speech and evidence of planfulness and "intelligent" behavior. There has been much recent interest in this stage from the standpoint of mental retardation, because it is thought to reflect the kind of thinking that is found in individuals with the more serious degrees of intellectual impairment. This segment of the retarded population presents especially difficult challenges to educators. Curriculum based on the sensorimotor period has been employed with persons classified as "profoundly" retarded; it is also used in instructional programs for retarded infants and preschoolers, irrespective of level of impairment (see Chap. 7).

Preoperational Intelligence

This period covers years 2–7. It is the time of the full flowering of language and the development of concepts of size, number, color, and beauty. But the transition from action-oriented sensorimotor intelligence to the rationality of formal operations is only gradual. Though often highly verbal at this stage, the child is indifferent to logic and consistency, is unable to view the world from any perspective than his or her own ("egocentric" thought), and is unable to consider the effect of more than one element at a time in understanding outcomes. The difficulty in considering multiple determinants is illustrated in children's errors on "conservation" problems. Transfer of liquid from a smaller but fatter container to one that is taller and thinner is perceived by the preoperational child as increasing the amount of the fluid. The child can only take account of the increase in the vertical dimension and ignores the change in the horizontal one. In Piagetian terms the child is "centering" on height as the determiner of volume.

Concrete Operations

During the years from 7 to 11, the child begins to show greater logic and consistency in the quality of thinking. The child can now look at events from the perspective of others; the egocentric quality of the younger child's perception of reality wanes. A very important development is the growing recognition that events may be influenced by more than one determinant. The kind of "conservation" error made by the preoperational chld diminishes. The concrete operational child can recognize equality even though its appearance has altered. The child is clearly less "suggestible"—less influenced by the "appearance" of things.

Another aspect of the growth in logical thought and reasoning is that the concrete operational child can begin to order the world in terms of hierarchies or groupings. On intelligence tests this is reflected in being able to tell how things that are different are also alike—for example, orange and banana. We will say more about this kind of cognitive function in a later discussion on the nature of mental retardation.

Formal Operations

The fourth and final stage in mental development for Piaget begins at about age 11. For the first time the child can begin to deal with abstract logical relationships. During the concrete operations period, the child's logic is tied to the "real" world, the world we can know through our senses. But the formal operations youngsters can now consider involve possibilities that are only theoretical. With regard to any problem the youth can entertain multiple possibilities and, importantly, more or less systematically explore their relative correctness. It is at this age that we begin to see formal planning and "strategizing" in problem solving and the use of formal reasoning. One of the important developments in mental retardation has been the attempt to *teach* planning and strategizing to retarded youth since they do not ordinarily reach the level of formal operations in their mental development.

INFORMATION-PROCESSING THEORISTS

Apart from Piaget, until 1960 research on the nature of intelligence was dominated by the factorial approach. But in the 1960s the focus of research shifted from the factor analysis of the "products" of intelligence test performance to one of attempting to identify the "processes" of test performance (Sternberg, 1981). The adoption of an information-processing approach is not regarded as a rejection of the factorial one; rather is it seen as an attempt to understand why individuals differ in these basic abilities.

Information-processing theorists have been particularly active in mental retardation, and in Chapter 8 we discuss how they have attempted to improve "problem solving" in retarded youth. This has consisted of teaching more effective "strategies," the element first referred to in the "formal operations" domain. One "process" long accepted as characterizing mental retardation but heretofore little studied is that of *speed of response*. Indeed we use the word "slow" to describe children with serious learning difficulties. Hunt (1976) has shown that brighter individuals are quicker in making even simple judgments (e.g., time to recognize the identity of letters that may differ in shape [e.g., *Aa*]. Other researchers (Lally & Nettelbeck, 1977) have found a correlation between "inspection time" for a simple visual discrimination judgment and the Performance Scale IQ on the Wechsler Adult Intelligence Scale. Those individuals who took less time to make a judgment had the higher scores. Speed of judgment does seem related to intelligence.

Of the various processes, the *inferring* of relationships has been seen as central to intelligence not only by Spearman but by others as well. Resnick and Glaser (1976) assert that intelligence is largely the ability to *learn in the absence of direct or complete instruction*—that is, to fill in or infer what is not directly given. Sternberg and Powell (1983) also give a prominent role to *inferred* understanding. They see it as the central *process* underlying the factorial ability—Verbal Comprehension. With regard to vocabulary tests, one of the standard measures of the verbal comprehension factor, the meaning of most words is learned *not* by going to the dictionary or by having them explained but rather by their repeated occurrence in particular contexts. As a result of repeated experience with a word, its meaning gradually becomes apparent (is "inferred").

Where factorial theories use the "factor" as the unit of analysis, information-processing theories tend to use the "component." The *component* is an elementary information process that acts on our internal (mental) representation of experience. The *component* may translate a sensory impression into a conceptual one (e.g., visual image of a tree [sensory impression] converted into its verbal equivalent [the word "tree"]). This alteration of the raw sensory experience is called *encoding*. The component may transfer one conceptual representation into another (e.g., some trees as evergreen and some as deciduous), or it may translate a conceptual representation into a motor response. Recognition that the tree is falling leads to the motor response "getting out of the way." The research related to "speed of response" also refers to "thought" leading to action.

Components may be distinguished by the functions they perform. In the model of Sternberg and Gardner (1982), five kinds of functional components are proposed: metacomponents, performance components, and the components of acquisition, retention, and transfer.

Metacomponents

These are higher-order control or "executive" processes used for *planning* and *decision making*. It is this part of our mental apparatus that "manages" our behavior when it "sizes up" a situation, considers alternatives, and then chooses. It does this by being aware of both its own problem-solving capabilities (i.e., knowledge of its other components—"self-awareness") and the situation that is to be addressed. It is this component that is thought to most nearly approximate g and to be most highly correlated with measures of general intelligence (Sternberg, 1981). It is the metacomponent that considers appropriate *strategies* for facilitating problem solving, a topic addressed in Chapter 8. It is apparent that a deficiency in the metacomponent is regarded as one of the major impediments to memory in persons with mental retardation (Belmont & Butterfield, 1971; Borkowski & Cavanaugh, 1979; Campione & Brown, 1977; Ellis, 1970). The metacomponent appears to reflect Guilford's cognitive operation of "evaluation."

Performance Components

These are the information processes actually used to carry out the plan or strategy conceived by the metacomponent. Each is now illustrated in the carrying out of the solving of a simple analogy $1:3 = A:\_\_$. At the metacomponent level there is first recognition of the nature of the problem—that it is an "analogy." The performance components now come into play. Up to seven have been proposed in the solution of this analogy. They are *encoding* (retrieval from memory of relevant information about each term), *inferring* the relationship between each term, *mapping* the higher-order relationship between the first and second halves (recognizing that one deals with the numbers and the other with letters), *applying* the relation inferred and selecting an answer, *comparing* answer options (as in a multiple choice question), *justifying* the choice if there are other potentially correct choices, and, finally, *responding* with the chosen answer.

The performance components incorporate the Reasoning factor of the Thurstones and the Cognition, Convergent Production and Evaluation operations of Guilford. They also appear to correspond to Cattell's "fluid intelligence."

Acquisition Components

These are processes used in learning new information. They involve the "encoding" or transforming of raw sensory experience (commonly in verbal form), the association of that coded event with other information, and the strengthening of association through such procedures as contiguity and reinforcement. This is certainly one of the major problem areas in mental retardation. Retarded persons learn more slowly and are limited in the complexity of the knowledge they can grasp.

Retention Components

This is the "memory" aspect of the system and refers to the processes involved in retrieving information from memory storage. Short-term memory has been much studied in persons who are retarded, and their memory deficiency has been attributed to a failure to spontaneously employ strategies that would aid retention, for example, simple rehearsal or continuous repeating to oneself what one seeks to remember (Ellis, 1970). This represents a failure on the part of the metacomponent to strengthen one of its other components probably because of lack of awareness of the nature of "strategy" as a means of "fixing" what has been previously learned and leads to a deficit in recall. The retention process relates in factorial terms to the Thurstones' primary mental ability of memory and to Guilford's cognitive operation of memory.

Transfer Components

These are the processes involved in "generalization"—in the applying of understanding gained in one context to that of another. If most of our learning is inferential rather than the product of direct instruction, most of the transfer of what we have learned to other settings occurs through generalization. This is another area of major deficiency seen in retarded individuals. Their knowledge tends to be tied to the situation in which it was acquired. They are less able to recognize underlying commonalities between nonidentical but similar situations. Not recognizing the underlying similarity, there is not cue to transfer or generalize, and this gives their thinking a highly specific or concrete quality. This element is elaborated later in the chapter as we look at the thinking of retarded individuals.

Relating Factors and Processes to Common Conceptions of Intelligence

Thus far we have (a) identified behaviors commonly regarded as manifestations of intelligence and (b) considered the elements that underlie the outward manifestations of intelligence—factors and processes. An integration of the outward and underlying aspects has been offered by Sternberg (1981).

ABILITY TO LEARN AND TO PROFIT FROM EXPERIENCE AND TO ACQUIRE KNOWLEDGE IN THE COURSE OF THAT EXPERIENCE

This outward manifestation depends on crystallized intelligence; the factors of Verbal Comprehension, Reasoning, and Number; and on the components of acquisition, retention, and transfer as controlled and driven by the metacomponents. "An intelligent person learns from his interactions with the environment and uses his experience to a greater advantage than does a less intelligent person. As a result, the intelligent person tends to know more . . ." (Sternberg, 1981).

ABILITY TO REASON

This outward manifestation of intelligence rests on fluid ability, the factor of reasoning, and the processes of the performance components as driven by the metacomponents. "An intelligent person can infer relations between events, apply these relations to new situations, integrate information, and otherwise exploit given information to a greater advantage that the less intelligent person" (Sternberg, 1981).

ABILITY TO ADAPT ONESELF
TO CHANGING CONDITIONS

This particular outward manifestation is relatively little measured on tests of intelligence, but it appears to rest most heavily on the cognitive operation of Evaluation and on all of the information processes with particular emphasis on the metacomponents (e.g., sizing up a situation). As characterized by Sternberg, this dimension also clearly depends on the acquisition of the Piagetian stage of concrete operations—the capacity to consider multiple elements in decision making. "An intelligent person is a better practical problem-solver. . . . In making a decision as to whether to consummate an important purchase, for example, such a person is likely to consult more sources of information (concrete operational—as against preoperational thought), . . . in particular those . . . that are most . . . critical, to evaluate (Guilford's evaluation) and integrate the information, . . . and to investigate more fully the alternatives that are available."

ABILITY TO MOTIVATE ONESELF
TO ACCOMPLISH WHAT ONE NEEDS
TO ACCOMPLISH

"An intelligent person is more highly motivated to accomplish the things that matter. . . ." This is not an aspect measured on tests of intelligence and in the author's view is, perhaps, better addressed in a nonintellective facet of the person—"personality." Indeed, David Wechsler, the author of the Wechsler intelligence tests, noted that individuals with similar test scores were not necessarily equal in their coping ability and that such personality traits as anxiety, persistence, and goal awareness interact with cognitive capacities in producing behavioral outcomes (Wechsler, 1981).

ISSUES RELATED TO CLASSIFICATION
AS "MENTALLY RETARDED"

Behavior Relevant to a Diagnosis
of Retardation

Although intelligence is equated with learning ability, knowledge, reasoning, and coping with new situations, definitions of mental retardation usually refer to the *adaptive* problems created by intellectual limitations. Traditionally, retardation has been identified with impairment in the capacity for *personal responsibility*— that is, for assuming the degree of independence appropriate to one's chronological age (Benda, 1954; Doll, 1941; Tredgold, 1937). Since incapacity for prudent self-management may also be due to emotional or physical problems, definitions of retardation always relate it to intellectual impairment.

RETARDATION AND IQ

Though definitions of mental retardation are couched in terms of personal responsibility, the actual determination of retardation has traditionally been based on performance on an intelligence test. Scores on these tests are expressed in IQ (intelligence quotient), with the IQ range representing retardation beginning at least 2 standard deviations[2] below the mean or average of the general population. This is the bottom 2–3 percent of the population (see Fig. 2). The upper limit of this range is approximately IQ 70 (Terman & Merrill, 1960; Wechsler, 1949). In 1959 the American Association on Mental Deficiency (AAMD), the main professional organization in the field, promulgated a definition of retardation that extended the range of retardation to within 1 standard deviation of the mean (Heber, 1959). Under it persons with IQs of 70 to 84 were classifiable as "borderline" retarded. The upward extension was unwarranted, and, in the 1973 revision of the AAMD definition, this category was eliminated (Grossman, 1973).

At this point the reader will begin to recognize the "man-made" quality of our definitions of retardation and that what one does one may undo. The "arbitrary" nature of who is classified as retarded is elaborated further in this section. There are at least two reasons why the earlier inclusion of the "borderline" category was inappropriate. First, it brought under the rubric of retardation individuals whose adjustive problems were primarily limited to school achievement; they did not manifest the wider range of adaptive difficulties typically associated with retardation. Second, it had the undesirable effect of multiplying nearly eightfold those who could be stigmatized with the label "mentally retarded." Since the epithet "retard" is a part of our vocabulary of ridicule, it will be appreciated that one seeks to avoid being so labeled. But it has been "special education" programs in our schools, classes serving children with poor acacdemic achievement and IQs below 70, that have particularly fired controversy over the IQ and over intelligence testing itself. Much of the concern stems from finding disproportionately large numbers of black and other economically disadvantaged youth in classes for retarded children (Dunn, 1968). Thus the definition of mental retardation has

---

[2]A statistical measure of the variability of a group.

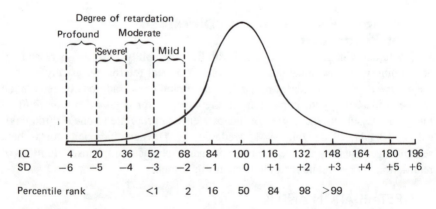

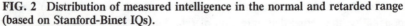

FIG. 2 Distribution of measured intelligence in the normal and retarded range (based on Stanford-Binet IQs).

become enmeshed in racial issues, and this has had enormous consequences for the field of special education.

IQ AND BEHAVIOR

One of the most complex issues surrounding the use of the IQ in mental retardation pertains to the distinction between performance on an intelligence test and general competency. Though subaverage intelligence unquestionably impedes school progress, it does not necessarily preclude adequate functioning in other areas. Thus even very limited reading and arithmetic skills will not, in and of themselves, prevent an adult, for example, from achieving an independent adjustment—a level of adaptation that is not only attained by those with IQs in the 70–84 or "borderline" range but also by many in the below-70 range (Cobb, 1972). Is it meaningful to classify someone as retarded who, in spite of a below-70 IQ, is able to function independently?

IQ, ADAPTIVE BEHAVIOR, AND THE AAMD
DEFINITION OF RETARDATION

In attempting to address this issue, the 1959 AAMD definition of retardation specifically distinguishes between IQ and overall adjustment by incorporating within it the concept of "adaptive behavior." By this is meant the adjustive difficulties commonly associated with significant intellectual impairment. Classification as retarded would now require the presence of adaptive impairment as well as subaverage intelligence. Thus far the effort to link the two criteria has had only limited success, largely because retardation has traditionally been so strongly equated with intelligence alone. Another important reason is that no measures of adaptive behavior have won the same degree of acceptance as have intelligence tests. In any case, in the below-50 IQ range, the distinction becomes largely academic because some difficulties in *all* aspects of living can be expected.

THE CULTURAL RELATIVISM
OF INTELLECTUAL IMPAIRMENT

Nowhere is the distinction between IQ and adaptive behavior more apparent than in the effect of low measured intelligence on members of different cultural and socioeconomic groups. The impact of intellectual impairment is determined by the kinds of coping demands our culture places on us. In less technologically advanced societies, persons with some intellectual limitation can still meet the culture's criteria for a grossly normal level of adjustment. Thus, in the largely rural milieu of underdeveloped countries, the lack of good reading and arithmetic skills will have a lesser impact than they would in more industrialized societies. The implication is that each culture will determine which individuals are to be considered retarded. This distinction is relevant only for persons who would fall within the mildly retarded IQ range because, below this, the degree of impairment would ordinarily preclude normal adaptation in any society.

The issue of cultural relativism is at the heart of criticisms of intelligence testing of Mexican-American and black youths in California. Mercer (1973), a sociologist, has shown that the number of Mexican-American children who are perceived by their community as retarded are far fewer than those so designated by intelligence tests and academic performance. Clearly, the school and the child's community are using different criteria. The school's criteria are academic impairment and IQ, but the same youngster who fails in school may function in an essentially normal fashion outside of school. This is the origin of the designation of such youngsters as the "6-hour retarded child." While recognizing the significance of this distinction, it would be the height of naïveté to ignore the postschool implications of poor academic achievement associated with low intelligence. As will be shortly seen, mental retardation assures poor academic achievement, and, in an increasingly technological 20th-century America, the lack of functional reading and arithmetic skills constitute severe limitations on job potential. It is, in fact, the concern for functional literacy and its occupational implication that have sparked the national quest for tying a high school diploma to basic reading and number competencies.

Prevalence[3] or Frequency of Mental Retardation

The cultural relativism of intellectual impairment has obvious implications for who and therefore how many people will be considered retarded within a given population. Both age and residence influence prevalence, especially in those with milder degrees of impairment. With reference to chronological age, the highest rates are at school age, when academic difficulties are certain to be manifest (Farber, 1959; Kott, 1968; Levinson, 1962). Both before and after the school years, the rates are lower, because intellectual limitations, at least those that are not severe in degree, will be less disabling relative to the developmental expectations for those two periods of life.

The variation in prevalence associated with place of residence really relates to general economic status, as higher rates are found among rural (Conley, 1973; Reschly & Jipson, 1976) and inner-city populations. Within these sources of variation, the most widely used prevalence rate is 3 percent (Luckey & Neman, 1976). This is probably a good estimate within the general population of the number of persons with IQ below 70, but a much fewer number would necessarily meet the dual AAMD criteria of subaverage intelligence *and* adaptive impairment (Mercer, 1973; Tarjan et al., 1973). A number of studies suggest that the proportion of persons meeting both criteria would be closer to 1 percent than 3 percent (Baroff, 1982; Birch et al., 1970; Heber, 1970; Mercer, 1973). With regard to the 3 percent rate, it is important to understand that it is a purely statistical extrapolation from the so-called normal curve. It merely roughly corresponds to that point on the curve that marks 2 standard deviations below the mean, and it has absolutely no behavioral correlate. Here we pick up the thread of the somewhat arbitrary nature

---

[3]"Prevalence" refers to the frequency of a condition either at a given moment in time or over a period of time. "Incidence," another commonly used term, refers to the number of *new* cases per unit time.

of who is called retarded, since no one would seriously claim that there is a meaningful difference in intelligence between a person with an IQ of 69 and one with an IQ of 71.

LABELING

Nowhere has the controversy over who is to be classified as retarded been more evident than in issues surrounding the educational placement of poorly achieving, disadvantaged minority youth. The controversy has come to be called "labeling," and its flavor is caught in "label jars, not people." The storm of concern here, as earlier noted, is the disproportionate representation of such youths in classes for retarded children, especially those for mildly retarded or, in educational parlance, "educable" children. The argument is made that such classes tend to stigmatize the children and, of course, the minority group they represent, and to adversely affect their self-image or self-esteem. The relevant research reveals that viewing labels and labeling as either *necessarily* bad or good represents a gross oversimplification (Gallagher, 1976; Hobbs, 1975; MacMillan, 1977).

In the following chapter, which deals with personality factors in mental retardation, this research is presented in some detail. Here it is sufficient to state that, contrary to the statements of the more impassioned opponents of labels and labeling, there is neither research evidence to support the notion that labels are the *cause* of academic difficulties nor evidence indicating that these labels in and of themselves result in either rejection by nonretarded peers or serious damage to self-esteem. This is not to say that labels have no effect but rather that it is the *academic* and *social* behaviors of these children that call attention to them and are their primary problems.

Whether labeled or not, the difficulties are there and can neither be ignored nor wished away, as they have extraordinary consequences for future employability and economic security. Whether these children should continue to be designated retarded is another question. It has been suggested that such youths might be included in a broader, nonspecific ("noncategorical") grouping—for example, "children with special learning needs." Such a category could also include so-called "learning disability" children as well as those with visual or hearing problems. Another alternative is more specific grouping within the educable or mildly retarded range (MacMillan, 1971).

CAUSATION

It has been common to include causation (etiology) in mental retardation diagnostic systems, and it is clear that there are two distinct groups who comprise the mentally retarded: (1) relatively mildly impaired and physically grossly normal persons who come from lower socioeconomic backgrounds and families in which other members are likely to be similarly affected, and (2) usually more severely impaired individuals who are visibly different from other family members and who are found with about equal frequency at all socioeconomic levels. In Aberdeen, Scotland, the site of long-term investigations of the intellectual status of the population, the former group, those with cultural-familial retardation, constituted 46 percent of all retarded individuals, the remaining 54 percent falling in the second category and in whom retardation is clearly associated with some biological abnormality (Birch et al., 1970). The term "cultural-familial" is now in disfavor presumably because of its past association with genetic as well as environmental causation. From a genetic standpoint this group was seen as simply representing the lower extreme of the normal range of intelligence in the general population, but increasing weight is now being given to environmental deprivation as an important factor in their intellectual impairment.

CURRENT AAMD DEFINITION OF MENTAL RETARDATION

The current AAMD definition of mental retardation is its 1983 version (Grossman, 1983) and is identical to the 1977 revision (Grossman, 1977) except for slightly greater specificity with regard to one of its elements, the "developmental period." The definition and its "commentary" is quoted from the 1983 manual and is followed by a detailed elaboration of each of its three components.

Definition

"Mental retardation refers to significantly subaverage general intellectual functioning existing concurrently with deficits in adaptive behavior and manifested during the developmental period" (Grossman, 1983).

Meaning of Its Major Components

"General Intellectual Functioning" This refers to an IQ, the score obtained on an individually administered intelligence test.

"Significantly Subaverage" This is an IQ of 70 or below though in educational settings the upper limit is commonly extended to 75.

"Deficits in Adaptive Behavior" These are significant lags in general maturation or major limitations in academic learning, personal independence, and social responsibility.

"Developmental Period" Though in earlier AAMD definitions this period was defined as birth to 18 years, the current version extends it backward to conception. The author is unaware of how you can measure general intelligence and adaptive behavior prior to birth! In the absence of such procedures, it can be presumed that the more traditional period will be honored, though some biological abnormalities typically *associated* with retardation are detectable prenatally. The best known of these is the chromosomal disorder, Down syndrome.

The AAMD definition refers only to behavior manifestitations and has no implications for causation. Indeed it represents itself as a description of current behavior and avoids a prediction of future status.

It departs from earlier traditional ones in its conceptualization of retardation in terms of adaptive behavior as well as general intelligence. Prior to the first AAMD definition in 1959 (Heber, 1959), only measured intelligence or IQ had been considered the relevant dimension. The inclusion of "adaptive behavior" implies that IQ alone will not perfectly predict general adaptation. Persons with identical IQs may be quite different in adaptive behavior and this will be especially apparent at lesser levels of intellectual impairment. Individuals with IQs in the 50+ range, for example, may be functioning in a fashion not grossly distinguishable from nonretarded persons while others with the same IQ may be operating at much lower levels. The distinction between IQ and adaptive behavior appears to diminish as the level of intellectual impairment increases.

The Relevant Domains of Adaptive Behavior   Since adaptive behavior expectations vary with chronological age, our standards for academic achievement and personal and social responsibility for a 16-year-old are very different from those of a 6-year-old; they're here spelled out in terms of age groups, albeit broadly.

Infancy and Early Childhood   During this period the focus is on general "maturation" and the acquisition of basic sensory and motor skills, language, self-help skills, and socialization.

Childhood and Early Adolescence   The focus now shifts from maturation-related functions to cognitive and social ones. There is concern with school learning, with appropriate social judgment, and with peer and adult relationships.

Late Adolescence and Adulthood   Increasing independence is the hallmark of this period. It should eventuate in the capacity to maintain a fully independent existence—to work, to fulfill the social roles of friend, spouse, and parent, to conform to community mores, and to participate as a "citizen."

Critics

Although the current AAMD definition has no serious challengers, it also has no "official" sanction, and workers may use it or not, guided only by the practices of their own state or local agencies. But the AAMD definition is not without its critics. Even its drafters recognize the complexity of measuring adaptive behavior relative to general intelligence, and it is likely that the diagnosis of retardation continues to be made largely, if not entirely, on the basis of IQ. In fact, Clausen (1967, 1972) has argued for limiting the concept of retardation to IQ alone, at least until we have widely accepted measures of adaptive behavior. While agreeing with Clausen regarding the lack of adequate measures of adaptive behavior, Mercer (1973) rejects the IQ as an exclusive criterion, contending that retardation is a *sociological* label which refers to particular role expectations and is culture-specific. She would reserve the classification "retarded" for persons who both score below 70 IQ and fail to meet the behavior norms of *their own cultural group*. Thus Mercer would make "adaptive behavior" culture-specific and she and her colleagues have begun to develop such norms in what is referred to as "pluralistic assessment" (Mercer & Lewis, 1975). While it is clear that culture-specific adaptive behavior assessment will reduce the number of disadvantaged minority youths classified as retarded in terms of adaptive behavior, it seems to ignore the fact that, at least economically speaking, there is but one culture in America and that, irrespective of one's cultural background, job potential—the key to economic self-sufficiency—is closely tied to basic reading and number skills. If the effect of pluralistic assessment is to *minimize* minority youth academic limitations by showing that it is "normative" within their particular subculture, the result is to do a disservice to them by assuring perpetuation of economic disadvantage in their adult lives.

ELABORATION OF EACH COMPONENT OF THE AAMD DEFINITION

"Subaverage General Intellectual Functioning . . ."

LEVELS OF RETARDATION

The current AAMD definition continues to distinguish four levels or degrees of retardation—mild, moderate, severe, and profound. These are purely statistical correlates of a population which, at least theoretically, can be divided into 6 standard deviations above and below the mean. This was shown in Figure 2. In such a population distribution, the proportion of individuals at each standard deviation level diminishes as we move away from the mean in either direction. While the prevalence of retardation does lessen as one moves from mild to profound, the actual number in the below-mild range far exceeds that predicted on the basis of statistical normality (Dingman & Tarjan, 1960). This "excess" in the moderate to profound ranges is recognized as reflecting the organic or biologically abnormal part of the retarded population—persons who have been displaced downward from where they would have fallen had they not been biologically impaired. It should be added, however, that biologically impaired individuals are also found in the mildly retarded range. In the earlier cited Aberdeen study, 24 percent or nearly one-quarter of those in the 50–70 IQ range had organic involvement (Birch et al., 1970). In spite of the statistical deviation from normality, the standard deviation model is as close as we have to an official classification scheme in retardation and is so regarded here. The four levels of retardation, their respective IQ ranges, and the proportion of retarded persons in each are shown in Table 1.

In the prior discussion of classification issues, reference was made to the controversy over intelligence testing and the use of IQs. The stigmatizing consequence of low intelligence is undeniable—we value good intelligence and demean persons who are lacking in it. The terms created by Goddard in 1910 (Kanner, 1964) to designate the levels of subnormality—moron, imbecile, and idiot—are not

TABLE 1   Levels of Retardation by IQ and Proportion of Retarded Persons at Each Level

| Level of retardation | IQ ranges[a] | | Approximate percent of all retarded persons[b] |
	Stanford-Binet and Cattell tests	Wechsler scales	
Mild	52-67	55-69	89
Moderate	36-51	40-54	7
Severe	20-35	25-39	3
Profound	0-19	0-24	1

[a]Two separate IQ distributions are given to accord with standard deviation equivalents of the tests on which they are based. Since the corresponding IQ ranges for each level vary slightly from each other, some scores would produce a different classification depending on the test used. Thus an IQ of 52 on either the Binet or Cattell test would fall in the range of "mild retardation" while the same score on the Wechsler scales would be in the "moderately retarded" range. This variation has the "virtue" of calling attention to mental retardation as a purely arbitrary designation based, in part, on one's score on an intelligence test

[b]President's Committee on Mental Retardation (1967).
Source: Grossman (1977).

only scientific anachronisms, they are also part of our everyday vocabulary. But there are other concerns about intelligence testing, and we address them now.

SCHOOL ACHIEVEMENT, IQ, AND TEACHER EXPECTANCY

One of the fears about intelligence testing is that eventual teacher knowledge of a child's IQ will create achievement expectancies that will be communicated to the child in the teacher's attitude and which the child will tend to confirm (Meyers et al., 1974). The so-called Pygmalion effect, first reported by Rosenthal and Jacobson (1968), has not been confirmed in subsequent research (Dusek & O'Connell, 1973; Fleming & Anttonen, 1971a; 1971b; Mendels & Flanders, 1973; Sorotzkin et al., 1974). While it is certainly true that expectancies may influence the teacher when there has been no prior contact with the child (Meyers, 1974; Yoshida, 1974), there is no evidence that the major academic difficulties of children with subnormal intelligence are the *result* of teacher knowledge of such information. In fact, present testing practice would dictate that intellectual assessment *follows* rather than precedes the appearance of school difficulties and would be done precisely for the purpose of attempting to understand the cause of a child's learning problems. It is the *effect* of subnormal intelligence on academic performance that is the primary problem, not the IQ score itself or teacher knowledge of it.

Finally, whatever expectancies are created by either test scores or labels are not fixed in the teacher's mind; rather are they subject to modification on the basis of the child's actual performance (Salvia et al., 1973; Yoshida & Meyers, 1975). In this regard, the author requires that each student in a course on the "exceptional child" be intimately involved with a handicapped youngster over a full semester in the belief that prolonged contact permits modification of whatever expectations and stereotypes the students initially bring with them.

VARIABILITY IN IQ

Since a diagnosis of retardation rests so heavily on measured IQ and the label "retarded" is an unwanted designation, it is important to know how much faith can be put in the accuracy of a given IQ score. In psychometric parlance this is called a test's *reliability* and refers to the degree to which repeated examination with the same test over a short time interval (e.g., 1 week) will produce the same score. There are numerous factors that can influence reliability, one of which, testee motivation, is often cited as a reason for reduced scores in minority youths, especially when the tester is a member of the dominant culture or of another race.

Undoubtedly, attitudes of examiner and examinee *can* influence test score (e.g., Zigler & Butterfield, 1968), but studies of intelligence testing of black children have usually found no effect of race difference alone (Sattler, 1974). Nevertheless, wide variation in IQ on the same test at different times is not uncommon and can occasionally exceed 30 points or more.[4] It is these instances of unusually wide individual variability, though not always referring to the same test, that are noted by those who distrust intelligence testing and the usefulness of IQ scores. Paradoxically, it is within the retarded range that there appears to be the *least* variability (Anastasi, 1964); McNemar, 1942). In a study of the long-term stability of IQ in normal children who were tested, in part, during ages 6 to 18 years, more than one-half (59%) showed changes of at least 15 points; 37 percent changed by 20 or more, and 9 percent by at least 30 (Honzik et al., 1948). Among retarded children, however, less IQ change over time is seen although variation of at least 10 points is found in nearly one-half of mildly retarded individuals (Alper & Horne, 1959; Clarke & Clarke, 1954; Collmann & Newlyn, 1958; Elwood, 1952; Stott, 1960; Walker & Gross, 1970). Even given this degree of variation, challengers of the accuracy of IQs in retarded persons will find little solace, since the changes that do occur are twice as likely to be in a downward as in an upward direction (Stott, 1960). This is particularly true in younger retarded individuals; after age 16 some increase in IQ is commonly found in mildly retarded persons (Bayley, 1970; Clarke & Clarke, 1975; Satter & McGee, 1954).

Whether one takes either comfort or anxiety from the research literature, the evaluation, diagnosis, and consequent labeling of a child are an individual phenomenon, and there can be no substitute for a competent examiner—one who knows the test(s) and the conditions under which they can be validly applied.

DO INTELLIGENCE TESTS MEASURE "INTELLIGENCE"?

Perhaps the most important question raised about intelligence tests is whether, indeed, they measure intelligence! This has been a special concern of those who see the apparent "street sense" of minority youths as belying the impli-

---

[4]The expected variation of a Binet test IQ is 5 points. This is its *standard error*.

cations of a low score on an intelligence test. Tests have been challenged as too narrow in the abilities sampled (Dingman & Meyers, 1966; Sarason & Doris, 1969), as too "verbal" and not including items relevant to the life experience of disadvantaged minority children (Anastasi, 1961; Mercer, 1973; Sarason & Gladwin, 1958; Williams, 1970), as offering little educational guidance to teachers, and as concerned only with answers, penalizing unconventional ones (Sigel, 1965) and ignoring the process by which they are achieved. The last mentioned, a product-versus-process controversy, is possibly the most significant of the criticisms, since it has led to attempts to incorporate process in the method by which intelligence is measured. So-called "learning potential assessment" varies from the traditional one-step testing method by adding two additional steps—*training* following original testing, and then *retesting* after training (Budoff & Corman, 1976; Feuerstein, 1970). The focus is not on the initial level of performance but rather on the degree to which that level can be raised following training. It is a procedure in which the tester also assumes the role of teacher. Its rationale lies in the assumption that inferior intellectual performance in some disadvantaged youths can be explained by their method of going about solving problems—that is, in their *cognitive styles* or *conceptual tempo*. These refer to tendencies to use certain kinds of logical relationships in "categorizing" tasks or to attack problems in an either reflective or impulsive manner (Kagan et al., 1964; Kagan & Kogan, 1970, Keogh, 1973). Impulsivity, for example, is an obvious deterrent to effective problem solving, though it may itself have been conditioned by prior failure in comparable situations. If one has come to expect failure, there is the tendency to "give up"—that is, to exert minimal effort and to terminate a painful situation as quickly as possible. In any event, there is yet only suggestive evidence regarding the efficacy of this method in significantly elevating general intellectual functioning (Budoff & Corman, 1976; Carlson & Wiede, 1978).

ON THE VALIDITY OF INTELLIGENCE TESTS

The question whether intelligence tests do measure intelligence—that is, the question of their *validity*—is, in a sense, unresolvable. Intelligence is not a "thing"; it has not tangible reality, and an IQ is merely the score on a test that has been identified by its developer as an intelligence test! But the test developer does not have unlimited freedom to represent his instrument as a test of intelligence, since its acceptance as a valid measure depends on its fulfilling consensually established criteria. For intelligence tests the primary criterion has been *school achievement* (Anastasi, 1961; Cleary et al., 1975), and a test that is a good predictor of this is, by definition, valid.

The use of school achievement as *the* criterion for intelligence tests has its basis in the very origin of the testing movement. The original Binet intelligence test, first published in 1905 and then revised in 1908 and 1911 (Binet & Simon, 1911), was specifically designed (interestingly enough in terms of this book) to identify children in the Paris school system who were not expected to make normal academic progress and for whom such identification was to lead to special instruction: These were retarded children! Future workers continued to relate intelligence test score (IQ) to school achievement and have reported correlations ranging from +.4 to +.7 (Anastasi, 1961). It must be acknowledged, of course, that the magnitude of this range of correlation is not remarkable, as it indicates that, at best, not more than one-half of the source of individual variation in school achievement is attributable to IQ. We are all very aware of the importance of motivation in academic success.

Regarding the tests themselves, in the prior section it was indicated that one of the criticisms of them is that they are too heavily "verbal" and that this unfairly penalizes disadvantaged minority youth. In fact, black children tend to score higher on the Binet, a verbally loaded test, than on the Wechsler Preschool and Primary Scale (WPPSI), and, even on the Wechsler Intelligence Scale for Children (WISC), there is some suggestion that their Verbal Scale scores will exceed those of the Performance Scale—all nonverbal tasks (Sattler, 1974). Both the Stanford-Binet and the WISC are considered to be good predictors of school grades in minority children (Sattler, 1974), though this was not the case in one study of elementary school–age black, Mexican-American, and "Anglo" children (Goldman & Hartig, 1976). While the WISC was a good predictor of the Anglo children's grades, it did not predict those of the other two minority groups. It appears that teacher grades rather than actual grade achievement level were used, and this could have reduced the correlation in the minority children. In any case, whatever the limitations of the WISC with disadvantaged youngsters, there is no doubt that although a high score does not assure academic achievement, a low score precludes it. As the author has watched the turmoil over intelligence testing, it appears that much of the controversy generated by cultural and racial differences might be lessened if intelligence tests were called what they really are—measures of *scholastic aptitude*.

CULTURE-FAIR INTELLIGENCE TESTS

Criticisms of the content of intelligence tests have led to efforts to develop so-called "culture-fair" ones. Two such tests are the Davis-Eels Games (Davis & Eels, 1953) and the Culture-Fair Intelligence Test (Cattell, 1959). The former requires no reading (there is little on the Binet and none on the Wechsler scales), its content is wholly pictorial, and it consists entirely of problem situations drawn from urban life. In spite of these modifications, economically deprived minority children are as equally disadvantaged as on standard tests (Anastasi, 1961). Nor has the Cattell shown any advantage over the Binet (Sattler, 1974).

An oft-heard complaint about the standard intelligence tests is that they are "middle class" in their orientation and that they do not tap the kinds of skills found in disadvantaged youths. To the degree that it is recognized that intelligence tests are measures of such basic cognitive functions as abilities to remember, reason, and calculate, such criticisms seem unjustified. In *all* cultures these skills are needed, although each culture will determine the frequency and kind of problems to which they are applied. Furthermore, if one realizes that intelligences tests are really measures of scholastic aptitude, is it reasonable to suggest that school achievement is only important to the middle class? Economically disadvantaged persons in our society, whatever their subculture, recognize that academic achievement is crucial to job success at skilled and technical levels, and it is *this* dimension that is the key to breaking the poverty cycle and achieving upward mobility.

INTELLIGENCE AND RACE

The particularly strident tone of recent criticism of intelligence tests and of testing itself pertains primarily to black-white differences in measured intelligence. With a general population mean of 100, the black mean is 90, but variations both above and below 90 have been found in populations that differ geographically and, probably, socioeconomically (Dreger & Miller, 1960, 1968; Kennedy 1969; 1973; Kennedy et al., 1963; Mercer, 1971). The lower black IQ is accompanied by a lesser level of academic achievement and though our schools have been much maligned for this, especially those in the inner city, it has been found that the relative deficit in IQ and academic status is already evident at the beginning of first grade and is not appreciably different at the end of 12th grade (Cleary et al., 1975; Kennedy, 1969). Although the mean IQ difference between blacks and whites is clear, the reason for it is not. Not only did the assertion of the psychologist Arthur Jensen (1969, 1972) that the basis for the difference is largely genetic create a storm of protest, but his claim that intellectual capacities could not be materially altered has been challenged by some indication that "reasoning," for example, can be improved with training (Budoff & Corman, 1976; Carlson & Wiedl, 1978). In any event, the current mean racial differences cannot be safely ascribed exclusively to either genetic or environmental factors. The powerful role of environment in affecting mental development is presented in detail in Chapter 5, and, in light of an already existent black lag in IQ by age 4 (Kennedy, 1973), the extreme importance of the early childhood years seem inescapable.

But a role for environment does not preclude a genetic influence as well. The possibility of a genetic effect depends only on the assumption that the biological basis for intelligence, the brain, is somehow influenced by genes and that marriage patterns in which race is a major determinant will necessarily lead to some differences in racial gene pools. Thus sickle cell anemia is a recessively inherited disorder largely confined to blacks, whereas Tay-Sachs disease, another recessively inherited condition, is found only in whites, specifically among Jews of Eastern European origin. In Chapter 5 we will try to show how both genetic and environmental factors interact to produce variation in intelligence; at this point, it is enough to state that intelligence test scores tell us little about the origin of individual differences in intelligence. We can, perhaps, think of the intelligence test as somewhat analogous to an X ray in that an X ray may reveal a problem without necessarily indicating its cause. The usefulness of intelligence tests depends on their ability to predict academic achievement, *whatever* that rests on.

ON THE NATURE OF INTELLECTUAL FUNCTIONING IN MENTAL RETARDATION

To this point in the elaboration of the first component of the AAMD definition, subaverage general intelligence, the cognitive impairment in retarded persons has been characterized only in respect to an IQ at least 30 points below the population average of 100. But what does it mean to be "retarded" in terms of thinking? To begin to answer this question, we must first define IQ and one of its elements— *mental age*.

Mental Age and IQ

The construct mental age derives from the original Binet test and is simply the sum of all items correctly answered on the test as expressed in years and months. Each item is associated with a particular chronological age, and, except for those in the preschool age range, all carry a weight of 2 months. A total score of 65 months, for example, would be expressed as a mental age of 5 years and 5 months or 5–5. Initially, Binet and Simon had proposed that a child be considered retarded if the mental age was at least 2 years below chronological age (Ingalls, 1978). But another early worker (Stern, 1914) pointed out that a 2-year lag in mental age was a much more serious deficit in a 4-year-old than in a 14-year-old, and he suggested that retardation be determined by a *ratio* rather than by simply subtracting mental age from chronological age. This was the origin of the IQ, and it first appears in the 1916 American revision of the test (Terman, 1916).

$$\frac{\text{Mental age (MA)}}{\text{Chronological age (CA)}} \times 100 = \text{Intelligence quotient (IQ)}$$

A child was considered normal if his mental age was the same as his chronological age, at least during the preadolescent years. Thus a child who, on his sixth birthday (CA 6–0) had a mental age of 72 months (MA 6–0) would have an IQ of 100.

$$\frac{\text{MA } 6}{\text{CA } 6} = 1 \ (100) = 100$$

A child who at age 6 had a mental age greater than 6 years would have an IQ of more than 100 (e.g., an MA of 8 years: $\frac{8}{6} = 1\frac{2}{6} = 1\frac{1}{3} = 1.33 \times 100 = 133$), but a mental age of less than 6 years would yield an IQ of less than 100 (e.g., an MA of 4 years: $\frac{4}{6} = \frac{2}{3} = .67 \times 100 = 67$).[5] We can think of mental age as a measure of our mental *power*; IQ tells us how that power compares with that of other persons.

The interpretation of mental age is straightforward in childhood and early adolescence. Thereafter, its meaning is complicated by a slower growth rate and an eventual cessation of growth in young adulthood. Moreover, the same mental age score among different individuals is unlikely to mean identical performances on the test, since the final score does not distinguish the particular items on which

---

[5]The *ratio* IQ, as shown above, has been supplanted by the *deviation* IQ. (Pinneau, 1961). This creates greater comparability both within a test from one age level to another and between tests with comparable *standard deviations* (Robinson & Robinson, 1976).

success was achieved. In spite of these and other limitations (Sattler, 1974), mental age is widely accepted as an index of school readiness and is probably the single most valuable piece of information that intelligence tests offer teachers.

Mental Age and Mental Retardation

But what does mental age tell us about retardation itself? It tells us nothing of the particular *pattern* of strengths and weaknesses in cognitive abilities by which it was obtained, nor does it imply that the mental functioning of a 12-year-old with a mental age of 7 years is just like that of a normal 7-year-old (Tansley & Gulliford, 1960). The 12-year-old retarded youngster may be much like a normal 12-year-old in his physical development, self-help skills, and interests. On the other hand, his reading and arithmetic skills may lag behind that of the normal 7-year-old. He may also appear less curious, spontaneous, and creative.

PATTERN OF STRENGTHS AND WEAKNESSES

To learn more about the cognitive abilities of retarded persons we need to look at their relative strengths and weaknesses. On intelligence tests a fairly clear picture emerges of relative strength on *nonverbal* tasks—those that involve some motor or manual response but do not require the use of verbal skills. Thus on the Stanford-Binet and Wechsler tests, retarded individuals tend to succeed on such tasks as copying geometric designs, solving jigsawlike puzzles, creating block designs from a visual pattern, and identifying missing parts in pictures. Not only do these problems not require a verbal response (as for example, in "What should you do if you see a train approaching a broken track?"), but the problem is always before the person in visual form. Contrariwise, tasks that are primarily verbal in nature and require reasoning and judgment tend to be more difficult. Examples of these are defining words, solving arithmetic problems, finding similarities among things that are different (categorizing), and demonstrating general knowledge. We may conclude that, relative to their own pattern of strengths and weaknesses, and in comparison with normal children of the same mental age, retarded individuals will tend to perform well on practical and concrete types of tasks and less well on those that are primarily verbal in nature. This pattern is particularly evident in mildly retarded and non-brain-injured children; those with brain injury may have somewhat greater difficulty in the copying of designs (Achenbach; 1970, Baroff, 1959; Magaret & Thompson, 1950; Sattler, 1974; Silverstein, 1968; Thompson & Magaret, 1947; Witkin et al., 1966).

THE QUALITY OF THINKING IN RETARDED PERSONS

Given this pattern, how do we "experience" the thinking of retarded individuals? What qualities do we perceive in persons who tend to have much difficulty on tasks of verbal reasoning and judgment?

Suggestibility

Retarded individuals are perceived as more suggestible ("outer-directed")—that is, as more easily influenced by external cues (Green & Zigler, 1962; Turnure

& Zigler, 1964; Zigler, 1966). This behavior appears to reflect both the "centering" quality of preoperational thought and a learned distrust of one's own abilities. It is intensified when coping skills are least available (Balla et al., 1971; Yando & Zigler, 1971). It is certainly not peculiar to retarded individuals, as it is also seen in normal children (Turnure, 1970a, 1970b; Turnure & Zigler, 1964). In association with the greater suggestibility one also recognizes a kind of passive quality in their thinking.

Passivity, Strategizing, and Memory

The quality of passivity is also evident in problem-solving situations where solution is aided by *spontaneous* initiation of appropriate strategies. The failure to initiate such strategies has been seen in tasks involving memory and verbal abstractive (categorizing) abilities and has already been described as a metacomponents deficit.

The recall of material that one seeks to remember is facilitated by its conscious repetition, or *rehearsal*. As noted earlier, retarded persons are less likely to use rehearsal *spontaneously* (Anders, 1971; Ellis, 1963, 1968), but this is not unique to individuals who are retarded. In fact, this is a mental age–related phenomenon since normal children of the same mental ages also do not spontaneously use rehearsal to help them remember (Corsale, 1977). Memory is also enhanced by the reorganization or restructuring of the material to be recalled, the effect being to create links between items. Independent elements may be combined in an image (Segal, 1971), in a sentence, or in a category or concept. The last mentioned has the advantage of reducing the total number of initially separate items into categories with each category subsuming two or more items (e.g., the category "breakfast" would be a good cue for items as orange, cereal, coffee, and bread—one item standing in the place of four). Where memory entails the recall of a series of numbers, the combining of them into smaller units—so-called "chunking" (Dember, 1974)—makes the task easier. Thus the last four digits of a telephone number ending 1-9-2-6 can be reduced to a group of two numbers 19-26. In each of these instances the learner *actively* engages the material that is to be memorized and shapes or reorganizes it so as to aid in its retention. But retarded individuals do not *spontaneously* generate the kinds of strategies that accomplish this (Jensen, 1965; MacMillan, 1972; Martin, 1967; Rohwer, 1968; Spitz, 1966). To what extent strategy-initiation is teachable will be discussed in the chapter on the education of school-age retarded youth.

Verbal Abstraction Ability

An example of this kind of cognitive skill is solving "similarities" problems (e.g., "In what way are a mouse and an elephant the same?"). The task involves the finding of likeness among nonidentical entities and requires the ignoring of the perceptual or associational differences conjured up by them—in this case, size and shape. The most common solution for an older child would be "animals," an answer that incorporates the use of a *category*, or *concept*. It has been suggested that incorrect categorizing by retarded persons is at least partly due to a failure to test out the appropriateness of the categories that come to mind (Griffith et al., 1959; McIvor, 1972), and training in this process has been helpful as has the actual teaching of concepts to retarded individuals (Bean, 1968; Corter & McKinney, 1966; Katz, 1962). This cognitive problem also illustrates another important quality in their thinking, a lack of *criticality*. While inadequate testing of possible solutions may be a factor, the main difficulty, in our view, is in generating the kinds of concepts that could solve it. This, too, seems to be a mental age–related phenomenon and explains both the initial difficulty in categorizing relative to nonretarded persons of the same age and the apparent lack of transfer of instructional gains into nonresearch settings (Bilsky et al., 1972; Gerjuoy & Alvarez, 1969; Gerjuoy & Spitz, 1966; Rossi, 1963; Stedman, 1963).

Concreteness

In attempting to solve similarities problems, there is indication that one of the major difficulties for retarded individuals, and for normal ones as well, lies not in the lack of the concept necessary to solution but rather in bringing to awareness concepts already possessed (Blount, 1968; Bortner & Birch, 1970; Milgram & Furth, 1963; Zigler & Balla, 1971). Thus, although a retarded youth and his normal mental age counterpart might both know that a mouse and an elephant are both animals, they could be diverted from reaching that answer by the impact of the size difference. But preoperational centering seems to be a lingering influence in retarded persons even when they are functioning in some respects at the concrete operational level. They continue to have difficulty in paying attention to more than one dimension at a time.

As the difference between things to be grouped increases, retarded persons seem more prone to reject the possibility of similarity and to assert only the obvious difference ("A mouse and an elephant cannot be the same because a mouse is small and an elephant is big"; or "A ship and an automobile are not alike because a ship rides on water and an automobile rides on land"). In the latter example, the retarded youth was unaware of his own use of "ride" in both contexts. Though "ride" is not often applied to ships, the intent is clear, but for this young man it is the *difference* between where they ride rather than that they both "ride" which dominates his thinking. In retardation there seems to be particular difficulty in acknowledging that difference and similarity can coexist. It is this tie to the obvious that gives their thinking the quality of concreteness and rigidity. This also, of course, relates to the previously noted quality of suggestibility. The retarded person is more influenced by surface cues; he's less likely to look behind things. His knowledge also tends to be specific to the situation in which it was acquired rather than generalizing to related ones. The result is that there is need for a greater repetition of experiences (more practice) and for more frequent explanations before a principle is grasped. For example, the retarded child who has learned to await his turn in a classroom game will need to have that same type of experience repeated numerous times before there is real understanding of the personal and social benefits of "waiting one's turn."

Limited Foresight and Planfulness

In comparison with normal children of the same mental age, retarded persons tend to perform less adequately on tasks requiring planfulness and foresight (Byrnes & Spitz, 1977; Spitz & Borys, 1977; Spitz & DeRisi, 1978; Spitz & Nadler, 1974; Spitz & Winters, 1977). Here we deal with the metacomponents and the cognitive operation of "evaluation." Planning involves "if-then" kind of thinking and also reflects the kind of hypothesis-making that characterizes Piaget's stage of "logical operations." It will be recalled that it was earlier stated that retarded individuals generally do not achieve this developmental level, their mental age at maturity usually falling short of 11 years.

Lesser Imagination and Creativity

Still another aspect of concreteness seen in retardation is a relatively weak ability for *imaginative* and *creative* activities. To imagine or to create is to go beyond that which is given to our senses (that which "is") and to produce something new. Creativeness requires either a restructuring of current reality or its use as a stimulus for generating a new one. But the situation-specific quality of retarded thought seems to bind it to what *is* and to make more difficult the creation of what might be.

"Adaptive Behavior: Deficits and Potential"

Much attention has been devoted to the nature of the intellectual impairment in mental retardation, because this is its central feature. Our focus now shifts to the second element of the current AAMD definition—*adaptive behavior*, that which refers to the impact of retardation on general adjustment. The elaboration of this part of the definition involves (a) an overview of the behavioral difficulties of retarded persons, and (b) a detailed presentation of them within a developmental framework, from the preschool years to adulthood.

OVERVIEW OF ADAPTIVE IMPAIRMENT IN MENTAL RETARDATION

The effect of mental retardation is seen in accomplishing the "developmental tasks" expected for one's chronological age. These tasks or age-appropriate developmental skills involve processes of *maturation, learning,* and *social adjustment.* In the preschool years a slower rate of *maturation* is reflected in lags in acquiring *motor skills, language, cognitive skills, self-help,* and *socialization.* At school age, the *learning* difficulty inherent in retardation is expressed in *poor academic achievement.* This is also the period, especially with the beginning of adolescence, of *increasing social isolation* from normal peers. Together with growing physical size and burgeoning sexuality, this can lead to the kinds of social pressures that we equate with adolescence. In adulthood, retardation may affect capacities for self-management (independence), employment, and fulfillment of adult interpersonal roles.

Relating subaverage general intellectual functioning to its developmental consequences not only provides us with age-appropriate criteria for evaluating adaptive behavior, but it also calls attention to the environment or cultural milieu as the medium through which the effect of retardation is measured. Subaverage intelligence will surely preclude age-appropriate school achievement, but its consequence for nonacademic tasks is less certain. As already stated, the person of limited intelligence who cannot adequately perform the role of student may be a reasonably effective adult because of a change in role expectations. The adult is no longer judged by classroom learning standards but rather by the ability to function independently, to work, to fulfill various adult social roles, and to conform to community mores. Many mildly retarded people achieve this level of adaptation and disappear from the rolls of the retarded. This is the issue of cultural relativism that was presented earlier.

The age-related criterion of the AAMD definition also directs our attention to *current* behavior. It does not presume to predict future adaptive status, a criticism made of earlier definitions, particularly that of Doll (1941). In his concept of mental retardation, Doll included the notion of incurability, and, to the extent that retardation in a given individual is caused by biological abnormality (e.g., Down syndrome), this is still largely valid. But Doll's definition was formulated before much research had been done on the possibility of modifying intelligence in nonorganically and even organically impaired infants and young children (See Chap. 7). Nevertheless, while the AAMD stresses current behavior, it is during the early childhood years that major changes in mental ability seem most realizable, though it has been suggested that we have underestimated potential change in adolescence and young adulthood (Clarke & Clarke, 1975). While the "current" focus helps us avoid self-fulfilling prophecies, it would be unrealistic to pretend that the presence of retarded mental development in school age, for example, does not imply some adaptive behavior problems in the future. Certainly, there is no question about this for those with more than a mild degree of retardation.

ADAPTIVE BEHAVIOR DEFICITS
DURING THE PRESCHOOL YEARS

Motor Development
During the preschool years mental retardation may be associated with a noticeable delay in the speed with which gross motor and fine motor skills develop (Malpass, 1960; Molnar, 1978). The infant who is developing normally will, during the first year of life, usually be sitting alone by 8 months, standing alone at 14 months, and walking alone at 15 months (Frankenburg et al, 1970). In the retarded child, however, especially one whose retardation is apparently of organic origin, these gross motor skills and developmental milestones will be delayed. In one survey of Down infants, for example, the average age of sitting alone was 11–12 months, standing alone 23 months, and walking alone 26 months (Share, 1975). This represents a 30–40 percent delay relative to normal infants, or a corresponding rate of development of about 60–70 percent of normal. A similar rate of

development is reported in another study (Dicks-Mireaux, 1972). It is a goal of "early intervention" programs for retarded infants to modify the delay through intense training and stimulation (e.g., Hayden & Dmitriev, 1975; Nielsen et al., 1975). In a parent survey, delayed or abnormal motor development was the second most common cause of suspicion of retardation (32%), obvious physical complications or abnormalities being the first (58%). In this study, incidentally, the average age when retardation was first suspected was 6 months (Abramson et al., 1977). After infancy (birth to 2 years), impaired motor development will be reflected in poor hand-eye coordination, reduced dexterity, and a lesser grace and agility in body movement. These motor lags will slow the acquisition of such dexterity-related self-help skills as feeding and dressing (e.g. buttoning and tying) and affect the child's play activities.

Motor Delay Not Associated with Retardation

Though delayed motor development may signify retardation, this is not always the case. In the infant, for example, slowness in reaching motor milestones may reflect only *normal variation* from the usual ages of appearance. These ages are only rough averages and, within a population of children, a deviation of 2–3 months is not inconsistent with later normality (Birch et al., 1962; Fishler, 1971). Two of the most variable milestones are "crawling" and "pulling to standing." In addition to variations within the normal range, there are conditions of true motor lag that are not necessarily related to retardation. *Hypotonia* is a motor delay due to muscle deficiency, and in *cerebral palsy*, a condition originating in the motor cortex of the brain, there can be severe motor involvement without accompanying intellectual impairment (Kirk, 1962). Motor development may also be affected by blindness. The blind infant is usually slower to walk, presumably because of fewer opportunities to move about safely and because objects do not attract the child's interests unless they emit sound (Holdon, 1972; Lowenfeld, 1950, 1971). The motor lag in blindness illustrates how the environment can affect even behavior wholly governed by biological maturation.

Language Development

In the normally developing child, the preschool years see the full flowering of language, and the average first grader is already fluent in his native tongue. In retardation, however, there are likely to be major abnormalities in *expressive language* (speech).[6] Again, as in the case of motor area, this is especially evident in children whose delayed development appears to have an organic basis. Speech develops more slowly, and that which is acquired is often marred in intelligibility (Kirk, 1964; Spradlin, 1963). In the language sphere, too, caution is needed in attributing delayed speech to retardation. Other sources of language delay are aphasia, deafness, and autism.

---

[6]"Language" may be characterized as *expressive* or *receptive*. Expressive language refers to speech; receptive language refers to the capacity to understand language. Receptive language is treated in this book as a part of general intelligence rather than of language per se.

Self-Help

During the preschool period the normally developing child moves from a condition of total dependency to one in which a considerable degree of self-care is exercised. By school age the child has most of the basic self-help skills of feeding, dressing, toileting, and grooming. The retarded youngster, however, is going to be delayed in the acquisition of these skills, in part owing to the aforementioned lag in motor development. Of these basic self-care skills, slowness in toilet training (especially in gaining bowel control) is likely to be particularly stressful to the child's caretakers. Where parents have had difficulty in adjusting to the child's slower rate of training, attempts to teach will be stressful for parent and child and can lead to the negativism and anxiety often exhibited by retarded children in later learning situations. On the other hand, slowness to learn may cause the oversolicitous parent to make too few demands on the child "because he's handicapped." This child fails to accomplish those things that are within his capability. The condition of mental retardation inherently creates a greater degree of dependency, but this needs to be kept at a minimum. Paradoxically, the oversolicitous parent may inadvertently add to rather than minimize the child's handicap.

Cognitive Skills

The normally developing preschooler has acquired many cognitive skills by school age. He has mastered the basic structure of his language and through it comes to be able to understand the world. He has knowledge of things related to himself, of common objects in his environment, of experiences, of concepts, and he has beginning reading, writing, and number skills. The normal 6-year-old has long since mastered concepts of size, shape, color, number, texture, sound, and smell. A retarded preschooler, however, will not have the same degree of understanding. A 6-year-old child who is at least moderately retarded might not recognize two of something, or identify the color red, or indicate which of two things is bigger, or which shape is square. It is not that the child perceives these things differently but rather that he has not yet learned the properties by which they are known and understood. What the retarded child is able to comprehend will roughly correspond to his mental age. The cognitive limitations of the child are a manifestation of his learning difficulties and a direct consequence of the impairment in general intelligence.

Social Skills

The quality of relatedness to other persons of the preschool-age retarded child is a function of both the degree of retardation and the extent of his acceptance by parents and sibs. Retardation itself will cause the child to appear immature, because at any given age his overall level of functioning will be more like that of a younger child. One can, in fact, think of retardation as a condition of permanent immaturity. At age 5, for example, the retarded child may still need much help in dressing and not yet be toilet-trained. The child's speech is likely to be much impaired, his general coordination poor, his understanding of situations not like that of a 5-year-old, and his emotional behavior marked by easier emotionality, greater impulsivity, and manifestations of affect appropriate to a child younger than himself. The immaturity that is built into retardation also affects the child's ability to relate to others. In selecting playmates he'll seek out children who are younger than himself—children whose developmental levels are closer to his own. Without the assistance of adults or access to nursery school or day care experiences, the child's immaturity is likely to lead to social isolation by other children and to foster clinging to parents long after other children have begun to develop meaningful peer relationships. In our view, retarded children are in particular need of preschool socialization experiences, and, wherever possible, these should be integrated with day care programs for normal children. Within such a setting the retarded child will have normal youngsters whom he can emulate, and the latter will be early exposed to the child who is "different" in a setting where attitudes of acceptance can be encouraged.

We have also said that family acceptance will affect the quality of the child's interpersonal relationships. Out of his early affectional experiences with parents and sibs will emerge attitudes toward himself (self-concept) and others which will shape his general responsiveness to people and to tasks. Where the family-child interaction is positive and the child feels wanted and loved, a sense of trust and confidence is generated that fosters attitudes of openness and approach to new people and experiences. Contrariwise, where the child has not been adequately loved and there is the feeling of covert if not overt rejection, the child's unconditional need for love and for persons on whom he can depend is frustrated, and he becomes fearful and antagonistic. People become a potential source of pain rather than pleasure, and behavioral styles are learned in which avoidance rather than approach predominates.

Another important determinant of the child's attitude toward himself and thus toward others is the degree to which there is some expectancy of success in coping with developmental tasks. Though the behaviors that grow out of the widespread human need to feel some sense of adequacy may be more apparent in older children and adults than in preschoolers, their roots are likely to lie in the early years. Retarded children come to anticipate difficulty rather than success in coping with new tasks. The nature of the child's disability makes coping difficulties inevitable, but, paradoxically, except when the degree of retardation is severe, the mental handicap is not so great as to prevent the child from ultimately becoming aware of his limitations. If this self-awareness has not occurred during the preschool years, it will certainly be achieved once the child is in school. It is in school as nowhere else that the retarded child's learning difficulties relative to other children will be manifest to him. One commonly hears adolescent retarded youth saying, "It's hard for me to learn." While frustration of the need to feel some sense of adequacy is itself painful, it is especially so if self-esteem has already been lowered by limited parental acceptance. Avoiding expected criticism becomes a means of protecting whatever acceptance is felt, and this leads to a restriction of activities to those with little risk of failure. We see this reflected in the retarded child's zealous preference for the familiar—for that which has already been mastered. But the achievement of some measure of security through the restriction of experiences is self-defeating because it precludes the learning of new skills and higher levels of adaptation.

We have discussed at some length a few important social and personality factors in mental retardation. Though introduced in the context of the preschool years, they operate, of course, throughout life; it is only that the early years seem to be important in setting their direction. We shall also return to these same personality variables in the next chapter.

ADAPTIVE DEFICITS
DURING THE SCHOOL YEARS

The school years are a crucial period for the retarded child because the intellectual impairment precludes normal educational progress. Mentally handicapped children are especially limited in the learning of basic academic skills, and it was this difficulty that led to the development of the first noninstitutional programs for these youths—special classes or special education in the public schools. Within the range of retardation only the mildly retarded (educable) youngster is likely to achieve any usable reading and number skills. Even here, however, the average level of attainment is only about third grade (Bilsky, 1976; Gunzburg, 1968), and this is hardly functional for the reading and number tasks involved in activities of daily living. One needs about a sixth-grade reading level to read a newspaper, and at least a fourth-grade arithmetic level for anything beyond simple addition and subtraction. Moderately retarded (trainable) children usually do not achieve beyond first-grade level; their educational experience is likely to be nonacademic in emphasis, with stress on strengthening of self-help, social, language, and motor skills (Campbell, 1968).

The school years are also an extremely significant period in social development. In the normal youngster it is a time of loosening ties with parents as peer relationships assume growing importance—first same-sex relationships and then, in puberty, opposite-sex relationships. The same pattern is seen in retarded youth though at a much slower rate. Mildly retarded youth, in particular, will manifest social behaviors that parallel those of normal youngsters, though their behavior will appear immature relative to their chronological age. Moderately retarded school-age youth are less likely to demonstrate the same degree of opposite-sex interest as those with mild retardation. Even through the high school years, their social behavior has a childlike quality. At severe and profound levels of retardation, the school years are at a time when social skills are still only slowly developing, and many of these youth, especially those with profound handicap, will show little interest in interpersonal relationships at any level.

The latter part of the school period is a time of vocational preparation, and the retarded youngster is going to be at a serious disadvantage because of the pronounced academic limitations. In spite of this, most mildly and moderately retarded youths are eventually employable, the former in regular unskilled jobs and the latter in sheltered workshops. In either setting success will depend heavily on the presence of good work habits (e.g., reliability, persistence) and the ability to cooperate with others. The fostering of these personality characteristics becomes an important educational goal as does instruction in the practical activities of daily living—safety, shopping, money management, household skills, use of leisure time, and so on. Mainstreaming of mildly retarded (educable) children into regular classes should not result in a diminished effort in these areas. This is accomplished by continued access of mildly retarded students to supportive services, through so-called "resource" teachers.

Identification of the Retarded Child in the Classroom

In the school setting the academic learning problem created by mental retardation is certain to call attention to these children. The process by which they are identified and, hopefully, served is now indicated. The focus here is on the intellectual part of the assessment.

The child with serious learning problems will eventually be referred for initial assessment as a means of trying to understand the cause(s) of the child's poor academic progress. It must be stressed here that assessment *follows* academic difficulties (Ashurst & Meyers, 1973; Meyers, 1971); it is neither their cause nor their cure! Consider, for example, a 6-year-old first grader who was, initially, much behind his classmates in so-called "readiness" skills and who, over a lengthy period, continues to function far behind them. Let's also assume that there are adaptive deficits in other areas as well as in the academic one. Thus in self-help, social, language, and motor skills, the child also functions at a level well below that of his classmates.

Intelligence Testing

The intellectual assessment of this child would likely be done with any one of three tests—the Stanford-Binet, the Wechsler Preschool and Primary Scale of Intelligence (WPPSI), and the Wechsler Intelligence Scale for Children–Revised (WISC-R). In this hypothetical evaluation we shall use the Stanford-Binet because, in addition to an IQ, it derives a "mental age," a score that is important in understanding the mental development of retarded children. Let us assume that on the Binet the child achieves a mental age of 4 years. The child was successful on all test items at the 3-year level (basal age) and had some successes at the III-6-, 4-, and 5-year levels before missing all items at the 6-year level (ceiling age).

To give some flavor of the test, the child's patterns of successes and failures are shown in Table 2 and are grouped in categories suggested by Sattler (1975).[7] Test items are described and shown as either correct or incorrect. The age at which each appears on the test is given in Roman numerals.

In conjunction with other assessment data related to the child's general developmental level, the examiner can now begin to understand something of the youngster's learning problem. In essence, the immaturity of the child in all areas of adaptive behavior appears to reflect a degree of mental development that is 2

---

[7]The reader might also wish to characterize the test item groupings in terms of "factors" and/or "processes."

TABLE 2   A Probable Pattern of Successes and Failures of a Retarded Child on the Stanford-Binet Test

Language

Correct	Incorrect
Size Comparison (III-6)	Giving verbal definitions of common objects (V)
Naming common objects in pictures (III-6)	Defining words (VI)
Labeling pictures (IV)	
Labeling by function (IV)	

Reasoning

Correct	Incorrect
Putting two halves of a picture together (III-6)	Recognizing similarities and differences in pictures (V)
Finding a particular animal in a group of them (III-6)	Putting two triangular pieces together to make a rectangle (V)
Sorting by color (III-6)	Showing what is missing in a picture (VI)
Finding like forms (IV)	
Recognizing similarities and differences in pictures (IV-6)	

Memory

Correct	Incorrect
Naming objects that were hidden (IV)	Following three directions (IV-6)

Numerical Reasoning

Correct	Incorrect
None	Number concepts to 10 (VI)

Visual-motor

Correct	Incorrect
Imitating the folding of a piece of paper (V)	Completing a drawing of a man (V)
Copying a square (V)	Tracing a simple maze (VI)

Conceptual thinking

Correct	Incorrect
None	Opposite analogies (e.g., "In daytime it is light, at night it is _____" (IV)
	Opposite analogies (IV-6) (VI)
	Giving verbal differences (VI)

Social intelligence

Correct	Incorrect
Giving details about a picture (III-6)	Telling why we have houses; why we have books (IV)
Telling what to do when thirsty; why we have stoves (III-6)	
Recognizing the prettier of two people (IV-6)	
Telling what things are made of (IV-6)	
Telling function of our eyes and our ears (IV-6)	

years behind that expected for the average child of 6. The reason for the poor school progress is now very apparent. The youngster is expected to cope with the academic tasks typically presented to a 6-year-old when mental development is much more like that of a 4-year-old. We do not expect the average 4-year-old to function like a first grader, but this is the situation in which this retarded child is placed. Continued failure is inevitable unless the program is adjusted in accordance with the child's current level of academic readiness. If this does not occur, school will come to symbolize failure, a setting that breeds low self-esteem, and one to be avoided wherever possible.

Mental Age and Intelligence Quotient

In describing this 6-year-old child, reference has been made only to mental age, not to IQ. It is the mental age that indicates the age equivalent of cognitive development and provides us with some specific educational guidelines. But now we look at IQ. The IQ not only tells us how this child's mental development compares with that of classmates, it also has *some* predictiveness for *future* mental age.

To further illustrate the meaning of IQ and MA and to better understand the relative deficit of the retarded youngster in comparison with children of the same age, now and in the future, let us look at the mental status of three first graders:

$$\text{Superior } \frac{\text{MA } 8}{\text{CA } 6} = \text{IQ } 133$$

$$\text{Average } \frac{\text{MA } 6}{\text{CA } 6} = \text{IQ } 100$$

$$\text{Retarded } \frac{\text{MA } 4}{\text{CA } 6} = \text{IQ } 67$$

Assuming that the two children representing superior and retarded mental functioning are at the extremes of the class, we quickly see that there is a 4-year mental age difference between its brightest and dullest pupil. The youngster with superior intelligence has a mental age of 8 years, which means a readiness to handle third-grade work. This child, too, may present problems in the classroom if the level of the educational experience is insufficiently challenging. Educational needs of the very bright child require no less attention than do those of a retarded classmate. Although the difference between the children at the extremes is enormous, it is the comparison between the average and retarded child that is most relevant. The retarded child at MA 4 years is, as we have noted, not intellectually ready to master academic material appropriate to the child with a mental age 2 years higher. But not only is this child *currently* 2 years behind normal classmates; if mental development continues at the level indicated by the present IQ, the difference will increase over time. One can also think of an IQ as a measure of *rate* of mental development, with an IQ of 67 reflecting a rate that is two-thirds of normal. The mental age implication is that while the child with an IQ of 100, for example, gains 12 months in mental age over a year, the child with an IQ of 67 gains only two-thirds of that amount—8 months of mental age. Assuming a relative constancy in IQ, there will be a cumulative deficit that increases by 4 months each year during the mental age growth period. This is shown in Table 3 and also, graphically, in Figure 3.

At age 6 there is a 2-years mental age difference; it increases to 4 years at age 12 and to 6 years at age 18. Note that the mental age corresponding to IQ 100 at age 18 is 17 rather than 18. This is because the rate of increase on the Binet decreases after age 14. Thus over the 4-year period from 14 to 18, the youth with an IQ of 100 gains 3 years in mental age. This slowing in mental age growth signals the impending termination of the mental age growth period.

The Mental Age Growth Period

We come now to a very important aspect of intelligence and mental development and one that can be confused by the ordinary meaning of the term "retarded." The word "retarded" in its usual sense connotes delay rather than arrest, and parents may interpret their child's retardation as a condition of slow mental development which, given enough time, eventually is overcome. But this is not the case. Mental growth like physical growth occurs only during a limited time period. The notion of a limited time period for physical growth is accepted without a second thought. It is understood that we grow in height from infancy to adolescence and that by late adolescence we've ordinarily attained our maximum height. Whatever our attitude toward our height, the fact that it is fixed for the rest of our lives is accepted as part of the nature of physical growth. The principle of growth seen in physical stature also applies in the mental sphere. Analogous to growth in inches, we grow in mental age from infancy on into adolescence with a virtual completion of that growth process by age 18 (Terman & Merrill, 1973) (See Fig. 3). By this is meant that in the years up to 18 there is continuous growth in mental age and at a rate reflected by IQ. At age 6 we can solve problems we could not solve at 3, at age 9 we can solve problems we could not solve at 6, and so on. Our mental powers grow from year to year and are reflected in increases in mental age.

TABLE 3   Approximate Mental Ages and Mental Age Differences at Three Chronological Ages

			CA			
	6 years		12 years		18 years	
IQ	MA	MA difference	MA	MA difference	MA	MA difference
100	6	2	12	4	17	6
67	4		8		11	

Based on 1972 revision of the Stanford-Binet (Thorndike, 1973).

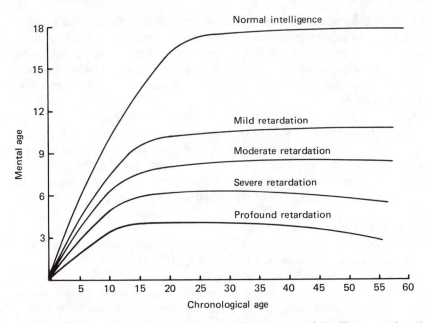

FIG. 3 Mental age growth curves corresponding to normal intelligence and to the four levels of retardation. Adapted from Fisher & Zeaman (1970).

But after age 18, mental age scores on the Binet generally no longer increase. That this is, in part, a function of the test rather than of a basic biological process is reflected in a somewhat longer growth period for raw scores on the Wechsler Adult Intelligence Scale (Wechsler, 1955). On this test, raw scores increase up to age 26 (Bayley, 1970). Beyond age 26 on the Wechsler Adult Intelligence Scale, raw scores remain fairly constant until old age, and even then very little decline is noted in persons who are in good health (Bayley, 1970; Birren, 1968).

The existence of a limited mental age growth period applies to all persons, retarded as well as normal. The retarded child does not catch up to the normal one because he,[8] too, operates within the same general developmental time frame. His rate of growth in mental age is slower, and his growth period is similar though there is some indication of a longer growth period in mildly retarded persons (Bayley, 1970; Clarke & Clarke, 1975; Fischer & Zeaman, 1970) and a shorter one in profoundly retarded ones (Fischer & Zeaman, 1970). The increase in mental age score in mildly retarded individuals is accompanied by an attendant increase in IQ because the Binet norms use 18 as the maximum denominator for chronological age. Based on changes in normal populations (Bayley, 1970), it is likely that these gains reflect increasing verbal skills such as defining words. Cattell has reported that growth in crystallized abilities (including verbal skills) continues long after growth in fluid abilities.

---

[8]The author will try to avoid "sexist" language but occasionally the use of such words makes life simpler!

Mental Age Growth and Learning

It is extremely important to distinguish between a limited mental age growth period and the capacity to learn. To say that out mental powers have largely reached their limit by young adulthood is not to say that we stop learning after this time. We can learn throughout our lives, retarded or normal; it is only that mental age roughly defines the complexity of that which we can understand.

ADAPTIVE PROBLEMS IN ADULTHOOD

We resume consideration of the adaptive problems associated with intellectual impairment by considering its impact on the developmental tasks of adulthood. We have reference to capacities for (a) self-management (independence, personal responsibility), (b) employment, (c) fulfillment of adult social or interpersonal roles, and (d) community adjustment. As is true in the preadult years, the quality of adaptation in each of these areas is closely tied to the degree of retardation.

Self-Management

Although the adaptive impairments created by mental retardation are often visible in early childhood and, inevitably, during the school years, the designation as retarded has always been at least implicitly associated with difficulty in functioning independently in adulthood. Through childhood and adolescence, a dependent status on the family is normative in our culture but, with the termination of formal education, the adolescent or young adult is expected to stand on his own two feet, to make his own way in the world. In this respect how have retarded persons fared?

It is clear from reviews of numerous long-term studies that they have done far better than was anticipated (Cobb, 1972; Goldstein, 1964; McCarver & Craig, 1974; Tizard, 1974). Whether first coming to the attention of investigators as former special class students in "educable" classes (Baller et al., 1966; Kennedy, 1966), as former institutional residents (Bell, 1976; Edgerton & Bercovici, 1976), or through a citywide survey (Richardson, 1978), the evidence is overwhelming that between 50 and 80 percent of mildly retarded adults can be expected to achieve an independent adjustment. It is true that the quality of that adjustment is probably more marginal than one would hope; problems are commonly cited with regard to handling money (McDevitt, Smith, Schmidt, & Rosen, 1978), utilizing leisure time, and finding employment (Bell, 1976). But the dire predictions of early workers with regard to this population have not been borne out.

Early in this century, retarded individuals were seen as a basically parasitic group (Fernald, 1919) who were not only crime- and pauper-prone but also a reproductive menace (Goddard, 1912; Kostir, 1916). Family studies that purported to show generations of retarded and otherwise physically or socially deviant persons led to the belief that retardation was largely hereditary (Dugdale, 1877; Goddard, 1912) and that retarded parents would only produce retarded children (Davenport, 1911). It was also feared that the families created by retarded parents would be larger than those of nonretarded individuals with the effect being to lower the general intelligence of the population and to actually threaten the quality of mankind! These fears led to the enactment of state sterilization laws in the period between 1910 and 1930 and to a change in the role of institutions. Formerly training- and education-oriented, they began to be used as custodial settings for the sexual segregation of retarded youth (Kanner, 1964). The fears of the early years of this century have been largely allayed, although their effects linger on in continuing controversy over sterilization and the rights of retarded persons to marry and to have children. The author's thoughts about this issue are presented in Chapter 9.

The at least marginally adequate adjustment of the majority of mildly retarded adults is an important antidote to our inherently egocentric view of the rest of humankind. We are not surprised that other who are like us can function reasonably well, but can these people whom, if we knew at all, we knew as school failures, also make out fairly adequately? The answer in many cases is "yes" even though, as will be indicated, there are some real differences in the quality of their general adjustment, especially in the work and social realms.

While independence is achieved by a majority of mildly retarded adults, this is not true for those with more severe degrees of retardation. In a follow-up study of a very large number of former students in classes for trainable children (usually IQ range of 30–50), about one-quarter had been institutionalized, and the remainder resided with their families (Saenger, 1957). Although few at that time were productively employed or had much of a life outside the home, parents were generally positive about their relationship with their retarded "adult-child." A similar picture of almost total family dependency is found in a former trainable class group followed up, even if only 3 years after school completion (Stanfield, 1973).

Although persons with more than mild retardation do not achieve independence, they can function in such nonfamily community residential settings as group homes. It is these community-based alternatives to the family that will help the more severely retarded individual avoid eventual institutionalization when access to family support is no longer possible.

Employment

As with self-management, all levels of employability are seen in retardation. Mildly retarded adults are capable of regular employment, typically in unskilled jobs (Heber & Dever, 1970), although those with good manual aptitude can aspire to a "helper" or to semiskilled status (DiMichael, 1964). Academic limitations preclude the attainment of full "skilled" status. While the proportion of unskilled jobs has sharply declined with the growth of technology (Goldstein, 1964), about one-fifth of all jobs are still classified as unskilled (Nixon, 1970), and these are increasingly found in the "service" rather than the "manufacturing" sector of the economy (e.g., motels, restaurants, laundries [Strickland & Arrell, 1967]). These are, of course, the lowest-paying jobs (Gozali, 1972; Heber & Dever, 1970); they provide little security and are particularly vulnerable to economic recession. But it has been noted that, with the growth of public assistance programs, retarded persons, like others who are economically disadvantaged, have learned how to survive when jobs are scarce (Edgerton & Bercovici, 1978). When we drop below mild retardation, the quality of employment changes, with a heavy concentration in "sheltered" rather than regular employment—sheltered workshops and work-activity centers. Here one finds some mildly retarded and many moderately retarded individuals productively employed. It has been suggested that gainful employment is possible for persons with IQs as low as 40 (Conley, 1976), but special training procedures indicate that even this may not be the necessary minimum (Bellamy et al., 1975; Crosson, 1969; Gold, 1973). In the case of severely and profoundly retarded persons, however, without special training there is unlikely to be the kind of task persistence that is essential to some degree of productive employment, and for them "activity" centers becomes the means of offering out-of-home daily activities of a meaningful nature.

Fulfilling Adult Social Roles

Throughout our lives each of us simultaneously fulfills a number of social (interpersonal) roles: student, worker, child, sibling, friend, friend to the opposite sex, spouse, and parent. Each of these roles carries with it culture-specific behavioral expectations, and the extent to which these can be fulfilled is at least partly related to general intelligence. Mildly retarded individuals function in all of these roles—they are members of families, they have friends, they marry, they have children. Nevertheless, their social lives seem to be more isolated, and fewer of them have opposite-sex friends, marry, or have children (Bell, 1976; Bowman & Hoffman, 1969; Edgerton & Bercovici, 1976; McDevitt et al., 1978). With regard to their role as parents, the author has some reservations, and these are discussed in Chapter 5 and again in Chapter 9.

One role that appears to be somewhat unique is that of "advisee." There is some indication that retarded adults, though living independently, still seek out "benefactorlike" relationships with normal persons, often neighbors (Edgerton, 1967). It is to these individuals that retarded persons turn for advice during periods of stress. And the life of the person whose social and economic adjustment is likely to be marginal does present special stresses which give to it a measure of instability and to the person, perhaps, some degree of stoicism. Happily, with time and a growing sense of confidence in one's ability to survive, the dependence on benefactors appears to diminish (Edgerton & Bercovici, 1976; Edgerton, Bollinger & Herr, 1984).

Although mildly retarded individuals function in all adult social roles, this is usually not true at more severe degrees of impairment. Moderately retarded adults do have friends and may have opposite-sex interests, but the latter are not likely to lead to marriage. They also seem to be quite isolated socially, as most of their leisure time is spent in solitary activity such as TV, card playing, looking at pictures in magazines, or walking alone in the neighborhood (Stanfield, 1973). Where the retardation is severe or profound, there may be difficulty in entering into even "friend" relationships, the person continuing to relate to normal adults in a childlike manner or showing little or no interest in others.

Community Adjustment

The focus here is on the general adjustment of the retarded persons in their home community. We noted that, during the early decades of this century, retarded individuals were perceived as a threat to society because of assumed excessive levels of dependency (pauperism), family size, and criminality. The dependency fear was early laid to rest, as have been the concerns about family size and criminality. With reference to family size, an interesting paradox obtains. Although it is true that average family size is increased among retarded people, the fact is that far fewer of them have children (Reed & Reed, 1965). Thus the high risk of retardation in these families, whether due to biological and/or psychological factors, is more than offset by a reduced frequency of marriage and childbearing. With regard to criminality, too, it is clear that early fears were grossly exaggerated, although the proportion of retarded persons in prison is in excess of their numbers in the general population—9 to 10 percent (Brown & Courtless, 1967; MacEachron, 1979). But there is good reason to believe that at least part, if not all, of the excess is attributable to a greater vulnerability of the retarded person to the vicissitudes of the criminal justice system. Thus retarded individuals are more prone than the general population to confess to crimes they have not committed (this caused by suggestibility and fear) or through their lawyer to plea bargain as a means of expedience. And once convicted and imprisoned, the retarded offender is more likely to receive no rehabilitation services, to suffer some abuse by other inmates, and to serve longer terms than nonretarded persons convicted of the same crime (Biklen, 1977). It would be incomplete, however, not to acknowledge that the offenses for which more severely retarded persons are imprisoned tend more frequently to be crimes against persons than is true of nonretarded offenders. In the below-55 IQ range, 57 percent were of such a nature as compared with 27 percent among nonretarded offenders. Undoubtedly, the presence of retardation reduces the likelihood of becoming involved in "white-collar" crime.

Apart from these special concerns, the hopes and aspirations of retarded adults do not seem very different from our own. In a second follow-up study of a group of 30 formerly institutionalized persons (Edgerton & Bercovici, 1976), we're told that their primary interest was in enjoying life, that what seemed uppermost to them was neither work nor an earlier-felt stigma associated with having once been institutionalized but rather the desire for recreation, hobbies, good times, friends, and family. And though more susceptible to the stresses of a marginal economic adjustment, the majority seemed reasonably content and happy.

"Impact of Onset in Developmental Period"

We come now to the third element in the AAMD definition of mental retardation; it identifies the period in life during which retardation originates or becomes manifest. The developmental period presumably refers to the time during which virtually all mental growth occurs. While there is certainly brain growth prenatally, we have no way of measuring either general intelligence or adaptive behavior prior to birth. To be consistent with the essence of the definition, return to the birth to 18 age range would seem appropriate even though measures of mental ability in the *infant* are regarded with caution.

One of the consequences of the traditional association of retardation with an origin in the early years, especially childhood, is to exclude from the classification persons who become intellectually impaired in the adult years. Thus intellectual deficit associated with head trauma or illness following a period of normal development has typically led to the designation as "brain-injured" rather than as retarded. Although it is doubtful that this distinction could be justified in terms of the services provided to the two groups, they are clearly different in how they were perceived by others and by themselves during the growing-up years. Apart from the mildly retarded, nonorganically impaired segment of the retarded population, the remainder are clearly different from parents and sibs and are so perceived by them. Their "difference" leads to a variety of special reactions and, sometimes, to problems of acceptance only rarely seen in nonhandicapped children. It is this aspect of the "developmental period" that seems at least as important as its equation with the period of growth in mental age. Thus the developmental period is also the time during which the basic personality characteristics of the retarded child are formed, and these will have significance for future adjustment and happiness. In the next chapter a picture of personality in mental retardation is presented; here we want only to address what is perhaps the most important shaper of that personality, the short- and long-term impact of retardation on the child's parents.

INITIAL IMPACT OF THE RETARDED CHILD

Shock and Grief

Whether the child is perceptibly different at birth, as is commonly the case in Down syndrome, or the retardation is not recognized until later in childhood, typically by age 2, the effect on the parents of learning the nature of their child's difficulty is devastating (Gardner et al., 1965; Hay, 1951; Koegler, 1963; Wolfensberger & Kurtz, 1969; Zwerling, 1954). Unless there has been a previously abnormal birth, no parent is psychologically prepared for anything but a normal one. For some, the experience is so overwhelming that they abandon any intention of fulfilling the parental role and seek immediate placement of the newborn outside the home. Until quite recently such decisions were often encouraged by physicians; they saw the child as only a future burden on the parents and one for whom the development of any parental attachment would lead only to future grief and disappointment. In effect, parents were frequently encouraged to "place the child and forget him" (Spock, 1961).

The physician's recommendations can be understood as a general reflection of our culture's negative attitude toward retardation and may also stem from both an awareness that there was no medical means of altering the child's condition and the assumption that the child could never bring happiness to himself or to others. In light of the tremendous proliferation of services in retardation, from infancy to adulthood, and the actual experiences of parents and sibs, some moderation of this sense of despair is appropriate.

Guilt and Isolation

Apart from the degree of support that parents may or may not receive from those who first identify the child's condition, another very stressful aspect of the initial impact of the diagnosis is that the parents, because of a frequent sense of guilt and shame (Wolfensberger, 1967), are constrained from reaching out to their usual sources of emotional support (Murray, 1959). Rather than feeling free to share their burden, they seek to hide it, and this only adds to their emotional tensions.

CONTINUING IMPACT OF THE RETARDED CHILD

Unending Parental Concern

The nature of the adaptive difficulties produced by major intellectual impairment is such that coping problems occur at all points in the child's life (Adams, 1971; Beck, 1969; Bryant & Hirschberg, 1970; Schild, 1971). For the parent of the young retarded child there is a prolongation of the normal period of infancy and of the intense dependency, typically on the mother, that is inherent in it. Later there will be concerns for playmates, possibly undue pressures on sibs to assume other playmate or surrogate-parent roles, and, in school, concerns for proper education, a social and recreational life, and a growing awareness and anxiety about the child's developing sexuality.

If sexuality in the normal teenager is a source of anxiety for parents, imagine the fears it evokes in parents of retarded youth. These are commonly fears of exploitation; on the other hand, many parents pretend that their "child" is not changing into an adolescent or adult and continue to treat him as if he really were a permanent child. In the adult years, the termination of school experience fosters parental concerns about finding meaningful activities to fill their child's day. And with the loss of school and relationships with teachers and classmates, there will be increased pressures on parents and sibs to meet the retarded person's social and recreational needs. For some, the sexuality of their now retarded "adult-child" can no longer be denied, and they experience fear because they regard the retarded youth as unable to manage these impulses judiciously. Finally, the mortality of the parents themselves is an ever present reminder that, eventually, someone else will need to provide a home for their child. In the past, the large state institutions assumed this care role, but with the recent development of such community-based residential services as "family care" and "group homes," the range of parental options has been considerably widened.

Each of the concerns constitutes a potential source of emotional stress for parents and sibs and, if chronic and severe, can jeopardize their capacity to provide the degree of love, acceptance, and stability needed by the retarded person— needs also shared by the rest of us. The nature of these needs is spelled out in the next chapter. While the problems that have been described make the role of parenting a retarded child seem hopelessly difficult and unrewarding, this is clearly not the case. Let us listen to some real parents as they describe their experiences. In them we will encounter both the sorrows and joys and the emotional growth that seem to be a common outcome of this kind of family experience.

First, the story of Roger, now in his early 30s, as told by his older brother. It originally appeared in a newspaper series on mental retardation (*The Washington Post*, August 22, 1977) and is quoted extensively because it gives the flavor of the impact of retardation on the affected person and his family.

The preschool years

Our parents did not begin to wonder about Roger's physical and mental capabilities until some six months after he was born. "He was a quiet baby in the daytime, but he cried and cried at night. . . . He could sometimes be lethargic or extremely active." He looked to them like "the sweetest baby in the world." [Roger's mother recalls a visit of her mother] "My mother came to visit her grandchild and she thought Roger was weak, that he didn't have any strength for finger pulls. I didn't know what to say."

For the next 18 months, our parents hoped and prayed that Roger's responses would speed up, that his strength would increase. . . . They compared his progress to mine—I was five years older—and it became apparent that Roger was not developing as he should.

When Roger was 2 they took him to a leading . . . neurologist. His conclusion was that "some retardation may be indicated." [Roger's father recalls his first thought] "Oh my God, where do we go, what do we do?" [Shock and bewilderment] My mother said, "I felt *guilty*, I had carried this baby, what had I done wrong? I felt lost and hopeless. People—even doctors told me not to worry, that things would be alright, but they weren't. . . . It was so devastating to be told that there was nothing wrong, or not very much wrong, when you KNOW, you just KNOW. . . ." [Parents do seem to want to know the full truth (Carr, 1974), though it is natural for the diagnostician to be both cautious and somewhat reassuring].

At the same time, the idea that a drug, or a procedure, or even just the passage of time would solve their problem was the kind of emotional carrot that led our parents on, though they were frustrated repeatedly over the years. [Hope does spring eternal.]

They were "terrified, terrified," that he would end up in a state mental institution—then the primary repositories of both the severely and mildly retarded [and the most visible of retardation services]. They saw pictures in newspaper exposés of people there with bent and broken bodies lying half-naked in their own filth, abandoned by everyone except the flies. . . .

[Commenting on the family pressures engendered by retardation, the noted psychiatrist in mental retardation, Dr. Frank Menolascino is quoted] "Having a retarded child does not have to be the end of the world, but you've got to be able to handle stress well. You've got to have good support systems—brothers, sisters, cousins you can turn to—and you've got to have good professional service, which just didn't exist then" [and still really doesn't].

Neither parent knew anyone with a retarded child and social stigmas kept them from asking too many questions. . . . "I was so alone, so isolated," my mother said [re the earlier reference to shame and the sense of isolation. . . . Some of the professional advice that they received was also not helpful. One doctor recommended megavitamins, another brain surgery, while a third assumed that Roger would never develop any reading or writing skills and that television would be his chief means of getting information. While of the three observations, the last is probably closest to the truth, in fact, mildly retarded persons, of whom Roger is one, do acquire some academic skills, though admittedly, often quite limited].

Roger's behavior as a child varied widely. He could be bright and alert and at other times lethargic, his gaze wandering and his head drooping. He had a soft bone structure and before he was 5 he had broken both collarbones in falls from bed. . . . He had a speech impediment and it was often impossible for my parents to understand him [speech intelligibility is a common problem]. At such times I would be the translator, telling them what he had said. Roger would often wake up screaming during the night, and frequently walked in his sleep. . . . "He was so highstrung, trying to keep up with others, trying to make himself understood . . . [emotional problems added to his intellectual and physical ones. The stresses of caring for Roger were almost totally borne by his mother as his father had immersed himself in his work, a common pattern, and mother sought to ease her tensions through alcohol.] "We'd be walking along [says the mother], the two of us, and I felt like we were two rejects, him and me. Society had rejected him and I was rejecting myself."

It was at this time that two new strains developed in her life, my mother said. One was what she called The Search. It was a 17-year-long attempt to find a residential facility to which the family could afford to send Roger. [Until recently only private residential (institutional) facilities were available as an alternative to the large state institutions and these were, and are, very expensive. Now, as already noted, group homes are increasingly available, and it was in such a facility that Roger was eventually placed.] The other [strain] was what she described as a reliance on alcohol to ease the pain and frustration and which also ended when she joined Alcoholics Anonymous.

The school years

Roger's first school was a private school . . . followed by public schools, often supplemented with private tutoring. They believed he had more ability than showed up on any of the tests he was given—

which, in a Catch 22 situation, they were never permitted by school authorities to see. [This is no longer true as the federal Education for All Handicapped Children Act (P.L. 94-142) gives parents the right to see all such materials.] . . . They attempted to give him as many "real-life" experiences as possible.

[His father speaks] "I took Roger to the rodeo, to the circus and took him to work with me on Saturdays [the father was in advertising]. I taught him to say 'L'addition, s'il vou plait' ['the check, please'] just like I did with you" [encouragement of at least a facade of normality].

My mother spent hours with him on his school work and socialization—making sure he knew the importance of and method for brushing his teeth, combing his hair, taking care of his appearance.

There were problems in school. Roger was teased and taunted. He'd always say, "Well Mom, I hate to tell you this, but they're making fun of me again." . . . Other children laughed at him when he couldn't keep up with them, or they mocked his speech impediment. [Why are we so cruel to each other?]

There was an incident . . . when a man tried to assault him sexually. "I got so hysterical I couldn't even dial the police. Roger called them himself, and I didn't think he knew how."

[Following several family moves due to economic dislocation] our father had found a job . . . and the family moved to a nice apartment with Roger enrolled in a nearby junior high school. [his mother was also working now as a secretary]. There his problems with so-called "normal" kids continued: a gang made him sing and dance in the schoolyard to their jeers. Roger, glad to have the attention, said "I thought they liked my singing." A neighborhood tough forced Roger to stand on his shoulders and knock out street lights. A bunch of kids cornered him at a park and made him take some clothes off.

My mother asked the school guidance counselor for help. His answer was to recommend that Roger be warehoused [undoubtedly mother's expression] in a state facility [that *would* resolve the teasing problem at school!]

"That made me so angry. I just can't tell you. . . . All of the work I'd done with him, every book I taught him to read [the earlier prediction of no reading ability was inaccurate] all of his manners—to throw everything away in some place where he'd be taunted and sexually abused and placed in a corner—never, I never for one minute considered it. I wouldn't have been able to live with myself. I could barely live with myself as it was."

Roger was becoming a young man, really very handsome, with light brown hair which he combed over his forehead, and a willingness to tell everyone he met that he was retarded. He likes to watch movies and sports on television, especially golf, perhaps because it is a game of understandable moves. Horror movies were particular favorites, perhaps because he could watch them without fear, a sign that he had overcome the nightmares of his youth. . . . He spent most of his time at home.

He was becoming interested in girls: teeny-bopper princesses with long blond hair. He put their pictures up on the walls and talked to the ones who walked by his house on their way to high school. But beyond that, he had little social life [the problem of finding out-of-school friends in adolescence]. "He was lonely, I think that's why he wrote his poetry. He needed to know other kids like himself, but didn't, our mother said [a role for local recreation departments]. He knew about sex, and often used a then-popular phrase that something was 'very sexy' but pronounced the words as if they were 'sax' and 'saxy.' "

But the real world could not forget that Roger was retarded, and our family was swiftly reminded of the fact on one painful occasion.

The postschool years

When he was 19, Roger wrote a Valentine's Day poem to a girl he met at the local YMCA, at the same time as someone else wrote her an obscene letter filled with sexual references. The girl's parents called the police, who because the mails were involved, called the FBI. Although the most explicit line in Roger's poem is "A Valentine is sweet, because it's sharing warm, affectionate love," Roger was tagged as the prime suspect in the case. An armed police officer went to the sheltered workshop where Roger was employed . . . [an extremely important resource for physically and mentally handicapped people] and took him into another room for interrogation. "The policeman showed him the letter but Roger had to ask him what the (obscene) words meant," my mother said. Roger was frantic with fear that he would lose his job. The policeman then showed the letter to my mother, covering up the dirty words. "I screamed that my son couldn't even *write* script (which the letter was written in), that he could only print." Roger's poem—decorated with large and small hearts—and the obscene letter were both sent to the FBI for analysis. The analysis determined that the real culprit was a "normal" 11-year-old boy who sat next to the girl in school. An FBI agent involved in the case later apologized saying, "I couldn't control the local cop. He thought Roger must have done it, because since he's retarded he's supposed to be 'different.' "

[When Roger was 20 The Search ended with Roger moving into a group home with other retarded youth. His mother recalls, "There wasn't a good-looking kid there. . . . But they all looked clean and happy. And the way they followed the director around, it was like they were following Jesus. I felt Roger could be happy there."]

The facility was not the perfect solution, because Roger was one of the smartest ones there. Initially, he was not challenged enough to live up to his potential [a common problem]. But times were changing, and so were the traditional attitudes toward the responsibility of government to provide help. With more and more government money available, there were more and more newly trained counselors, bringing more and more ideas to challenge the residents to think and act for themselves. They went bowling, hiking, held discussion group meetings. Roger eventually moved into . . . individual living units . . . , then into his own apartment, and was married [at age 24 . . . work, poetry, marriage—all of this was possible for Roger in spite of early prophets of doom. In his own words, "People are retarded by what they don't know. That's why I work so hard to learn the things I don't know and become more normal."]

The story of Roger has been fraught with family stresses, but in his young adult years he appears to have surmounted them, as have his parents. He has insight into the nature of his difficulty as does his wife, Virginia, who is also mildly retarded. Asked how it is to be retarded she replied, "How is it with us? It is no different than it is with anyone else, except we're slower."

Before ending this section there is one more parental experience that should be shared with the reader. Roger's story conveyed nothing but a sense of travail and would lead one to believe that there can be little joy in the rearing of a retarded child. Let us listen to the mother of an 8-year-old Down syndrome child as she describes her experience in a letter to a newspaper.[9]

If this turns out to be a Pollyanna-like story I hope no one reads it, or else reads it and writes a nasty letter. Being a Pollyanna can be tolerated in some instances I suppose, but never in regard to retardation. And that's what this is about, mental retardation, or more precisely, certain feelings I have toward my eight-year-old son who is mentally retarded.

Now believe me, I have had my moments of weeping and despair. When I first learned that our baby, that rosy, dimpled infant was retarded I almost died of agony. The doctors were wrong [grief and denial are common initial reactions to catastrophic events] . . . Our Ben couldn't be what they said, a child with Down's syndrome . . . a mongoloid. But he was, and he is, and that's a primary fact of his life and ours [ultimate acceptance of reality]. Today Ben is a sturdy eight-year-old. And I sometimes find tears in my eyes at the sight of him trying to keep up with his neighborhood peers who are so brightly normal, but I more often find myself smiling, sometimes even belly-laughing at the sheer exuberance with which this child faces life. The very idea for writing this at all is that not an hour ago I witnessed the most ecstatic, uninhibited reaction to a fried chicken TV commercial

[9]Originally published in *The Washington Post* and reprinted in *Mental Retardation News*, 1976, 25, No. 3.

that any sponsor could hope for in his wildest dreams. Who else can raise his arms in gustatory triumph over a dancing chicken and shout, "Wow!" in such a way as Ben? What an ability to translate the mundane into something terrific! It gives his life an added flavor at every turn.

He is lucky, this little boy of mine. He will not conquer the worlds of the academic, the scientific, or the great doers. But he has a unique appreciation for those ordinary rites of life that seem only dull and jaded to the rest of us. And it goes way beyond fried chicken. The neighbor's dog comes loping by covered with mud from a nearby creek and all we see is one big messy mutt. But Ben sees a friend, and they sit on the walk together, Ben's arms around the dog's neck, dog licking Ben's face; sheer joy in one another. We go to the ocean and contemplate its vast magnificence. The ocean fills a hole Ben has dug in the sand. "Beat it, Ocean," says Ben. Around 3:20 every afternoon the front door bangs open and various articles are dropped on the floor. "I'm back, Mommie," shouts Ben and comes to give me my home-again hug. . . .

One recent Saturday morning the whole family had slept late and as my husband and I were struggling awake Ben came into our room to say good morning. He looked at his stubble-chinned, disheveled father and in the tone of a true believer announced, "Daddy is Prince Charming." At that moment I could see more of a resemblance to Godzilla but Ben saw Prince Charming. And then he turned to me—a half-unconscious Phyllis Diller—and said, "Mommie is The Sleeping Beauty." How wonderful to wake to laughter. And how wonderful to live with someone who can look at a couple of creaky parents and see a prince and a princess.

Pollyanna, go fly a kite.

But, Ben . . . , oh how I love you!

ADAPTIVE POTENTIAL, CHRONOLOGICAL AGE, AND DEGREE OF RETARDATION

In our elaboration of the definition of mental retardation we have identified major adaptive behavior deficits of retarded persons. To recognize them as deficits is to call attention to the fact that impaired intelligence leads to behavior patterns that differ from what is expected of the average individual of that age. While these differences are viewed as limitations, limitations as such are not unique to retarded persons. All persons are limited in the sense that we can always find others whose capacities in one form or another exceed our own. The bright student sees others with even greater academic ability, the talented musicians hears a virtuoso whom he does not expect to equal, the pretty girl sees another with even greater beauty, and the outstanding athlete encounters other athletes who outdo him. It is in the nature of things that our individual capacities are limited relative to others, but as long as our abilities are grossly normal the individual differences we recognize are not perceived as pathological or deviant. Let us now change our perspective of the retarded person from one of adaptive deficits to one of adaptive potential: what he can do, as well as what causes him difficulty. There is now given a detailed description of the adaptive potential of retarded persons from infancy to adulthood. It is presented in the form of rough norms which offer behavior expectations as a function of mental age, chronological age, and degree of retardation. The norms themselves are based on an integration of earlier summarized ones (Robinson & Robinson, 1965), general developmental data (Hurlock, 1964), and norms offered in the 1973 and 1977 AAMD manuals (Grossman, 1973, 1977). In presenting them it should be understood that the intent is only to offer a rough approximation of what might be expected as a function of chronological age and degree of retardation. The offering of such norms may be viewed by some as creating undesirable expectancy attitudes in workers by relating behavioral expectation to degree of retardation and to implying limitations as well as potential. It is true that we cannot know what is ultimately possible for any human being, but within the constraints of present pedagogy and medical science such limitations do exist, and awareness of them cannot be ignored in the planning of services to retarded persons.

The norms are divided into two parts—the first covers the developmental period, the years to 18; the second covers the adult years. The norms for the period to 18 years are organized around mental age, individuals with the same mental age having similar behavorial expectancies although differing in chronological age and degree of retardation. In fact, mental age is most predictive of cognitive and academic potential and less so of self-help and motor skills. In the latter areas, chronological age would make a difference, with the older child ordinarily functioning at a higher level than a younger one of the same mental age. This results from greater opportunities for "practice" in the older child simply because he has lived longer. Practice effects also seem more attainable on tasks involving motor skills. The second part of the norms, those for the adult years, are organized on the basis of degree of retardation as changes in mental age are not expected after age 18.

Mental age 1 year, chronological age 4 years and older, profoundly retarded

Self-help: Opens mouth for feeding, drinks from cup with help; beginning attempts at finger-feeding. *Motor:* Sits alone; may pull self to standing briefly; reaches for and manipulates parts of body, e.g., toes, objects; has thumb-finger grasp. *Language* (expressive): Imitates sounds, laughs, or smiles in response; may say "mama" or "dada"; expressive language will be at a pre-speech level—crying, vocalization, and gesture; *Language* (receptive): Some understanding of gestures and of very familiar words, e.g., "no." *Social:* Recognizes familiar persons and interacts with them but not verbally.

Mental age 1–2 years, chronological age 3–6 years, severely retarded; chronological age 8 years and older, profoundly retarded

Self-help: Finger feeds, may show beginning use of spoon; passive cooperation in dressing, bathing, and toileting; may have some bowel movements when placed on toilet, may remove simple articles of clothing, e.g., hat and socks. *Motor:* Stands alone; may walk though needing help; performs simple motor tasks, e.g., turning, pulling, grasping. *Language* (expressive): May use one or two words but pre-speech forms continue to predominate. *Social:* May respond to others in predictable fashion; plays "patty cake" or plays imitatively with others; may play by self briefly.

Mental age 2–3 years, chronological age $3\frac{1}{2}$–5 years, mildly retarded; chronological age 5–7 years, moderately retarded; chronological age 6-9 years, severely retarded; chronological age 10 years and older, profoundly retarded

Self-help: Some use of spoon but with spilling; uses cup; more active cooperation in dressing and undressing; some use of toilet; may begin to indicate when pants are wet. *Motor:* Walks alone steadily; may run, jump in place, and climb stairs with help; may be able to turn single pages, open boxes, unscrew lids, string beads; may be able to imitate vertical and horizontal lines. *Language* (expressive): May use several words; if pronouns are used they're often used incorrectly; still using gestures. *Cognitive:* May recognize different shapes; possibly beginning number concepts, e.g., distinguishing between "one" and "many." *Social:* May play with others for short periods but play is "parallel" rather than interactive; recognizes other people and shows preferences.

Mental age 3–4 years, chronological age 5–7 years, mildly retarded; chronological age 7–10 years, moderately retarded; chronological age 9–12 years, severely retarded; chronological age 12–16 years; profoundly retarded

Self-help: Uses spoon with little spilling; beginning use of fork; can remove some clothing, e.g., coat or dress, can partially dress self; attempts to help in bathing and in washing hands; may indicate toilet accidents and need to use toilet. *Motor:* Can go up and down stairs; can run, jump, and balance on one foot; can pass a ball, transfer objects; will need much assistance in "fine motor" activities, e.g., buttoning, using zipper. *Language* (expressive): May use two- and three-word phrases, e.g., "where daddy?" "mommy go bye-bye"; beginning to use pronouns correctly and to refer to self by pronoun rather than by name; in pronunciation is usually correct on beginning and ending consonants, e.g., *mom, bib*; beginning to use "what," "where," and "who." *Cognitive:* Can identify own sex, recognize primary colors; beginning "time" concepts, e.g., today, tomorrow, yesterday; beginning "position" concepts, e.g., on top of, under, inside; number concepts through "two"; simple size concepts; may be able to print a few capital letters. *Social:* Can spontaneously engage with others in interactive play, usually with only one or two others; can be guided into play with larger groups; showing preferences among children.

Mental age 4–5 years, chronological age 6–9 years, mildly retarded; chronological age 10–12 years, moderately retarded; chronological age 12–15 years, severely retarded; chronological age 16 years and older, profoundly retarded

Self-help: Can feed self with spoon and fork; beginning to use knife for spreading; gets drink unassisted; can undress self; can put on clothing but needs help with zippers and small buttons; attempts to bathe self but needs assistance; washes and dries hands but not carefully; usually uses toilet when placed on it but may still have accidents (daytime training precedes nighttime control). *Motor* (gross-motor skills): Can climb stairs in alternating fashion; can hop, skip, balance on toes, walk balance boards, ride tricycle (over 8 years—bicycle); may climb trees or jungle gym; can play dance games; can throw ball at target; *Motor* (fine-motor skills): Can grasp pencil in manner resembling adult position; can button and lace. *Language* (expressive): May have considerable speaking vocabulary though speech will be particularly impaired in youngsters with more than mild retardation—if non-verbal, as in severely and profoundly retarded youth there may be use of gestures to communicate needs; *Language* (receptive): Understands simple verbal communications, e.g., following directions, responding to questions. *Cognitive-academic:* Has size concepts, can match pictures of identical objects, can answer simple "why" questions; beginning to be able to match geometric forms; some elementary reading skills—may recognize common printed words, e.g., STOP, GO, BOY, GIRL. *Social:* Can participate in group activities and games; can engage in simple play with other children, e.g., "store," "house."

Mental age 5–6 years, chronological age 8–10 years, mildly retarded; chronological age 11–13 years, moderately retarded; chronological age 13–15 years, severely retarded

Self-help: Adequate use of spoon and fork; can use knife for buttering though needs assistance with knife in cutting; can dress self including buttoning and zipping; may tie shoes; bathes self with supervision; washes and dries hands and face; brushes teeth; toiled-trained though there may be bladder accidents at night. *Motor:* Can run, hop, skip, and dance, can use skates, sled, or jump rope, can march to music. *Language* (expressive): Mildly retarded child may be using fairly normal sentence structure and have speech of good intelligibility; at more severe levels of retardation language may be at the phrase or single-word level and also be indistinct in pronunciation. *Cognitive-academic:* Can match geometric forms; has concepts of texture and weight; some idea of beauty, beginning concept of laterality, right-left; able to give differences between some common objects; may have number concepts up to "thirteen"; may be able to print name in large letters; may show frequent letter reversals; can print some numbers. *Social:* May participate spontaneously in group activities; can engage in simple competitive games, e.g., tag, races, dodge ball; may have true friendships (more likely in children who are not more than moderately retarded). *Community:* May be able to perform simple errands; make purchases with a note; understands that money has value but doesn't know how to use it (except in coin machines). *Household:* May prepare simple foods (sandwiches); perform simple household tasks, e.g., bedmaking, sweeping, vacuuming; can set and clear tables. *Self-direction:* May seek things to do; can pay attention to a task for at least 10 minutes; attempts to be dependable and to carry out responsibilities (more likely of mildly retarded youth).

Mental age 6–7 years, chronological age 10–12 years, mildly retarded; chronological age 14 years and older, moderately retarded

Self-help: Can feed, dress, and bathe self: may choose daily clothing, combs and brushes hair; may shampoo and roll hair; may wash and/or iron. *Motor:* Adequate motor skills especially in mildly retarded youth. *Language* (expressive): May be able to carry on simple conversation and use complex sentences (more true of mildly than of moderately retarded youth). *Cognitive-academic:* Beginning reading skills, can recognize simple words or read brief sentences (reading skills are likely to lag relative to mental age and its equivalent grade-age expectancy). *Social:* May interact cooperatively or completely. *Community:* May be able to perform simple shopping errands without notes; can make small purchases, some beginning money skills—understands values of coins; can do simple coin counting; can add and subtract up to ten. *Household:* Can prepare simple foods, e.g., sandwiches; perform simple household chores, e.g., dusting, dishwashing, garbage. *Self-direction:* May initiate much of own activities; can attend to tasks for at least 10 minutes; may be conscientious in assuming responsibility.

Mental age 7–11 years, chronological age 13–18 years, mildly retarded

Self-help: Cares for self in feeding, dressing, toileting, bathing, and grooming; may need health or personal care reminders; may need some assistance in selection and purchase of clothing. *Motor:* Essentially normal motor skills in "cultural-familial" retarded adolescent;

may be some impairment in motor skills in adolescent with "organic" retardation. *Language* (expressive): Essentially normal fluency though pronunciation problems may persist. *Cognitive-academic:* Reading and arithmetic achievement will closely correspond to mental age though often lag behind it somewhat; range in reading and number skills will be from first to sixth grade. *Social:* Can relate as friend to same sex and opposite sex; can participate in recreational activities enjoyed by adolescents but may have problems in complex games or competitive sports. *Community:* Some mobility in community, able to use public transportation; may drive; can do some independent shopping; can handle simple change-making but will have difficulty in money management; number skills will ordinarily be limited to addition and subtraction. *Household:* Can perform most routine household chores. *Self-direction:* Initiates most of own activity; relatively normal attention span; can perform routine tasks with only nominal supervision.

The Mentally Retarded Adult

Mildly retarded: IQ range 52–68 (Binet),[10] mental age range 8–11 years

Self-management: Full self-help skills; often function independently in the community though some will need assistance in managing activities of daily living; benefits from a person who can serve as an advisor. *Language:* Adequate for ordinary purposes of communication at both the expressive and receptive levels. *Academic:* May be able to read simple materials for information; unlikely to read for pleasure; number skills will tend to be limited to simple addition and subtraction and much assistance is needed in budgeting and general money management. *Vocational status:* Capable of regular employment in unskilled jobs though some can achieve "helper" status in trades. *Social roles:* Can fulfill all adult social roles: have friends, marry, become parents. *Community adjustment:* Some increased rate of delinquency in cultural familial group.

Moderately retarded: IQ range 36–51, mental age range 6–8 years

Self-management: Have basic self care skills but do not achieve an independent adjustment; will always require some degree of supervision. *Language:* Language is generally functional for purposes of communication but intelligibility of speech may be much impaired. *Academic:* Do not achieve functional reading and money skills. *Vocational status:* Do not ordinarily work at the level of regular employment but can work productively in sheltered workshops. *Social roles:* Usually do not fulfill roles of spouse and parent though capable of friendships

---

[10]The Binet IQ ranges are being used in preference to the Wechsler Scales because the latter does not provide a means for distinguishing between levels of retardation below the mildly retarded range.

with same and opposite sex. *Community adjustment:* Do not fulfill ordinary "citizen" functions and are unlikely to get into difficulties with the law.

Severely retarded: IQ range 20–35, mental age range 4–6 years

Self-management: Do not function independently though can acquire some self-help skills e.g., feeding, dressing, and toileting; will need assistance in complex acts of grooming and personal hygiene. *Language:* Understanding of language is likely to be much better than the ability to express it; speech may be very poorly articulated and difficult to understand. *Academic:* No functional reading or number skills for activities of daily living. *Vocational status:* May be capable of performing some useful work at either the sheltered workshop of work-activity levels of productivity; more likely to be attending an activity center. *Social roles:* Do not fulfill adult social roles; can have some peer relationships; relate to adults in childlike fashion. *Community adjustment:* Perform no "citizen" roles; do not get into difficulties with the law.

Profoundly retarded: IQ range 0–19, mental age range 0–4 years

Self-management: Will always require much supervision though some self-help skills may be acquired. *Motor:* Mobility may be impaired due to physical or sensory problems; a large proportion of so-called "non-ambulatory" retarded persons fall in this range of retardation. *Language:* Ability to understand is likely to far exceed ability to speak; there may be little or no speech; capable of following simple directions. *Academic:* No academic skills. *Vocational status:* May be unable to perform any useful work though with training in an activity center some may achieve a work-activity level of productivity. *Social roles:* Fulfill no adult social roles; may appear as a social isolate, paying little attention to others except as it relates to own needs; commonly shows "stereotyped" behavior. *Community adjustment:* Fulfill no community roles and commonly institutionalized.

Personality, Mental Retardation, and Related Developmental Disorders

OVERVIEW

In Chapter 1 the nature of mental retardation was detailed with particular emphasis on its cognitive side—that is, the character of the intellectual impairment and its effect on general adjustment. In this chapter the focus shifts to the affective or emotional side as we look at the retarded individual as a person who, like ourselves, can be understood in terms of the things that make for happiness or unhappiness.[1] It will be recalled that in the follow-up study of formerly institutionalized persons by Edgerton and Bercovici (1976), the primary interest of those retarded adults was in "enjoying life." Work had declined in importance for some, but there was widespread desire for recreation, hobbies, good times, friends, and family. These desires are not different from our own and reflect something of the nature of the human condition—of what it means to be a "person." In this chapter the personality of the retarded individual is examined through a personality model which focuses on the psychological needs of all of us, normal as well as retarded, and considers how these needs may be met or frustrated by the condition. The model presented bears some similarity to Maslow's (1954) and incorporates a strong emphasis on self-esteem (Epstein, 1973) as a factor that motivates our behavior. Following presentation of (a) the model and (b) a consideration of what it means to be retarded through its major "need" constructs, our attention is directed to (c) common personality characteristics and behavior problems in retardation, (d) the related disorders of autism and learning disabilities, and (e) the role of psychotherapy, counseling, and behavior modification in the management of behavior problems. With regard to behavior modification, many illustrations of its

[1]For general review of personality in mental retardation, the reader is referred to Heber (1957), Cromwell (1963), and Zigler (1966).

behavioral and educational application are found in the "management" chapters. The use of psychotropic drugs in the treatment of behavior problems is discussed in Chapter 10.

ON PERSONALITY ITSELF

The personality model offered views humankind in terms of three major dimensions—*resources, needs,* and *values.* Each is briefly defined and then integrated in a summary which seeks to provide the reader with an organized way of looking at all people, normal and retarded.

Resources

"Resources" refers to our capacities or abilities and can be grouped into such broad categories as (a) intelligence, (b) communication skills, (c) health and physical skills, (d) temperament, emotions, and character (commonly equated with "personality"), and (e) esthetic appreciation.

INTELLIGENCE

As elaborated in Chapter 1, intelligence is equated with behaviors that reflect learning ability, knowledge, reasoning, and coping with new situations.

COMMUNICATION SKILLS

This refers to our ability to make ourselves understood, most often through speech, but also including the written word, gesture, sign language, and the artistic modes of literature, poetry, art, dance, and music.

HEALTH AND PHYSICAL SKILLS

This refers to our general state of health; the intactness of our senses, typically vision and hearing; the functionality of our limbs—hands, arms, and legs; and such physical characteristics as strength, endurance, speed, and coordination.

TEMPERAMENT, EMOTIONS, CHARACTER

Temperament

This refers to behaviors in the infant and young child that appear to be relatively independent of parental child-rearing style and are presumed to be biological in origin. Behavioral differences between children are observable in infancy and give to each child his "individuality." The behaviors subsumed under temperament are activity level, rhythmicity, approach-withdrawal tendencies, adaptability, threshold of responsiveness, intensity of reaction, mood, distractibility, and attention span and persistence (Thomas, Chess, & Birch, 1968). Another behavior in this category, though not detectable until after infancy, is the degree to which children are reflective or impulsive in their problem solving (Kagan, 1971).

Emotions

Emotions refer to affective or feeling states that are classifiable qualitatively as to pain or pleasure and quantitatively as to degree. Common painful emotions are fear, anxiety, aggression, and sadness; common pleasurable ones are satisfaction, pride, and joy.

Character

This refers to consistent patterns of behavior shown over a fairly wide spectrum of situations (Cofer & Apley, 1967). These are patterns of relatedness to people, objects, and events. At the "people" level, these patterns reflect such behaviors as assertiveness, sociability, and empathy. At the "object" level, they refer to such behaviors as orderliness and possessiveness.

ESTHETIC APPRECIATION

This refers to our capacity to enjoy beauty in all of its manifold forms—nature, art, music, dance, literature, and poetry.

Needs

"Needs" refers to the forces or drives that give direction to or motivate our behavior. Psychologists have commonly held that our primary (first-order) need is to avoid pain or to terminate it as quickly as we can and to obtain pleasure. In terms of the personality model presented here, this is accomplished by the meeting of our biological and psychological needs (second-order needs). Thus "needs" are also closely tied to emotions. When needs are met, we experience states of comfort or pleasure. When unmet, we experience various states of tension and unpleasant feelings. Biological needs are those that are essential to our survival—food, water, and temperature regulation. Sex, too, would fall within this category. Generally, the meeting of biological needs is not a critical problem in retarded persons, although those in whom the retardation is organic in origin often have such major health problems as epilepsy, paralysis, and visual and hearing loss. The greater concern in retardation is with meeting psychological needs, and these are here defined as structure, self-esteem, and self-expression.

STRUCTURE

This refers to our need for predictability, congruity (Osgood, Suci, & Tannenbaum, 1957), the absence of cognitive dissonance (Festinger, 1957), continuity, and a sense of the familiar as against the strange. In our child-rearing behavior, structure refers to limits, discipline, and the expectations they create (Coopersmith, 1967); in our games, it refers to rules. To the degree that there is structure, events have a predictable cause-and-effect relationship; things make sense to us. In its absence we experience anxiety and, in severe degree, bewilderment.

SELF-ESTEEM

This refers to our "self-concept," our sense of worth or "goodness." The fulfillment of the need for self-esteem is regarded as central to mental health (Strupp & Hadley, 1977), and much of our happiness, pleasure rather than pain, is tied to activities that are designed to maintain or enhance it. The significance of the self in terms of worth is recognized by all personality theorists (e.g., Coopersmith, 1967; Epstein, 1978; Maslow, 1954; Rogers, 1951), though the material presented here, as elsewhere in the model, represents the author's own thinking and attempt at integration. The first example of this integration is in treating self-esteem as a complex need which is the outgrowth and reflection of three subneeds: intimacy, success, and autonomy.

Intimacy

This refers to our "affiliative" behavior—to our condition as "social" creatures. Our need to relate to other human beings was attributed by Plato to our dependence on them for survival, by the psychologist McDougall to instinct, and by modern theorists to the creation of an "affectional reward system" which results from our early child-rearing experiences and which can only be fed by other people (Severy, Brigham, & Schlenker, 1976). Intimacy is the need to receive and give love. It encompasses the whole range of experiences that constitute mutually positive interactions with others. At the "receiving" end it includes experiences of attention, recognition, acceptance, approval, and love. At the "giving" level, it consists of all behaviors that reflect a concern for the well-being of others. It is also presumed that the ability to give love depends, in part, on our having first received it. Intimacy is regarded as the most important determinant of self-esteem. To the extent that we have it, we feel secure, protected, loved. To the extent it is lacking we may feel a wide range of painful feelings—anxiety, depression, anger, and a general state of inadequacy.

Success

This refers to our sense of accomplishment as we tackle the significant tasks in our daily lives, tasks whose outcome is perceived as due to our own efforts. Related terms used by psychologists are a need for *achievement* (McClelland, Atkinson, Clark, & Lowell, 1953) and for *effectance* or *competence* (White, 1959). Success produces in us feelings of satisfaction, pride, and, in some cases, unmitigated joy. Failure carries with it feelings of disappointment, sadness, and sometimes shame and humiliation.

Autonomy

This is our need to feel some control or power over our individual lives. It is the sense that we are the "cause" of our own behavior, and at least one psychologist (DeCharms, 1968) has suggested that this is our most fundamental motivating force. With autonomy there are feelings of pride and confidence; without it there can be rebellion, a feeling of futility, and, ultimately, apathy.

SELF-EXPRESSION

This is that third of the group of major psychological needs and refers to our desire to engage in activities that are pleasureful. Our leisure pursuits fall into this category, but it can also include work or other "required" activities that are experienced as pleasurable or gratifying for their own sake. Access to such activities can provide a wide variety of positive feelings; their absence can lead to states of boredom and frustration.

Values

The concept of "values" has been an elusive one in psychology. Values are regarded as more than "interests," being seen as pursuits which are highly prized (Wenar, 1971). In our own definition values refer to that which we come to prize—activities, people, objects, and ideas—because they are the medium through which biological and psychological needs are met. Since values are tied to needs, like needs they give direction and specificity to our behavior. Though we all share the same biological and psychological needs, the particular ways in which these needs are met reflect our individual tastes. At the recreational level, for example, one person may highly value the pursuit of a quiet, nonvigorous indoor activity such as stamp collecting while another particularly enjoys vigorous outdoor activities such as shooting baskets on the playground. Obviously, our preferences will consist of a blend of all kinds of activities; it is only that their specific nature (e.g., basketball vs. softball) and order of preference within our hierarchy of values are a very individual matter.

Putting the Pieces
of the Person Together

A model of a "person" has been presented that incorporates three major dimensions: resources, needs, and values. Resources are our capacities or abilities (intelligence, communication skill, health and physical skills, temperament-emotions-character, and esthetic appreciation). They are the raw material of behavior; they are what we use when we "behave." For example, in reading these lines the reader is using his vision (health and physical skills) and his capacity for comprehension (intelligence). Our resources are not employed in a random manner; rather they are directed toward activities that are *valued* because they lead to the satisfaction (reduction) of basic biological and psychological *needs*. To the extent that needs are met, we are relatively free of tension, and our prevailing feeling states are pleasant. To the extent that needs are unmet, and they are never permanently met—only temporarily sated—they make themselves known through our emotions, and these impel their own discharge so as to end unwanted feeling states (e.g., Young, 1961). Our ability to manage our feelings and the actions (impulses) they impel in an adaptive manner depends on two factors—our capacity to foresee the consequences of our actions (reality testing) and the intensity of our needs. The former has particular relevance for retarded persons.

APPLYING THE PERSONALITY MODEL
TO RETARDED PERSONS

Resources

INTELLIGENCE

Within this model handicapping conditions are viewed as resource deficiencies with retardation seen as a deficit in intelligence (e.g., deafness and communication skill, cerebral palsy and health and physical skills, mental illness and temperament-emotions-character). Most major handicaps involve multiple resource impairments, with cerebral palsy, for example, primarily affecting health and physical skills but also commonly impairing speech (communication skill) and intelligence. While retardation also frequently affects other resources as well as intelligence, it is the latter that is the primary impairment.

COMMUNICATION SKILL

In describing the adaptive behavior problems associated with retardation in the preschool years, it was noted that delay in the acquisition of language is typical. In retardation, speech (expressive language) tends to be simpler in structure, less clearly articulated, and, where the degree of retardation is either severe or profound, limited to brief phrases or single words. In many who are profoundly retarded, no speech at all is present.

HEALTH AND PHYSICAL SKILLS

In retardation we often encounter health and physical problems especially in those with organic etiologies and more than mild impairment. Thus among those with IQs of less than 50, about 30 percent have major sensory (visual and/or hearing), motor (e.g., spasticity), or general health problems (e.g., epilepsy and congenital heart defect) (Payne, 1971).

TEMPERAMENT, EMOTIONS, CHARACTER

Temperament

In terms of temperament there are commonly extremes in "activity level," particularly overactivity or *hyperactivity*, a behavior also frequently seen in children with "learning disabilities" (described later in this chapter). The hyperactive child seems to be in constant motion—always getting into things, restless, and fidgety. These children are also said to be unable to restrict their activity on command, to appear capable of only one speed of response, and often to show other physiological and behavioral problems (Ross & Ross, 1976). Although hyperactivity is presumed to be biological in origin, it is much affected by psychological factors. When the hyperactive child is exposed to stress, little structure, and high stimulation, the behavior intensifies. This type of child benefits from routines and setting firm limits (maximizing structure) and from avoiding overstimulation (Cruickshank, Bentzen, Ratzeburg, & Tannhause, 1961; Haring & Phillips, 1962; Ross & Ross, 1976). Stimulant drugs have been widely used, a controversial treatment procedure (Wender, 1971; Werry, 1970), but evidence regarding the likelihood of developing a drug addiction is lacking (Ross & Ross, 1976). It is clear, however, that caution in the use of drugs is in order and that they should not be used before there has been a careful medical assessment and a remedial behavior program is under way.

Some of the other behaviors of hyperactive children relate to two other dimensions of temperament—*distractibility* and *attention span and persistence*

(Lerner, 1971; Van Osdol & Carlson, 1972). These behaviors, like hyperactivity, are subject to psychological influences. The retarded or even normal youth who seems unable to concentrate and to stick to a task can show surprising persistence when provided with activities that are both within his ken and of interest to him. Thus the retarded adolescent who manifests little interest in a third-grade reader, one that is at his comprehension level but not his interest level, can be expected to demonstrate much greater enthusiasm when offered reading materials that are appropriate to his interests as a teenager as well as to his level of reading comprehension. Fortunately, such educational materials are available.

Further indication of the role of motivation in behaviors traditionally tied to retardation is seen in "attention span and persistence." Though typically depicted as deficient in this behavioral dimension, one also finds retarded persons characterized as "perseverative!" There is a body of research (Zigler, 1966) which reveals that retarded youth will persist at mastered tasks longer than nonretarded ones. One interpretation of this kind of persistence is that retarded youngsters have a higher threshold of boredom and are therefore more accepting of nonchallenging activities. Another explanation (Zigler, 1966) is that, in at least some situations, this behavior reflects implicit assumptions regarding task expectancies of adults and a strong need to please them because of prior histories of social deprivation ("intimacy" deprivation).

Another type of perseveration is observed in profoundly retarded individuals. When asked to copy a simple figure such as a vertical or horizontal line, the response may not be limited to correctly reproducing the line, for example, but rather the person continues to draw more lines of the same kind. The author has speculated that this kind of perseveration reflects very limited or absent number concepts (Baroff, 1974). Since this same behavior is seen in normal children who are less than 3 years of age, it is clearly a mental age–related phenomenon. When you or I are shown a single line and asked to copy it, we do so by drawing another single line. Without explicit awareness, we understand that the task involves only one line and that to add more lines would be an incorrect representation of the stimulus. But the very young normal child or the retarded person with a mental age of less than 3 years does not make this implicit numerical distinction. At this cognitive level, copying a line is not to copy *a* line, it is to copy a *line*. Only the shape of the stimulus is relevant; its number is not.

Emotions

The second component of this resource is emotion. Do retarded people have the same feelings or emotions we do? This question is not ordinarily posed, as such, though all textbooks in the field devote some portion to "personality disorders"—behaviors that are viewed as reflective of *emotional* disturbance. Appendices group personality disorders under such headings as emotional problems (Ingalls, 1978), emotional disturbance (Robinson & Robinson, 1976), and emotionally disturbed (MacMillan, 1977). It is simply assumed that one need not underscore the obvious—that retarded people are *people* and that people have emotions. But in my experience with students, I have been struck by the importance to them of coming to recognize that retarded people do have feelings. Prior to their contact with them they carry whatever stereotypes our culture teaches, and this, typically, has the effect of creating psychological distance between them and the retarded person. Retarded individuals, like others who are handicapped, are perceived as "different" and almost in the most profound sense—as if they were members of a different species. Undoubtedly, much of the neglect that has characterized our treatment of retarded persons reflects this kind of "subhuman" perception of them. One of the keys to achieving recognition of the humanness of retarded individuals is to discover that they, like you and me, also have feelings. This is a very powerful means of reducing psychological distance, achieving some degree of identification, and developing compassion for those who, on superficial encounter, may seem very different from the rest of us. Thus it is that we stop a moment to make explicit what is usually only implied and to do it by taking advantage of one of literature's great soliloquies. Do retarded people experience the same emotions that we do? The answer is clearly "yes," and Shylock's magnificent statement about the sense of difference created by being a Jew in a Christian land could equally be spoken for retarded persons or for any other group of individuals who, within a given culture, are perceived as "different." It is here quoted substituting only "retarded" or "retarded person" for "Jew":

> I am [retarded]. Hath not a [retarded person] eyes? Hath not a [retarded person] hands, organs, dimensions, senses, affections, passions; fed with the same food, hurt with the same weapons, subject to the same desires, healed by the same means, warmed and cooled by the same winter and summer . . . ? If you prick us do we not bleed? If you tickle us do we not laugh? If you poison us do we not die? (Shakespeare, *The Merchant of Venice*).

Yes, retarded persons love, and hate, and fear. They know the same hungers, feel the same pains, and share the same longings. The experiences of Roger and Ben described in the first chapter make this poignantly clear. Recall Roger's Valentine poem about "sharing warm affectionate love" and little Ben's exuberance and love of his neighbor's dog.

Character

The third component of this resource is the one that most closely approximates what is generally meant by "personality." It is addressed in two ways. First, the findings with regard to two behaviors are reviewed—anxiety and aggression; later we look at the effects on personality of the degree to which basic psychological needs are met.

    1. Anxiety. The research literature suggests that retarded individuals will generally show higher levels of anxiety than nonretarded ones (Gardner, 1968; Silverstein, 1970), and, in light of the stresses experienced by the aforementioned Roger, this is hardly surprising. As a further example of how retarded persons are like rather than different from us, their response in experimental settings designed to evoke anxiety parallels that of

their normal counterparts, On well-mastered tasks anxiety does not impair performance (Feldhusen & Klausmeier, 1962), but on more difficult ones it does (Lipman & Griffith, 1960). Retarded children, too, like nonretarded ones, are adversely affected by "test" anxiety (Wrightsman, 1962; Silverstein, 1966). Those with chronic anxiety also appear to have poorer self-concepts (Cowen, Zax, Klein, Izzo, & Trost, 1965). That chronic anxiety is associated with a poorer self-concept is just what would be predicted from the personality model. Anxiety is one of the painful emotions experienced when basic needs are not met. If retardation results in rejection rather than acceptance (intimacy) and in failure rather than achievement (success), two of the subneeds essential to self-esteem are unfulfilled.

2. Aggression. The research on aggression has been largely limited to institutionalized persons and has illumined the conditions of institutional life that are most likely to foment it. Little privacy, crowding, and a lack of a meaningful daily program of activities can all encourage aggressive behavior. This is particularly apparent in those with very limited communication skills as in severely and profoundly retarded populations (Talkington, Hall, & Altman, 1971). It is these individuals who may experience physical closeness in day-room settings as an encroachment on their living space (territorality) and a source of conflict with other residents (Paluck & Esser, 1971). Since the range of social interactions among nonverbal, profoundly retarded individuals appears to be quite limited and often aggressive in nature, with "action" serving as a substitute for nonexistent verbal skills, residential settings that reduce "crowding" will also reduce aggression (Boe, 1977).

As to the aggressive propensities of retarded people as such, we know little except that those who get into chronic difficulty seem never to have learned to control anger when frustrated. In Chapter 5, retarded sisters are described who as adults continue to show the kind of tantrum associated with the young child. Chronic acting-out behavior in retarded youth is likely to be the result of family experiences that were either lacking in appropriate role models or where there was inconsistency or surrender to the child's demands. The effect is an "unsocialized" human being. (In Chap. 10, an entire section is devoted to the management of aggression.)

ESTHETIC APPRECIATION

Mental retardation per se does not appear to adversely affect the capacity to enjoy a variety of esthetic experiences (Van Osdol, 1972), though the quality of what is enjoyed is related to mental age. Music, dancing, drawing, poetry, arts and crafts—all of these are sources of pleasure to retarded persons. Indeed, many learning situations are enhanced in their appeal to retarded (and nonretarded) individuals by incorporating activities that are "inherently" pleasurable (e.g., teaching "following directions" by playing a game of musical chairs).

Of particular interest in this area are those retarded persons who manifest an unusual gift in a highly specific artistic or cognitive ability. The term *idiot savant* has been applied to individuals who, except for this one ability, function in the retarded range. These abilities are not merely exceptional in comparison with their other skills, they are unusual for the normal population as well. The most common areas of idiosyncratic excellence are "calendar calculating," memory, music, and art (Hill, 1974 Hoffman, 1971). "Calendar calculators" are able to tell the day of the week on which a particular date falls for past and future as well as for current calendar periods. Most are unable to explain how they do this, although one appeared to have memorized a series of base dates from which the number of days in each month were used to count forward or backward to the desired date. These operations are performed without the use of pencil and paper and, in spite of their remarkable mental ability in this area, when not calendar calculating they are unable to carry out even simple arithmetic operations beyond the retarded level (Hoffman, 1971; Horwitz, Kestenbaum, Person, & Jarvik, 1965; Rubin & Monaghan, 1965). In the musical area the case is reported of an adult, IQ 67, who was an outstanding pianist and who performed with renowned musicians in rehearsal. He had a remarkable memory and was capable of repeating, word for word, two and a half pages of print after reading them once silently (Anastasi & Levee, 1959). In art, several instances of unusual painting and drawing ability have been observed. According to Hill (1974), the most famous was Gottfried Mind, a person whose retardation was due to congenital hypothyroidism (cretinism) and who was famed in Europe for his paintings of children and animals. In recent times, unusual painting and drawing gifts have been observed in two Japanese youths, one of whom is autistic as well as retarded (Morishima & Brown, 1976, 1977). (The nature of autism is spelled out later in this chapter.) Retardation in the nonautistic individual is associated with hydrocephaly, and, apart from his special talent, language, cognition, and general behavior is in the retarded range. His work, too, is said to be highly regarded and has been exhibited at art shows in Japan and America.

Thus far, explanations for the special abilities of these retarded individuals are entirely speculative and really descriptive rather than explanatory. Hoffman (1971) points out that these abilities are not unique to the retarded and that their special development seems to be associated with the capacity to funnel all of one's interest and energy in this one area—a kind of obsessional preoccupation. This is particularly apparent in the artists (Morishima & Brown, 1976, 1977). But such an explanation explains neither the rarity of the condition in retarded persons nor how these abilities can be so circumscribed within a given individual (LaFontaine & Benjamin, 1971).

"Needs" and Personality

We looked earlier at anxiety and aggression as two behaviors studied in retarded individuals. But these behaviors and the emotions they represent are a response to the frustration of basic needs, particularly psychological ones. We resume our description of personality characteristics in mental retardation, but now as they relate to the degree to which retardation affects the meeting of needs for structure, self-esteem, and self-expression.

STRUCTURE

There is no doubt that retarded persons have more intensive needs for structure. Their cognitive difficulties limit comprehension of what is expected or appropriate in a given situation. Moreover, as noted in Chapter 1, there is less transfer (generalization) of what *is* learned in one setting to comparable new ones. The effect is to create stress when the retarded individual is confronted with a psychologically new (unmastered) situation and to cause a more zealous clinging to that which is familiar (known, mastered). There is greater readiness to seek guidance and direction from others. This is the quality of suggestibility or "outer directedness," referred to in Chapter 1. The overall effect is to foster in retarded individuals an exaggerated degree of *dependency*. Together with the dependency is the just-mentioned greater caution (anxiety) when encountering unfamiliar settings. Two of the important consequences of this intensified need for structure are (a) the necessity to make *explicit* ordinarily implicit expectations, and (b) the need to minimize anxieties about the "new" by building "bridges"—that is, providing for *gradual* movement from the known (mastered) to the unknown (unmastered). This is to apply the behavior modification principle of "successive approximation."

SELF-ESTEEM

Intimacy

Of the three subneeds that determine self-esteem, intimacy is regarded as the most important. It touches on the extraordinary intensity and pervasiveness of our need to be accepted, liked, admired, and loved. The primary obstacle to the fulfillment of this need in retarded (or otherwise handicapped) persons is that they possess characteristics that are viewed as undesirable (unattractive). Their mental and often physical abnormalities evoke fear, derision, and, sometimes, repulsion. Recall the teasing of Roger and our own teasing of others who are "different" in undesirable ways. "Pity" is often the most "positive" feeling engendered. The consequence of these unwanted characteristics is to produce in us attitudes of avoidance and rejection rather than attraction (Bialer, 1970; Efron & Efron, 1967; Fine, 1967; MacMillan, 1974; Ricci, 1970; Wolfensberger, 1967; Wong, 1969), although less antipathy toward the disability on the part of the general public seems evident (Gottlieb & Siperstein, 1976; Latimer, 1971).

1. Parents and sibs: These unwanted or negatively valued characteristics not only create distance between the retarded individual and general society, they can also affect the degree to which parents and sibs provide the normal degree of family affection (Hurley, 1965; Ricci, 1970). In Chapter 1 there was reference to the kinds of problems in retardation that are potential sources of stress to parents and sibs. Now we specifically address the psychological consequence of being either the parent or sibling of a retarded child.

As parents, we see our children as psychological extensions of ourselves

(Ryckman & Henderson, 1965); the same is true for sibs although, perhaps, to a lesser degree (Kaplan, 1969; Grossman, 1972). *Our* self-esteem is affected by how other members of our family are perceived by those whose approval (intimacy) we seek. Children of whom parents can be proud because they possess culturally valued characteristics will elevate parental pride (self-esteem). Conversely, if the child or sib has unwanted characteristics, parents and sibs cannot, at least initially, avoid viewing their family member as an unfavorable reflection of themselves. They will react with painful feelings of shame, hostility, and then guilt at these feelings, all contributing to a diminished sense of self-esteem (Roos, 1963).

But the psychological discomfort that attends states of low self-esteem is not easily borne, and "defenses" are erected to mitigate it. In fact, defensive behavior is merely the way in which we protect ourselves from acknowledging realities about ourselves which would produce anxiety and a fall in self-esteem. Parental reactions to the threat to self-esteem can lead to such inappropriate behaviors as the *denial* of the reality of the condition, zealous *overprotection*, or *rejection*. Where parental attitudes reflect either covert rejection as in denial or, more rarely, overt rejection, the child's need for intimacy is unmet. The child feels unloved and, later, unlovable (a chronic state of low self-esteem), and this leads to prevailing emotional states of anxiety, hostility, and sadness. Such children are driven to seek approval (intimacy) and are very sensitive to criticism. Overprotection, too, can sometimes reflect rejection, with the apparent excessive concern for the child's welfare serving to disguise one's true feelings. Such parents are likely to vacillate in their attitudes toward the child, thus adding "unpredictability" (lack of structure) to the emotional pressures created by ambivalence. Unfavorable parental attitudes are most often seen in parents who place a very high value on academic achievement. They will have greater difficulty in fully accepting the child and can add personality problems to the coping burdens that the child's retardation itself presents. Since these personality problems will interfere with the child's ability to respond appropriately to other adults or children, their prevention through family counseling is a very important though still largely unmet need (Ross, 1964).

Sibs, too, may have negative as well as positive feelings toward a brother or sister whose deviance is, by association, perceived as a threat to *their* need for peer acceptance and self-esteem. This is especially prominent during adolescence, when, for some youths, a main concern is to avoid being identified with the retarded sib (Kaplan, 1969). Other concerns are the degree to which the retarded sib understands his own impairment, appropriate methods of discipline, and the family's freedom to talk about retardation. In a study of the impact of a retarded sib on college-age youths (Grossman, 1972), equal numbers appear to have either benefited or been hurt by the experience. Those who had benefited seemed to be more tolerant and compassionate and more aware of prejudice and its consequences. Others were bitterly resentful, were guilty about their rage at parents and sib, and were fearful that they themselves might somehow be defective or tainted. Of particular importance in determining sib attitudes were those of the parents. In families where parents were seen as accepting the child, the sibs seemed able to cope more effectively with the meaning of the handicap for them.

2. Peer acceptance: another tremendously important source of intimacy is one's peer group. Peer acceptance is, undoubtedly, one of the main reasons why adolescent sibs seek to avoid being identified with their retarded brother or sister. But the age mates of retarded children or youths, like the rest of society, are more likely to "avoid" than to "approach" or, in the classroom, to regard with neutrality if not to actively reject (Goodman, Gottlieb, & Morrison, 1972; Gottlieb & Davis, 1973; Guskin, 1963; Johnson, 1950; MacMillan, Jones, & Aloia, 1974; Meyerowitz, 1967; Miller, 1956; Monroe, 1968; Rucker, Howe, & Snider, 1969; Wilson, 1970).

We all know how children can be cruel to another, to ridicule, to tease. This ubiquitous need to call attention to the limitations of others seems to be a disguised way of asserting our own self-worth. In effect, we say, "See, I'm not like that" or "I'm stronger [or smarter, or more attractive] than you." Though we are usually unaware of our motives for teasing, a former student once expressed pleasure that there were handicapped people on the campus so that he could see others with whom he could favorably compare himself! Concerns about unfavorable peer attitudes of school age youth and their teachers also lie behind the effort to avoid permanent and day-long placement of at least mildly retarded (educable) children in so-called self-contained special classes, and, instead, to integrate them as fully as possible in regular classes ("mainstreaming"). "Mainstreaming"[2] has also been justified on the grounds that there were no apparent academic benefits from special-class placement that could compensate for the presumed adverse social ones (Cegelka & Tyler, 1970; Johnson, 1962; Sparks & Blackman, 1965).

Curiously, the original justification for self-contained special classes was at least as much "social" as "academic." It was viewed as a setting in which the retarded child would not have to compete, academically, with normal children. There would be fewer failure experiences and greater opportunities for peer acceptance. But the assumed social benefits have been overridden by the presumption that such placement unduly calls attention to limitations and, thus, lowers self-esteem. More recent studies of peer attitudes suggest, however, that irrespective of type of class placement, retarded classmates are less likely to be accepted as "friends" (Goodman, Gottlieb, & Morrison, 1972; Rucker, 1968), though age, sex, and social class differences can affect the degree of acceptance. For example, girls are more accepting than boys (Sheare, 1974; Siperstein, Bak, & Gottlieb, 1977; Siperstein & Gottlieb, 1977).

There is also indication that children who represent the same socioeconomic group from which the bulk of the *mildly* retarded derive are more accepting than children of higher socioeconomic status (Bruininks, Rynders, & Gross, 1974; Gottlieb, 1974). The level of intelligence also seems to affect peer attitudes, more positive ones tending to be directed to the least retarded children. Interestingly, this is also true *within* retarded populations. Though our words may belie it, it appears that intelligence is valued at all levels of ability (Dentler & Mackler, 1962; Diggs, 1963; Guskin & Spicker, 1968). While each of these factors influences the

---

[2]A special section on special education and mainstreaming is found in Chapter 8.

extent to which retarded children find acceptance, the most important determinant is the degree to which their general behavior is socially appropriate for their age (Johnson, 1950; Turner, 1958; Wilson, 1970). After all, historically, it was typically the mildly retarded child who was *also* a classroom behavior problem who was moved out of the regular class and into the "special" one.

3. "Mainstreaming" and peer attitudes: Although it is clear that intellectual differences between children do affect their acceptance of each other, especially when the intellectual impairment is of major magnitude, the hope of mainstreaming is that these attitudes can be modified in a positive direction. However, research does not indicate that mainstreaming has resulted in more favorable attitudes toward retarded children (Goodman et al., 1972; Gottlieb & Budoff, 1973; Gottlieb & Davis, 1973; Iano, Ayers, Heller, McGettigan, & Walker, 1974), although one notable exception to these findings is Sheare's (1974) study of the effects of integration on a large series of ninth graders. With integration restricted to nonacademic classes (e.g., physical education, health, art, etc.) and the number of retarded pupils limited to not more than two per class, clear evidence of a positive attitude change was found. Admittedly, this constitutes mainstreaming at its most minimal level, but it may indicate how desired attitude changes can be obtained.

4. "Labeling" and peer acceptance: As noted in Chapter 1, the controversy over the presumed stigmatizing nature of special-class placement has come to be equated with the term "labeling." Labeling refers to the outcome of the traditional diagnostic and evaluation process which follows the discovery of a child who is not making normal progress in school. Since the special remedial services such a child might receive have been traditionally tied to diagnostic or categorical labels (e.g., retardation, learning disability, visually impaired, etc.), the label came to be a vehicle for obtaining such services. But since, at least for the mildly retarded or educable child, the special class was seen as offering no academic advantages and was also disproportionately filled with disadvantaged minority youth, the label has come to be regarded as a means of maintaining unfavorable racial and cultural stereotypes.

On the labeled child is heaped the cultural disdain associated with the label, for example, "retard"! In addition to its adverse consequences for the child's self-esteem, it is also seen as assuring continued poor academic performance by lowering teacher expectations and, therefore, efforts to elevate the child's level of achievement. But research that seeks to specifically explore the influence of labels per se indicates that, at least for elementary school–age children, it is the *behavior* of the retarded child rather than the label that most affects perceptions of him. Children tend to prefer other children who are perceived as *competent* on a task irrespective of whether that child is labeled or not (Budoff & Siperstein, 1978; Gottlieb, 1974). When, however, the child is seen as incompetent on an academic task, the label seems to be protective, as the *labeled* incompetent child is regarded more favorably than the *unlabeled* incompetent one (Budoff & Siperstein, 1978). Other studies have also found that the label, by virtue of the expectations it generates, tends to lead to greater rather than lesser acceptance of negative behavior

(Gersh & Jones, 1973; Goodman, Gottlieb, & Morrison, 1972). Similarly, merely de-labeling educable mentally retarded children and reintegrating them in regular classes did not affect normal peer perceptions of them (Gampel, Gottlieb, & Harrison, 1974).

5. Retarded students' perceptions of their class placement: Opposition to labeling and to special class placement has, naturally, been an organized movement *for* rather than *by* retarded students. Their attitudes toward special-class placement seem much affected by *chronological* age. Elementary school–age retarded children do not appear to regard special–class placement unfavorably (Warner, Thrapp, & Walsh, 1973), but older children do (Gozali, 1972). Clearly, the age of the child affects his capacity to see himself as other do. Children who have been reintegrated in regular classes following mainstreaming express preference for the regular-class placement (Gottlieb & Budoff, 1972), although this does not necessarily imply previous unhappiness in the special-class setting. In a survey conducted by one of my students of integrated junior high school students who had formerly been in special classes, they expressed satisfaction with both settings, though their preference was for the integrated one.

6. Behavior of retarded children in integrated and special classes: Given that the most important determiner of peer attitudes is the general behavior of retarded children, are there differences between children that relate to the kind of setting in which they are placed? In the past this certainly was the case, since it was the behavior problem retarded child who was certain to be moved out of the regular class and into a "special" one. And research has found more aggressive peer interactions in special class children than in integrated ones (Gampel & Harrison, 1972). But does integration of former special-class students affect their behavior? In an interesting study of a number of classroom behaviors (Gampel et al., 1974), there is indication that the classroom behavior of former special-class students changed such that they displayed less aggressiveness than their special-class counterparts. More importantly, they were indistinguishable from other regular-class children in their behaviors. It would appear that the regular-class milieu and its "modeling" implications can affect the behavior of former special-class pupils in a positive way.

7. Labeling and self-esteem: We have explored the relationship between labeling, special-class placement, and their effects on normal peer acceptance because of the former's importance to self-esteem via "intimacy." To recapitulate, the presumption has been that the label that attached to special-class placement adversely affected self-esteem because of its negative effect on normal peers. But we have seen that it is the *behavior* rather than the *label* that carries the greatest weight and that the label may be protective as well as stigmatizing. We conclude that elementary school–age mildly retarded children will win a greater degree of peer acceptance by acquiring more socially appropriate classroom behavior, labels notwithstanding. In the adolescent years of junior and senior high, the label itself probably carries greater weight for peer acceptance and self-esteem.

8. Self-concepts of retarded youth: Apart from inferences to be drawn regarding peer attitudes and self-esteem, a number of studies have sought to directly

measure the effects on self-esteem of labeling and special-class placement. Here, as in the case of the effects of labeling on peer attitudes, the findings are complex rather than one-dimensional. The impact of special-class placement on self-esteem seems to depend on *which aspect* of self-esteem you are measuring. On self-concept scales that primarily tap perception of one's *scholastic adequacy*, special-class children actually tend to report *higher* self-esteem than their integrated counterparts (Schurr & Brookover, 1967; Schurr, Joiner, & Towne, 1970; Towne & Joiner, 1966). Moreover, they even compare themselves favorably, abilitywise, with normal children (Curtis, 1965; Fine & Caldwell, 1967, McAfee & Cleland, 1965; Ringness, 1961), though this is regarded as "defensive" in nature. While in some cases this may be true, positive academic self-concepts in elementary-age special-class children are not necessarily defensive in character. They may also be the product of perceived success in that more ability-appropriate class setting.

In a review of self-concept research in mental retardation (Schurr, Joiner, & Towne, 1970), two studies are reported that relate self-esteem to another highly controversial facet of the labeling issue, ability grouping. Both found that students of low ability tended to have more positive self-images in classes that were homogeneous, abilitywise (Drews, 1962; Goldberg, Passow, & Justman, 1961). Parenthetically, it appears that it is the more academically capable former special-class student who can most easily be mainstreamed (MacMillan, 1977), and one important measure of that may be the presence of some functional reading ability. In any case, the implication is that in self-evaluation, we tend to compare ourselves with members of our own group rather than with members of a different one. But when self-concept measures tap social rather than scholastic dimensions, a different picture emerges. Numerous studies have found negative effects of special-class placement on self-esteem (Borg, 1966; Carroll, 1967; Mann, 1960; Meyerowitz, 1962) and, as has been suggested, with an apparently more negative impact on adolescents (Gozali, 1972; Jones, 1972). Apparently, the reference group for "social" self-esteem is broader than just one's own classmates.

9. Summary. In summary, the effects on intimacy, and self-esteem, of special-class placement of educable children would appear to be negligible in the elementary school–age child and could provide the setting for the most intensive development of the child's academic and behavioral skills. Once in junior and senior high, however, special-class placement clearly has a mortifying component and is to be avoided, especially for students who have some functional reading skills. Of course, the integrated retarded junior and senior high student will continue to require special assistance, typically in "resource" classes, because the gap between his academic achievement and that of his normal classmates will necessarily increase year by year.

Success

This is the second component of self-esteem and one that has attracted much research in mental retardation. It is assumed that retarded people have more frequent experiences of failure (Bialer, 1970; Chess, 1970; Heber, 1957; Moss,

1958). Indeed, as noted in the prior section, one of the primary reasons for the establishment of special classes was to offer retarded pupils an educational setting in which they could experience success (Martin, 1940). As a consequence of pervasive adaptive difficulties, the retarded individual is viewed as coming to distrust his own judgment (Zigler, 1967), as having a lesser expectancy of success in new situations (Heber, 1957; Jordan & DeCharms, 1959), and as avoiding situations in which there is the possibility of failure (Guthrie, 1964; Moss, 1958). With reference to the last mentioned, a distinction has been made between motivation for achievement based on "success striving" as against "failure avoiding," and it is the latter that is considered to be particularly salient in retardation (Moss, 1958). The significance of this element of self-esteem in retardation is also reflected in related findings which report a greater sensitivity to failure and success (Bialer, 1970) and a more intense reaction to success than is found in nonretarded individuals (Gardner, 1958; Miller, 1961; Ringelheim, 1958). Still another consequence of the greater expectation of failure is its effect on the readiness to persist when frustrated. It appears that retarded learners are more likely to give up in the face of failure (Heber, 1964), and this has led to efforts to develop teaching situations that keep errors at a minimum.

Autonomy

Of the three ingredients of self-esteem, autonomy may not appear to be an important need to retarded persons. After all, autonomy refers to desires for self-determination, choice, and maximum independence. But it is dependence rather than independence that is a common consequence of retardation as well as of other handicapping conditions—for example, blindness. Indeed, research on the personality variable "locus of control" (Bialer, 1961; 1970), a measure of the degree to which we experience success or failure as related to our own efforts, indicates that retarded individuals are less likely to perceive themselves as "self-determining" or having an "internal" locus of control. In part this is a mental age–related phenomenon (Bialer, 1970), but it also probably affected by their typical experiences of success or failure. To suggest, however, that retarded people may show a lesser need for autonomy is not to say that they are indifferent to it. Like the rest of us, they have preferences and tastes and are as entitled as we to having them satisfied when appropriate. It is only that patterns of dependency and frequent lack of assertiveness may mask underlying autonomy needs. They are there, however, and can be easily recognized when opportunities for choice are given.

Mowatt (1970) has described a group of cerebral palsied adults, some of whom were also retarded, as being much incensed by restrictions placed on them by their parents. They wanted greater freedom for themselves—to ride buses, to visit friends, to date, to try to live away from home. Only one member of the group had experienced a nonrestrictive upbringing: a mildly retarded as well as cerebral palsied young woman. Her father had insisted that she learn to cook and to keep house, and he had deliberately sent her on difficult errands and bus trips to prepare her for as independent a life as possible. Now living in her own apartment, possibly a "sheltered" apartment,[3] as both parents are dead, she expressed genuine gratitude for what her father had taught her.

This group of handicapped persons felt much more confident in handling themselves than did their parents. (Recall Roger's mother's surprise when he dialed the telephone to call the police following the attempted sexual-assault episode. She did not think he knew how!) The group saw their parents, particularly their mothers, as too protective. As one wheelchair member of the group thoughtfully phrased it, "It's harder for us to get along by ourselves, so we need *more* not fewer chances to learn. . . ." (Roger communicated the same extremely insightful thought when he said, "People are retarded by what they don't know. That's why I work so hard to learn the things I don't know and become more normal.")

The problem of *overprotectiveness* or *excessive control* in parents of retarded children is of great importance (Cook, 1963; Kogan & Tyler, 1973) and was earlier referred to in the section on intimacy. Most often it is observed in parents of more severely impaired children and is presumed to usually reflects a genuine concern for the welfare of the child and the dangers that may befall him because of perceived limitations. And it is natural to be cautious about exposing a loved child to a situation that might prove dangerous. After all, it is only the parent and the child who must live with the consequences of such decisions. But if parents are governed *only* by the need to avoid any possible mishaps, then their protection serves only to prevent the kinds of learning experiences that could teach the very skills that would enable their child to cope safely with them!

Another consequence of overprotectiveness is the persistence into the adult years of behavior patterns and interests that are more appropriate to children. These often result from the perception of the retarded adult as a "child." Pearl Buck, the famous novelist, saw her severely retarded adult daughter as an "eternal child." While some of this "childishness" is tied to mental age and may not be easily modified, especially in those with severe and profound retardation, at lesser levels of impairment it can also reflect only continued exposure of the adult to things and activities enjoyed as a child. In this connection, the emphasis on "normalization" (Nirje, 1969; Wolfensberger, 1972) has been an important antidote because it proclaims that retarded people can most nearly approximate normality when they are encouraged to engage to the utmost in activities appropriate to their *chronological* age. Thus the retarded adult with an IQ of 50 and a mental age of about 8 years can be encouraged to participate in such atypical 8-year-old activities as working and as socializing with members of the opposite sex.

Sex

With reference to opposite-sex interests of retarded adults, it will be recalled that one of the areas in which greater autonomy was sought was "dating." We now address the sexual needs of retarded persons, and this is certainly an area in which demands for greater autonomy will produce the greatest resistance. It is a fact that retarded persons, like the rest of us, are sexual beings, although, as noted in

[3]One of the range of community nonfamily residential options.

Chapter 1, many parents would prefer not to think so. The free expression of one's sexuality becomes a problem if others are fearful that you may be exploited, as in the case of Roger, or behave in a socially unacceptable manner. Since marriage has been the traditional social vehicle for full sexuality, parents are unlikely to be sympathetic to evidences of sexuality in children who are seen as too immature to fulfill the role of spouse. In our view, assisting retarded youths in relatively non-conflictive ways of expressing their sexuality begins with teaching them what nonretarded persons learn naturally, the conditions under which sexual behavior can occur. This means the teaching of "discretion," the knowledge of the when and where of sexual behavior. Retarded persons also need to learn the relationship between sex and pregnancy; it is certainly the latter that creates and merits real concern. The author is comfortable with retarded individuals in dating and marital roles but is less sanguine about them as parents. While they may be able to fulfill the affectional side of parenting, it is the "teaching" role that would ordinarily be beyond them. (This is spelled out in Chapter 5, and a comprehensive treatment of sexuality and mental retardation is presented in Chapter 9.)

Summary

The need for self-esteem has been examined in terms of the effect of mental retardation on experiences of intimacy, success, and autonomy. Of these three ingredients of self-esteem, the greatest attention was given to intimacy. We explored (a) attitudes of parents and sibs, and of peers, especially in the school setting; (b) the role of regular versus special class placement in affecting peer attitudes, and (c) the impact of "labeling," inherent in special class placement, on how retarded pupils are seen by others and by themselves. Within families in which the functioning of the retarded child is very different from those of other family members, the retarded child is undoubtedly the object of much more ambivalent feeling than is likely to be true of other children (Roos, 1963). Nevertheless, most parents and sibs appear to come to love the handicapped child no less intensely than is true for nonhandicapped ones. While intimacy is ordinarily attained in the family, the establishment of satisfying peer relationships is much more difficult, particularly in the adolescent and postschool years. Though economically disadvantaged minority mildly retarded youths can be expected to achieve general acceptance among social-class peers, those with more than mild retardation will probably have to depend on other handicapped persons to meet social needs. The need for success can be met through the provision of learning experiences that are both age- and ability-appropriate. The challenge of mainstreaming is to continue to provide to the mildly retarded pupil a curriculum and educational setting in which there can be success. If the integrated student primarily experiences failure and peer rejection, it can be expected that the need to maintain self-esteem will lead to inappropriate ways of obtaining it. At the end of the school years the need for success will require access to meaningful work or work-related activities. Finally, a sense of worth can be affirmed by the avoiding of a too-zealous protection and control of the retarded person and by a conscious effort to provide experiences that encourage decision making, confidence, and greater independence. Since "not malization" calls for providing to the retarded individual that setting which most closely approximates that for nonhandicapped persons, it encourages exposure to the most complex rather than the least complex environment to which the person can adapt. It is this kind of milieu that will develop the highest level of adaptation the retarded individual can achieve.

Self-Expression

The last of the group of major psychological needs refers to our desire to engage in activities that are pleasurable. For the most part, these are our leisure time or recreational pursuits, and retarded individuals can participate in a wide variety of such activities (Carlson & Ginglend, 1961, 1968; Neal, 1970). While the range of their recreational interests is probably narrowed by cognitive and possible motor impairments, there are still an enormous number of indoor and outdoor games and arts and crafts they can enjoy. These pleasurable activities can also serve an educational purpose—providing experiences in which fun and learning go hand in hand. Bowling is one such activity (Fitzimmons, 1970). Not only does it offer a pleasant physical outlet, but aspects of the sport and the setting in which it occurs provide abundant cognitive and social learning opportunities. The sport itself can sharpen motor skills, and score keeping can help to develop number abilities. The milieu of a bowling alley offers opportunities for simple shopping and money management experiences, and the presence of nonhandicapped individuals can provide appropriate social models. Even the getting to and from a bowling alley can have an educational purpose—teaching "travel training" and thereby increasing mobility, self-reliance, and the sense of independence. (A special section on recreational programs is presented in Chap. 8).

MENTAL RETARDATION AND PERSONALITY DISORDERS

Common Characteristics of Retarded Children

To this point we have looked at personality in retardation as it would be affected by the degree to which the condition will frustrate basic "need" gratification. From the history of Roger and the research that relates to intimacy, success, and autonomy, we should not be surprised at the frequent presence of personality problems. The tendency toward anxiety has already been noted. Still the question may be put as to whether some personality disorder is *inherent* in retardation or whether retarded persons can be "healthy" personalitywise apart from their cognitive impairment. In a sense the posing of such a question implies a view of the disorder as different from most other kinds of handicaps. We recognize that one may be *physically* handicapped, for example with cerebral palsy, blindness, or deafness, but still have a "good" personality. And, within the framework of the personality model presented here, there is no a priori reason why a retarded person need also have a personality disorder. If basic biological and psychological needs are met, prevailing feeling or emotional states should be relatively tension-free. Psychopathology here and elsewhere (Martin, 1977) is viewed as the outcome of chronic tension (painful emotions) created by frequent frustration of those needs.

It *is* generally agreed that there is an increased frequency of personality disorders in retarded persons (Blatt, 1958; Chess, 1970; Menolascino, 1965, 1966; Richardson, Koller, & Katz, 1985) with reported frequencies varying from 30 to 70 percent, a prevalence rate that at its minimum is about twice that of the general population (Joint Commission on Mental Health in Children, 1969). And one worker, a child psychiatrist (Webster, 1970), suggests that there are some intrinsic personality characteristics in retardation which, when associated with stress, would lead to disturbed behaviors. Contrariwise, Chess (1970) and Bialer (1970) reject the notion that there are any emotional or behavioral characteristics peculiar to retardation and, in concert with other investigators (Cytryn & Lourie, 1967; Philips, 1966; Shaw, 1966), argue that retarded individuals can be free of personality disorder. We shall explore both of these positions.

Webster's assumption of inherent personality characteristics in retardation is based on a survey of 159 children who had applied for admission to a preschool for retarded children. They were 3–6 years of age, and approximately two-thirds had IQs above 50. They comprised a wide range of diagnostic groups with the large majority categorized as either "organic brain syndrome" or "Down syndrome" (mongolism). A major limitation of the study is the lack of data regarding the number of children manifesting each of the behaviors that Webster associates with retardation; we know only that their occurrence was correlated with the degree of retardation.

In spite of this limitation, the behaviors depicted are ones that workers in the field will recognize and add to our own effort to flesh out the picture of what retarded people are "really like." In essence, *Webster reported that there were no retarded children whose emotional behavior was wholly explicable in terms of mental age but rather that there were additional special features.* They were tendencies (a) to engage in *solitary* activity, (b) to be unduly *repetitive* in activities, (c) to appear *inflexible* with regard to change, (d) to be *passive* rather than active in seeking new experience, and (e) to manifest a *simplicity* in one's emotional life. Under stress these tendencies would lead to such problems as *impulsiveness, fearfulness, negativism, compulsiveness, excessive immaturity, easy regression* (loss of previously acquired skills), and *childhood psychosis*. Of this population, two-thirds were seen as either moderately or severely disturbed. Of interest was the absence of any relationship between behaviors and the cause of retardation. No characteristic behaviors were identified in the children with organic brain syndromes; the only description applied was that they were "erratic" in their behavior.

Chess and Hassibi (1970), two other child psychiatrists, studied the behaviors of another series of retarded children. These, too, were a school population, but they were older, varying from 5 to 12 years. Unlike the Webster series, they were all mildly retarded, IQs falling in the 50–70 range. On the basis of past experience, attention was focused on six behaviors with the intent of determining how characteristic they were in a (mildly) retarded population. Of the six only two were observed in at least one-half of the children—*restlessness or excessive motor activity* (58%) and *repetitive aimless motor activities* (52%). The latter differs from the "repetitiveness" described by Webster in that it refers to less purposeful behavior, specifically "stereotypy." This refers to a variety of odd, rhythmic, and repetitive motor activities that are commonly viewed as forms of self-stimulation (Baumeister & Forehand, 1973).[4] The most frequently seen stereotypy in these children was "rocking"; the other two were "arm movements" and "jumping."

What was particularly striking to Chess and Hassibi was the presence of these peculiar behaviors in children who were apparently relating well to others and who were considered to be free of psychiatric disorder. Of further interest was their presence in children who were not more than mildly retarded. Stereotypy is quite common in severely and profoundly retarded children, and in adults as well, and is also seen in many children classified as having "early infantile autism."[5] Parenthetically, the author is surprised that there was no mention of such behavior in the Webster study. Apart from the two behaviors noted by Chess and Hassibi, the only one that occurred in a substantial number of children was *speech impairment* (45%). In Chapter 1 there was reference to the language problems of retarded children, and the observations of Chess and Hassibi offer additional elaboration of its nature. The most general finding was that the child's speech resembled that of a younger child: Articulation defects were common, speech often took the form of a monologue directed at toys in play, and there was frequent reference to the self in the third person. All of these language behaviors are seen in young normal children but typically *at a younger age* than even the mental ages of these retarded children. Thus we have here another example of the special deficiency of retarded children in the language or verbal sphere, a problem area noted in Chapter 1 in connection with their common pattern of strengths and weaknesses on the Binet intelligence test.

The other three behaviors studied were (a) *obsessional behavior* (29%)—for example, the repetitive play activity referred to by Webster but also including eating and sleeping "rituals" and the carrying around of a particular object, (b) *unusual seeking of sensory experiences* (29%)—that is, activities in which the aim seems to be the experiencing of a particular sensation itself (e.g., masturbating, rubbing, hitting, and movement), and (c) *explosive activity* (8%). This last mentioned refers to apparently unprovoked and sudden episodes of shouting, screaming, or attacking objects or people. In light of its negligible frequency, this could not be considered a common behavior in retarded children.

In considering the two studies, the only area of obvious overlap was in the reference to tendencies to engage in repetitive behaviors. In view of Webster's assertion that there are some personality characteristics inherent in retardation, we might have expected a more similar descriptive picture, chronological age differences notwithstanding. Presumably, had Webster looked at his group of children in

[4]Stereotypies are discussed in depth in Chapter 10.
[5]Early infantile autism is discussed later in this chapter.

terms of the same behaviors studied by Chess and Hassibi, a more similar picture would have emerged. Nevertheless, what is striking is the *absence* of a uniform behavioral picture, even within no less than between these two groups. Recall that even the two most frequently seen behaviors by Chess and Hassibi occurred in only little more than half the children. Apart from the intellectual impairment and its effect on learning, the "typical" retarded child does not seem to exist!

Common Personality Disorders

While recognizing the variability of behavior in retardation, certain types of disorders are common. Especially prominent in the young child are *hyperactivity, short attention span* (distractibility), *low frustration tolerance,* and a *general impulsivity.* In adolescence or adulthood, if these behaviors are tinged with aggression, they produce some of the more difficult management problems.

In older children hyperactivity tends to diminish, and one is likely to see a variety of personality disorders. Common ones are *anxiety* (fears of the new structure), fears of rejection (intimacy), and fears of failure (success); *shyness* or *withdrawal* tendencies; *negativism;* and *compulsive behaviors.*

Psychotic disorders, too, are found: hallucinations, delusions, and major mood disorders have been described in retarded adults by the British psychiatrist, Reid (1972). Acute psychosis has also been observed in young children (Menolascino, 1965b). A $4\frac{1}{2}$-year-old Down syndrome child began to withdraw and to display catatonic posturing and bizarre speech following the hospitalization of the father, with whom there had been a very close relationship. The symptoms disappeared after a brief period of inpatient care.

Table 4 lists personality disorders diagnosed at a mental health center serving a community-based retarded population, chiefly adolescent and young adult (Reiss, 1982; Reiss & Trenn, 1984). Largely between the ages of 15 and 29 and two-thirds male, they were typically referrals from community programs. The most frequently diagnosed behaviors were "schizophrenic symptomatology," antisocial behavior, and personality disorders. Dealt with on an outpatient basis, a wide range of treatment modalities were employed—individual and group psychotherapy, cognitive-behavior therapy, behavior modification, family therapy, art therapy, and the use of psychotropic drugs. Let us look at each of the major diagnostic groupings.

SCHIZOPHRENIC SYMPTOMATOLOGY

This term referred to behaviors associated with schizophrenia, but only one individual was clearly "psychotic," hallucinating at the time of referral. Other behaviors included were social withdrawal, thought disorder (presumably a change in the quality of thought), flattened affect, paranoid tendencies (blaming others), autism, hebephrenia (especially, inappropriate silliness), and anxiety. These behaviors were more frequent in adults than in adolescents, 30 percent to 18 percent, predominant in those with severe and profound retardation (47%), and occurred equally among males and females. We would caution that the term "schizophrenic symptomatology" is not to be equated with "schizophrenia." Were persons with

TABLE 4   Mental Health Problems in Retarded Youths and Adults

Diagnosis	Age groups		
	Children/adolescents (6–20) (%)	Adults (21+) (%)	All (%)
"Schizophrenic symptomatology"	9.1	15.2	24.3
Antisocial behavior (aggression)	15.2	9.1	24.3
Personality disorder [a]	7.6	7.6	15.2
Depression	3.0	10.6	13.6
Hyperactivity	4.6	0.0	4.6
Enuresis/encopresis	4.6	0.0	4.6
Phobia/anxiety neurosis	1.5	3.0	4.5
Undetermined disease	3.0	0.0	3.0
Hysteria	0.0	1.5	1.5
Sex problems	1.5	0.0	1.5
Alcoholism	0.0	1.5	1.5
Dissociative state	0.0	1.5	1.5

[a]Poor self-concept with either problems of dependency or nonassertiveness.
Source: Reiss (1982).

severe and profound retardation experiencing hallucinations and delusions, the intellectual deficit would make their detection difficult. This population does show some of the stereotypic motor behaviors observed in catatonic psychosis and in early infantile autism; the overlap between the retarded and autistic populations is described later, in the section on autism.

ANTISOCIAL BEHAVIOR

This category consisted of problems of aggression, lying, stealing, and "oppositional" behavior. Occurring in the younger age group and almost entirely limited to males, it was found at all levels of retardation. A survey of behavior problems in the entire New York State community and institutional retarded population (Jacobson, 1982) found that physical assaults were prominent in the severely and profoundly retarded groups. In contrast, delinquent antisocial behavior is more common in those with less intellectual impairment (Koller et al., 1983).

PERSONALITY DISORDER

The behaviors classified here were problems of dependency and nonassertiveness in individuals with poor self-concepts (self-esteem). These behaviors were observable in persons with not more than moderate retardation, chiefly in adults, and equally among the sexes.

DEPRESSION

The behaviors included here are those typically associated with depression— crying, sadness, hopelessness, sleeplessness, and weight disturbance. Chiefly observed in mildly retarded women, the sex difference is consistent with findings in the general population (e.g., Coleman & Miller, 1975). Reid, to whom there was earlier reference, has described manic-depressive psychosis in retarded adults. He has also suggested that mood disorders can be diagnosed in those with severe and profound retardation on the basis of sudden changes in the usual level of activity and mood.

RELATED DEVELOPMENTAL DISORDERS: AUTISM AND LEARNING DISABILITIES

Autism

The largest area of behavioral overlap between mental retardation and other developmental disorders is found in young children diagnosed as having "infantile autism." Distinguished from childhood schizophrenia on the basis of an earlier age of onset, its chief characteristics are severe social isolation, failure to develop normal language, preference for ritualistic and compulsive behaviors, and occurrence by age $2\frac{1}{2}$ (Rutter, 1972).[6] Other behaviors include abnormalities of cognition, emotional response, play, sensory preferences, and motility (Creak, 1964; Goldfarb, 1970; Hingtgen & Bryson, 1972; Wing, 1976). The emotional withdrawal and speech deficit so characteristic of these children are captured in the following description of an autistic child:

> The child did not habitually stay near people, especially, other children. Eye contact was of short duration, and the child looked through people rather than at them. . . . He did not imitate their physical actions or play with other children even though he may have hovered at the edge of a group. He did not respond to other people's attempts to engage him in simple conversation, although he may at times have given a clear indication of understanding uncomplicated speech, especially when it related to food, a favored object, or a routine. Parents frequently described the child as one who stays in "his own little world" needing his parents only when in physical distress or if he wants or dislikes something. His signaling system under these conditions was rudimentary—only a cry, a tantrum, or leading the parent by the back of the hand. (Speech problems are characteristic with many such children never developing speech [mute] or limiting speech to parroting others [echolalia]. Even those with functional speech show a mechanical and computer-like quality in its quality and inflection.) He did not signal by pointing or by serial pantomine as an *aphasic*[7] child

---

[6]The diagnostic criteria adopted by the American Psychiatric Association in its 1980 manual "DSM-III" includes the same behaviors: "Onset usually prior to 30 months but up to 42 months; lack of responsiveness to other human beings ('autism'); self-isolation; gross deficits in language development; if speech is present, peculiar speech patterns; peculiar interest or attachments to animals or inanimate objects" (American Psychiatric Association, 1980).

[7]"Aphasic" refers to expressive or receptive language problems not explicable in terms of general intelligence and presumed to be due to organic impairment in the cortical language centers (Eisenson, 1965).

would. Between episodes of generalized and occasionally gross expressions of displeasure or pleasure, the child had flat affect described by parents as a "don't care" attitude. At times, he "did not want his mother out of sight," and sought physical contact at every opportunity (Allen, DeMyer, Norton, Pontius, & Yang, 1971).

Numerous studies reveal that the majority of autistic children test in the mentally retarded range (e.g., DeMyer et al., 1974; Lotter, 1966; Rutter, 1966). Even more significant is the degree of cognitive impairment. From one-half to two-thirds are more than mildly retarded (Lotter, 1966; Rutter & Lockyer, 1967). The more severe levels of retardation tend to be found in those with neurological abnormality, and these are the children with the poorest prognosis for major improvement. Some workers have challenged the validity of IQ scores obtained in this population, claiming that the child's personality disorder would preclude cooperating with the test procedure. While it is obvious that adequate assessment of intelligence will be impossible in a highly withdrawn or negativistic child, there is evidence that cooperation can usually be secured when the test tasks presented are *within their capacities* (Alpern, 1967; DeMyer, Norton, & Barton, 1971; Schopler, 1976).

Cognitive Characteristics

Autistic children, like their nonautistic but retarded counterparts, function better in nonverbal tasks, but the degree of their relative deficit in verbal ones is much greater (DeMyer et al., 1974). Autistic children tend to be extremely literal or concrete in their interpretation of the meaning of words. Here are some examples.

> Words are used and responded to in a very limited way. An autistic child who always referred to the dog's dinner plate as a "dish" was confused when asked to put some food in the dog's "bowl." She solved the problem by giving the food to the dog in the washing-up bowl. [For this autistic child, the word "bowl" was obviously tied to its usage in her home in connection with washing. She did not understand that it is a perfectly good synonym for "dish."]
>
> Slapstick comedy and very simple obvious jokes involving words may be much enjoyed, but humor depending on the multiple association of words ["double meaning"] is greeted by blank comprehension or by a totally literal interpretation without any realization that the anecdote was intended to be funny (Dewey, 1973). [Parenthetically, retarded individuals, too, often fail to appreciate humor based on a play of words—the same problem of concreteness but not to the same degree.]
>
> Idiomatic expressions can be very confusing for even the brightest autistic child, and parents and teachers learn through experience to choose their words with care. One child was terrified when her mother used the familiar phrase "crying her eyes out" [fear of losing her

eyes]. Another, when asked if he'd lost his tongue, started anxiously searching for it (Ricks & Wing, 1976).

Islets of Intelligence ("Splinter Skills")

Some autistic children, even those who are retarded, sometimes display abilities that are normal or even superior in their own right. The child may perform in age-appropriate fashion in the assembly of picture puzzles (DeMyer, 1976) or show good rote memory. The same child who is having tremendous difficulty in *understanding* language may, in parrot fashion, demonstrate rote recall for lengthy amounts of material (Ricks & Wing, 1976). The problem is that this capacity is nonfunctional for the child. It is a special skill, which operates outside the child's normal problem-solving abilities. This is similar to the *idiot savant* phenomenon described earlier in the chapter. The author once tested a pair of autistic twins who were calendar calculators. They could tell on what day of the week a particular date would fall but were unable, on the Binet test, to solve even simple addition and subtraction problems involving numbers of less than 10!

Intellectual and Speech Impairment in Prognosis

Retardation is not only a common finding in autism, it also has important prognostic implications. Those autistic children with IQs of less than 50 tend to show relatively little improvement (DeMyer et al., 1973; Gittelman & Birch, 1967; Goldfarb, Goldfarb, & Pollack, 1966; Mittler, Gillies, & Jukes, 1966). Parenthetically, those children who become sociable begin to manifest this around school age (Wing, 1972).

Another prognostic sign is the presence of some functional speech by age 6. These are the children who are likely to become less withdrawn. The importance of speech as a predictor of later development in autism was initially recognized by Kanner (1957), the child psychiatrist who first described the disorder and has been confirmed by later investigators (Rutter, 1970; DeMyer et al., 1973).

With regard to prognosis as such, the impact of infantile autism is likely to be seen throughout life. Again referring to a major follow-up study (DeMyer et al., 1973), at a mean age of 12 most of the children were educationally behind—consistent with the intellectual impairment—and nearly half (42%) had been institutionalized. On a more positive note the proportion who were severely withdrawn had diminished from 75 percent in early childhood to only 25 percent by adolescence. Again referring to speech, of the 25 percent who were still much withdrawn, most were either mute or only echolalic at age 5. Overall, only about 17 percent of autistic children appear capable of achieving an independent adjustment in later life; difficulty in social relationships is a persisting characteristic (Wing, 1976).

The Severely Retarded Autistic Child

The autistic child whose IQ is in the below-50 range is likely to be bereft of functional language. Either mute (producing sounds but not words) or echolalic (parroting what is heard), meaningful speech is generally limited to a few highly reinforced words—those that relate to favorite foods. But not only is functional language absent, unlike in the deaf or aphasic child or even in the prespeech normal infant, there is no use of gestures. It is these children who are now being taught simple sign language as a means of encouraging the development of some form of communication.

Together with the cognitive and speech deficits, these children also manifest other aberrant behaviors, notably in the motor domain—repetitive and rhythmic body movements (stereotypies) and hitting and biting oneself (self-injurious behavior). Both of these are dealt with in depth in Chapter 10.

CAUSATION

Earlier Perspectives

Kanner (1943, 1957) attributed autism to a biologically determined inability to form emotional attachments but in families where parents were viewed as emotionally distant.

Early workers tended to stress presumed *parental* aloofness and emotional detachment as the cause, but later studies of the personalities of these parents (Creak & Ini, 1960; Rutter, Bartak, & Newman, 1971) and of their child-rearing practices (DeMyer et al., 1972; Gillies, Mittler, & Simon, 1963; Pitfield & Oppenheim, 1964) have failed to distinguish them from parents of nonautistic children. If the parents were the primary cause, one would expect high levels of personality disorder in the sibs, but this does not seem to be the case. In a major survey, 5 percent of the sibs were classified as either retarded or psychotic by school age. The other 95 percent were free of psychiatric disorder (Lotter, 1967b).

Current Perspective

Current workers tend to view autism as caused by some form of organic brain abnormality (Rutter, 1972; Schopler, 1983; Wing, 1976). A striking neurological finding is the much increased risk of epilepsy, with about one-third so affected by adulthood (Deykin & McMahon, 1971; Rutter, 1970). This contrasts with a risk of approximately one percent in the general population.

A study of autism in twins, identical and fraternal, produced some provocative findings (Folstein & Rutter, 1977). Among discordant identical twin pairs, one affected, one unaffected, the autistic twin was much more likely to have had perinatal problems that often accompany brain injury. The study did not show any evidence of a strong genetic basis for autism. Of the 11 identical twin pairs only 3 were "concordant" (both affected) and 8 were discordant. All of the fraternal twins were discordant.

Of particular interest was the tendency toward some intellectual impairment and speech articulation problems in the nonautistic identical cotwins. Four were so affected. In an earlier study, the relatives of autistic children were found to show an increased frequency of *delayed language development* (Bartak, Rutter, & Cox, 1975) while two recent ones reported increased rates of mental retardation in nonautistic sibs (August, Stewart, & Tsai, 1981; Minton et al., 1982).

LOCALIZING THE PRESUMED BRAIN ABNORMALITY

While evidence for some brain abnormality is overwhelming, one that affects language, thinking, sensory perception, and emotions, there is, as yet, no indication of its specific nature.

Numerous brain areas have been proposed as possible sites. Earlier speculations of a *subcortical* abnormality (Gellner, 1959; MacCulloch & Sambrooks, 1972) have found later support in indications of a brain stem dysfunction in the auditory pathway (Fein, Skoff, & Mirsky, 1981). Another early brain stem-related finding was of a diminished lateral eye movement response (nystagmus) to stimuli that ordinarily cause dizziness (Ornitz & Ritvo, 1968). None of these findings means that the disorder *arises* in the brainstem, only that this brain area is affected (Fein et al., 1981).

Apart from the brain stem, the *left temporal lobe* of the cortex has evoked much interest (Hetzler & Griffin, 1981). It is this part of the brain through which speech is understood and it must also be involved at some level in the receptive language deficit.

Perhaps related to some deficiency in the left temporal lobe is evidence for an atypical pattern of *cerebral hemisphere specialization* in "dominance" (Dawson, 1982, 1983; Prior & Bradshaw, 1979). Autistic youth appear to be less "lateralized" for language in the left hemisphere. Language stimuli produce greater than expected electrical activity in their right hemisphere. That their right hemisphere enjoys a greater than normal between-hemisphere influence is suggested by their commonly better performance on visual-spatial tasks and in music; both are right hemisphere functions.

A tantalizing finding is a possible association between autism and the form of mental retardation caused by *Fragile X*, a chromosomal abnormality described in Chapter 3 (Brown et al., 1982). The excess of males is consistent with a possible X chromosome involvement and the Fragile X could account for the retardation.

Finally, numerous studies have sought to identify specific *biochemical* abnormalities in autism, thus far to no avail (Wing, 1976).

TREATMENT

Current treatment approaches tend to have an *educational* rather than psychotherapeutic emphasis, for example, those of Schopler (1976) and Wing (1972). These workers see the autistic child as "handicapped"—disabled by fundamental cognitive deficit of organic origin. Treatment goals as defined by Schopler have three main objectives: (a) to prevent or reduce troublesome behavior; (b) to circumvent the specific disabilities associated with the handicap (e.g., with sign language); and (c) to improve the child's general level of functioning. Wing (1972) offers a number of suggestions for parents with stress on the benefit of the "behavioral" approach. (This approach is described in Chap. 7 and then presented in detail in Chap. 10.)

Psychotropic drugs are also widely used with these children but side effects call attention to their hazards and the need for careful monitoring.

Language

A major focus of the education of autistic children is in language. Especially for those who at school age are either essentially mute or echolalic, the teaching of some communication skill is paramount.

Language training in autism has taken two forms, the teaching of speech through behavior modification (operant conditioning) and the teaching of sign language as an alternative to speech (Bonvillian, Nelson, & Rhyne, 1981). The behavioral approach has been able to train appropriate speech utterances, especially in echolalic children, but the youngsters do not progress to the *spontaneous* use of untrained speech. Sign language instruction is usually augmented by the simultaneous use of speech and virtually all autistic children learn to understand and to produce at least some signs. In addition to the signs trained one also observes the occasional spontaneous combining of single signs into the equivalent of two-word utterances. Still, the acquisition of some signs does not result in the kind of continuous and rapid growth in sign proficiency found in deaf children. Again, the language deficit in autism is not purely "mechanical"; the *desire* to communicate is also lacking.

In the teaching of signs it was also hoped that their acquisition would facilitate speech itself. While some growth in speech may occur, it will generally not be as great as in the learning of the signs themselves.

Social Skills

Within educational programs, particular attention is also given to "social skills," the teaching of appropriate social behaviors. Also much in vogue in mental retardation, it involves three elements—modeling of the appropriate behavior by the instructor, practice by the student, an feedback from the instructor (Mesibov, 1983). While such methods can create at least an approximation of normality in the situations trained, they cannot be expected to produce the kind of flexibility that characterizes the subtle adaptations inherent in normal social interactions. The social estrangement that epitomizes autism is a particular barrier to the teaching of more "social" behaviors. Interestingly, even high-functioning autistic adults, those who are aware of their "difference," recognize this as their problem in developing friendships and ask professionals for assistance with it (DeMyer, 1979).

Mental Retardation and "Learning Disabilities"

Another major developmental learning problem is the so-called *learning disabilities*. They are distinguished from retardation in two important ways: (a) the associated learning difficulties tend to be relatively specific (e.g., in reading, writing, or arithmetic) rather than generalized, and (b) they are not explicable in terms of general intelligence. Indeed, their hallmark is that, academically, the child performs more poorly than expected on the basis of general intelligence. Within the learning disabilities, the focus here is on reading.

READING DISABILITY (DYSLEXIA)

This is the most common of the learning disabilities. It consists of difficulties in word recognition, in the comprehension of written material, and in its retention. Dyslexic readers read laboriously, word by word, and the most severely affected may be unable to read virtually any words at all. A 15-year-old of average intelligence could only immediately recognize "stop," "no," and "yes." Fluent in speech and quite skilled in woodworking, he was simply unable to make an association between the *visual* symbol and its meaning.

The earliest examples of dyslexia in children and youth were described in the 1890s in Great Britain. They were called "congenital word blindness" to distinguish them from losses in the ability to read following organic brain disease.

One of the first described was an adolescent schoolboy, Percy, who despite apparently normal mental ability could not read. When he was given some material to read this is what was observed:

> He did not read a single word correctly with the exception of "and," "the," "of," and "that." The other words seemed quite unknown to him and he could not even make an attempt to pronounce them. Asked to write, he fared no better. He wrote his name "Precy." His schoolmaster said that if all lessons had been conducted orally he'd have been at the top of his class (Morgan, 1896).

In addition to impaired word recognition or even the sense of how visual symbols (letters) "group" to form words, there is much difficulty with spelling. Percy mispells his own name! Note that the error consists of incorrect placement of the letter "r," an error of letter *sequence*. Problems of sequence may not be limited to spelling and can be seen in difficulty in mastering the months of the year or the multiplication tables. Together with problems of word recognition, reading comprehension, spelling, and sequencing, also observed often are difficulties in attending (short attention span), rapid forgetting of what was seemingly learned, hyperactivity, easy emotionality, impulsivity, easy disorganization, and fine motor incoordination.

Some researchers have sought to distinguish forms of dyslexia on the basis of the kinds of errors made (Boder, 1971; Ingram, Mason, & Blackburn, 1970; Johnson & Myklebust, 1967). The majority of dyslexics make visual errors, although there is a group whose primary difficulty is in the auditory sphere.

Visual Dyslexia

It is the visual dyslexic who makes the kind of "reversal" errors so characteristic of the disorder (see Fig. 4). Letters with similar configurations are confused (e.g., b and d, b and p, p and q, n and u, and m and w). These confusions reflect an inattention to the differences between these letters in their *spatial* orientation. In the b/d and p/q confusions there is an ignoring of the difference in the

Poor drawing reproduction

Reversals of the letter "b"

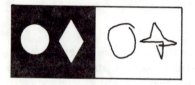

Dictated by teacher	Dyslexic responses
Body	Boby
Bug	Bug
Dad	Bob
Did	Bi'D

Female   Age: 6 years, 7 months
            Grade: 1.6
            IQ: 114 Stanford-Binet

Errors of omission and sequence in the alphabet

Lesli

ABCPFGHiJKLWhOPQ

r+4VMXYS

Spelling errors

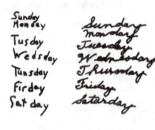

Reversals

Infantile drawing; improved
after 4 months of tutoring

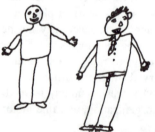

FIG. 4 Common problems in dyslexic children. From Johnson and Myklebust
(1967), *Learning Disabilities: Educational Principles and Practices,* by permission of
Grune & Stratton.

lateral plane, whereas the b and p confusion pertains to the vertical one. Reversals
are also seen in words (e.g., "saw" and "was") and may reflect difficulty in
maintaining a consistent left-to-right reading orientation. These errors do not represent a literal reversal of the perceptual experience (Vellutino et al., 1975); typically they are made when reading under the pressure of normal reading speed.
Indeed, they are commonly seen in normal 4- and 5-year-olds and do not disappear

in nondyslexic readers until about age seven (Gibson et al., 1962). Johnson and Myklebust (1967) explain letter and word reversals in terms of the child's way of viewing his visual world. For the child (and for the rest of us), a dog is a dog whether it is standing and its legs are down or it is on its back and its legs are up. The letters m and w and n an u share this same up-down relationship; it takes time for the beginning reader to understand that a difference in the vertical, or in the case of b and d the horizontal, relationship is important and that a b turned to the left is not a b at all but rather a d. Somehow, this distinction does not become automatic in the visual dyslexic.

Another major problem, indeed the primary one, is difficulty in learning the association between the letters as visual symbols and their sounds. While these associations are drummed in by teachers day after day, and on any given day are seemingly learned, on the next day they are forgotten. It is as if they were never "learned" in the first place, a great frustration to teachers and parents no less than to the student. Difficulty in remembering letters and words is also evident in their spelling. For the visual dyslexic, this is especially obvious in the kinds of errors made (Boder, 1971). Apart from the kind of sequence error in Percy's spelling of his name, there is particular difficulty in spelling nonphonetic words, words in which all of the letters cannot be heard, for example, the w in "sword" or the gh in "tight." In contrast, their spelling of phonetically regular words is much better (e.g., bind). The visual dyslexic speller simply does not remember how the correctly spelled word looks; he has to spell it by sounding it out.

Problems in the visual mode are also seen in their drawings. Drawings lack detail (e.g., in Fig. 4), and there may be difficulty with picture puzzles, reading maps, and building models—all tasks involving *visual-spatial* understanding.

Educational procedures focus on teaching reading through the auditory modality, since the visual dyslexic has particular difficulty at the visual level. Instead of a "sight word" or "whole word" approach to recognizing the printed word, the emphasis is on learning the letter sound equivalents for the individual letters and syllables, and reading words by sounding them out. This is the "phonics" approach and it is the most widely used method to teach reading to dyslexics (Johnson, 1978; Johnson & Myklebust, 1967).

Auditory Dyslexia

Letters and letter combinations have sounds as well as visual dimensions. Learning the alphabet and its use in reading involves the recognition of how the visual symbol is pronounced. For the minority of dyslexics whose problem is primarily auditory, the difficulty is recognizing the sounds that are associated with the visual symbol. The auditory dyslexic, unlike his visual counterpart, can recognize words visually and, necessarily as whole, but is unable to decode a word by its sounds. Unable to learn letter sound families, each word has to be learned as a distinct entity. The normally reading first grader may learn the word "cook." When the child hears the new word "took," there is recognition that the ending of the new word is identical to a word already known. It is merely necessary to change the sound of the first letter and to repeat the sound that ends both words and the word is correctly read. But the auditory dyslexic doesn't recognize the sounds conveyed by the letters, and the word has to be learned visually.

Difficulties in discriminating sounds are most evident in short vowels (e.g., pin, pen, pan). These words are understood by the context in which they are used; the differences between them are not perceived when heard only as single words. The apparent impairment in auditory discrimination interferes with the ability to appreciate poetry. There is no recognition of rhyme. Like the visual dyslexic, there is an analogous inability to remember sounds seemingly learned. This is compensated for when reading aloud by substituting words that fit the context of what is being read.

Sequencing problems here, apart from calendar and multiplication tables, are evident in errors made in word pronunciation. Where the visual dyslexic misplaces letters in writing, the auditory dyslexic errs in reading aloud. The word "enemy" for example is said as "emeny." The confusion of speech sound sequences is considered by one major researcher as a specific subtype of dyslexia ("dysphonemic sequencing difficulty"; Denckla, 1975).

Interestingly, the auditory discrimination problems here do not seem to be associated with any significant hearing loss. However, there is often a history of delayed speech and language development. And just as the visual dyslexic prefers to learn through hearing rather than seeing (recall Percy's teacher's comment about his skill at learning what was heard) the auditory dyslexic prefers to learn through the visual mode and often shows skills in crafts and athletics.

For teaching dyslexics who have special difficulty in analyzing words by their sounds, the phonics approach presents major problems. Auditory dyslexics learn best through a whole-word visual approach, and this is stressed during their initial reading instruction. However, phonics cannot be ignored, because it is the only way in which we can decipher unfamiliar words. Words first learned through sight become the basis for teaching sounds.

Mixed Dyslexia: Visual and Auditory

Some dyslexics are impaired in both perceptual modalities. They can learn words neither phonically nor through sight (Boder, 1971). For these, other sensory modalities must be employed—tactile and kinesthetic. The learner is taught what the shape of a letter feels like (as if blind) and practices the movements involved in writing it. The letter is also simultaneously verbalized and looked at, in an attempt to strengthen its auditory and visual impression. Needless to say, these are the most impaired of the dyslexic population.

Educational Outcome

Although dyslexia has been described here in terms of sensory modalities, this distinction is not evident in the literature on the effects of remediation. Studies are mixed with regard to eventual reading competency (Abbott & Frank, 1975; Balow & Bloomquist, 1965; Edgington, 1975; Frauenheim, 1978); Hinton & Knights, 1971; Howden, 1967; Kline, 1975). One's overall impression is of enduring difficulties in reading, especially reading aloud, persistent problems in spelling, even when reading is essentially normal; and difficulties in mathematics, not in calculating but in understanding *written* problems. The initial level of impairment seems to be the best indicator of ultimate reading accomplishment (Akerman, Dykman, & Peters, 1977a, 1977b; Gottesman, Belmont, & Kaminer, 1975; Hinton & Knights, 1971; Koppitz, 1976). In a study of change in reading level between grades 2 and 5 (Satz, Taylor, Friel, & Fletcher, 1978), only 3 of 49 children (6%) labeled "severe" at grade 2 were improved by the end of grade 5. In contrast, 11 of 62 "mild" cases (18%) showed significant improvement.

Adult Status

As implied in discussing "educational outcome," the effects of dyslexia are not necessarily limited to the school years. On the one hand there are autobiographical materials that dramatically shows the kind of gain that is possible (Simpson, 1979) as well as the enduring day-to-day difficulties (Hampshire, 1982), while on the other there are adults of normal intelligence who read at less than a 5th-grade level. The adult who reads with difficulty or not at all is isolated from an ever more technological world. Mail, newspapers, magazines, books, maps, timetables—all of these are obstacles to "keeping up" and "keeping in touch." Moreover, the dyslexic lives with constant fear that the disability will be discovered. Usually unaware of why they cannot do what is so easy for others, they try to hide or disguise their "weakness," and feel themselves to be stupid. Indeed, it would appear that their greatest fear is to be thought "retarded" (Hampshire, 1982; Simpson, 1979).

CAUSATION

Theories of the cause of developmental dyslexia, and of learning disabilities in general, have commonly pointed to some kind of neurological abnormality in brain function, especially as it relates to the *processing* or interpreting of auditory and visual stimuli and to the translating of stimuli experienced in one sensory modality into another—for example, reading aloud (verbal expressive) what one sees (verbal receptive). Early workers noted that specific language difficulties were seen in persons who had suffered brain injury, such as aphasias in stroke patients, and later ones observed in some brain-injured children behavior problems often found in learning disability youngsters, notably distractibility, hyperactivity, disorganization, awkwardness, and emotional lability (Strauss & Lehtinen, 1947). In spite of the presumed organic abnormality, as in autism, no specific ones have been found; in fact, these children are typically free of conventional neurological problems (Johnson & Myklebust, 1967).

Apart from an assumed biological impairment, those learning disability children with severe receptive language problems show some similarity to autistic and to the aphasic ones. These three groups have special difficulties in understanding or making sense of what is heard, although the learning disability child does not show the extraordinary aloofness, cognitive deficit, and ritualistic behavior of the autistic child or the severity of language impairment of the aphasic one.

MANAGEMENT OF PERSONALITY PROBLEMS IN MENTAL RETARDATION: OVERVIEW

In this final section of the chapter we begin to consider the treatment procedures applied to behavior problems in retarded persons. There are three major approaches—psychotherapy and/or counseling, behavior modification, and psychotropic drugs. In the material that follows, attention is directed primarily toward the psychotherapy/counseling approach with sections on behavior modification and drugs reserved for the later "management" chapters.

Psychotherapy/Counseling

This treatment modality refers to procedures that seek to improve personality adjustment by helping the individual gain a better understanding of the nature of his problems and how he may contribute to them. This is typically accomplished through verbal communication, though nonverbal means such as play (Leland & Smith, 1965), and music and art (Ludins-Katz, 1972) are also widely used. The heavy dependency on verbal skills as *the* communication mode between therapist/counselor and client as well as the focus on "understanding" have raised questions as to the appropriateness of this procedure in helping retarded individuals with their personality problems (Abel, 1953; Rogers, 1951; Sarason, 1949). While individual workers have reported successful psychotherapy with retarded clients, the fairly considerable research literature offers little scientific basis for drawing any kind of firm conclusions on its effectiveness with this population (Bialer, 1967; Browning & Keesey, 1974; Sternlicht, 1966).

In the author's view, the question of the appropriateness of psychotherapy and counseling with retarded persons ultimately depends on one's definition of a "therapeutic experience." In terms of our personality model, a therapeutic experience is one in which the basic psychological needs of structure, self-esteem, and self-expression are met. Since a common goal of psychotherapy or counseling is elevation of the client's self-esteem, we can ask ourselves whether the psychotherapeutic or counseling encounter can provide retarded individuals with experiences that enhance feelings of intimacy, success, and autonomy. If we examine the benefits seen by proponents of these procedures, at least for those who are not more than mildly retarded, elements are found that relate directly to our personality model. With regard to intimacy, the counselor or therapist can provide experiences of acceptance, warmth, and even affection (Gunzburg, 1958; Thorne, 1948; Weist, 1955). This is, of course, the essence of intimacy. It is vital to the mental health of all of us and particularly appreciated by persons whose disabilities have traditionally evoked rejection rather than acceptance. Given a relatively non-judgmental and accepting relationship, the client will be freer to express feelings, to ventilate frustrations, and to begin to discharge potentially troublesome impulses verbally rather than behaviorally.

Another extremely important element in counseling and psychotherapy, and one that relates to needs for structure and success, is the role of the therapist as an interpreter of reality. In behavior modification parlance, this is to help the client understand the "contingencies" associated with his behavior. This is of special significance in retardation, because the intellectual impairment interferes with both the client's awareness of general behavioral expectations and an understanding of how his own behavior gets him into difficulty. Even within these limitations, however, there is no doubt that mildly retarded youth and adults can recognize basic contingencies if these are presented in concrete terms and richly illustrated with examples from the client's own experiences (Rosen, Clark, & Kivitz, 1977). In this role, the therapist/counselor serves as a bridge to reality and as a teacher (Slivkin & Bernstein, 1970). By helping the client to better appreciate the contingencies his behavior evokes and by discussing alternative ways of dealing with sources of frustration, the therapist/counselor/teacher creates conditions for more effective self-management. To the degree that the client attempts to use this knowledge and finds it helpful, he has direct experiences of success. This also leads to greater autonomy as awareness grows that feelings can be controlled and that one can have some influence on how we deal with others and how they deal with us.

Given the possibility of these kinds of experiences in psychotherapy and counseling, undoubtedly these procedures can be therapeutic for the retarded individual. It is true that the activity of the therapist/counselor is likely to be modified in working with the retarded client. He is going to be more "active" and directive (Sternlicht, 1966) in seeking to enhance client understanding. He must build explanatory bridges that the normal client constructs for himself.

While our focus has been on the potential benefits of the therapist-client relationship, this need not be a one-to-one experience. In fact, group therapy appears to be the more widely used approach. It offers a controlled setting for examining interpersonal relationships and becoming aware of how our own behavior affects and is affected by others (e.g., Kaufman 1963; Slivkin & Bernstein, 1970).

Behavior Modification

Whereas psychotherapy and counseling strive to improve adaptation through increased understanding and self-awareness, in behavior modification the focus shifts away from the client to the contingencies or consequences his behavior evokes. Although in principle this is not different from interpreting reality to a client, the emphasis is less on what the client says or feels and more on what the client "does" and what his environment "does back." The latter refers to the kinds of positive and negative consequences (contingencies, reinforcers) that are meaningful to the person ("values") and through which he can be encouraged to increased desired behavior and to reduce undesired behavior. In the contingent use of positive and negative consequences, the behavior modification specialist is regarded by the author as simply applying in a very systematic manner the "first order" need in our personality model—that we are ultimately governed or motivated by the need to avoid painful consequences (negative reinforcers) and to obtain pleasurable ones (positive reinforcers). The behavior modification approach has had a profound impact on the education, training, and behavior management of retarded persons (Gardner, 1971; Matson & McCartney, 1981; Thompson & Grabowski, 1972, 1977), and examples of its application will be seen in the "management" chapters.

Biological Factors in Mental Retardation: Chromosomal and Genetic

OVERVIEW
Mental retardation may be caused by biological factors either operating fairly independently, as in the case of such clearly organic forms as Down syndrome (mongolism), or interacting with psychological ones as may be true in cultural-familial mental retardation. In the following two chapters the role of biological factors is explored beginning first with chromosomal and genetic ones. In this chapter we consider (a) some basic biological concepts necessary to the understanding of chromosomal and genetic disorders; (b) autosomal (nonsex chromosomes) abnormalities associated with retardation—Down syndrome (trisomy 21) (including its clinical, behavioral, and family aspects), Edwards syndrome (trisomy 18), and Patau syndrome (trisomy 13–15); (c) abnormalities of the sex chromosomes associated with retardation—Klinefelter, XYY, XXX; Turner, and Fragile X; and (d) gene-determined disorders—dominant, recessive, and presume polygenic.

SOME BASIC BIOLOGICAL CONCEPTS
There are instances of mental retardation that are determined at conception. These are due to chromosomal abnormalities, as in Down syndrome, or to gene-determined or hereditary disorders, as in phenylketonuria (PKU). The genes, the units of heredity, are carriers of biochemical information to the cell, patterning the kinds of proteins the cell will produce. Proteins serve as enzymes or catalysts of the body's enormous number of chemical reactions. A genetic defect is, in essence, a biochemical error resulting from failure to produce the enzyme necessary to a specific biochemical reaction. This is later illustrated with regard to PKU; first it is necessary to review some basic biology in order to have a general understanding of the mechanism of heredity.

Cells

All living things are composed of cells. Each cell has a nucleus, and within the nucleus is material called chromatin. Cells grow and divide, and during the process of division the chromatin arranges itself into pairs of threadlike structures called chromosomes (see Figs. 5–7). It is on the chromosomes that the hereditary units, the genes, are found.

To understand how nature assures the chromosomal and genetic integrity of living things, let us examine the process of cell division. Cells divide in either of two ways depending on whether they are sex cells (egg and sperm) or somatic cells (all other cells of the body—skin, hair, blood, muscle, bone, etc.). Somatic cells divide by the process called "mitosis" or "equal cell division." In mitotic divi-

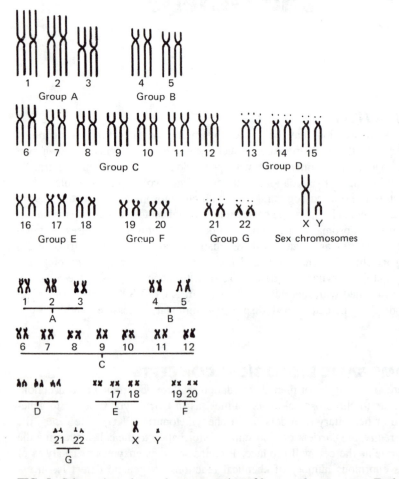

FIG. 5 Schematic and actual representation of human chromosomes. Each chromosome pair has its own numerical designation as well as a letter designation for the structural group of which it is a member. The seven "groups" are arranged in order of decreasing length.

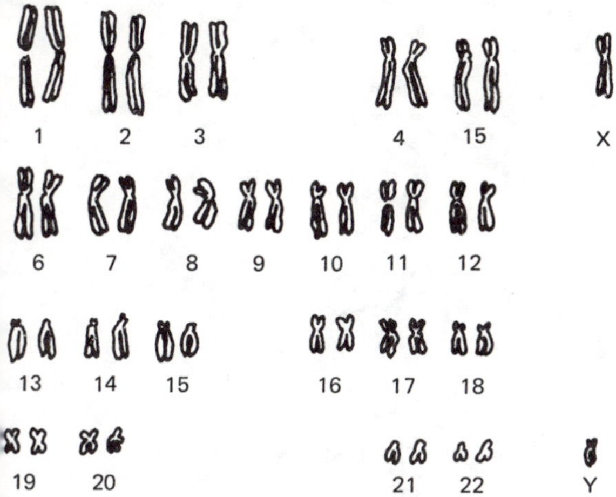

FIG. 6a   Chromosomes (karyotype) of normal male. Note the sex chromosomes, X and Y, on the right-hand side of the figure. The chromosomes are arranged in pairs so that they can be studied.

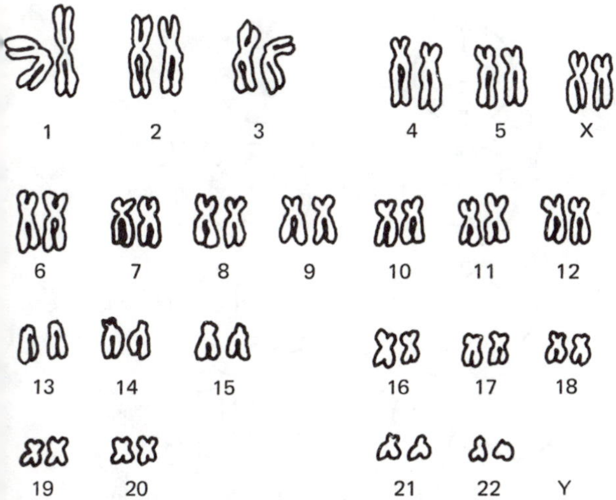

FIG. 6b   Chromosomes of normal female. Except for the absence of a Y chromosome and the presence of two X's, they are not distinguishable from those of a male.

sion, each chromosome in a cell duplicates itself (replication), resulting in a cell with double its normal number of chromosomes. The cell then divides, creating two cells, which have the same number of chromosomes as the mother cell prior to replication. In division of sex cells, however, replication is followed by *two* divisions, the second of which leads to a cell that contains only half of the chromo-

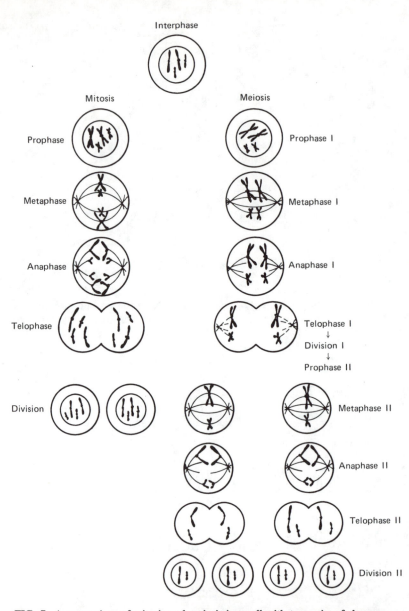

FIG. 7 A comparison of mitosis and meiosis in a cell with two pairs of chromo-somes. During interphase, and prior to prophase, the individual chromatids duplicate themselves. The duplicate chromatids then align themselves at their centromeres and thus give the appearance of one rather than two chromosomes. Separation of the chromatids and return to their appearance during interphase occurs during anaphase in mitosis and the second anaphase in meiosis. Change in the angle of each chroma-tid as between metaphase and anaphase is due to the force exerted on the centromere as the chromatid is pulled from the equatorial plane to the aster. From *Foundations of Genetics* by A.C. Pai, Copyright © 1974, McGraw-Hill. Used with permission of McGraw-Hill Book Company.

somes of the mother cell. This process by which sperm and egg cells are formed is called "meiosis," or "reduction division."

Chromosomes

Chromosomes exist in pairs, with each pair structurally and genetically distinct from all other pairs. Our chromosomes were literally given to us by our parents through their sperm and egg cells; thus there is a maternal and paternal chromosome for each chromosome pair. All human cells except the sperm and egg contain 23 pairs of chromosomes, or 46 chromosomes in all. The sperm and egg cells, however, as a result of reduction division, contain only 23 chromosomes in all, with each chromosome as the sole representative of each of the original 23 pairs. In human reproduction the union of sperm and egg creates a new cell—a fertilized egg, or zygote—which, combining the 23 chromosomes of the father with the 23 chromosomes of the mother, produces the correct human chromosomal complement of 46. Schematic representation of the chromosomes and of the processes of mitosis and meiosis for a hypothetical cell that contains two pairs of chromosomes is shown in Figure 7.

Genes

We have already referred to the genes as the basic unit of heredity. Because of their extraordinary importance in life processes and the remarkable knowledge about them gained in our own generation, some additional description of their two primary functions, self-replication and protein synthesis, is appropriate (Dobzhansky, 1962).

SELF-REPLICATION

This property refers to the capacity of the gene to organize the materials around it to duplicate its chemical structure. This capacity for self-copying, unique in living matter, is unaffected by changes that may occur in the gene, and future "copies" will incorporate these changes (mutations).

Gene Structure

The biochemical "instructions" on protein synthesis are encoded in chain molecules of nucleic acids, DNA (deoxyribonucleic acid), and RNA (ribonucleic acid). Each chain of DNA is a double spiral strand (helix) of four chemical substances called nucleotides (see Fig. 8). Thousands of these nucleotides are joined end to end to form these chains. Each nucleotide itself consists of several other chemicals, a phosphate, a sugar, and a nitrogenous base, and it is the last mentioned that represents the genetic code. In DNA, four of these bases are commonly found: adenine, guanine, thymine, and cytostine. The two chains or strands of the helix are held together by hydrogen bonds; one can think of the strand as a coiled ladder with the rungs of the ladder connecting the bases. The essential point is that an adenine base on one strand is always bonded to thymine on the other, and, similarly, guanine is always bonded to cytostine. The two chains are exact comple-

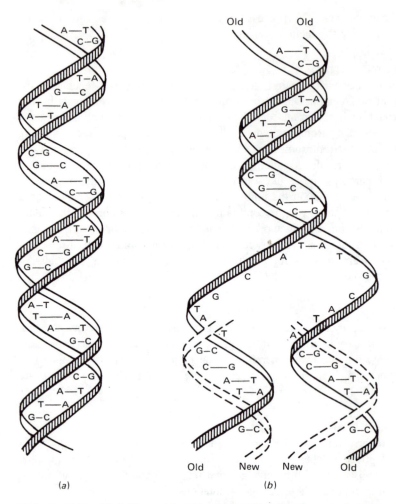

FIG. 8 *(a)* Double helix model of the gene (DNA). *(b)* Presumed manner of gene replication. Strands separate in zipperlike fashion and old strands serve as templates for new ones. Adapted from Watson (1968).

ments of each other. When they separate into two single strands during cell division, each separate strand can form an exact copy of the original double structure by the proper coupling of the four bases—adenine to thymine and guanine to cytostine.

Genetic Code

The genetic code can be conceptualized as a four-letter "alphabet," each letter standing for one of the bases—A (adenine), T (thymine), G (guanine), and C (cytostine). Just as an enormous number of words can be made up from the 26 letters of our alphabet or even just the two "letters" of the Morse code, so these four letters are capable of representing endless combinations. If we think of a gene as a "word" of n letters, the number of possible permutations of four letters in a word of n letters is 4^n. If a particular gene is a section of the double helix that contains 10 base pairs, for example, the number of possible sequences for the four "letters" is 4^{10} or 1,048,576. Thus within only 10 base pairs, more than a million genes are possible. While it is improbable that just any sequence of bases will make a functional gene, virtually an infinity of gene structures is possible if a gene contains hundreds or thousands of bases.

PROTEIN SYNTHESIS

The protein code originates in the nucleus of the cell, but protein synthesis occurs in the cytoplasm. The code is transferred from the nucleus to the cytoplasm via RNA. In the cytoplasm, RNA organizes amino acids, the chemical substrate of proteins. The genetic code determines the positions in the protein of each of the approximately 20 kinds of amino acids. For example, a molecule of insulin contains a total of 51 amino acids—comprising 15 (of the 20) different kinds. The insulin of different animals (e.g., cattle, sheep, and pigs) differs slightly but significantly by the substitution of only one or two amino acids. The importance of even one difference with regard to health or illness is illustrated in another protein, the oxygen-carrying component in our red blood cells, hemoglobin. In sickle cell anemia, hemoglobin is abnormal because of the substitution of only *one* amino acid out of the approximately 300 of which hemoglobin is composed!

How Heredity Works

Sickle cell anemia, a common disease in blacks, is an inherited disorder caused by a single gene. It is inherited as a "recessive," meaning that both parents are carriers of one normal and one abnormal gene but that the affected child receives only the abnormal gene from each parent (this mechanism is spelled out later in connection with PKU). The effect of the two recessive genes is to cause the child to be able to manufacture hemoglobin with only the one wrong kind of amino acid. The consequence is severe anemia with death often occurring by adolescence.

Types of Genes

It has been proposed that there are three types of genes: structural, operator, and regulator (Jacob & Monod, 1961). Structural genes, the kind we have been describing, determine the proteins; operator genes turn protein synthesis on and off in adjacent structural genes; and regulator genes suppress or activate operator and structural genes at the "systems" level (Jacob & Monod, 1961; Lerner, 1968; Martin & Ames, 1964). The structural genes are common to a wide variety of species and function in each in about the same way. This is what provides a fundamental identify among living things. It is the regulatory genes that are thought to cause diversity both within and between species by their control of the structural genes (Scarr-Salapater, 1975; Thiessen, 1972).

WITHIN-SPECIES GENETIC VARIATION

If regulator genes act in such a manner as to cause diversity among living things, they must influence the three known sources of variation among members of the same species—mutation, crossing over, and random assortment of chromosomes. Each of these is briefly described, though "random assortment" is treated in greater detail because its grasp is necessary to an understanding of the genetic risks borne by families in which genetic forms of retardation have a high probability of occurrence.

Mutation

Mutation refers to a change in the biochemical structure of a gene thereby producing a new or mutant gene. The mutant gene will alter metabolic functioning to a variable degree, and major changes are usually undesirable. All genes mutate but at a very slow rate, thus ensuring biochemical stability within a population. Radioactivity increases the rate of mutation and is one of the reasons the general level of radioactivity to which we are exposed is kept at a minimum.

Crossing Over

Crossing over refers to an exchange of chromosomal material (genes) between corresponding parts of a particular chromosome pair, resulting in the creation of two new modified members of that pair.

Random Assortment

Random or independent assortment is nature's chief means of generating diversity within sexually reproducing species by creating *variety* among the sperm or egg cells carried by each individual within that species. In humans there is an extraordinarily high probability that no two sperm or egg cells of the same person will be identical. "Identical" means that the sperm or egg cells share the same maternal or paternal member for all of the 23 chromosome pairs. Recall that reduction division is the process by which sex cells are formed. In man, for example, from an original 46 chromosomes (23 pairs), an egg or sperm is produced with 23 chromosomes, one member or representative from each of the 23 pairs. Each sperm or egg cell is likely to have a mix of maternal and paternal representatives of each of the 23 pairs that differs from the mix of other sperm or egg cells. The number of possible mixes or combinations that can be randomly drawn from 23 pairs is astronomical—2^{23}, or 8,388,608. But within this diversity there is also similarity. On the average, sperm or egg cells will be identical with regard to one-half of the 23 chromosomes, and this is what accounts for the similarities among siblings.

The concept of random assortment can be confusing, but to understand it will be helpful later as dominant and recessive forms of mental retardation are presented. Figure 9 illustrates the number of possible sperm cell combinations that could be generated from a cell that originally had three pairs of chromosomes. Since there are two possibilities for each chromosome pair, either drawing the maternal or paternal member of that pair, the total number of possible combina-

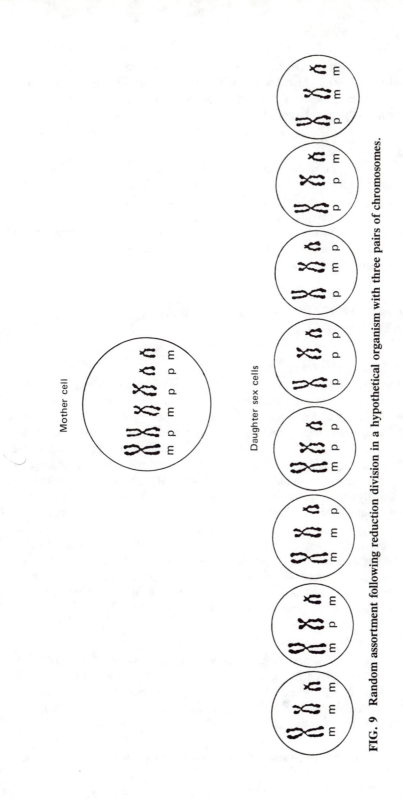

Mother cell

Daughter sex cells

FIG. 9 Random assortment following reduction division in a hypothetical organism with three pairs of chromosomes.

tions for a cell that contains three pairs of chromosomes is 2^3, or 8. Since the maternal and paternal chromosomes within a given pair are structurally indistinguishable, for purposes of diagrammatic illustration the maternal member is denoted by *m* and paternal member by *p*.

Summary

This survey of some basic biological concepts serves as a backdrop for a presentation of major chromosomal and genetic disorders associated with retardation. Human life begins with the union of egg and sperm cell, creating a fertilized egg to which both parents are equal contributors. The vital material of the fertilized egg is its 46 chromosomes on which are found, perhaps, as many as 3000 genes per chromosome (Asimov, 1962). The retardation-related problems produced by chromosomal and genetic errors now follow.

CHROMOSOMES AND MENTAL RETARDATION

A Little History

The basic principles of heredity were first enunciated by Mendel in 1866 and were rediscovered and confirmed about 1900, but this was long before the laboratory technology was available for the accurate study of human chromosomes (Engel, 1977). Human chromosome counts began in the 1920s, and, until the early 1950s, it was believed that we had 48 chromosomes. With improvement in techniques for studying chromosomes, the scientific world was startled to discover that the correct number was 46 rather than 48 (Ford & Hamerton, 1956; Tjo & Levan, 1956). Shortly thereafter, it was found that several major disorders were traceable to chromosomal abnormalities. Two of these are associated with mental retardation, Down syndrome (Lejeune, Gautier, & Turpin, 1959) and Klinefelter syndrome (Jacobs & Strong, 1959). These and other conditions are caused by such abnormalities as extra or missing chromosomes or loss of part of a chromosome (deletion). Chromosomal abnormalities are not rare. They are the single most important cause of spontaneous abortions, occurring in at least 20 percent of cases (Nyhan & Sakati, 1976) and in one in 200 live births (Engel, 1977).

Down Syndrome

The best-known and most common chromosomal disorder is Down syndrome. It occurs with a frequency of about one in 700 live births (Donnell, Alfi, Rublee, & Koch, 1975) and accounts for about 8 percent of the institutionalized retarded population.[1] Down syndrome is caused by an extra chromosome, there being three rather than two chromosome 21's—47 chromosomes in all.

---

[1] In 1977 and 1978, the proportion of Down syndrome residents in North Carolina's institutions was 7.8 percent.

HISTORICAL ASPECTS

The syndrome was first described in 1886 by Langdon Down, a London physician, who called it "mongolism" because of the facial similarity to Asians of Mongolian extraction (Warkany, 1975; Jarvik, Falek, & Pierson, 1964). In fact, the facial similarity is superficial, and the condition can be recognized in Asian children almost as easily as Caucasian ones (Kramm, 1963). Prior to 1959, the actual cause of Down syndrome was unknown, though its much increased occurrence in women over 35 led to speculations about "maternal exhaustion" or to consequences of pregnancies following long periods of sterility. It was also thought to be of endocrine origin (Warkany, 1975). On the basis of twin studies it had been concluded that the events causing the disorder had to occur very early in pregnancy (Allen & Baroff, 1955; Baroff, 1958), and this conclusion was soon confirmed with the discovery in 1959 of the presence of an extra chromosome. This meant that vulnerability to the disorder was set at conception itself. Though the nature of the chromosomal abnormality has been clear for more than two decades, we are only just beginning to discover some of the biochemical consequences of the presence of an extra chromosome 21.

CLINICAL FEATURES

The physical symptoms of Down syndrome include a variety of skeletal, joint, muscle, and organ abnormalities. Frequencies of the various symptoms have been noted by several workers (Oster, 1953; Smith, 1975), and Hall (1964) has specified those most often recognizable in newborns. In spite of the obvious physical similarities among affected persons, considerable individual symptom variability exists (Smith, 1975), with none of even the most familiar ones found in more than 90 percent of cases.

HEAD AND FACE[2]

The head is small (as is general stature) and flattened in the rear (occiput), ears are small with lobes often absent, and the nasal bridge is flattened. There is general underdevelopment of the nasal bones and of the upper jaw (Sanger, 1975). The most prominent of all external features are the slanting, almond-shaped eyes. Speckling of the iris is common (Brushfield spots) as is the presence of the epicanthus, a little fold of skin on the inner corner of the eye.

MOUTH

There are several major abnormalities in the oral cavity. There appears to be a high, arched palate; teeth are small and irregularly aligned, and the tongue appears large, furrowed, and often protruding. It has been suggested that the mouth is commonly open and the tongue protrudes because a narrowing of the

[2]Plastic surgery is now being performed to modify facial appearance and tongue size. Preliminary impression is of no benefit regarding speech or eating following tongue clipping, or of more than "modest" cosmetic effect following facial surgery (personal communication: Montefiore Hospital, New York, and Rhode Island Developmental Center, July 1984).

pharynx causes the person to breathe primarily through the mouth rather than through the nose (Donnell, Alfi, Rublee, & Koch, 1975).

HANDS

Characteristics of Down syndrome are short, broad, and spadelike hands. The little finger is shortened and curved, and there is a single palmar (simian) crease.

OTHER COMMON FINDINGS

Muscle and joint abnormalities are common. There is usually a reduction in muscle tone (hypotonus) and a hyperflexibility of the joints. This permits the unusual sitting positions often seen. Finally, there are frequent heart, lung, and eye problems. Congenital heart defects occur in at least one-third of Down newborns and produce a 43 percent mortality in the first year of life. Even among Down infants without heart defects, there is a 15 percent death rate during this period. A generation ago only about 40 percent of all Down children survived to age 10 years (Carter, 1958), but, with recent medical advances, life expectancy during the age range of 5 to 50 is only slightly below that of the general population, 6 percent (Lilienfeld, 1969) and not different from that of other persons with similar degrees of retardation (Forssman & Akesson, 1970; Richards & Sylvester, 1969). Seizure disorders also appear to be increased, especially after age 20 when the rate is about 8 percent (Coleman, 1978; Veall, 1974).

MEDICAL TREATMENT

A variety of medical therapies have had their adherents, but all have proved disappointing (Share, 1976; Smith, 1975). Extracts of the thyroid, pituitary, and thymus glands were ineffective in clinical trials as was glutamic acid, a much heralded treatment of some years ago. It has been suggested that the facies and neuromusclar function could be improved with dehydroepiandrosterone, but this could not be validated. Abnormalities in blood levels of serotonin, a neurotransmitter in the brain, have been reported in this condition as well as in other forms of retardation. Treatment designed to elevate and normalize serotonin (5-hydroxytryptophan) is said to have reversed the usual finding of very loose muscle tone (Bazelon et al., 1967), but a subsequent study failed to confirm this (Coleman, 1975). Still another investigation of the effects of serotonin normalization on general development showed only very slight effects that were regarded as clinically inconsequential (Weise, Koch, Shaw, & Rosenfeld, 1975). According to Smith (1975), very unusual combinations of drugs and vitamins, the so-called "V" series, were purported to be therapeutic (Turkel, 1963), but this was not confirmed in clinical tests (Bumbalo, Morelewicz, & Berens, 1964). Similarly, a treatment that involved both injection of embryonic cells into muscles (Siccacell) and a vitamin-mineral-hormonal preparation proved nontherapeutic (Bardon, 1964; Black, Kato, & Walker, 1966) as did the same regimen without Siccacell (White & Kaplitz, 1964). Freeman (1970) has been very critical of Siccacell treatment and offers general guidelines for evaluating reports of drug effectiveness. In summary, in a field where new treatments are often heralded, all appear to have failed to hold up under scrutiny (Smith, 1975).

MATERNAL AGE

Reference has already been made to the well-known relationship between Down syndrome and maternal age. The increased frequency in women over 35 is simply part of a broader risk for all kinds of chromosomal anomalies in babies born to older mothers. The rate of all chromosomal anomalies in mothers in the 35–40 range is 1.5 percent (Milunsky, 1976); it increases to 3.4 percent at age 40 and to as much as 10 percent at 45 (Sells & Bennett, 1977). For Down syndrome itself, with a general population frequency of about 1:700, the risk in women under 30 is less than 1:1000. In the age range 30–34, it rises slowly to 1:750, but thereafter the rise is dramatic. In the 35–39 range the risk is about 1:300; it increases to about 1:100 at 40–44, and from 3–6:100 at 45 and older (Donnell, Alfi, Rublee, & Koch, 1975; Mikkelsen & Stene, 1970; Smith & Wilson, 1973; Warkany, 1971).

HEPATITIS AND DOWN SYNDROME

In the 1960s Australian epidemiologic[3] studies noted increased frequencies of Down syndrome occurring 9 months after peaks of viral hepatitis (Kucera, 1970; Stoller, 1960; Stoller & Collman, 1965). Another study reported that viral hepatitis prior to pregnancy occurred more often in mothers of Down infants than in a control group of mothers (Pantelaskis et al., 1970). These findings suggested that hepatitis in pregnant women may induce the chromosomal anomaly. Epidemiologic studies in the United States and Canada have not confirmed the Australian findings (Baird & Miller, 1968; Madden et al., 1976; Stark & Fraumeni, 1966), although Down individuals do appear to have a greater susceptibility to one form of the disease (hepatitis B) (Blumberg, Sutnick, & London, 1970; Madden et al., 1976; Szmuness & Prince, 1971; Szmuness, Prince, Etling, & Pick, 1972).

FORMS OF DOWN SYNDROME

There are three chromosomal variants of Down syndrome—trisomy, translocation, and mosaicism. In trisomy each cell contains an extra chromosome 21; in translocation the extra chromosome is attached to another, typically 14; and in mosaicism some cells have the normal complement of 46 chromosomes and others have 47. Of the three variants, trisomy is by far the most common and, in a recent study of over 800 cases, accounted for 92 percent. Of the remainder, about 5 percent were translocations and 3 percent mosaics (Donnell, Alfi, Rublee, & Koch, 1975).

---

[3]Epidemiology is the study of the frequency (prevalence and incidence) of disease in a population and of the risk factors involved.

Trisomy

Trisomy usually results from an abnormality in the formation of the egg, although in about a quarter of the cases it is the sperm that is at fault (Magenis, Overton, Chamberlin, Braby, & Lourien, 1977). This process is shown in Figure 10b. Of the two types of abnormal sex cells (egg or sperm) shown, one is nonviable because of the absence of at least one of the autosomal[4] chromosomes of a pair, and the other contains two members of one pair rather than just one. When the latter is fertilized by a normal sex cell, the result is a fertilized egg with three members of a chromosome "pair" rather than just two. When that additional chromosome is a 21, the result is Down syndrome.

[4]The "autosomes" are the 22 pairs that are not the sex-determining chromosomes. The sex chromosomes are labeled "X" and "Y."

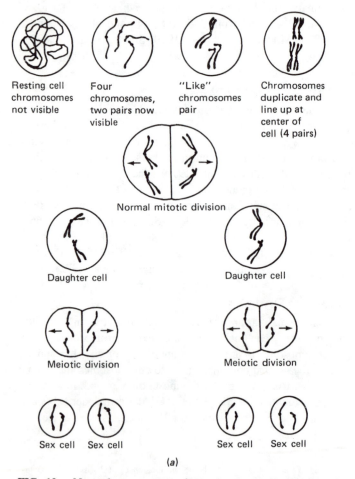

(a)

FIG. 10a Normal egg or sperm formation in a cell with four chromosomes (two pairs). The normal sex cells have one member of each of the two pairs.

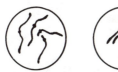

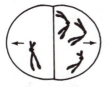

 Abnormal mitotic
divisions (both pairs
are not represented
in each daughter
cell to be)

Daughter cell   Daughter cell

Meiotic division   Meiotic division

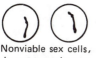   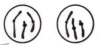

Nonviable sex cells,   Sex cell with extra
do not contain one   chromosome, two members
member of each pair   of one pair (trisomy)

(b)

FIG. 10b Abnormal egg or sperm formation due to error at first division stage
(mitosis). The daughter cells do not contain the proper number of pair 1. This error
is carried through in the second division (meiosis) and leads to abnormal sex cells.

Translocation

Translocation occurs when the extra (supernumerary) chromosome has been fused
to another, usually in the D (13–15) or G (21–22) groups. This is shown schemati-
cally in Figure 11. The most common translocation is 21/14, though 21/15 is
frequent and is also shown in Figure 11 (Donnell, Alfi, Rublee, & Koch, 1975;
Hecht & Kimberling, 1971). Though translocation accounts for only about 5 percent of Down cases, its occurrence has special significance because the risk of
recurrence in subsequent pregnancies is approximately 20 percent (Kaback &
Leisti, 1975). The increased risk results from the presence of the translocation in
one of the parents who are themselves unaffected because they do not have an
extra 21. It is only that one of their 21s is attached to another chromosome. In

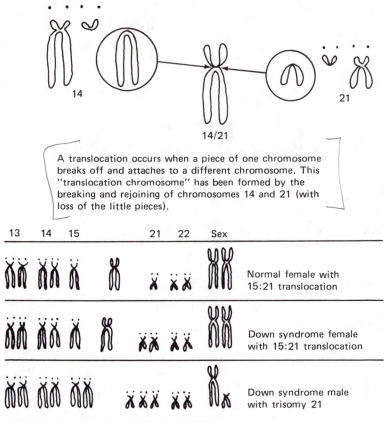

A translocation occurs when a piece of one chromosome breaks off and attaches to a different chromosome. This "translocation chromosome" has been formed by the breaking and rejoining of chromosomes 14 and 21 (with loss of the little pieces).

13	14	15	21	22	Sex	
						Normal female with 15:21 translocation
						Down syndrome female with 15:21 translocation
						Down syndrome male with trisomy 21

FIG. 11   Translocations 14/21 and 15/21.

genetic parlance, such unaffected individuals are characterized as normal "carriers" of the translocation. In this connection, the risk of a recurrence of trisomy was once thought to be no greater than that for all women of the same chronological age. It is now thought to be about twice that of one's age group (Kaback & Leisti, 1975).

Mosaic

The mosaic form is an example of "partial" Down syndrome. There are at least two cell lines present, one normal and one having the extra chromosome, and the individual may vary from virtually normal to typically affected. While earlier workers suggested that the degree of abnormality would be related to the proportion of trisomic cells (Valencia, Delozzio, & DeCoriat, 1963; Zellweger & Abbo, 1963), at least for measured intelligence, no such relationship has been found (Fishler, 1975; Shipe, Reisman, Chung, Darnell, & Kelly, 1968).

AMNIOCENTESIS AND PRENATAL DETECTION OF DOWN SYNDROME

Reference has been made to increased risks for additional cases of Down syndrome in translocation and in trisomy. There is now available a safe procedure for studying the chromosomes of the fetus in utero and thereby determining whether the child is affected. This prenatal diagnostic method is called amniocentesis.

The fetus grows within a sac of amniotic fluid into which are shed fetal cells. In amniocentesis, a thin needle is introduced thorough the pregnant woman's abdomen into the amniotic sac from which is drawn a small sample of fluid and fetal cells (see Fig. 12). The procedure is usually carried out between weeks 11 and 18 of pregnancy and is commonly preceded by ultrasound scanning of the amniotic sac to ensure that the needle penetrates neither the fetus nor the placenta. Ultrasound scanning can also provide a measurement of the fetal head and an accurate assessment of gestational age, and it can detect multiple fetuses such as twins (Sells & Bennett, 1977). Once the cells are withdrawn from the amniotic fluid, they are made to grow (cultured) in the laboratory and then studied to detect all chromosomal abnormalities, including Down syndrome and more than 60 genetic metabolic disorders.

Safety

In the 1970s, a major study of amniocentesis (1040 subjects and 992 controls) affirmed its safety. In about 2 percent of the women there was some vaginal bleeding or fluid leakage, but there was not statistically significant difference between the two groups in rate of fetal loss (3.5% in amniocentesis and 3.2% in the controls) or in complications of pregnancy or delivery. Examination of newborns found no differences in incidence of birth defects and, at 1 year of age, the two groups of children did not differ in physical, neurological, or developmental status. Diagnostic accuracy was 99.4 percent, and it was concluded that midtrimester amniocentesis is a highly accurate and safe procedure that does not significantly increase the risk of fetal loss or injury (NICHD, 1976). Still considered a safe procedure, current workers tend to see its use as adding a risk of 0.5 percent (1 in 200) to the possibility of pregnancy complication.

Prenatal Findings from Amniocentesis

In the 1040 women, 34 fetuses showed abnormalities—19 chromosomal and 15 metabolic. Of the 19 chromosomal defects, eight were Down syndrome—four trisomy and four translocation, a surprisingly even distribution considering the more than 90 percent trisomy found in Down populations. Of the 15 fetuses with metabolic diseases, four were Tay-Sachs, a recessively inherited condition causing mental retardation, blindness, and early death. Eight other metabolic disorders were also detected.

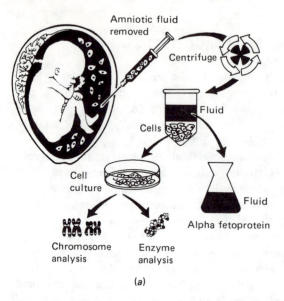

(a)

FIG. 12a Schematic representation of amniocentesis and of subsequent diagnostic studies for chromosomal and metabolic (enzymatic) abnormalities. Alpha fetoprotein study is diagnostic of spina bifida.

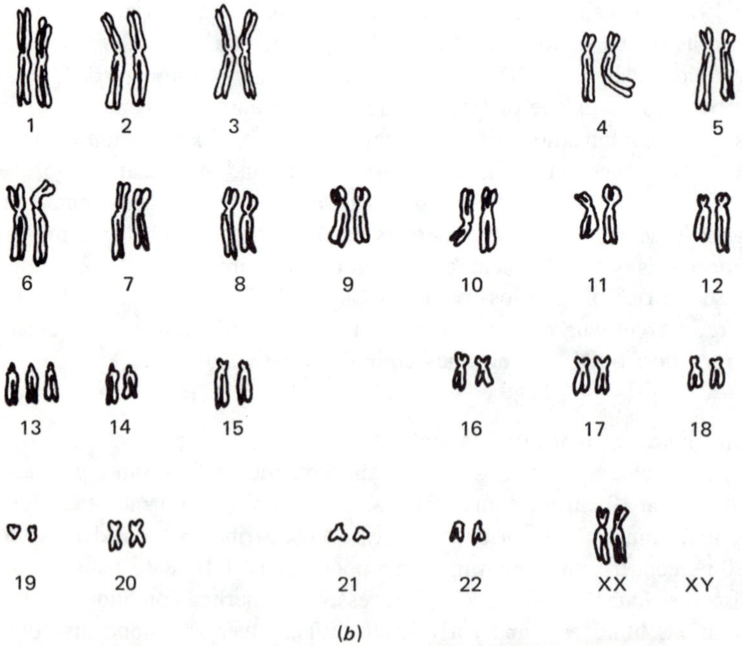

1	2	3			4	5
6	7	8	9	10	11	12
13	14	15		16	17	18
19	20		21	22	XX	XY

(b)

FIG. 12b Actual chromosomes drawing from amniotic fluid. The array includes an extra chromosome 13 and this almost always causes a spontaneous abortion. The two X chromosomes (bottom right) show that the fetus was female. From Fuchs (1980).

Parental Response to Findings

As a result of amniocentesis, elective abortions were performed in 16 of the 19 chromosomal abnormalities and in 11 of the 15 metabolic diseases. It is here that amniocentesis serves its purpose. It allows parents to elect to terminate abnormal pregnancies or to assure those who have an increased risk of abnormality that the fetus is apparently normal. Amniocentesis also permits parents who would avoid all future pregnancies because of increased risk to take that risk and to discover early enough in pregnancy what the outcome will be. Since the great majority of children born even to high-risk parents are normal, amniocentesis provides a means of reasonably assuring that those children will be normal. Kaback and Leisti (1975) present a very sensitive treatment of how amniocentesis encourages the birth of healthy children and offers parents options with regard to problem pregnancies.

A Cautionary Note

Although amniocentesis is clearly regarded as an accurate and safe diagnostic procedure, it is not completely error free. Two children were born with Down syndrome although their prenatal diagnosis had been normal, and one child who appeared to have galactosemia, a metabolic disorder causing retardation, was found at birth to be normal. The sex of the child was also incorrectly identified in three cases, but this, of course, does not constitute the same order of seriousness as diagnosis missed or incorrectly made. We repeat, the overall level of accuracy was 99.4 percent, and that is probably about as much assurance as we can expect from a major medical procedure.

CHORION BIOPSY: AN ALTERNATIVE TO AMNIOCENTESIS

This still experimental prenatal diagnostic procedure is a promising alternative to amniocentesis (Gosden et al., 1982). In chorion biopsy a plastic tube is inserted into the womb and tissue is snipped from the chorion, the outermost fetal membrane. Chromosomal study is then done with cells from the chorion. Its apparent advantage over amniocentesis is that the procedure can be done earlier in the pregnancy, during the first trimester rather than in the second, as is true for amniocentesis, and results are available in days rather than weeks. The "waiting" period is drastically reduced, and earlier and safer abortion is made possible if prospective parents so choose.

DEVELOPMENT

Developmental Status in Childhood

Intelligence: There have been a number of studies of the intellectual development of persons with Down syndrome, principally during infancy and early childhood (Carr, 1970; Cowie, 1970; Dameron, 1963; Dicks-Mireaux, 1972; Melyn & White, 1973; Morgan, 1979; Share, 1975; Share & French, 1974; Share, Koch, Webb, & Graliker, 1964; Share & Veale, 1974; Thompson, 1963). Workers differ as to how early developmental lag can be detected, but it will generally be recognizable during the latter half of the first year. Mental development in Down syndrome is characterized by a slow decline in IQ (e.g., Fishler, 1975; Melyn & White, 1973). Measures at 1 year are usually at the upper limit of the mildly retarded range. By age 4 they will have dropped to the range of moderate retardation and, at the end of the mental age growth period, they will commonly be at the level of severe retardation. Higher IQs, those in the moderate and even mildly retarded ranges, tend to be seen in children reared at home rather than in institutions (Carr, 1970; Centerwall & Centerwall, 1960; Melyn & White, 1973; Rynders, Spiker, & Horrobin, 1978; Shipe & Shotwell, 1965; Stedman & Eichorn, 1964), and this has encouraged both the avoidance of early out-of-home placement and the provision of educational experiences during the preschool years (Connolly & Russell, 1976; Hanson, 1976 [motor], Hayden & Dmitriev, 1975 [general]; Rynders & Horrobin, 1975 [speech]). Table 5 shows IQs for a very large number of children seen in an outpatient clinic; note the decline in IQ. This decline should not be interpreted as a kind of mental deterioration or loss of ability but rather a reflection of the disadvantage of Down children on intelligence test items that grow increasingly verbal in nature (e.g., Silverstein, Legotki, Friedman, & Takayama, 1982). The special language problem in Down syndrome, at least as it pertains to speech, will shortly be described.

Sex difference: Within the Down population there appears to be a sex difference in intelligence with females generally exceeding males by about five IQ points (Carr, 1970; Clements, Bates, & Hafer, 1976).

Developmental milestones: The developmental delay associated with Down syndrome is evident in all aspects of behavior. In Figure 13, a picture of the

TABLE 5   Actual and Predicted Average IQs for 14 Age Groupings of Down Syndrome Children

N	Midpoint (years)	Actual average IQ	Predicted average IQ	95% Confidence interval
70	0.5	58.28	58.23	54.84–61.62
75	1.5	58.10	56.43	50.51–62.35
75	2.5	54.46	54.63	48.71–60.55
73	3.5	54.40	52.83	46.91–58.75
76	4.5	49.35	51.03	45.11–56.95
76	5.5	48.26	49.23	43.31–55.15
66	6.5	45.36	47.43	41.51–53.35
36	7.5	44.25	45.63	39.71–51.55
34	8.5	45.36	43.83	37.91–49.75
28	9.5	43.38	42.03	36.11–47.95
15	10.5	41.53	40.23	34.31–46.15
9	11.5	37.40	38.43	32.51–44.35
6	12.5	33.66	36.63	30.71–42.55
4	13.5	37.66	34.83	28.91–40.75

Source: Melyn & White (1973). Copyright © American Academy of Pediatrics, 1973.

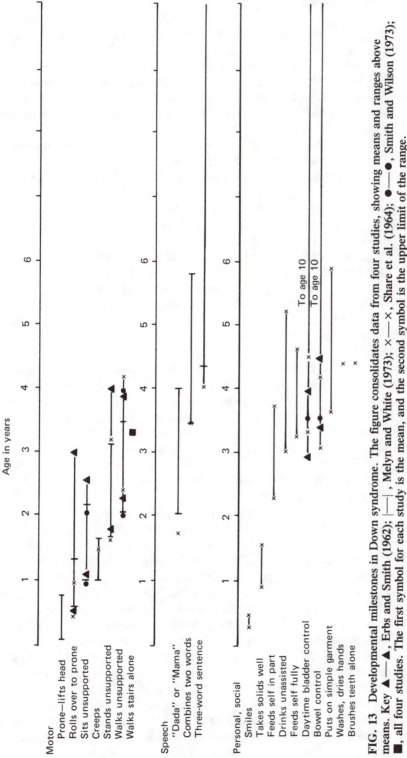

FIG. 13 Developmental milestones in Down syndrome. The figure consolidates data from four studies, showing means and ranges above means. Key ▲——▲, Erbs and Smith (1962); |——|, Melyn and White (1973); ×——×, Share et al. (1964); ●——●, Smith and Wilson (1973); ■, all four studies. The first symbol for each study is the mean, and the second symbol is the upper limit of the range.

development of the preschool-age Down child is presented in terms of motor, speech, and personal-social skills.

Gross motor skills: Within a common pattern of moderate to severe retardation, the Down child will generally appear to be most advanced in gross motor skills. By age 5, these children are able to walk, run, and negotiate stairs, and their hand-eye coordination is adequate to engage in such activities as stacking blocks and stringing large beads.

Self-help skills: One of the most stressful aspects of rearing a child who is at least moderately retarded is the slowness of the child in acquiring the basic self-help skills of feeding, dressing, and toileting. The child is likely to lag in their acquisition by from 1 to 2 years in comparison with normal children, and it is the delay in bladder and bowel control that is going to be most burdensome. Parents can anticipate, however, that toileting skills will ordinarily be acquired by age 3 to 4, though some help with the dressing aspects will still be needed. It also should be realized that these developmental norms probably do not include many individuals who have had the kind of intensive training reflected in the work of Azrin and Foxx (1971) and popularized in their book on achieving toilet usage in 24 hours. Their work does not relate specifically to Down children, but there is no doubt that, with intensive and systematic training, all of the developmental milestones can be hastened in their attainment.

Speech: The area of greatest developmental lag is in speech. Down individuals function at levels below that expected for their mental age (Thompson, 1963). Their articulation tends to be poor (Dodd, 1975), with imitation speech superior in intelligibility to that which is used spontaneously (Dodd, 1975; Lenneburg, 1967; Smith, 1975). In terms of complexity, while capable of using language that relates to past or future events, they, like other language-impaired children, tend to use more present-oriented utterances (Layton & Sharifi, 1978). Some perspective on the extent of the speech lag is gained by considering that of the average 6-year-old. He can ordinarily understand and communicate easily, although some sound blends may not yet be fully accomplished.

Speech will consist of phrases or sentences which in their grammar reveal mastery of the basic structure of the language. In contrast, while most Down syndrome children are at least combining words at age 6, some are not. Their speech may consist only of one-word utterances, more characteristic of the 1- to 2-year-old than of the first grader. Adding to the picture of extraordinary speech deficit is the poor quality of word intelligibility. Not only is articulation impaired, but many words consist only of their initial sound. Short sentences are often run together like a single word, and voice quality is harsh. The child's speech is best understood if the listener knows what the child is talking about or is thoroughly familiar with the child's vocabulary. The extent of this impairment in intelligibility becomes evident in comparison with an early study of normal children in whom by age $4\frac{1}{2}$ almost all utterances were understandable (McCarthy, 1930).

While speech is the most retarded aspect of development, brighter Down children attempt to overcome their verbal limitation through *gestures.* The less capable children make no efforts to find alternate modes of communicating. This use of gesture is the most striking example of the special nature of the speech problem in Down syndrome; some of the children employ the same means of nonverbal communication found in youngsters whose lack of speech is due to deafness! A greater reliance on gesture has also been noted when Down children are compared to normal youngsters at comparable developmental levels (Greenwald & Leonard, 1979).

The expressive language difficulties of the young Down child are later reflected in particular weakness in understanding and communicating at the verbal level and a relative strength in receptive and expressive abilities at the purely visual one (Bilovski & Share, 1965; Nakamura, 1965). The use of gestures to complement speech may be an example of reliance on the visual modality as may be of the oft-noted mimicry ability in these children. In a related finding, Silverstein et al. (1982) compared a large series of Down subjects with a matched population of non-Down retarded individuals in their relative strengths and weaknesses on the Stanford-Binet. The Down group was strongest on items involving nonverbal visual-motor tasks. The non-Down group did best on items involving verbal comprehension.

In commenting on the relative strengths and weaknesses of children with this condition, it might be added that they appear to be particularly deficient in interpreting stimuli presented at a purely tactile level (Belmont, 1971; Knights, Atkinson, & Hyman, 1967; O'Connor & Hermelin, 1961).

Fine motor skills: Another area of particular difficulty is in fine motor skills. Though gross motor skills are relatively advanced (standing, walking, etc.), tasks that require steadiness and relatively precise movements (e.g., buttoning and tying) are troublesome.

Developmental Status in Adulthood

To this point our focus has been primarily on the development of Down syndrome children in infancy and early childhood. It is here that higher IQs tend to be found—whereas in the young adult, when mental ability growth has ceased, they are usually somewhat lower. A cross-sectional study of the mental development of 44 Down young adults seen at a community mental retardation clinic is shown in Figures 14a and 14b.

In addition to showing the level of mental development (mental age and IQ) at various chronological ages from 4 to 17, these figures also indicate, for comparative purposes, adaptive behavior scores on the Vineland Social Maturity Scale. The Vineland scale is an indicator of the extent to which one is meeting the personal, social, and vocational expectancies for one's chronological age, and scores are given in social age and social quotient. With regard to intelligence, Figure 14a shows the fairly steady deciine in IQ noted earlier. Again, this decline should not be interpreted as a loss in intelligence per se. Previously acquired abilities, as measured in mental age, are not lost. It is only that the *rate* of their gain diminishes with age so that for each 12 months of chronological age the number of months of mental age added steadily lessens. A semilongitudinal study (the same person being tested at least twice) of mental-age growth in an institution-

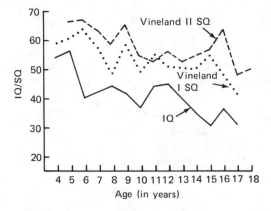

FIG. 14a Intelligence quotient and social quotient as functions of chronological age in Down syndrome. From Cornwell and Birch (1969).

alized population, ages 13–50 years, is shown in Figure 15. (Demaine & Silverstein, 1978). It actually reveals a very slow but continuous growth in mental age all the way to age 40, and it is only after age 40 that mental age scores decline. Curiously, the continued growth in mental age beyond age 18, the upper limit set on the Binet, would mean that IQ scores would actually *increase* during the adult period, dropping off only after age 40 with the fall in mental age. Perhaps earlier-reported studies discontinued their mental testing prematurely!

Figure 14a shows the average social quotients obtained (Vineland I) when first seen at the retardation clinic and those obtained following 2 years of clinic service (Vineland II). Social quotients appear to follow the same pattern of decline seen in IQ, although social quotient scores are consistently higher than IQs by about 10 points. Higher social quotients have also been noted by Pototzky and

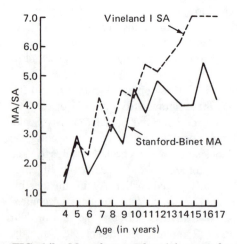

FIG. 14b Mental age and social age as functions of chronological age in Down syndrome. From Cornwell and Birch (1969).

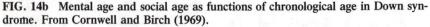

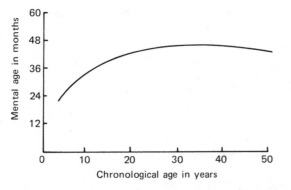

FIG. 15 Mental-age changes in a series of 189 institutionalized Down syndrome individuals tested at least twice during the chronological-age period. Adapted from Demaine and Silverstein (1978).

Grigg (1942) and Quaytman (1953). The impact of clinic services is seen in comparing the Vineland I SQ with the Vineland II SQ. Though some effect is suggested by typically higher social quotients at the end of the 2-year period, the amount of gain was considered disappointing: "Progress in the development of social skills was slow and eventually ceased when the demands of social situations required higher level verbal and abstract capacities than our population reached" (Cornwell & Birch, 1969).

Figure 14b gives a picture of the mental age and social age development of this population. Although the number of individuals at each chronological age from 4 to 17 is necessarily very small, the relative lack of variability in the growth curve gives it a fair degree of reliability. The pattern is one of more or less steady growth in social age and mental age to about age 10. After 10 there is divergence between the two ability measures because of the previously noted near cessation in mental-age growth. The upper limit in mental age in this group is about 4 years, very close to the ceiling shown in Figure 15. There also appears to be an upper limit in social age of about 7 years.

Young Adult Status

As young adults these individuals were most adept at motor-skill tasks that could be practiced daily. They had achieved some degree of independence in self-help skills and no longer required constant assistance in feeding, dressing, and toileting. A similar picture of partial self-sufficiency emerges from a study of over 2000 institutionalized Down individuals (Johnson & Abelson, 1969). As young adults, approximately half dressed themselves, brushed their teeth, and used all utensils. About two-thirds managed themselves at the toilet and rarely had nighttime bladder incidents.

These young adults were most impaired on tasks requiring planning, initiative, responsibility, and the use of language and academic skills; tasks closely related to general intelligence. It would be incorrect, however, to infer from the social age data that these young adults could not perform tasks beyond those ordinarily expected of a 7-year-old child. Many Down adults can be helpful at home and are employable in nondemanding work settings. In the home they can perform simple household chores, and they can learn to move freely about their immediate neighborhood. Many also achieve a worker role if only in a well-supervised and non-production-oriented facet of a sheltered workshop. Nor are these severely retarded adults necessarily dependent on others for transportation to their place of employment. In no less a complex urban environment than New York City were Down workers in a sheltered workshop able to learn to use public buses to travel the specific route from home to job.

PHYSICAL FINDINGS AND INTELLIGENCE IN DOWN SYNDROME

While environmental factors associated with home or out-of-home placement and access to preschool programs appear to have a genuine impact on mental development in Down syndrome, perhaps most clearly in the realm of expressive language (Kugel & Reque, 1961), there has been considerable interest in the possible relationship of physical aspects of the condition and intelligence.

Interest in a possible association between physical signs and intelligence may have peaked in the 1960s. A review of the literature in the late 1960s (Baumeister & Williams, 1967) failed to reveal any relationship between the number of physical symptoms and intelligence (Benda, 1960; Domino & Newman, 1965; Johnson & Barnett, 1961; Kaariainen & Dingman, 1961; Oster, 1953; Shipe, Reisman, Chung, Darnell, & Kelly, 1968), though one study (Gibson & Gibbons, 1958) did report a positive finding.

The existence of three chromosomally distinct subgroups with Down syndrome provides another biological dimension that might have a behavioral correlate. Two kinds of studies have been done here—those relating chromosomal variant to IQ and those relating the proportion of normal and abnormal cells to IQ in the mosaic form.

Chromosomal Forms and IQ

The research indicates that there are some differences between the three chromosomal variants. The translocation form appears to be associated with higher IQs than is true of trisomy (Gibson & Pozsonyi, 1965; Johnson & Abelson, 1969; Shipe et al., 1968) and the mosaic type clearly shows the highest IQs of all (Fishler, 1975). The mosaic form may also be the most variable of the three, but this remains to be confirmed (Rynders, Spiker, & Horrobin, 1978). Mean IQs in mosaicism appear to fall in the mildly retarded range 57–67 (Fishler, 1975; Rosecrans, 1968; Rynders et al., 1978; Shipe et al., 1968), and, perhaps, from 15 to 20 percent of these individuals may have IQs of from 80 to 100 (Fishler, 1975; Rynders, et al., 1978).

Proportion of Abnormal Cells and IQ in Mosaicism

At first blush the possibly greater variability in IQ in the mosaic form would suggest an explanation in terms of the proportion of normal to abnormal cells, but, as noted earlier, no such relationship has been found (Fishler, 1975; Shipe et al., 1968).

BIOCHEMICAL FINDINGS

We appear to be beginning to unravel the *biochemical* consequences of an extra chromosome. An extra chromosome should mean an extra dosage of the genes on that chromosome and extra amounts of the proteins associated with those genes. Two gene proteins have thus far been traced to chromosome 21 (superoxide dismutase and phosphoribosyl glycinamide), and levels of these enzymes have been found to elevated 50 percent in Down syndrome (Francke, 1981). This is just what would be predicted on the basis of an increase of from two chromosomes to three: an increase of 50 percent!

Other investigators have reported a so-called Down syndrome protein found with increased frequency in mothers of Down children (Kerkay, Zsako, Cotton, & Kaplan, 1975; Kerkay, Zsako, & Kaplan, 1971; Miles, Gnezda, & Kerkay, in press).

OTHER BEHAVIORAL CHARACTERISTICS

Of all of the subgroups within retardation, none has been so clearly stereotyped as the Down syndrome child. The behavioral picture presented in the first description of the syndrome by Down in 1866 and reported by Kanner (1964) has a very contemporary ring. "They have a considerable power of imitation, even bordering on being mimics. They are humorous, and a lively sense of the ridiculous often colours their mimicry. They are usually able to speak; the speech is thick and indistinct. . . ." (Down, 1867). Belmont (1971) reviewed the historical and contemporary literature on the behavioral aspects of Down syndrome and notes that affected persons tend to be seen as cheerful, good-natured, happy, and sometimes indiscriminate in their show of affection. The author would regard this as a mental age–related phenomenon rather than as peculiar to Down syndrome. They are also considered to have good imitative ability, as responsive to music, as occasionally obstinate, and as showing diminished sexual interest.

Contemporary research has generally confirmed the impression of a relatively good adjustment at both institutional (Decker, Herberg, Haythornwaite, Rupke, & Smith, 1968; Tarjan, Dingman, Eyman, & Brown, 1960) and community (Ellis & Beechley, 1950; Lyle, 1960; Menolascino, 1965) levels. Several studies have compared Down and non-Down populations on personality scales, and these indicate that the former are usually viewed more favorably (Domino, Goldschmid, & Kaplan, 1964; Moore, Thuline, & Capes, 1968; Silverstein, 1964). In one study, however, a Down group was not distinguishable in terms of either positive or negative behaviors (Blacketer-Simmonds, 1953).

The behavioral picture is not always positive. There is clearly no uniformity of personality (Belmont, 1971), and one sees a variety of behavior problems (Rollin, 1946; McIntire, Menolascino, & Wiley, 1965; Menolascino, 1967) including psychosis (Menolascino, 1967; Neville, 1959). Menolascino (1967) studied a series of 86 Down children who were part of a much larger group seen for diagnostic evaluation in a mental retardation clinic. Of the 86, 11 were regarded as having a significant psychiatric problem. This represents 13 percent of the Down group and compares very favorably to a 30 percent prevalence rate in the non-Down children. This is further evidence for the generally positive stereotype. The problems that were seen were of three kinds: (1) short attention span, hyperactivity, and low frustration tolerance; (2) nonpsychotic emotional distress in response to new family conditions—for example, birth of a sib; and (3) a brief psychotic episode in response to stress. The last-mentioned was catatonic posturing in a $4\frac{1}{2}$-year-old and was described in Chapter 2.

The general confirmation of the behavioral stereotype is not paralleled in the musical and sexual spheres (Belmont, 1971). Regarding sexuality, masturbation, at the very least, is not unknown in this group, and there have been some pregnancies in Down women. It is probably true that Down adolescents and adults do not exhibit the degree of sexual interest expected for their chronological age, but this is also the case in other retarded persons, especially in those with more than mild impairment. The tendency to deny sexuality in dependent, retarded persons is simply a way of denying a reality that is extremely difficult for parents and other caregivers to deal with. Finally, within a population of severely retarded and institutionalized Down adults, no superiority in imitative behavior relative to a control group could be demonstrated (Silverstein, Aguilar, Jacobs, Levy, & Rubenstein, 1979).

PREMATURE AGING: DOWN SYNDROME AND ALZHEIMER DISEASE

An apparent early onset of aging has long been noted in Down individuals, although, as earlier reported, life expectancy after age 5 is not different from that of other retarded individuals with similar degree of impairment. In any case, autopsy studies have consistently found evidence of Alzheimer disease (Jervis, 1948; Malamud, 1964), the dementing brain disorder that has achieved high visibility in our general aging population. One set of investigators claim that the full development of the cerebral neuropathology of Alzheimer (senile plaques, neurofibrillary degeneration, and neurondegeneration) is found in Down individuals by their 30s (Burger & Vogel, 1973).

In spite of the presumed high frequency if not universality of Alzheimer disease in Down syndrome, the behavior changes and eventual dementia associated with the disorder are usually not found (Owens, Dawson, & Losin, 1971; Solitaire & Lamarche, 1966), though some memory loss (Dalton, Crapper, & Schlotterer, 1974), personality changes (Wisiniewski, Howe, Williams, & Wisiniewski, 1978), and behavioral deterioration (Miniszek, 1983) may be observed that are greater than in nonDown adults.

SOME FAMILY ASPECTS

There are numerous problems that confront parents of retarded children. Some of these were indicated in the description of the childhood and adolescent years of Roger as presented in Chapter 1. Here we want to address two issues that are particularly relevant to children whose abnormality is usually observable at birth or shortly thereafter: (1) the "informing encounter" and (2) the question as to whether the child should be reared at home or placed in an out-of-family residential setting.

THE "INFORMING ENCOUNTER"

One of the most difficult tasks life presents is to be the bearer of bad news. To inform new parents that their baby is abnormal in some not insignificant manner must be extremely painful. The "informing" interview is labeled an "encounter" in order to magnify its importance for the new parent(s). Indeed it may be the greatest emotional crisis they have ever faced (Raech, 1966). This means that the informer, typically the physician, must be both professionally and emotionally prepared to help the parents deal with the inevitable trauma.

Current practice stresses informing the parents and *both* parents as soon as the condition has been diagnosed. While the trauma is inescapable, parents of Down children, at least retrospectively, strongly state a preference for being told as soon as possible (Drillien & Wilkinson, 1964; Gayton & Walker, 1974; Tizard & Grad, 1961). The initial pain is seen as clearly preferable to the anxiety of prolonged uncertainty. A small proportion of those who were informed before the mother left the hospital wished that the doctor had waited until the mother left confinement, but none really wanted any prolonged delay in learning the truth about the child's condition.

But *how* that truth is conveyed is also very important. Wolfensberger and Menolascino (1975) call attention to the need for a "gentle, undramatic interpretation of the facts in an atmosphere of maximal emotional support." Since the degree of expected retardation is not predictable from the physical signs, the approach recommended by them is one that is "fact-oriented" but with a "reasonable balance of caution, uncertainty, and positive elements." The last-mentioned can focus on the generally desirable behavioral characteristics of these children as well as on the services that are increasingly available to them in their preschool, school, and adult years. This requires that the physician be knowledgeable about the range of development seen in these children and about habilitative services now being offered. In this way, there can be a moderating of what Coleman (1975) has referred to as the depression and despair created by informing parents at birth of the coming disability of their child. Again, if we are to believe what parents tell us in retrospect, they are not asking that we delay informing them, only that we be sensitive to their needs at the time. What will also be crucial for the parents is the assurance of *future* opportunities to talk about the child's development and potential, as the initial encounter will raise such emotion as to allow only a small proportion of the child's condition to be "heard." We shall return to family concerns as they relate to the diagnostic process in Chapter 5.

WHERE SHOULD THE CHILD LIVE?

According to one group (Koch, Fishler, & Melnyk, 1971), the question most frequently asked by parents of a newborn Down infant concerns the choice of home care or out-of-home placement. While parents usually want to keep their

baby, some physicians routinely recommend immediate placement, either in a foster home or in an institution. The proportion of physicians making such recommendations has diminished with the increased awareness of a wider range of community services to infant and family, but in the 1970s about one-third still followed
this practice (Gayton & Walker, 1974). In any case, parents who have allowed
others to make this decision for them have often regretted it. In one series, fully
one-quarter who had originally acquiesced to the physician's recommendation for
placement in infancy changed their minds when they had an opportunity to recon-
sider after the shock and trauma of the early postnatal period had passed (Giannini
& Goodman, 1963). The great weight given by parents to physician's recommendations for out-of-home placement has been noted by another important group of
workers (Kugel, Fedge, Trembath, & Hein, 1964). They point out that the recommendation is usually based neither on medical nor educational considerations but,
rather, on social ones. Numerous reasons are given to parents, virtually all of
which are clearly rationalizations for justifying a recommendation that is really
based on negative attitudes toward the condition and a wish to achieve a kind of
"out-of-sight, out-of-mind" outcome. Some parents, on the other hand, have such
strong feelings of guilt or shame (lowered self-esteem) that they seek to conceal
the reality of an abnormal baby and separate themselves from the infant as soon as
possible.

Present practice clearly calls for the rearing of the child in the family home.
We have already indicated some of the developmental advantages in language and
in IQ of home-reared Down children. Moreover, health problems are common in
Down syndrome and are much better dealt with at home than in even the best of
institutional settings (Koch, Fishler, & Melnyk, 1971). Under certain circumstances, of course, early placement may be the only alternative, but even here
parents will ordinarily need an opportunity to express fully whatever guilt or
misgiving such a drastic action may evoke.

Other Autosomal Abnormalities

There are three trisomies of the nonsex chromosomes commonly found. We
have looked at one of them, Down syndrome, with some depth, and we now
briefly describe the other two—trisomy 18 and trisomy 13. Of the three, Down
syndrome is the least severely disabling, presumably due to the small size of
chromosome 21, the number of extra genes present being less than in the other two
trisomies (Melnyk & Koch, 1971).

TRISOMY 18 (EDWARDS' SYNDROME)

This is the second most common of the trisomies. It occurs with a frequency
of about one in 5000 live births (Carswell, 1973; Conen & Erkman, 1966), and
only about 10 percent survive the first year (Weber, 1967). The symptom picture
includes severe mental retardation, skull malformation, and abnormalities of the
heart, kidneys, and nervous system (Edwards, Harndon, Cameron, Cross, &
Wolff, 1960; Smith, Patau, Therman, & Inhorn, 1962). The child has a long and

narrow head, low-set and pointed ears, a small mouth, and a receding chin. The face often has a triangular appearance. At birth the newborn appears undernourished because of a low birth weight and "loose" skin (Warkany, 1971). The occurrence of trisomy 18 appears to increase the likelihood of future trisomic births, especially Down syndrome, the risk being comparable to a prior Down birth itself (Hecht, Bryant, Gruber, & Townes, 1964).

TRISOMY 13-15 (D) (PATAU SYNDROME)

In 1657, the following birth was described in Copenhagen.

Monster without eyes.

In our town a monster was born of honest parentage. In the parturition everything passed off well. But the child had no eyes. There was a wide, open void of red colour. The nose broad and oblong, from which a tumor protruded, one part bony, the other part fleshy, without nostrils. The mouth wide and deformed. The upper maxilla (jaw) seemed to consist of one bone. Either hand had six fingers, as had the left foot (polydactyly). By pitiable and continual howling it attracted everybody's compassion until it breathed its last. (Translation from Warburg, 1960.)

This rare but striking combination of congenital anomalies has been identified with a trisomy of one of the three chromosomes in the D group (illustrated in Fig. 12b). Its main symptoms are the absence of eyes, cleft lip and palate, extra fingers and toes (polydactyly), and cerebral malformations (Patau, Smith, Therman, Inhorn, & Wagner, 1960). This is the rarest of the trisomies, occurring in about one in 10,000 live births (Carswell, 1973). Only about 18 percent survive the first year, and these show severe retardation, seizures, and growth defect (Smith, 1970). Like the other two trisomies, the occurrence of trisomy 13 is associated with an increased risk of either 21 or 18. Clearly, the vulnerability is to the general property of trisomy rather than to a specific form itself. Some instances of trisomy 13 are due to translocation, and, because of the much increased risk associated with that phenomenon, determination of the chromosomal variant is important.

PARTIAL DELETIONS

In addition to the presence of extra chromosomes, there are abnormalities of single chromosomes. Sometimes a portion of a chromosome is missing, a so-called "deletion." If the deleted part is large, the loss of the genes associated with it is likely to prove lethal, but small deletions are compatible with life (Melnyk & Koch, 1971). Two partial deletions associated with retardation are the *short arm of chromosome 5*, the "cat cry" (cri-du-chat) syndrome (Lejeune et al., 1963), and the *long arm of chromosome 18* (Wertelcki, Schindler, & Gerald, 1966). The former takes its name from a high-pitched cry in the child. Considerable variation in terms of both degree of retardation and life span have been observed in it (Jarvik, 1976). The latter condition commonly includes visual and hearing defects, structural anomalies of the face, microcephaly, and at least moderate retardation.

"SEMIDELETION"

More recently another kind of chromosomal abnormality has been found. It involves a *constriction* of one of the regions on the X chromosome arm. It is a constriction of the X chromosomes in *males* that is of particular interest in mental retardation. The abnormality is called "Fragile X" and is discussed later in this chapter.

RELATED ETHICAL DILEMMAS

In describing such severe physical and mental disorders as trisomy 18 and 13, one cannot but be aware of the extraordinary ethical dilemmas these conditions may present to physicians and others responsible for the care of these individuals. We deal here with fundamental attitudes toward the "quality of life" and the degree to which lives should be sustained which in no sense would we seek for ourselves. It is here also that we confront our negative attitude toward mental retardation as such. We value and esteem intelligence, competence, and achievement and tend necessarily to devalue their opposites. This presents an ambivalence that cannot be avoided. Continued physician recommendations for immediate placement of Down infants reflect the negative valuation of the disorder, and this is even more dramatically seen in physician attitudes toward the preservation of life itself in severely affected individuals. A survey of obstetricians and pediatricians in the San Francisco area revealed that from 22 to 53 percent favored active or passive euthanasia, depending on the anomaly. Although "only" 22 percent favored such measures for Down syndrome, the proportion rose to 50 percent when the Down infant also had an intestinal obstruction. This much increased rate was seen as allowing more negative attitudes to surface since the operation itself is regarded as a relatively simple procedure. It is interpreted as revealing "their subconscious feeling against prolonging the life of an abnormal conceptus." For trisomy 18, 53 percent favored euthanasia. The influence of a religious affiliation is reflected in lower proportions favoring such measures, but, even among them, 43 percent would support such actions with regard to hydrocephalus at birth. Among those professing no religious affiliation the proportion increases to 57 percent. Clearly, even in physicians with a religious affiliation, a substantial proportion favor such measures (Mental Retardation News, 1976).

"Quality of life" issues are presumed to underlie the 1982 Baby Doe episode. A Down newborn with an esophageal obstruction had treatment and sustenance withheld at the request of the parents, and, presumably, with the acquiescence of the medical staff. The baby died. In 1983, the U.S. Department of Justice intervened on behalf of an infant born with hydrocephalus, an open spine, and other severe defects. The parents had declined treatment, but the intervention of the federal government had the effect of requiring it. After much national debate about the appropriate response to the birth of such babies, the issue was addressed in the 1984 Child Abuse and Treatment Act. It includes under its definition of "child abuse" the denial of food, water, or medical treatment for such newborns.

While the author supports this action, it is also recognized that parents should have the right to choose not to rear such a child, if that is their wish, and instead to allow that child to be cared for by other means. Neither should they nor foster or adoptive parents be required to suffer the extraordinary medical expenses that the treatment and care of such children may entail. If the law insists that the baby has a right to life, it should also share the economic burden of supporting that life.

Abnormalities of the Sex Chromosomes

Three trisomes of the nonsex chromosomes (autosomes) have been described, but abnormal numbers of the sex chromosomes are also found. It will be seen that the number of extra X chromosomes can vary of from one to three and that there appears to be some relationships between the number of extra Xs and intellectual impairment.

KLINEFELTER SYNDROME (XXY)

This is a condition in which a person who is biologically male has an additional X chromosome. The typical chromosomal complement is 44 + XXY. Its major effects are hypogonadism and infertility (Myhan & Sakati, 1976; Smith, 1976). In preadolescence body proportions are slim, with relatively long legs and small testes. Personality problems are common, and some intellectual impairment may be present. In adolescence there are likely to be enlarged breasts (gynecomastia) and underdeveloped secondary sexual characteristics. This condition is the most common single cause of hypogonadism, occurring with a frequency of about one in 600 live male births. While most affected persons appear to have only one additional X chromosome, two or three additional Xs may also occur. Some also have an extra Y—that is, XXYY. The usual form of the disorder, XXY, illustrates that biological maleness is determined by the Y chromosome. Irrespective of the number of Xs, a single Y causes the sexually undifferentiated embryonic gonad to differentiate into testes and maleness. With regard to cognitive impairment, several studies indicate that IQs in the 80–90 range are common (Nielson, 1970; Pasqualini, 1957; Valentine, 1966) with approximately one-quarter functioning in the below-70 range. The latter are usually not more than mildly retarded. The most extreme variant, XXXXY, is associated with much more severe retardation. The IQ range in one series of 30 cases was 19–57 with a mean of 34 (Zaleski, Houstin, Pozsonyi, & Ying, 1966). Treatment for Klinefelter syndrome and its most extreme variant involves testosterone replacement in early adolescence.

XYY MALES

This has been a somewhat sensationalized chromosomal anomaly in males with the extra Y chromosome thought to increase aggression and antisocial behavior. The condition occurs in about one in 700 male births (Leonard, Landy, Ruddle, & Lubs, 1974), but its prevalence in prison populations is, perhaps, ten times greater (Nyhan & Sakati, 1976). It should be noted, however, that among all XYY males in the general population only about 1 percent are actually imprisoned (Hood, 1973). Thus virtually all such males are grossly normal. Physically, the only findings are tendencies to tall stature and to elbow abnormalities, but these are group differences only, as many are without any distinguishing features. Intellectual functioning is grossly unimpaired although an average reduction in IQ of about 10 points is indicated (Baker, Telfer, Richardson, & Clark, 1970; Nielson, 1970). Studies of the behavioral histories of XYY males suggest that their aggressiveness may be better defined as an increased impulsivity (Hook, 1973; Money, 1970, Noel, Duport, Revil, Dussuyer, & Quach, 1974).

XXX SYNDROME

In females are also found individuals with from one to three extra X chromosomes. The additional X chromosome does not produce any abnormality in physical development, and mental retardation may or may not be present (Nyhan & Sakati, 1976). It occurs in about one in 850 births. Variants of these are the XXXX syndrome in which retardation is the only regular feature; IQ range is 30–80 with a mean of 55 (Smith, 1976; see also Howard-Peebles & Markiton, 1979), and XX-XXX, where there is a growth deficiency as well as greater retardation (Smith, 1976).

TURNER SYNDROME (XO)

This is a condition in which the female has only one X chromosome. Presumably, this is the only chromosome whose complete absence is compatible with life. Turner syndrome occurs in about one in 2200 female live births (Leonard, Landy, Ruddle, & Lubs, 1974), but approximately 96 percent of Turner conceptions die in utero (Hecht & MacFarlane, 1969). About 30 percent are mosaics (XO/XX), and, in these, the condition is usually less severe (Ferguson-Smith, 1965). The most consistent features are small stature and sexual infantilism—the latter due to incomplete ovarian development. Treatment consists of cyclic estrogen replacement in adolescence. Because of ovarian dysgenesis, Turner women are unable to conceive (Smith, 1970). Other common findings are webbing of the neck, elbow deformity, and congenital heart disease (Nyhan & Sakati, 1976). Intelligence is usually in the normal range, although some specific cognitive deficits have been reported on tasks involving space-form perception and visual-motor representation (Alexander, Ehrhardt, & Money, 1966; Alexander & Money, 1965; Money & Alexander, 1966).

FRAGILE X

An increased frequency of mental retardation in males has been frequently noted (e.g., Lehrke, 1972; Penrose, 1938; Turner & Turner, 1974). On this basis and observation of families where males were predominantly affected, Lehrke (1972) hypothesized a relationship between the X chromosome and intelligence.

His prediction appears to have been borne out with the recent discovery of an abnormality of the X chromosome called "Fragile X" (Gerald, 1980; Lubs, 1969; Sutherland, 1977; Turner, Daniel, & Frost, 1980). In 1974 a study of all retarded children born in New South Wales, Australia, over a 10-year period revealed an excess of males of 32 percent. This excess was considered to be unrelated to social factors, and significantly, affected males more often had affected brothers than affected females had affected sisters (Turner & Turner, 1974). The findings suggested that one or more yet unrecognized forms of X-linked mental retardation might account for the abnormal sex ratio.

Earlier Lubs (1969) had described a family where four brothers and the mother had an X chromosome anomaly. The chromosome was constricted near the end of the long arms, producing either separated pieces of chromosome or a small extension (Fig. 16). All of the brothers were retarded, and the mother was normal. No physical abnormalities were seen, and no causative relationship was posited between the chromosomal anomaly and the retardation. The significance of the Lubs finding was unrecognized for nearly a decade, and then, in 1977, an Australian cytogenetics laboratory confirmed its importance with the discovery of eight families in which males were retarded and had the same chromosomal aberration (Harvey, Judge, & Wiener, 1977). The work that led to the rediscovery of the anomaly first seen by Lubs seems to have been the result of an accidental change in the medium used to culture and study the chromosomes. At the time of the Lubs finding, other methods began to be used to culture chromosomes, and the constricted region appears to be invisible in it! Fortuitous use of the older method revealed what had been seen earlier.

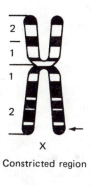

X
Constricted region

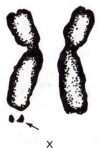

X
Fragile X and normal X
in carrier female

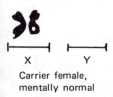

X   Y
Carrier female,
mentally normal

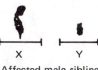

X   Y
Affected male sibling
of carrier female

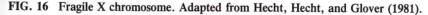

FIG. 16   Fragile X chromosome. Adapted from Hecht, Hecht, and Glover (1981).

Clinical Features

Among males the most characteristic features are mental retardation and much enlarged testes (macroorchidism). Though the testicular enlargement is usually not seen until after puberty, it has been reported in some infants (Cantú et al., 1976). Interestingly, endocrine and germinal function are normal, and the size increase is thought to reflect excess fluid. Not all affected males have enlarged testes, and in some this increase is unilateral in nature (Turner & Opitz, 1980). Some facial characteristics have also been reported—a prominent forehead and jaw and protruding ears. Females appear to be free of any physical abnormalities.

Retardation

The literature suggests that some degree of intellectual impairment is an invariant feature in males and that the degree of retardation is usually more than mild (Turner & Opitz, 1980). This is in contrast to females, where perhaps only about one-third show retardation and its degree is usually mild.

Prevalence

The frequency of this disorder is estimated at about 0.01 percent (1/1000) of the general population (Hecht, Hecht, & Glover, 1981) but in at least 2 percent of retarded populations (McBride, 1981).In one study of 72 mildly retarded girls in whom there were no physical abnormalities, 7 percent had Fragile X (Turner, Daniel, & Frost, 1980). Among the chromosomal disorders causing retardation, it ranks second only to Down syndrome.

Prenatal Detection

Prenatal diagnosis through amniocentesis has yet to be reliably demonstrated (Turner & Opitz, 1980), though genetic counseling in the case of a normal carrier mother would seem feasible.

GENES AND MENTAL RETARDATION

Our focus shifts now from the chromosomes to the genes. Although chromosomal disorders have been here considered under the rubric "genetic," they are not heritable in the same way as gene-determined conditions. Three kinds of gene mechanisms will be illustrated, two of which, dominant and recessive, are clearly associated with mental retardation syndromes. The third gene mechanism, multifactor or polygenic inheritance, is discussed because of its possible role in cultural-familial mental retardation.

Dominant Inheritance

Conditions inherited as "dominant" are likely to recur in successive generations. Typically, one of the parents is affected, and each child bears a 1-in-2 risk of inheriting the condition. The affected child then through parenthood may transmit the trait to his offspring and so on. Tuberous sclerosis and neurofibromatosis are two examples of dominantly inherited conditions.

TUBEROUS SCLEROSIS

This syndrome is caused by one member of a pair of genes. For purposes of illustration (see Fig. 17), let each gene be designated by the letter which stands for the name of the condition and also let that letter be either capital or lowercase depending on whether the gene it represents is dominant or recessive. Thus the dominant gene which causes tuberous sclerosis is denoted T, and the recessive gene, in this instance the gene for "health," is t. (Note that the members of the gene pair are located on corresponding parts of chromosomes that make up a pair [homologous chromosomes].) It is not known on which chromosomes the genes for tuberous sclerosis are found except that they are not on the sex chromosomes. Each person has some combination of these two genes, and this combination is designated as their *genotype*. The possible gene combinations and their significance for tuberous sclerosis are (1) TT the person has two dominant genes and has tuberous sclerosis, (2) Tt the person has one dominant gene and has tuberous sclerosis, (3) tt the person has two recessive genes and does not have tuberous sclerosis.

Genotype 2, where the person has one gene for tuberous sclerosis and one gene for "health," illustrates the meaning of dominant inheritance. The two genes do not have equal weight. One gene, here the gene for illness, masks the effect of the gene for health and is designated a "dominant" gene.

Most readers of these lines, but not all, are tt—that is, free of tuberous sclerosis. Some of us may actually be Tt—that is, carriers of the dominant gene but essentially unaffected by it because dominant conditions tend to be quite variable in the degree to which they manifest themselves (variable expressivity). An individual may be only very mildly affected or may have the full-blown syndrome. The nature of this variation in symptoms will be made explicit in the clinical description that follows.

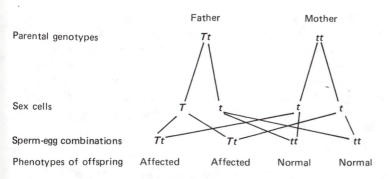

	Father	Mother
Parental genotypes	Tt	tt
Sex cells	T t	t t
Sperm-egg combinations	Tt Tt	tt tt
Phenotypes of offspring	Affected Affected	Normal Normal

FIG. 17 Mechanism of dominant inheritance.

First let us see how the dominant gene is transmitted from parent to child. Assume the father to be affected but only mildly so. He has married, he works, and he has raised a family. His genotype is *Tt* (*TT* would be a much less probable combination), and the mother who is unaffected would be *tt*. Figure 17 shows (1) the genotypes of the father and mother, (2) sperm and egg cells formed by reduction division, (3) the possible sperm-egg combinations at conception, and (4) the phenotypes of the children. Step 4 shows a distribution of half affected and half normal. It should be understood, however, that the 50 percent or 1:2 risk among children is only a statement of statistical probability. By chance all children could be affected or none, the probability of each of these events being the same, $\frac{1}{2}^n$ (where *n* is equal to the number of children). The statistical probabilities for a dominantly inherited condition are identical to those that hold for the sex of a child. Approximately half of all children are males, and half are females. Your family may have equal numbers of sons and daughters or more of one sex than the other, or all of only one sex. By way of prediction what *can* be said in the case of a dominant condition is that each child bears a 50 percent risk of inheriting it.

Let us now look at the condition itself. An excellent overview has been provided by de la Cruz and La Veck (1962), who characterize tuberous sclerosis or *epiloia* as one of a group of diseases associated with abnormalities of the skin and nervous system. In its full-blown form its symptoms comprise sebaceous adenoma, which appears as a butterfly rash on the face, cerebral calcifications, epilepsy, and mental retardation. The calcium deposits in the brain are presumed to cause the epilepsy and retardation. In addition to these primary symptoms, abnormalities of the retina, heart, kidneys, and lungs are commonly found. Retardation is said to occur in about two-thirds of affected individuals (Lagos & Gomez, 1967).

Though a variety of causative factors have been proposed, the condition is considered to be caused by a dominant gene with the ultimate symptom picture influenced by a pair of so-called "modifying genes" (Penrose, 1954). Though seen as a dominantly inherited disorder, the expected family distribution is often not found, and this has been thought to be due to the extreme variability in symptoms. A high mutation rate has also been suggested to account for nonfamilial cases.

Tuberous sclerosis is a very rare disorder with an incidence in the general population from 1:200,000 (Ross & Dickerson, 1943) to 1:300,000 (Dawson, 1954). Affected individuals appear normal at birth, but subnormal mental development is usually evident during infancy. The amount of mental retardation varies greatly, though it increases with age and is usually severe in degree. Seizures ordinarily begin by age 6, nonspecific in type, and skin symptoms usually appear by age 13. Most patients do not live beyond age 25 (Chao, 1959), but some show normal longevity and good intelligence.

A family with tuberous sclerosis

Wallace and Jean are a young rural couple with four children. Wallace is 27 years old, had a second-grade education and is employed as a farm laborer. His health is good. His wife Jean is 25; she's had a fourth-grade education and is a housewife. Her general health is also good. Their eldest child is Martha who at age 5 is severely retarded. Martha has no speech, but hearing is intact. Martha had developed normally until $1\frac{1}{2}$ years of age when she began to have grand mal seizures. Her seizures have been fairly well controlled through medication but some mental deterioration is said to have occurred. At age 5 she presents the tuberous sclerosis symptom triad of adenoma sebaceum on cheeks, chin, and forehead; epilepsy; and mental retardation. Although her epileptic seizures are controlled, the electroencephalograph is diagnostic of epilepsy with evidence of a right midtemporal epileptogenic focus in the brain. In addition to Martha, there are three other children, ages 4, 2, and 5 months. Four-year-old John is in good health but 2-year-old Stanley began to have seizures during his second year. He has started to fall behind in his general development and some degree of retardation is expected. He, too, has been diagnosed as having tuberous sclerosis. The fourth child is only 5 months old and it is too early to know whether she also has the disease. In addition to at least two of the four children being affected, the father, Wallace, also has one of the symptoms of the disease, the facial adenoma. He has never had seizures and, though somewhat limited in mental ability, he's not retarded. It has been recommended to the family that they have no more children and the mother has been accepting of this.

NEUROFIBROMATOSIS
(RECKLINGHAUSEN DISEASE)
This disorder consists of areas of abnormal skin pigmentation (café-au-lait spots), tumors (neurofibromas) of the central and peripheral nervous system, bone changes, and endocrine and growth disturbances. It is quite variable in its manifestation. It occurs with an incidence of about one in 3000 births, and in about half the cases affected relatives are also found. Inheritance through at least four generations has been repeatedly observed (Borberg, 1951). It is estimated that from 10 to 25 percent of affected persons have some degree of intellectual impairment, presumably due to tumors in the brain, but the degree of deficit is usually not more than mild (Borberg, 1951; Crowe, Neel, & Schull, 1956).

Etiology Obscure
but with Occasional Dominant Mode

STURGE-WEBER SYNDROME
(NEVOID AMENTIA)
This disorder is characterized by facial angioma (a port wine–colored nevus), seizures due to brain calcifications (as in tuberous sclerosis), and mental retardation of variable degree. Less frequent findings are hemiparesis and glaucoma. Familial occurrence is rare (Warkany, 1971).

CRANIOSTENOSIS

Premature closure of the sutures of the skull results in deformities of the head and frequently in damage to the brain and eyes. The most severe abnormalities result if closure precedes birth. When growth, usually lateral, is inhibited by premature suture closure, the head tends to be elevated in its vertical dimension, cerebral convolutions are flattened, and internal hydrocephaly, optic neuritis, and atrophy may develop. To make room for the expanding brain, the prematurely closed skull must be opened by surgical means; more than one operation may be needed because the healing bone tends to reunite itself (Warkany, 1971). Two of the craniostenoses are associated with variable retardation—Crouzon syndrome (craniofacial dysostosis) and Apert syndrome (acrocephalosyndactyly). In the latter, skull and facial abnormality is combined with fusion (syndactyly) of fingers and toes. In Crouzon, dominant inheritance is found in two-thirds of the cases, whereas in Apert, heredity is only rarely seen. In the absence of family history it is assumed that conditions that are at least apparently dominant represent instances of new mutations. As in the case of most of the conditions described in this section, intellectual impairment is extremely variable (Blank, 1960; Smith, 1970).

Recessive Inheritance

In contrast to conditions inherited through dominant genes, with affected persons found in successive generations and where the risk for each child is 1 in 2, in recessively inherited ones the parents are typically unaffected, and the risk for each child is 1 in 4. Examples of recessive disorders associated with retardation are listed in Table 6. Description of several of the major forms now follows with particular emphasis on phenylketonuria (Milunsky, 1975).

PHENYLKETONURIA (PKU)

In dominant inheritance, the condition is ordinarily caused by one member of a pair of genes; in recessive inheritance it is caused by both members of the gene pair. As before, let each gene be designated by the letter that corresponds to the name of the condition. In the case of PKU, a recessive trait, let the gene for the disorder be p and the gene for health be P. These genes are located on corresponding parts of a chromosome pair, and, as in the case of tuberous sclerosis, the actual pair on which they exist is unknown except that they, too, are not on the sex chromosomes. Again, as in the case of a dominant condition, there are three possible genotypes: (1) PP the person has two dominant genes and does not have PKU, (2) Pp the person has one dominant gene and does not have PKU, (3) pp the person has two recessive genes and has PKU.

Genotype 2 illustrates the recessive nature of PKU. When one is a carrier of the recessive gene, genotypically a heterozygote, there is no effect, because the gene for health is dominant to the gene for illness. Phenylketonuria can occur only in the absence of the gene for health and in the presence of two recessive genes.

Recessive disorders illustrate how a condition can be inherited that is not present in the parents. Assume both parents to be normal but carriers of the recessive gene. Their genotypes would be Pp. Figure 18 shows (1) the parental

TABLE 6 Biochemical Disorders Associated with Retardation

Disorder	Gene mechanism	Clinical features	Detectable via amniocentesis	Detectable in carrier
Argininemia	Autosomal-recessive (Shih, 1978)	Spastic diplegia, seizures	yes	yes
Arginosuccinic aciduria	Autosomal-recessive	Seizures, enlargement of liver and spleen (hepatomegaly), ataxia	yes	yes
Citrullinemia	Autosomal-recessive	Episodes of vomiting, hyperammonemia	yes	yes
Cystinosis, infantile form	Autosomal-recessive	Rickets, hypopigmentation, growth retardation, photophobia, death by late childhood	yes	yes
Galactosemia	Autosomal-recessive (Soriano, 1977)	Cataracts and visual impairment treated by dietary exclusion of galactose (see text)	yes	yes
Gaucher disease, infantile	Autosomal-recessive	Opisthotonos, rigidity, death by 1 year	yes	yes
Glycinemia, nonketotic	Autosomal-recessive (Nyhan, 1978)	Seizures, spasticity, opisthotonos; dietary exclusion of glycine of uncertain value (Milunsky, 1975)	Not as of 1975	Not as of 1975
Glycogen storage disease	Autosomal-recessive	Hepatomegaly, growth retardation, hydoglycemic seizures (Sidbury, 1977)	II and IV yes	Not as of 1975
Hartnup disease	Autosomal-recessive	Ataxia, photosensitive rash	yes	yes
Histidinemia	Autosomal-recessive	Speech retardation, possible growth retardation (Nyhan, 1977)	yes	yes
Homocystinuria	Autosomal-recessive	Variable retardation; lens dislocations; elongation of legs, feet, and fingers; blood vessel disease	yes	yes
Hunter syndrome A and B	Sex-linked recessive	Hurler variant: stiff joints, dwarfing, enlarged liver and spleen (hepatomegaly), deafness (Danes, 1977)	A yes; B Not as of 1975	yes
Hurler disease	Autosomal-recessive	Dwarfism, humpback, large bulging head, cloudy corneage, clawlike hands, deafness (see text)	yes	yes

TABLE 6 Biochemical Disorders Associated with Retardation (*Continued*)

Disorder	Gene mechanism	Clinical features	Detectable via amniocentesis	Detectable in carrier
Hyperammonemia	Unclear (Shih, 1978)	Vomiting, lethargy, episodic coma in early infancy; seizures, hyperammonemia (Taft & Cohen, 1977)	Not as of 1975	Not as of 1975
Hyperlysinemia	Autosomal-recessive (Nyhan, 1978)	Seizures, hypotonia, growth retardation (Nyhan, 1977)	Not as of 1975	Not as of 1975
Hyperprocinemia and hydroxyproliemia	Autosomal-recessive (Scriver, 1978)	Abnormal kidneys, deafness (Nyhan, 1977)	Not as of 1975	Not as of 1975
a-Methyl-B-hydroxybutyric acid	Autosomal-recessive (Rosenberg, 1977)	Intermittent acidosis, ketosis, hyperglycinemia syndrome (Nitonsky, 1977)	Not as of 1975	yes
Maple syrup urine disease, sev. inf.	Autosomal-recessive	Maple syrup odor of urine, hypertonia, seizures (Taft & Cohen, 1977)	yes	yes
Niemann-Pick disease	Autosomal-recessive (Brady, 1978)	Enlargement of liver and spleen (hepatomegaly), severe generalized weakness, emaciated (Brady, 1977)	yes	yes
Phenylketonuria	Autosomal-recessive	Seizures, eczema, reduced stature and head size, lighter coloring, musty odor of urine, treated by dietary restriction of phenylalanine (see text)	Not as 1975	yes
Sanfilippo A and B	Autosomal-recessive	Moderate skeletal abnormalities similar to but less severe than Hurler; severe MR (Danes, 1977)	A yes; B Not as of 1975	yes
Tay-Sachs disease	Autosomal-recessive	Early blindness, seizures, hypersensitivity to sound, spasticity, death by about age 3 years	yes	yes

Source: Milunsky and Atkins (1975), Stanbury et al. (1983).

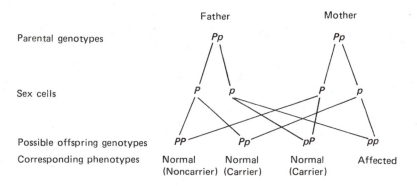

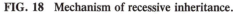

FIG. 18   Mechanism of recessive inheritance.

genotypes, (2) the kind of sperm and egg cells that can be formed from these genotypes, (3) the possible sperm-egg unions at conception, and (4) the phenotypes of their offspring. Step 4 shows three children normal and one affected. This illustrates the famous Mendelian 3:1 ration associated with recessive inheritance. Once again it should be understood that this is only a statement of statistical probability; any combination of affected to unaffected persons is possible. We can tell parents who are carriers, however, that each pregnancy bears a 1-in-4 risk of producing a phenylketonuric child. With such information parents have the opportunity to make decisions regarding children, which should make for healthier children and happier families.

Biochemical Error

What is phenylketonuria? It is a form of mental retardation caused by excessively high levels of an amino acid called phenylalanine. The abnormally elevated level is itself caused by a deficiency of an enzyme (phenylalanine hydroxylase) which metabolizes or converts phenylalanine into another substance called tyrosine. Widespread screening programs to detect newborns with PKU have uncovered several variants that are also characterized by elevated blood phenylalanine levels, the most common of which is called "atypical phenylketonuria" (Menkes, 1974). The nature of the biochemical deficiency in "classical" PKU is shown at point *A* in Figure 19. This is a so-called "inborn error of metabolism." Figure 19 also illustrates three other recessive conditions associated with phenylalanine-tyrosine metabolism. One of these, albinism, is well known to all of us. None of the other conditions are associated with retardation.

Prevalence

Phenylketonuria is a relatively rare condition with a range of incidence in newborn screening programs of 1:4500 to 1:20,000 and an overall incidence of 1:11,500 (Levy, 1974). On this basis, the number of normal carriers of the recessive gene in the general population is estimated at about 1 in 54. As a non-sex-linked trait, equal numbers of males and females would be expected, but a higher

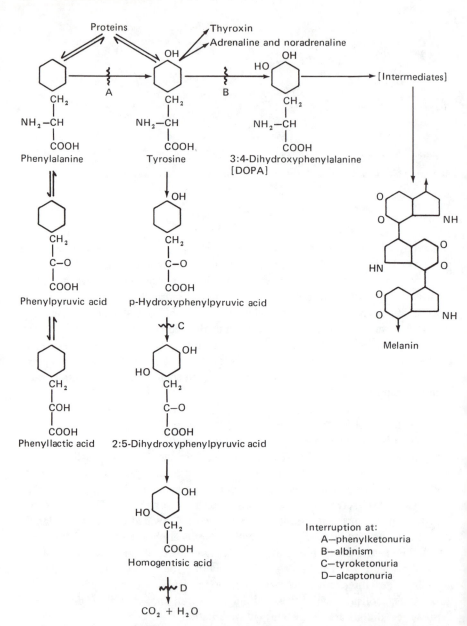

FIG. 19 The probable phenylalanine-tyrosine metabolic sequence in man. The points at which this sequence appears to be interrupted by known inherited metabolic defects in man are indicated by }. The key to the specific defect involved is given in the lower right-hand corner of the figure. (With modifications after Crowe and Schull, Folia hered. et path., 1:259, 1952, and reprinted from Neel and Schull, 1954. Copyright 1954 by The University of Chicago. All rights reserved.)

frequency of males was noted in one major study (Dobson & Williamson, 1970; Dobson, Williamson, & Koch, 1970). This sex difference was not confirmed by another investigator (Berman, 1970).

Behavioral Aspects

The primary symptom of PKU is mental retardation. If untreated it is usually severe to profound in degree, although atypical cases are not uncommon and untreated phenylketonurics of normal intelligence are found (Perry, Hansen, Tischler, Richards, & Sokol, 1973). On the basis of what has been learned from dietary control of this disorder, the PKU infant is normal at birth, but the process of intellectual impairment begins as the newborn ingests protein, a food essential that contains about 5 percent phenylalanine. If the deterioration is neither prevented nor arrested, the retardation is likely to be very severe. The average IQ of untreated phenylketonurics is from 20 to 25 (Baumeister, 1967b; Jervis, 1963; Paine, 1957; Partington, 1962) with about one-quarter functioning in the 25–50 range (Paine, 1957; Partington, 1962). The behavior of PKU children is frequently autisticlike and sometimes misdiagnosed as childhood schizophrenia. Such children are often hyperactive, unpredictable, and they show stereotypic movements (e.g, rocking and hand-posturing) (Koch, Acosta, Fishler, Schaeffler, & Wohlers, 1967). Other investigators have noted that they tend to exhibit greater activity, aggressiveness, and general upset than other retarded persons of comparable mental age (Johnson, 1969; Wright & Tarjan, 1957). The description of a phenylketonuric woman follows.

A mentally retarded woman with phenylketonuria

Jane is a 20-year-old who was placed in a State institution for the retarded at age 16. She is one of two children, the other an older brother who is in his last year of pharmacy school. There was one other pregnancy but it ended in miscarriage. Jane's family history is unremarkable. Her father had 2 years of college and is employed as a mail carrier. He is in good health. Her mother completed high school and nurse's training. Her health is only fair.

Jane's early development indicates some lag in the acquisition of motor and language skills but she was said to have been fully toilet trained by age 2. Institutionalization was sought because of behavior problems. Jane had been in the same trainable class for 7 years and was no longer interested in attending it. At home she had become increasingly unmanageable and was said to have terrific temper tantrums both at home and in public. She also is said to have an intense need for the "immediate and undivided attention of adults." The mother was becoming increasingly depressed over her inability to deal with Jane and the family doctor recommended institutionalization. Psychological testing at age 15 showed a mental age of 4 years, 8 months, and an IQ of 34. She was described as a neatly dressed but rather dull-looking girl whose speech was unclear though usually understandable. She was cooperative during the examination and appeared to enjoy the test situation.

At age 15, Jane had fairly good self-help skills—she was able to use a fork and spoon, to dress herself though she had difficulty with buttons and zippers, and she was toilet trained. She was described as hyperactive and taking medication for control of hyperactivity. It was the feeling of the institutional staff that some of Jane's behavior problems were due to the parents' failure to set any limits on her behavior during the growing-up years. Now, in adolescence, for the first time they were trying to set limits and Jane was reacting very negatively to this.

The diagnosis of phenylketonuria was made after Jane was institutionalized. Physically she is tall, thin, and has the blond hair and fair complexion often seen in PKU. She has made only a marginal institutional adjustment. She does not relate well to other girls and devotes most of her energies to trying to gain the attention of her cottage parents. She does this by resorting to such infantile behavior as talking like a baby. Her parents continue to be very interested in her and in her institutional adjustment.

Physical Aspects

The phenylketonuric child is reasonably well developed physically and does not present the kind of obvious physical anomalies seen in Down syndrome. Fairly characteristic, however, are very light coloring and blue eyes (Langdell, 1967). This fairness actually reflects a deficiency in pigmentation and is caused by the reduced amount of tyrosine. As shown in Figure 19, tyrosine is a product of one of the steps in the chemical chain that leads to melanin, the body's source of dark pigmentation. Other common symptoms of PKU are seizures and eczema (Paine, 1957), reduced stature and head circumference, and a musty odor in the urine. It was this urine odor that led Fölling in 1934 to first identify the disorder and then to discover that it was due to an excessive amount of phenylalanine.

Preventability

The most interesting feature of phenylketonuria is its preventability. There is the tendency to think of our genetic constitution as a fixed "given" about which nothing can be done. In fact, genetic problems are not necessarily untreatable. One of the forms of diabetes, diabetes mellitus, has a hereditary component, but the genetic defect can be circumvented by providing the body with the insulin that the biochemical error has prevented the body from manufacturing. In phenylketonuria, prevention and treatment consist of placing the newborn on a low phenylalanine diet (Lofenalac). An excellent review of the effects of the diet on the prevention of retardation (Baumeister, 1967) reveals the importance of the time of its initiation (see Table 7). Intelligence is least impaired in children who began the diet before 15 weeks of age, but after 36 weeks of age response to it is unpredicta-

TABLE 7   Age of Diet Initiation and IQ in
Treated Phenylketonurics

Age diet initiated	Average IQ
1–13 weeks	89
14–26 weeks	74
27–156 weeks	50
After 156 weeks	26

ble. Several groups of workers have suggested that even a delay of a few weeks is detrimental (Berman, Graham, Eichman, & Waisman, 1961; Centerwall, Centerwall, Armon, & Mann, 1961; Kang, Sollee, & Gerald, 1970), though one study reported no such effect (Sutherland, Umbarger, & Berry, 1966).

Initial enthusiasm for the diet has waned, however. Some degree of intellectual impairment, though only mild, is common, and the maintenance of the child on the diet is very difficult. Moreover, the diet has apparently been unnecessarily provided to children with the variants of classical PKU. It is only the child with classical PKU who requires it. Problems of maintaining children on the diet have created such stresses for child and family that it has been customary to terminate it at school age.

While some workers had noted physical and personality changes in children following its termination, it was assumed that the child was no longer vulnerable to the cognitive impairment associated with high blood phenylalanine. But recent studies indicate some adverse cognitive and/or educational effects of diet termination at age 5 or 6 (Berry, O'Grady, Perlmutter, & Bofinger, 1979; Brown & Warner, 1976; Cabalska et al., 1977). IQ declines averaging 9–12 points have been found. One study found no difference between diet-continued and diet-terminated children after a 2-year interval (Holtzman, Welcher, & Mellits, 1975), but those reporting a difference tended to be evaluating children at more than a 2-year interval. Other problems that have been reported in off-diet children are hyperactivity, difficulties in concentrating, and the development of abnormalities in brain wave (EEG) (Cabalska et al., 1977).

The findings of continued vulnerability to the deleterious effects of high levels of phenylalanine, at least until age 12, can create a severe dilemma for parents and physician if there is major child resistance to diet continuation. A more palatable diet has recently been developed, Phenylfree, which may ease the problem.

Untoward Genetic Consequences

Although the dietary prevention of serious mental handicap is an obvious blessing to the phenylketonuric child and to his family, there are some undesirable genetic consequences. The effect of preventing retardation is to increase the number of recessive genes for PKU in the general population. The *untreated* phenylketonuric is usually so severely retarded as to be sexually inactive. The affected individual is unlikely to reproduce and thus to transmit recessive genes. The *treated* and normally functioning phenylketonuric, however, is, a potential spreader of recessive PKU genes. Since the normal phenylketonuric has only recessive genes for PKU, all of the children would at least be carriers. If the phenylketonuric should produce children by a carrier, the risk of PKU for each child would be 1:2. Figure 20 shows the outcome of matings between a normal phenylketonuric female and noncarrier and carrier males. In step 2 note that only one sperm and egg cell is shown for the homozygous parents (*pp, PP*), because all sperm cells will be alike (*P*) and all egg cells alike (*p*) with regard to the kind of gene carried for phenylketonuria. Fortunately, there are biochemical tests for identifying carriers (Griffin & Elsas, 1975) and fixing the risk of producing affected children.

Maternal-Induced Retardation

Another untoward consequence for both normal phenylketonuric women and those whose retardation is not severe enough to preclude pregnancy is the likelihood of inducing retardation in a genetically non-PKU fetus by exposing it during pregnancy to the mother's high level of phenylalanine. The placenta is not a barrier to phenylalanine, and fetal exposure appears to carry a very high risk of retardation (Mabry, 1965). In one family in which there were four normal PKU women, nine of their 12 children were either retarded or "slow learners" (Farquhar, 1974). The clinical picture of "induced PKU" is one of reduced stature, microcephaly, and retardation (Fisch, Conley, Eysenbach, & Chang, 1977), and recommendations to prospective PKU mothers comprise avoiding pregnancy, therapeutic abortion, or returning to a low phenylalanine diet (Forbes, Shaw, Koch, Coffelt, & Straus, 1966; Farquhar, 1974; Koch, 1967; Mabry, Denniston, & Caldwell, 1966). The diet's low palatability and propensity for causing nausea during pregnancy seem to raise serious question as to the feasibility of the third option, and one worker has suggested that phenylketonuric women might remain on at least a modified diet during youth and their childbearing years so as to reduce the trauma of its full reinstatement during pregnancy (Farquhar, 1974). Again, the new diet may be helpful here as well.

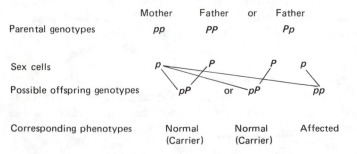

FIG. 20 Two types of matings in the phenylketonuric female.

OTHER WELL-KNOWN
RECESSIVE DISORDERS

Galactosemia

This disorder results from the inability of the newborn to metabolize galactose, a milk constituent. Milk consumption causes a failure to thrive, and frequent vomiting and diarrhea. Damage to the liver results in jaundice and, if untreated, death. The lens of the eye is also commonly affected, causing cataracts and visual impairment. Cataracts are reversible if treatment is begun by age 3 months. Galactosemia also affects the brain and causes mental retardation (Nyhan & Sakati, 1976), although, with very early recognition and milk restriction, intellectual impairment appears preventable.

The disorder is immediately responsive to elimination of milk from the diet. In several studies, the IQ of treated children ranged from 91 to 94, somewhat below their unaffected sibs, though a subsample of second-born galactosemic children had a mean IQ of 102. In the case of the latter, forewarned by the first affected child, a diagnosis was made before symptoms were evident. Apparently, in those who are unrecognized before symptoms appear, some slight impairment relative to unaffected sibs is found (Kalckar, Kinoshita, & Donnell, 1973; Nadler, Inouye, & Hsia, 1969; Nyhan & Sakati, 1976).

Poor visual-motor drawing performance is commonly seen as are general academic difficulties (Gershen, 1975). The heterozygous state in prospective parents is detectable, and dietary treatment in the infant consists of the substitution of casein hydrolysate (Nutromigen) for milk formulas. The condition itself is quite rare—for example, 1 in 200,000 births in Massachusetts (Shih et al., 1971)—but several states have added galactosemia to their PKU screening programs (Sells & Bennett, 1977). A complicating problem in attempting to screen for galactosemia and PKU simultaneously is that by the time blood is taken for PKU analysis (4th to 14th day of life), galactosemia may have taken so fulminating a course that death would occur prior to the receiving of test results! Ideally, cord blood should be tested, and this is done in the Massachusetts Metabolic Disorders Screening Program (Chitham, Starr, & Stern, 1976; Levy, 1974).

Tay-Sachs Disease

This is an extraordinarily lethal disorder that results from the inability of the infant to metabolize fats (lipids). Gradual accumulation of lipids in many tissues, including the retina and the brain, leads to early blindness, seizures, hypersensitivity to sound, spasticity, and mental deterioration. Death eventuates at about age 3.

Tay-Sachs occurs with a particularly high frequency among Jews of Eastern European origin. Fortunately, the heterozygous or carrier state can be detected biochemically in prospective parents, and the condition itself is diagnosable prenatally through amniocentesis. This allows for the exercise of the option of therapeutic abortion (Sells & Bennett, 1977).

Hurler Syndrome

Also known as gargoylism, this disorder results from the accumulation or "storage" in cells of mucopolysaccharides, substances associated with carbohydrate metabolism. Its primary symptoms are dwarfism, humpback, large bulging head, cloudy corneas, clawlike hands, deafness, and retardation. Affected infants appear normal at birth, but symptoms begin to be apparent by 1 year (Warkany, 1971). The complete disease picture develops during childhood, and most die within the first decade. There is no treatment at present. Hurler syndrome is inherited as a simple autosomal-recessive, but there is a milder form, *Hunter syndrome*, which is inherited as a *sex-linked* recessive. This means that the gene for the variant is found on the X chromosome (see Fig. 21). Since the female has two X chromosomes, a carrier female ($X^H X^h$) would be unaffected because the gene for the disease is recessive. If the male happens to inherit the X chromosome with the recessive gene (X^h), he will be affected, because he has no other chromosome that could carry the normal gene. In sex-linked conditions, on the average half of the males will be affected and half unaffected. For a female to have any sex-linked disorder, she must carry the recessive gene on both X chromosomes. The frequency of sex-linked conditions is thus much higher in males than in females. Other sex-linked conditions, though unrelated to mental retardation, are color blindness and chondrodystrophy.

Lesch-Nyhan Syndrome

This is another sex-linked recessive condition which is best known because of its association with self-mutilative behavior. Occurring exclusively in males and caused by an abnormality in nucleic acid metabolism, its main symptoms in addition to self-mutilation are retardation and cerebral palsy. The disease is expressed biochemically in high amounts of uric acid (hyperuricemia).

Affected children appear normal for the first 6 to 8 months. Motor symptoms then appear; there is loss of previously acquired head and trunk control. Later the motor problem (spasticity) will be of such severity as to prevent sitting unassisted or standing. Retardation is a prominent feature and is usually at least

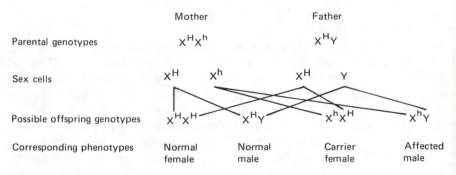

FIG. 21   Sex-linked inheritance on the X chromosome.

moderate in degree, although a few individuals of normal intelligence have been observed. Even here, however, the motor abnormality is severe.

The self-mutilative behavior causes these children to be perceived as bizarre and aggressive (Nyhan & Sakati, 1976), the aggressiveness usually taking the form of self-directed biting of the lips and fingers. The biting can actually cause tissue loss, and partial amputations of fingers have occurred. There is no indication of an impairment in pain perception, as apparent screaming in pain is said to accompany the biting. In this respect, Lesch-Nyhan children differ from many other retarded individuals who engage in self-mutilation or self-injurious behavior. The later usually show no discomfort at self-hitting. They are also generally free of gross motor abnormality. Self-injurious behavior was mentioned in Chapter 2 in connection with the "severely retarded autistic child" and is dealt with in depth in Chapter 10.

This extraordinary disorder can be detected in the heterozygous state in normal "carrier" females and can also be diagnosed prenatally through amniocentesis. While there is medical treatment for the hyperuricemia and also gout, which commonly accompanies it, this does not reduce the self-mutilative aspect (Lesch & Nyhan, 1964; Nyhan & Sakati, 1976).

Cloning of the Lesch-Nyhan Gene

In 1982 scientists reported the first cloning of a gene on the human X chromosome (Brennard, Chinault, Konecki, Melton, & Caskey, 1982; Jolly, Esty, Bernard, & Friedman, 1982). The gene produces the enzyme HPRT (hypoxanthine/guanine phosphororiboxyltransferase), and it is this enzyme that is deficient in Lesch-Nyhan syndrome. This work is seen as a first step in understanding the nature of the specific defect in the gene and would lay the basis for future diagnosis and treatment.

Disorders of Multiple Etiology but Including a Recessive Form

CONGENITAL HYPOTHYROIDISM (CRETINISM)

The earlier term used for this disorder (cretinism) gives it a very special place in the history of mental retardation; the first formal programs for retarded children were developed in Switzerland for youths with this disorder. Congenital hypothyroidism is an endocrine disease caused by lack of development of the thyroid gland and was endemic in areas deficient in iodine, such as in parts of Switzerland. With the development of iodized salt, the endemic form is wholly preventable. The nonendemic or sporadic form occurs in about 1 in 6000 births (Sells & Bennett, 1977) and may be variously caused by (a) agenesis or dysgenesis of the thyroid gland, (b) an inborn and genetic enzymatic error, or (c) maternal ingestion of antithyroid drugs during a pregnancy (Warkany, 1971). The genetic form has several variants and is associated with a goiter (enlargement of the thyroid gland) which either is present at birth or develops in childhood.

The primary symptoms are growth and intellectual retardation. There are characteristic facial features and the child appears dull and apathetic and has a hoarse cry (Villee, 1975). A major diagnostic problem is that the infant may appear normal at birth with symptoms developing only very insidiously during the first 6 months. Treatment consists of thyroid hormone replacement. As in the case of PKU, intellectual development is closely related to the time of treatment initiation. In a series of 31 children diagnosed as having severe congenital hypothyroidism (athyreotic and goitrous) by age 3 months and in whom treatment was variously begun in the periods 0–3 months, 3–7 months, and after 7 months, the respective mean IQs were 89, 71, and 54 (Klein, Meltzer, & Kenny, 1972). Of those treated by 3 months, 78 percent had IQs of 85 and above, in the 3- to 7-month range, only 19 percent had IQs greater than 85; and in the post-7-month group, none had an IQ greater than 80. These findings are similar to those of another study (Smith, Blizzard, & Wilkins, 1971) where less than 10 percent of those whose therapy began after 6 months of age had IQs in the normal range. Nevertheless, as in earlier described conditions, even treatment begun very early does not assure perfectly normal mental development. Of the three children whose treatment began at 1 month, one had an IQ of 105 and the other two had IQs of 89 and 86. Similarly, the mean IQ of the six children who commenced treatment at 2 months of age was 86 (range 64–107). It would appear that congenital disorders of metabolic or endocrine origin that affect the brain carry at least 5- to 10-point IQ reduction risk at the very least.

MICROCEPHALY

This is a generic term which refers to an abnormally small brain and skull. Early workers attributed the small brain to premature closure of the cranial sutures, a problem earlier referred to in craniostenosis. Here, however, the small skull is merely a response to reduced brain size.

In the nineteenth century, with popularization of Darwin's theory of evolution, malformations were often considered "atavisms" or regressions to earlier phylogenetic stages, and microcephaly was identified with the simian brain. In fact, the microcephalic brain is much more human than simian and resembles that of the human fetus. The condition is now attributed to arrested fetal development.

Microcephaly may be of either genetic or nongenetic origin. The former is inherited as a simple autosomal-recessive, whereas the nongenetic or environmental form is secondary to various disease processes that arrest brain development. The majority of cases are environmental in origin.

The microcephalic head shows a narrow and receding forehead, small cranium, and flattened occiput—all of which gives it a conical appearance. As the child grows, the diminished head size becomes more apparent, though the entire body is commonly dwarfed and underweight. Developmentwise, cognitive, motor, and speech functions are delayed; the children are often hypertonic, and about one-third have seizures. Retardation is likely to be severe to profound (Warkany,

1971). Normal intelligence is also found, though there are commonly signs of minimal brain dysfunction (Martin, 1970).

MACROCEPHALY

This a generic term for an abnormally large head. The enlargement may be due either to increased free fluid in the cranial cavity (hydrocephaly) or to a large brain (megalencephaly).

Hydrocephaly

This is a condition of diverse origins and includes both genetic and nongenetic forms. It may be present at birth in conjunction with a variety of malformations of the brain and spinal cord, most notably spina bifida (gaps in the spine). Congenital forms are seldom compatible with normal delivery and postnatal life. In hydrocephaly arising in the postnatal period, associated malformations are also not rare (e.g., spina bifida and harelip and cleft palate), and it may also accompany infectious conditions that were prenatal in origin (e.g., congenital syphilis and congenital toxoplasmosis). The incidence of hydrocephalus is about 1 in 1000 births but its frequency doubles when it is included with spina bifida (Alter, 1962).

The symptoms typically arise from a *blockage* in the circulation of cerebrospinal fluid in the ventricles of the brain, although *overproduction* of cerebrospinal fluid has been established in some cases. Advanced forms of hydrocephaly are immediately recognizable. The head can become enormous—there is bulging of the forehead, parietal, and occipital areas. The eyes are directed downward, and, with the white of the eye (sclera) visible above the cornea, they give the appearance of setting suns. Other eye-related abnormalities are strabismus (cross-eyed), nystagmus (involuntary movement of the eyeball, usually in a lateral direction), and optic atrophy. Blindness may ensue. Ultimate physical and mental development depends on many factors—rapidity of onset, intracranial pressure, compensatory growth of the head—the nature of the basic malformations leading to excessive cerebrospinal fluid and the progress or arrest of the process. In one series of patients who received no treatment, about half showed a spontaneous arrest of the process, and, of these, about 40 percent had grossly normal intelligence. The remaining 60 percent showed all degrees of retardation (Lawrence, 1960). Treatment is limited to surgical intervention (Warkany, 1971).

Megalencephaly

This head size anomaly is due to a brain of excessive size and weight. It can be demonstrated only by special diagnostic procedures during life (e.g., pneumoencephalography) or at autopsy. Though the term tends to be limited to pathologic conditions, excessively large brains (over 450 g in the neonate and over 1600 g in the adult) have also been found in persons of normal or superior intellect. Megalencephaly is an extremely rare condition and was diagnosed in only 7 of 550 cases of "hydrocephaly" (Almeida & Barros, 1964; Rubenstein & Warkany, 1976).

In the form in which there is no underlying disease, *primary megalencephaly*, the head appears large at birth and grows rapidly but is often not grossly abnormal in shape. While intelligence may be unimpaired, retardation of all degrees is more often the case. The etiology of megalencephaly is obscure. Some cases appear to be genetic and inherited as autosomal-dominants, but a recessive mode is also indicated in at least one family history. *Symptomatic* or *secondary megalencephaly* may also be seen in some of the recessively inherited metabolic disorders and in brain neoplasm. There is no treatment for primary or even secondary megalencephaly, and, in the absence of signs of disease, the affected person should be reassured, observed, and protected against unnecessary medical procedures (Rubenstein & Warkany, 1976).

Polygenic Inheritance

The polygenic mode of inheritance differs from the so-called "major gene" effects of dominant and recessive heredity in that it refers to cumulative or additive effects of one or more pairs of genes. Polygenic inheritance is attributed to hereditary traits that exist in degree or gradation as contrasted with the more or less discrete or "all-or-none" quality of hereditary conditions caused by major genes. It must be added, however, that recessive conditions much more than dominant ones display an all-or-none character.

Phenylketonuria illustrates a discrete or all-or-none effect in that, typically, one either has or does not have the condition; you are either affected or normal with respect to PKU. Polygenic inheritance, on the other hand, is applied to such hereditary traits as height and hair color. Each of us has some degree of height, for example, and we differ only in the degree of height that we possess. Another "trait" that exists in degree and which appears to have a very significant genetic component is intelligence (Scarr-Salapater, 1975; Scarr & McCartney, 1983).

Polygenic inheritance is thought to play an important role in what was called "cultural-familial retardation" (Allen, 1958, Jensen, 1970; Roberts, 1952) but which, in the recent AAMD diagnostic nomenclature, is referred to as "psychosocial disadvantage" (Grossman, 1973, 1977, 1983). The change in terminology now places this diagnostic category under "environmental influences" and appears to reject the possibility of a genetic component. In its traditional usage, the term "cultural-familial" retardation referred to retardation that was not attributable to any obvious biological abnormality and where similarly affected persons were found in parents and sibs. The degree of retardation was usually mild. Familial patterns of mild retardation were the focus of late nineteenth- and early twentieth-century studies of the Jukes (Dugdale, 1877) and Kallikak families (Goddard, 1912); modern studies of such families are represented by those of Roberts (1952) and Reed and Reed (1965). The earlier workers, especially Goddard, tended to view the familial pattern as evidence of a genetic causation; what was ignored was that the mildly retarded children emerging from these families tended to be exposed to the most adverse of environments. The quality of life in such homes is presented in Chapter 6, wherein the influence of the environment on intellectual development is explored.

The polygenic mode of inheritance as applied to intelligence is illustrated in Figure 22 adapted from Gottesman (1963). For purposes of simplicity, a two-gene

Step 1

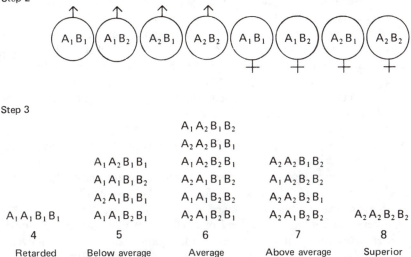

Step 2

Step 3

FIG. 22   Theoretical distribution illustrating two gene pair polygenic model.

pair model is shown, although a 12-gene pair model is necessary to account for all IQs that fall within the so-called "normal intelligence" range. Assume then that intelligence is determined by two pairs of genes, pair A and pair B, and let each of the genes within a pair be labeled as either 1 or 2. Genes designated as 1 will stand for dullness, and those designated as 2 for brightness. The genotype of a person with cultural-familial retardation would carry only genes for dullness—$A_1A_1B_1B_1$— and would have an additive weight of 4. An individual of superior intelligence would have only genes for brightness—$A_2A_2B_2B_2$—and would have the additive weight of 8. The genetic contribution to the difference in intelligence between two individuals is based solely on the weights of each of the genes, as there is no difference between the effects of genes A and B per se. Assume now a marriage of persons with average intelligence—that is, a genotype weight which is exactly intermediate between the extremes of 4 and 8, or a weight of 6. In Figure 22, step 1 depicts the parents' genotypes, step 2 indicates all possible sperm and egg cells, and step 3 shows all of the genotypes that can be derived from this marriage. Note that marriage of two parents of average intelligence can produce children with all possible genotype weights from 4 to 8 but that the proportion of different geno-types varies somewhat. Of the 16 possible genotypes, the largest group has a weight of 6, the value that corresponds to that of the parents. Thus the largest grouping within this hypothetical family of 16 children would have average intelli-gence, as do their parents. The proportion of other genotypes diminishes as we move into the above-average and below-average ranges, and the reader may recognize that the distribution represents expansion of the binomial.

In proposing a polygenic inheritance mode as at least a partial explanation of cultural-familial mental retardation, the assumption is made that persons with this form of retardation represent an integral part of the so-called "normal" range of intelligence. Just as polygenic factors are presumed to contribute to intelligence in the average and superior ranges, so are they thought to account for functioning in the below-average and retarded ranges. The intelligence range to which we refer represents IQs varying from about 50 to 150. IQs below 50, that is, those in the moderately, severely, and profoundly retarded range, are not ordinarily seen as reflecting normal variation (Penrose, 1954; Roberts, 1952) but rather as the consequence of the impairment of a higher potential resulting from genetic abnormalities or from prenatal, natal, or postnatal disease.

But if environment as well as heredity affects mental development, then it is necessary to include a consideration of its role in cultural-familial retardation, because it is this very group that is most likely to be subjected to the least favorable of environments. The concept that seeks to relate heredity and environment is that of *reaction range* (Dobzhansky, 1955). As applied to intelligence, reaction range or norm of reaction refers to a range of IQs each of which could be found in the same person according to the kind of environment to which that person is exposed. Heredity and environment are often thought of as opposites with events construed as *either* hereditary or environmental in origin. Fuller (1954), however, has defined these two concepts in terms of each other; heredity is seen as the capacity to respond to environment in a particular way. The definition implies that each person will respond to events in a manner that reflects his own unique genetically determined capacities (Scarr, 1985; Scarr & McCartney, 1983). Genetic uniqueness would be seen as accounting for differences among individuals sharing a similar environment (e.g., same-sex fraternal twins) but would not preclude commonality among genetically different persons exposed to similar environments (e.g., behavioral similarities among unrelated members of a particular cultural or ethnic group). One problem in attempting to apply the definition is that it is not always clear to what the term "heredity" should refer. Complex behavior such as intelligence represents not only gene-determined central nervous system response capacities but also how that biological potential has been shaped by experience (environment). The developing child's response capacities become the inextricable product of hereditary *and* environmental influences, which can only begin to be separated through the medium of twin studies, reference to which will be made in the next chapter. Most easily identified as hereditary are physical characteristics associated with major gene effects such as phenylketonuria or sickle cell anemia (also a recessive) or even such a polygenic characteristic as height.

Definitions aside, the concept of reaction range is illustrated in Figure 23, which shows hypothetical reaction ranges for four individuals. Each one reflects potential IQ in three different kinds of environments. The three environments are denoted I, N, and E; I refers to a relatively impoverished environment for that individual, N to his usual environment, and E to a relatively enriched environment for him.

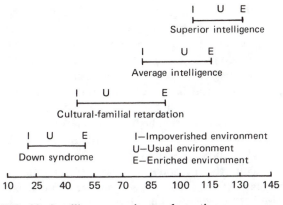

FIG. 23   Intelligence quotient and reaction range.

Each of the reaction ranges has some overlap with another—the overlap resulting from either enhanced or depressed intellectual functioning associated with relatively enriched or impoverished environments. Thus the individual with cultural-familial retardation could conceivably function in the low-average intelligence range and actually achieve a higher IQ than a person who, on the basis of his parents, is presumed to have the biological potential for average intelligence but whose environment has been impoverished. A somewhat greater degree of overlap is projected for individuals of average and superior intelligence, because the difference between their IQs under normal environmental conditions is only 20 points as compared with an expected 40-point difference between persons with average intelligence and cultural-familial retardation in their normal environments.

In addition to overlap, the model proposes reaction ranges that differ somewhat in magnitude. In the case of Down syndrome, the model suggests that under the best of possible environments the likelihood is small that the affected individual would exceed an IQ of 50. The constraints created by biology are not easily circumvented. On the other hand, wider ranges of potential functioning are proposed for persons who are free of major biological abnormalities except for those of superior intelligence. The largest benefit is proposed for the cultural-familial person, and the smallest is indicated for individuals of superior intelligence. The reaction ranges projected here differ from those proposed by Gottesmen (1963) in that the latter show a positive relationship with IQ, the widest reaction range being given to persons of superior intelligence. Gottesman also proposes an upper limit of about IQ 80 for individuals with the cultural-familial form of retardation. Our own estimate based on studies to be presented in Chapter 6 would suggest that that "limit" extends into the normal range itself. *Within* the model presented here, the projected reaction range differences are attributed to the nature of the normal environment for each range and to possible species limitations, as such.

The normal environment for the child born into a family in which one or both parents is retarded is likely to be one that does not foster mental growth-producing psychological experience. The quality of life in the cultural-familial family is described in the chapter that follows. For the moment accept impoverishment, at its minimum, as an environment that provides the child neither with a *mother-teacher* person who consciously seeks to encourage the child's mental development nor with the kinds of verbal experience that somehow facilitate later academic success. If the child born into poverty and retardation is provided early with the kinds of physical and psychological nourishment that foster growth, for him an enriched environment, retardation may be prevented. This is not to suggest that all children born into such families function in the retarded range. From one-third to one-half of children from families in which both parents are retarded and in which there has been no special enrichment operate in the borderline to average intelligence range (Halperin, 1945; Penrose, 1938; Reed & Reed, 1965). This finding also seems to support, indirectly, the notion that polygenic factors are important determiners of intelligence. If one chooses to attribute the retardation of the cultural-familial child entirely to environmental deprivation, then how are the nonretarded children who emerge from such families to be explained?

In contrast to the relatively impoverished quality of the normal environment of the cultural-familial retarded child, the milieu of the child born to bright parents and siblings is much more likely to offer models and experiences that tend to encourage mental growth. His normal environment is already enriched, at least in terms of providing stimulus to intellectual development. This, of course, in no sense implies that the child's needs for love and competence will also be met. Some bright parents fail miserably to meet the affectional needs of their children. The relatively small allowance for enrichment gain in this child is based on the notion that our biological endowment sets limits on our response capacities. Living creatures differ in capacities between and within species. The kangaroo jumps farther than man, the leopard runs faster, the lion is stronger, and so on. Within man there are differences in capacities—one man can outjump another or run faster. A track coach, for example, can help an athlete make full use of his potential, but that potential is determined by the athlete's biology. It was also suggested that potential is not unlimited. The best track coach may not be able to produce a sprinter who can run the hundred in less than 9 seconds or the mile in less than 3 minutes. The unique biological properties of man, as of all creatures, provide both abilities and limitations. This probably applies to intelligence as well as to more "physical" characteristics. The child of superior intelligence is by definition already functioning toward the upper extreme of the population intelligence scale. The child whose IQ is 120 is surpassed by less than 10 percent of his peers. It is true that there are geniuses whose IQs have been estimated at more than 200, but normal man is represented by an upper limit of about 150, with only a tiny fraction exceeding IQ 130. What is being suggested is that the bright child is already receiving and taking a great deal from his environment, that he is already operating closer to his potential, and that enrichment will not add as much to his abilities as to children who function at lesser levels.

4

Nongenetic Biological Factors: Prenatal, Perinatal, and Postnatal

OVERVIEW

In this chapter we move, timewise, from those retardation-producing disorders that are determined at conception to those that occur thereafter. We have reference to the 9-month prenatal (gestational) period, to events at birth and in the early neonatal weeks, and to postnatal life. This chapter depicts forms of retardation associated with (a) exposure of the fetus to an adverse intrauterine environment, (b) hazards of prematurity and of the birth process, and (c) postnatal biological events that can arrest mental development. A listing of these "acquired" forms, most of which are described in the text, is shown in Table 8. The chapter concludes with a description of two major disorders, of diverse origin, and often associated with retardation—cerebral palsy and epilepsy.

PRENATAL HAZARDS

Although the role of prenatal biological factors in the cause of mental retardation is relatively well understood, their specific influence is complicated by (a) the time period that may intervene between the precipitating event and its actual detection, and (b) a likely interplay of causative factors (Masland, 1958). The latter is illustrated in such conditions as hemorrhage during pregnancy and prematurity, both of which increase the likelihood of abnormality, but the abnormality may also be the cause rather than the effect of maternal illness.

Embryological Timetables

Among the guides that assist in determining the significance of prenatal events are embryological timetables. The anatomical growth of the fetus is fixed in sequence and time, and specific anatomic abnormalities provide clues to the time

TABLE 8   Nongenetic Biological Causes of Mental Retardation

Prenatal

Infection: rubella, toxoplasmosis, syphilis, cytomegalovirus

Maternal-fetal blood incompatibilities: Rh and ABO

Drugs and alcohol: Heroin, methadone, antiepileptic, alcohol

Maternal-fetal irradiation: microcephaly

Chronic maternal health problems: diabetes, hypertension

Perinatal

Prematurity: types I, II, and III

Asphyxia (hypoxemia): birth, injury, hypoglycemia, prolapse of umbilical cord

Head trauma: hemorrhage, infection

Infection: herpes, encephalitis, meningitis

Kernicteris

Postnatal

Infection: encephalitis, meningitis, brain abscess, postimmunization encephalopathy

Cerebral trauma: head injury, cerebrovascular accidents, hemorrhage from coagulation defects, thromboses, ruptured aneurysm

Poisons and environmental toxins: lead, mercury

Anoxia: cardiac arrest, hypoglycemia, respiratory distress syndrome

Hormonal deficiency: hypothyroidism

Metabolic: hypernatremia, hypoglycemia

Brain tumors

Epilepsy

Nutrition

Source: Milansky (1975), Taft and Cohen (1977).

period during which the biological insult occurred. Cleft palate, for example, is known to result from an event that occurs prior to the 11th week of gestation, because the palate is ordinarily closed after that time (Fulton, 1957; Warkany, 1967). Warkany (1967) has reviewed the role of critical periods in the dating of causative occurrences and suggests that organ growth termination periods are precise enough to exclude alleged causal events that occur after the termination period for that particular growth process. The same degree of precision in organ vulnerability will be associated with a time *period*, rather than with a single *moment* in time. Cleft palate in the rat can be induced before the 16th day of gestation (termination period), but it can be produced only from the 11th day on—a vulnerability period of 5 days. Erroneous application of growth timetables was reflected in speculations regarding the cause of Down syndrome prior to the discovery of the chromosomal abnormality. Some of the specific anatomical defects of Down syndrome are associated with growth processes that are completed by the eighth week of life. It was presumed that the cause of the condition was to be sought in an event that occurred during the eighth week. In fact, the event was determined 8 weeks earlier, at conception itself. Attempts at precise retrospective dating are further bedeviled by the fact that each fetus does not respond to the same biological insult in exactly the same manner—another example of the heredity-environment interaction. Warkany cites a pair of fraternal twins whose mother had taken thalidomide during the first 4 months of pregnancy. One twin showed the typical symptom picture of malformed arms and hands, but the other had essentially normal arms and hands although the thumbs were abnormal and other nonskeletal defects were present. Here, perhaps, is an example of how two different genotypes responded to the same environment.

A similar kind of caution has been expressed by Birch (1956) with regard to the tendency to oversimplify the behavioral consequences of brain injury. Reference has been made to our still primitive understanding of the relationship of the brain to behavior; Birch notes that persons with brain injury will differ behaviorally according to such factors as site of injury, extent, the degree to which it is additive (provides a focus for seizures) or subtractive (causes central sensory deficit), and the time of its occurrence.

Infections

The most common prenatal infections associated with mental retardation are rubella, toxoplasmosis, syphilis, and cytomegalovirus. In absolute terms, these infectious diseases are small contributors to the population of retarded persons. Over a 25-year period, they accounted for only 0.3 percent of an institutionalized population (Yannet, 1966). Postnatal infections were a much heavier contributor, accounting for about 4 percent of all admissions during that time.

CONGENITAL RUBELLA

This disease in newborns is caused by a virus[1] that infects the pregnant woman during the first 3 months (first trimester) of pregnancy. The virus may produce few symptoms in the prospective mother, but it can have grave effects on the fetus. The placenta, ordinarily a protective shield for the fetus, is not a barrier to the rubella virus. So serious are its complications that, in a study of 333 rubella pregnancies, only 25 percent went to term. Of the 75 percent that did not, two-thirds were ended by elective abortion, and spontaneous abortion accounted for the remainder (Cooper, 1977). The origin and course of the disease have been described by Cooper (1968, 1977). Viral infection of the pregnant female may persist for 1 week and lead first to placental and then to fetal infection. The embryological timing of the viral insult is crucial, as the fetus is especially vulnerable during the first 3 months of pregnancy. The symptoms are varied and unpredictable; rubella pregnancies may lead to spontaneous abortion, to stillbirth, to live birth with one or more abnormalities (about 25% have multiple defects), or to a perfectly normal child.

The major clinical symptoms in a large series of infants followed to age 18 months were congenital heart defect (52%), hearing loss (52%), visual impairment due to either cataracts or glaucoma (40%), and hemorrhaging (31%). The infant mortality rate (death by age 1 year) was 13 percent. Unhappily, some infants who

---

[1]A virus is the smallest of human living organisms; about 1/25,000,000 of an inch. It reproduces itself only within living susceptible cells and causes a wide range of infectious diseases in humans, plants, and animals.

appeared unaffected at birth later showed full-blown symptoms. This is presumed to result from persistence of the rubella virus in the child.

Symptom Picture and Fetal Age

The symptom picture of congenital rubella is closely related to the time of fetal infection (Cooper, 1977; Sever & White, 1968; Wright, 1971). Approximately half of the fetuses affected in the first 2 months do not survive while, of the remainder, about 50 percent will show serious abnormalities. Fetal infection during the third and fourth months will not cause death, and the frequency of malformation drops to 20 percent. There appears to be no fetal risk in the last trimester.

Within the variability of fetal response to the rubella virus, the ultimate symptom picture illustrates the embryological timetable. The heart has been described by Koch (1967) as in a fairly critical stage of development throughout the first 3 months of life. Infection during the first 5 weeks of gestation particularly damages the valves and septa of the heart—that which forms its chambers and assures proper blood flow through it. Another heart defect, but one that appears to result from infection at any time during the first trimester, is an abnormal ductus arteriosus. This is a shunt between the aorta and the pulmonary artery which is normally closed at birth but remains open owing to the rubella virus. The visual defects of rubella are associated with the developmental period for the eye, the fourth to 10th weeks of life. Dental anomalies of crown morphology and of tooth composition are also found and are caused by viral invasion during the sixth to ninth weeks. Hearing loss and heart defeats are the two most prominent symptoms of rubella, with the hearing defect primarily due to damage to the organ of Corti in the inner ear. The hearing mechanism, like the heart, is vulnerable throughout the first 3 months, but it is also susceptible to damage during the fourth month.

The brain is another major target of the rubella virus, with some effects later seen as mental retardation. Of the 64 rubella infants followed to age 18 months, 44 (69%) had some degree of neurological impairment. The spectrum of neurological symptoms included motor abnormalities (cerebral palsy), seizures, and such behavioral deviations as delayed and sequentially disordered motor development, lag in adaptive behavior (mental retardation), hyperactivity, restlessness, and stereotyped movements. The last mentioned was particularly evident in children with sensory deficit—hearing and/or visual loss—and consisted of body rocking, head banging, hand waving, and so on. Although rocking and head banging are seen in infants who are clinically normal, these activities are more commonly found in retarded or emotionally disturbed children. Other unusual mannerisms, principally seen in children with eye lesions, were lengthy staring at the hand, waving of spread fingers before the eyes, and intentional poking of fingers into the eyes. The writer has seen all of these symptoms in severely retarded children and especially in those in whom retardation is combined with blindness. The author has also seen rubella children with blindness *and* deafness as well as retardation.

Regarding intellectual impairment, some degree, varying from borderline to profound, is present in about half of affected children (Chess, Korn, & Fernandez, 1971; Cooper et al., 1969).

On the other hand, a number of children with multiple disabilities are said to eventually make excellent adjustments, and Cooper (1977) considers that the developmental potential of rubella children is often significantly underestimated during their preschool years.

The relatively destructive impact of the rubella virus on the embryo, in contrast to its generally mild effect on the mother, illustrates critical periods of vulnerability and the immunologic mechanism. With regard to the latter, once an organism has been infected, antibodies are produced that can destroy the invading virus during subsequent reinfection. The adult either will have created a reservoir of antibody protection or is unaffected by the virus because the period of greatest danger is confined to the first 3 months of prenatal life. The fetus, however, is vulnerable on both counts—in terms of age and in lacking antibodies to combat the virus.

Preventability

Congenital rubella is now wholly preventable through a vaccine that has been available since 1969. The vaccination of children is of special concern because they are often the spreaders of the viral infection to previously unexposed mothers. About 80 percent of all children had been immunized by the mid 1970s, and this is reflected in about an 80 percent reduction in new cases. Schools now require such vaccination as a condition of admission, and this should eventually lead to complete elimination of the disease. For the present, it continues to be important to identify prospective mothers who have not been immunized by an earlier rubella infection (Orenstein & Greaves, 1982), and a special test permits this determination. Following such vaccination, pregnancy should be delayed for at least 2–3 months.

CONGENITAL TOXOPLASMOSIS

This is a protozoan infection that, like rubella, is typically noninjurious to the pregnant woman but devastating to the fetus. Also, as in rubella, fetal vulnerability is largely confined to the first 3 months of prenatal life. The congenital form of the disease is characterized by ocular and neurologic lesions and brain calcification. Microcephaly or hydrocephaly are common sequelae. The acutely ill newborn usually dies in the first month of life, and the great majority of survivors show retardation of variable degree, complete or partial blindness, and psychomotor disturbances. The writer has known three such individuals. Their IQs varied from 25 to 45, they had fairly good self-help skills and good speech, could perform simple chores, but, as indicated by their IQs, lacked functional academic skills.

Treatment for the newborn consists of chemotherapy which is designed to at least arrest the infectious process. The protozoan parasite that transmits the infection is found in raw meat and in cat feces. The newly pregnant female will want to avoid both eating uncooked or rare meats and physical contact with sources of cat feces contamination (e.g., litter boxes and flower beds)(Eichenwald, 1969; Wittner, 1977).

CONGENITAL SYPHILIS

Syphilis is caused by a spirochete bacterium[2] that is transmitted through sexual contact and which affects a number of organ systems. Syphilis was a fairly common disease in the prepenicillin era, and, in 1947, the number of cases reported to health services was 100,000. With the condition being extremely responsive to penicillin, the number of reported cases had declined to only 6,250 by 1957 but has been rising again to a current rate of about 25,000 per year. The increase in the general incidence of syphilis is paralleled by a twofold rise in the congenital form of the disease, and it is the latter that is associated with retardation. Unlike in rubella, the fetus is vulnerable only during the latter part of a pregnancy, because it is only after the 18th week of gestation that the so-called Langhans cell layer of the early placenta atrophies and permits the spirochete to cross the placenta and infect the fetus. Treatment of the mother before the 18th week will prevent any future fetal infection, and treatment after it will cure both mother and fetus because penicillin also crosses the placental barrier. Congenital syphilis is divided into an early and a late stage. The early stage is characterized by symptoms before age 2 years, and these chiefly include lesions of the skin, bones, and central nervous system; anemia; and hepatosplenomegaly (an enlargement of liver and spleen). The late stage refers to the persistence of the disease beyond age 2 years. In about 60 percent of cases the disease does not progress beyond age 2; in the remainder there are visual and hearing impairments and anomalies of the teeth. The neurological sequelae are usually not observable in infancy, but intellectual impairment becomes evident in childhood, and there may also be seizures (Finberg, 1977; Holmes et al., 1972; U.S. Department of Health Education, and Welfare, 1968). Retardation is rarely seen in postnatally acquired syphilis, but long-untreated persons may show the form of mental illness called paresis.

CONGENITAL CYTOMEGALOVIRUS

This is the most common of fetal infections and is found in about 1 percent of all newborns. Fortunately, about 95 percent of affected infants are asymptomatic, whereas among the remainder there is enlargement of the liver and spleen, jaundice, skin hemorrhages (purpura), microcephaly, chorioretinitis, and cerebral calcification. Neonatal death is common, and about 75% of survivors show neurological abnormality, blindness, deafness, spastic quadriplegia or hyptonia, and variable degrees of mental retardation (Hanshaw, 1977). Only recently has the first effective treatment of the disorder been reported.

Maternal-Fetal Blood Incompatibilities

Retardation may occur when the mother acquires what is, in effect, an allergic reaction to her unborn baby's blood. Rh disease (erythroblastosis fetalis) is the

---

[2]Bacteria are one of the types of unicellular microorganisms that cause infectious diseases. Others are Rickettsiae (Rocky Mountain spotted fever), viruses (rubella), yeasts and fungi (ringworm and thrush), and protozoa (toxoplasmosis).

well-known example of the phenomenon. ABO blood group incompatibility is also a potential though lesser cause of fetal central nervous system damage.

RH INCOMPATIBILITY

Rh incompatibility occurs when mother and fetus have different Rh blood group factors. The Rh factor is an autosomal hereditary trait; Rh-positive is dominant to Rh-negative. The maternal-fetal incompatibility arises *only* when an Rh-negative mother (Rh—Rh—) bears the child of an Rh-positive father (either Rh+Rh+ or Rh+Rh—). Where the father is homozygous dominant (Rh+Rh+), all of the children would be Rh-positive and potentially vulnerable to the incompatibility. Where the father is a carrier (Rh+Rh—), only the Rh-positive offspring would be vulnerable, the remainder being Rh-negative like the mother (Rh—Rh—).

Although the precondition to Rh disease is an Rh-negative mother and an Rh-positive fetus, problems arise only if there has been some previous mixing of fetal and maternal blood. If this has occurred, the mother's Rh-negative blood will have responded to the baby's foreign blood—that is, Rh-positive blood—by producing antibodies that have the capability of destroying fetal red blood cells. Such antibody effects are more likely to be found in later-born children but, fortunately, only about 10 percent of vulnerable mothers so react. Sensitization (immunization) of the Rh-negative mother to Rh-positive blood usually occurs at childbirth, when some mixing of maternal and fetal blood is common. It can also happen during pregnancy from leakage of fetal blood into the maternal circulation, or after an abortion. Following sensitization of the mother, she begins to produce antibodies against the Rh-positive blood. If this occurs during a first pregnancy, there are usually no ill effects on the fetus. But if during succeeding pregnancies mixing recurs, an enhanced maternal store of antibodies can destroy red blood cells, causing fetal anemia and setting the stage for possible postnatal damage to the brain. It is the latter that has implications for mental retardation.

In the destruction (hemolysis) of the oxygen-carrying red blood cells, there is released a pigment called *bilirubin*, a breakdown product of hemoglobin that is usually metabolized (conjugated) by the liver, and which in high amounts is toxic to the brain, especially the basal ganglia. Interestingly, during pregnancy the fetus is protected against high levels of bilirubin by its passage through the placenta into the maternal bloodstream, where it is subsequently metabolized by the mother's liver! When the infant with erythroblastosis fetalis is born, however, the neonatal liver cannot adequately metabolize the bilirubin, and, unless its level is controlled, damage to the brain ensues. This postnatal disorder is called *kernicterus*, and its symptoms can include motor abnormalities, intellectual impairment, and hearing loss. Prevention of kernicterus in the newborn may be accomplished through either phototherapy (exposure to light) and/or exchange blood transfusions.

The ultimate answer to erythroblastosis fetalis and its postnatal complication of kernicterus is to prevent Rh-negative mothers from exposure and sensitization (immunization) to Rh-positive blood in the first place. In about 98 percent of cases this is now feasible through the administration to Rh-negative women of RhoGAM within 72 hours after delivery. RhoGam provides a store of *externally* derived antibodies against Rh-positive blood and eliminates the fetal red cells from the maternal circulation *before* the mother has an opportunity to develop her own antibodies (becomes "sensitized"). In cases of unusually large fetomaternal "transfusion" or where the newborn shows evidence of extensive intrauterine hemorrhage, a larger dose of RhoGAM will be needed to prevent sensitization. Where sensitization has already occurred, RhoGAM is of no value. In an already sensitized women, prevention will involve careful observation during pregnancy to see if fetal red blood cell destruction is taking place. Prior to about 34 weeks of gestational age, treatment will take the form of an intrauterine blood transfusion of the fetus; after this time, the fetus will be of sufficient maturity to be delivered from the adverse maternal environment through cesarean section. Intrauterine transfusion can be done beginning about the 25th week and is usually reserved for fetuses that are so severely affected that they are unlikely to live long enough to be able to be delivered with a reasonable chance of survival (Phibbs, 1977).

ABO INCOMPATIBILITY

This is one of the commonest causes of neonatal jaundice and, in severe degree, can cause kernicterus and its associated mental and motor problems. The incompatibility is limited to mothers who are blood group O and whose fetuses are A or B. The disease is usually mild, the level of red blood cell destruction typically resulting in little or no anemia at birth. Postnatal hyperbilirubenimia is milder than in Rh incompatibility and can be controlled through phototherapy, exchange transfusions being unnecessary (Phibbs, 1977).

Drugs, Alcohol, and Tobacco

There are some 20 drugs that are known to produce adverse fetal effects, so-called "teratogens." In the late 1950s and early 1960s we became aware of thalidomide, an antinauseant used during pregnancy and a cause of limb malformations (phocomelia). In the 1960s, with the flourishing of "hard" drugs, we were alerted to chromosomal breakage in connection with LSD and to fetal abnormalities of heart, skeleton, and central nervous system associated with maternal use of amphetamines. Also in the 1960s it was found that drug-addicted women delivered babies who were themselves addicted ("passive" addiction). In the 1970s and 1980s, attention has been called to the adverse effects on the fetus of alcohol and tobacco during pregnancy. Marijuana usage during pregnancy has yet to be conclusively linked to any teratogenic effects. Of perhaps greatest significance, in the long run, are teratogenic dangers created by drugs that are used for purely medical purposes!

NARCOTIC ADDICTION

The use of heroin and methadone throughout pregnancy appears to have two fetal effects. Babies tend to be smaller (e.g., $\overline{X}$ 2500 g vs. 3200 g), and about 80 percent are born addicted. There is, however, no evidence that these drugs increase the frequency of congenital anomalies in the fetus (Blinick, Wallach, Jerez,

& Ackerman, 1976). With reference to size, 25 percent of one series showed retarded growth (4% in control group), and they were also much more prone to infection (26% vs. 3%) (Pelosi et al., 1975).

Addiction is seen in the appearance of withdrawal symptoms within 4 days after birth. In order of frequency, they involve the central nervous system (tremulousness, incoordination of sucking and swallowing, and seizures), the gastrointestinal system (vomiting and diarrhea), the respiratory system (rapid breathing), and the autonomic nervous system (high fever, yawning, sneezing, sweating, and lacrimation). Recognition of the syndrome and its treatment have dramaticaly reduced earlier high infant mortality rates. These withdrawal symptoms are usually confined to the first few weeks, although hyperirritability, hyperreflexia, tremulousness, and reduced social responsiveness may last for up to 6 months. Withdrawal symptoms can be prevented either by drug discontinuation a month prior to delivery or by a lowered methadone maintenance dosage (Madden et al., 1977; Phibbs, 1977).

At least two potentially "beneficial" effects have been reported. Addicted prematures appear to be less susceptible to respiratory distress than nonaddicted ones, and addicted infants show an accelerated maturation of the bilirubin system, about which we spoke in the last section. They are less likely to have high bilirubin levels (Kendall, 1977).

There have been several small studies on the later childhood status of antenatal heroin-exposed children (Sardemann, Madesen, & Friis-Hansen, 1976; Wilson, Desmond, & Verniaud, 1973; Wilson, McCreary, Kean, & Baxter, 1979). The two Wilson studies indicate that neonatal growth effects continue to be seen. The children tend to be smaller and appear to run an appreciably higher risk of a small head. In the later Wilson study, 14 percent (4 of 22) had a head circumference below the third percentile in contrast to only 2 percent of the controls. No other physical or health differences have been found. Studies of cognitive functioning indicate grossly normal mental ability. Slight differences in favor of non-heroin-exposed children may be explicable in terms of a greater instability of the parent-child relationship, since heroin-exposed children were much more likely to be separated from their mothers and placed in foster care.

Studies of methadone-exposed children seem to show lesser effects (Finnegan, 1981), though the neonatal withdrawal symptoms are actually more severe (Rosen & Pippinger, 1976). But methadone-exposed babies are at increased risk for a respiratory disorder (bronchopulmonary dysplasia), which makes them more vulnerable to sudden infant death syndrome. Fear of the latter is discouraging doctors from moving heroin patients to methadone (personal communication).

MARIJUANA

The effect of marijuana smoking during pregnancy is unclear. Women who use marijuana during pregnancy *are* at greater risk for babies with low birth weight, shorter gestation periods, and major malformations, but this appears to be related to *other* health-related characteristics of users rather than to the effect of marijuana itself (Shia et al., 1983). Other risk-related factors in these women are alcohol use, tobacco smoking, the quality of prenatal care, and general health history. One pregnancy complication found in both marijuana users and tobacco smokers is a higher frequency of bleeding in the third trimester associated with premature detachment of the placenta (abruptio placenta). This exposes the fetus to interference with oxygen supply and to possible severe hypoxemia. Among marijuana smokers, abruptio placenta was slightly more frequent among those who were daily or weekly users than among infrequent users.

A study of the neonatal status of marijuana-exposed infants found diminished responsiveness to light, less success in self-quieting, and increased tremors and startle. About one·third also had a high-pitched cry similar to that of neonates undergoing drug withdrawal (Fried, 1982). These problems appear to resolve by 1 month of age. Neither the animal nor the very limited human data currently indicate any adverse effects from marijuana use per se (Gal & Sharpless, 1984).

ALCOHOL

The most commonly abused drug, alcohol, has been clearly tied to fetal abnormalities, including retardation. The clinical picture in the neonate has been termed the *fetal alcohol syndrome* (Jones & Smith, 1975). In the United States it occurs in about 1–2 of every 1000 births, a rate comparable to that of Down syndrome, according to a 1983 report from the National Institute on Alcohol Abuse and Alcoholism. Its symptoms are retarded physical development (especially height), microcephaly, micrognathia (small jaw); microphthalmia (narrow eyes), cardiac defects, and mental retardation (Jones, Smith, Ulleland, & Streissguth, 1973; Ouellette, Rosett, Rosman, & Weiner, 1977; Ulleland, 1972; Umbreit & Ostrow, 1980). Some workers have questioned the existence of a "syndrome" as such, although there is no disagreement that these symptoms, either singly or in combination, are found with an increased frequency in the offspring of alcoholic mothers.

In a large study of women who were seen for routine prenatal care, heavy drinkers (average of about 5 oz of alcohol per day) had twice the risk of having a child with congenital anomalies as women who either drank moderately (average of 1 oz per day) or not at all. Most importantly, of the 42 children born to the women who drank heavily throughout their pregnancy, nearly one-third (32%) were found to have some congenital abnormality. Among moderate drinkers the risk was 14 percent, and in nondrinkers it was 8 percent. There were no differences between the three groups of newborns in infant mortality or in Apgar score—a screening measure of neonatal respiratory state. Nor could the high rate of abnormality in the mothers who drank heavily be attributed to nutritional deficiencies, a common problem in alcoholism, as all three groups of mothers were comparable in their nutritional status. Neuropediatric examination of these babies by physicians who were unaware of the drinking history of the mother ("blind" diagnosis to assure objectivity) revealed higher frequencies of jitteriness (29%), small size for gestational age (27%), hypotonia and prematurity (17%), and diminished sucking ability (12%).

The growth deficiency noted in connection with heroin and methadone addiction is also seen here. Babies of heavy drinkers were smaller in length and head size. Of the 42, five (12%) had microcephaly itself whereas only 1 in 274 of the remaining infants (0.4%) was so affected. As in the case of heroin or methadone use, reduction in alcohol intake during pregnancy appeared to have real benefits. Of the 15 women who reduced their drinking while pregnant, 10 bore healthy babies (67%), and only two of the 27 babies of the women who did not alter their drinking were unaffected (7%).

Heavy drinking during the first trimester was seen as producing the greatest risk. Indeed, the very earliest period of pregnancy, even prior to awareness that one *is* pregnant—up to the first 6 weeks—seems to carry the greatest risk (Clarren & Smith, 1978; Landesman-Dwyer, Ragozine, & Little, 1981). One study found that reduction of alcohol intake during this period was more predictive of future status than the amount consumed during pregnancy (Landesman-Dwyer et al., 1981).

A study was conducted of the children of moderate drinkers (2–4 oz per day) in the immediate neonatal period and at age 4 years. In the newborn one saw increased body tremors, a lowered activity level, and a dazed expression. At age 4 the only residual effects were a slightly shorter attention span, a little more fidgetiness, and a little less compliance (Landesman-Dwyer et al., 1981).

There is no doubt that heavy drinking during pregnancy much increases the risk of major fetal abnormality and that even the moderate drinker seems to bear a slightly higher risk (Clarren & Smith, 1978; Hanson, Streissguth, & Smith, 1978; Landesman-Dwyer et al, 1981).

Intellectual Impairment

While research indicates that retardation will be found in at least those children with microcephaly, a larger series of children is necessary to assess the impact on mental development of maternal alcoholism during pregnancy. In studies reported to date, children with the full-blown syndrome are likely to fall in the mildly retarded range (IQ ~ 55), whereas those with lesser degrees of physical abnormality average about IQ 80 (Jones & Smith, 1975; Streissguth, Herman, & Smith, 1978). There is no question that heavy drinking during pregnancy increases future risk of impairment in intellectual functioning.

Learning Problems in Children of Normal Intelligence

Even in children with fetal alcohol syndrome and normal intelligence, school learning difficulties seem to be prominent (Shaywitz, Cohen, & Shaywitz, 1980). In a series of 15, ages 6–18, all had histories of hyperactivity, short attention span, and distractibility. These are behaviors commonly associated with organic brain disorders in children (Strauss & Kephart, 1947) and with "learning disability" (Johnson & Myklebust, 1967; Bannatyne, 1974). They also all had some degree of fine motor incoordination.

OTHER TERATOGENIC DRUGS

Drugs used for medical purposes may also damage the fetus. Reference was made earlier to thalidomide. Quinine can cause deafness, and anticonvulsant drugs (e.g., Dilantin) can produce abnormalities. The so-called *fetal hydantoin syndrome* occurs in about 10 percent of the offspring of epileptic women and, like the fetal alcohol syndrome, includes growth impairment at both the physical and intellectual levels (Hanson, Myrianthopoulos, Harvey, & Smith, 1976; Hill, Vermand, Horning, McCulley, Morgan, & Houston, 1974). Since the drug cannot be discontinued, management involves informing the woman of the risk and ensuring that she is receiving the minimum dosage necessary to control her seizures. The drug appears to increase the risk of spontaneous abortion, and in one study half of the surviving children had some features of the syndrome (Smith, 1983).

Other anticonvulsants with teratogenic effects are trimethadione or paramethadione (Gal & Sharpless, 1984; German, Kowal, & Ehlers, 1970; Zackai, Mellman, Neiderer, & Hanson, 1975). More than 80 percent of fetuses exposed to trimethadione either have been spontaneously aborted or were born malformed (Moss, Wyatt, & Flora, 1982). A commonly used anticoagulant, warfarin (Coumadin), has been strongly linked to fetal defects (Bonnar, 1981; Hall, Pauli, & Wilson, 1980; Smith, 1976) and aspirin, that most widely used of medications, poses some risks of lung disorders in neonates.

TOBACCO

Although there is no direct evidence of an adverse effect of maternal tobacco smoking during pregnancy on later mental development, research does indicate increased pregnancy risks that could be associated with neurological abnormality and cognitive impairment.

The initial study on the effects of cigarette smoking during pregnancy (Simpson, 1957) found an increased risk of prematurity in the newborn (birth weight of less than 2500 g). Numerous studies reveal that birth weights are reduced in proportion to the number of cigarettes smoked (Meyer & Tonascia, 1977).

There is now evidence that maternal smoking also indirectly increases the risk of early fetal death and of neonatal death due to prematurity. These deaths are associated with smoking-related increases in several complications of pregnancy: bleeding, abruptio placentae, placenta previa, and premature and prolonged rupture of the membranes (Meyer & Tonascia, 1977; Naeye, 1978).

Interestingly, the adverse effects of smoking are thought to generally relate less to nicotine than to hypoxia (diminished oxygen supply) (Meyer & Tonascia, 1977). Cigarette smoke contains about 4 percent carbon monoxide, and hemoglobin, the oxygen-carrying cell, has a much greater affinity for carbon monoxide than for oxygen. The overall effect is to diminish the oxygenating capacity of hemoglobin.

Studies on the long-term effects of fetal exposure have found conflicting results, some finding none (Hardy & Mellits, 1972), others reporting reduced growth, school learning problems (Butler & Goldstein, 1973), and increased behavior difficulties (Dunn, McBurney, Ingram, & Hunter, 1977). Effects that have been found tend to be limited to low–birth weight children of smoking mothers, but even here reported growth retardation appear to be limited to weight and length and *not* to head size (Holsclaw & Topnam, 1978; Naeye, 1981). Gal and Sharpless (1984) conclude that direct evidence of fetal damage caused by smoking has yet to be shown. What is clear, however, is that the increased risk of growth retardation and low birth weight renders the fetus more vulnerable to other biological hazards.

Radiation

The teratogenic effects of radiation have long been known. Early studies found that women who were receiving therapeutic pelvic irradiation for cancer during early pregnancy have an increased risk of having children with microcephaly and mental retardation (Murphy, Shirlock, & Doll, 1942; Rugh, 1958). The same clinical picture was seen in pregnant women exposed to radiation in the atomic bombing of Hiroshima (Wood, Johnson, & Yoshiaki, 1967). It is now recognized that even low levels of radiation during pregnancy, especially in the first trimester, can be harmful. It also increases the risk of leukemia and other cancers in children (National Research Council, 1972). There is evidence that radiation prior to pregnancy can increase the likelihood of later spontaneous abortion associated with chromosomal abnormality (Alberman, Polani, Roberts, Spicer, Elliott, Armstrong, & Dhadial, 1972). Since most of our radiation exposure is through medical treatment, prevention of these problems requires careful use of X ray in pregnancy and throughout the childbearing years (Sells & Bennett, 1977).

Chronic Maternal Health Problems

We earlier described a series of maternal infectious disorders that can be injurious to fetal development, such as rubella. But there are also at least two noninfectious and chronic health problems that can threaten the health of the fetus—hypertension and diabetes.

HYPERTENSION

In hypertensive disorders, high blood pressure affects the circulation to the uterus and may either interfere with the development of a normal placenta or cause it to undergo degenerative change. In either case, the fetus is deprived of adequate blood supply, either causing in utero death or impairing general growth and development. Hypertensive disease is a particular problem in the *last* trimester of pregnancy and is a major cause of maternal death and fetal loss.

DIABETES

The diabetic mother, whether the diabetes is chronic or gestational in nature, also creates fetal risks. She is much more susceptible to hypertension and to its potential placental circulatory problems. Diabetic women also tend to bear babies who are very large and yet have physiologically immature lungs. Their large size and immaturity can lead to problems of brain damage. This will be discussed later in a section on the "overgrown infant." Apart from brain damage itself, there is some indication that diabetic women who are not adequately controlled during pregnancy will bear offspring whose general level of intellectual functioning is reduced by an average of about nine IQ points relative to children of well-controlled ones (Churchill, Berendes, & Nemore, 1969).

OTHER HAZARDS

Together with these disorders, poor maternal nutrition during pregnancy increases the risk of a premature baby and, as will be seen in the following section, carries special vulnerability to serious health problems. Finally, maternal stress has been suggested as a possible noxious influence on the fetus, and at least one study has linked chronic and severe stress during pregnancy to physical and psychological problems in childhood (Stott, 1973). At this point, there is no evidence that the transient episodes of stress that we all experience are detrimental to the fetus.

PERINATAL HAZARDS

In terms of health, the first 28 days of life are the most important period in childhood. This is the time of greatest infant mortality, but it is also a period during which sublethal damage from perinatal events is frequent. Brain injury suffered during labor or delivery or neonatally causes a large proportion of the neurological problems which later manifest themselves as cerebral palsy, deafness and/or mental retardation (Phibbs, 1977b).

Prematurity

Of the factors associated with either neonatal mortality or chronic brain injury, abnormalities of birth weight and gestational age, typically prematurity, are of particular importance. The premature infant has been traditionally defined as either born before 38 weeks of gestation or having a birth weight of less than $5\frac{1}{2}$ pounds (2500 g). About 7–10 percent of births are "premature" but its frequency varies with the sex of the child and with race and socioeconomic status of the mother. Prematurity is twice as frequent in nonwhites as in whites—14 percent versus 7 percent. This difference is largely attributable to prenatal care, the risk being three times greater in those with no or inadequate[3] prenatal care (Levine, Carey, Crocker, & Gross, 1983). Although this population has been declining, it still constitutes about 15 percent of pregnant women in poverty areas (Gortmaker, 1979). Maternal health problems and dietary deficiency are specific major causes of prematurity. Other factors for which at least a statistical risk have been identified are heavy cigarette smoking and extremes of maternal age—either under 18 or over 35. Interestingly, too little weight gain during pregnancy can be a problem, indicating undernutrition of the fetus.

---

[3]Failure to have a medical examination in the first 13 weeks of pregnancy and to have less than five such visits subsequently.

GENERAL VULNERABILITY

Of neonatal deaths, 75 percent are prematures; they also have a threefold greater risk of suffering neurological damage (Niswander & Gordon, 1972). Even in prematures without obvious signs of abnormality, some trend toward depression of intellectual function has been reported (Weiner, Rider, Oppel, Fischer, & Harper, 1965). The health problems of the premature neonate tend to be proportional to the degree of prematurity. For example, among children whose birth weight was less than 3 pounds (1300 g), 58 percent later had IQs of less than 80, and 70 percent were educationally handicapped (Drillien, 1967). The outlook for normal development improves with birth weight for any given gestational age and is also enhanced by greater gestational age at any birth weight (Lubchenko, Delivoria-Papadapolous, & Searls, 1972).

The vulnerability of the premature infant lies in the fact that it must adapt to extrauterine conditions with some organ systems that are not physiologically ready to do so. The premature neonate may be unable to maintain body temperature or to suck and swallow adequate amounts of food. The infant will grow more jaundiced and will be increasingly susceptible to the neurotoxic effects of unmetabolized bilirubin. This is the substance discussed earlier in terms of hemolytic disease and can be injurious to the brain. The premature newborn is also more prone to oxygen deprivation during the birth process (intrapartum asphyxia) and to respiratory failure after birth because of immature lung structure or function. Cardiac abnormalities may also be present. Some of these problems demand oxygen therapy, but the incompletely developed blood vessels in the retina of the eye are vulnerable to the effects of oxygen. Prior to the 1950s, premature infants were inadvertently blinded (retrolental fibroplasia) by the oxygen given in incubators intended to sustain them. The brain of the premature is also subject to hemorrhage because of structural weakness of cerebral blood vessels and coagulation abnormalities. Finally, the premature infant is more susceptible to infections (Phibbs, 1977).

TYPES OF PREMATURITY

There are actually two kinds of premature infants: those who are small only because of a gestation age of less than 38 weeks but whose weight is appropriate to their age and those who are small in weight for gestion age per se. It is the latter who are of special concern, as their small size reflects inadequate intrauterine growth.

There are two primary causes of intrauterine growth retardation: (a) impairment of the potential for normal growth associated with earlier-described chromosomal abnormalities, exposure to toxins, and intrauterine infection, and (b) restriction of a normal potential due to such factors as multiple pregnancies or placental vascular disease as in diabetes or hypertension. The former, so-called type I prematurity, is particularly associated with neurological abnormality and mental retardation. Here, either the abnormality has been present since conception, as in the case of a chromosomal defect, or a normal fetus has been exposed to a noxious environment (e.g., rubella infection) during the period from conception to 24 weeks of gestation age. The decreased potential for growth in these prematures is reflected in an *actual reduction* in the number of cells in most organs. At birth these infants are more than 2 standard deviations below the mean for their gestational age in weight, length, and head circumference. It is the much-reduced head size that indicates abnormal brain development.

Types II and III prematurity are less dangerous and are associated with a normal growth potential exposed to an adverse environment *after* 24 weeks of age. In type II, there is chronic fetal malnutrition which occurs during the 24th to 32nd weeks of gestation. This results from abnormal blood supply in the placenta caused by such maternal conditions as toxemia, hypertension, severe diabetes, and renal disease. In type III, the fetal malnutrition is limited to the period after the 32nd week of gestation and may be caused by a blockage in the placenta (placental infarction) or a lowered oxygen level in the mother (hypoxia) resulting from such factors as exposure to high altitude or from cyanotic cardiac or pulmonary disease. Here the fetal deprivation is acute rather than chronic. Type II and III prematures have normal numbers of cells, though these may be reduced in size. After birth these infants usually have normal physical growth and mental development. Although they are small for gestational age, unlike type I prematures, head size is usually close to average for gestational age. They do have an increased risk of infection in both infancy and early childhood. Type III prematures, the least affected of the three, show average length but are underweight. Their scrawny appearance is said to suggest recent weight loss (Gaston, 1977).

The Overgrown Newborn

Although it is the very small infant who is of major concern among newborns with abnormal birth weights, some neonates present problems due to very large birth weight. The "overgrown" newborn is one whose weight exceeds the 90th percentile for gestational age. Interestingly, many such infants are also born prematurely. Some of these large-for-gestational-age infants are perfectly normal. Their size derives from large parents, size having a considerable genetic component. Others, however, combine large size with abnormalities of organ systems and tissue, especially the lungs. The most common cause of abnormal size is maternal diabetes, either specifically associated with pregnancy (gestational diabetes) or chronic in nature. Prior to insulin, diabetic women seldom produced viable offspring, and spontaneous abortion, stillbirth, and neonatal death were common. The current outlook is, of course, much brighter. Nevertheless, a mild or moderate degree of diabetes leads to a large fetus and to increased risk of perinatal death. Where the diabetes is severe and is associated with serious vascular placental disease, one is likely to see a small-for-gestational-age newborn—the type II form of prematurity. From a retardation standpoint, the major risk is of too low blood sugar in the infant (hypoglycemia). This is presumed to result from prenatal exposure to at least intermittent episodes of high maternal blood sugar levels (hyperglycemia) to which the fetus responds with an overproduction of insulin. Hence, too little blood sugar may be present in the newborn, and this can lead to brain damage and retardation (Ballard, 1977).

Asphyxia and Physical Trauma

ASPHYXIA

While the roles of perinatal asphyxia (oxygen deprivation, or hypoxemia) and physical trauma as causes of brain damage have probably been exaggerated in the past, these hazards are still important (Chamberlin, 1975). Asphyxia is a leading cause of death in very small infants, those with birth weights of less than 1000 g ($\sim$ 2 lb) (Behrman, 1973). On the other hand, the healthy newborn is said to be remarkably resistive to it *if* there has been no prior brain damage. It is evident, however, that prolonged perinatal asphyxia can produce either brain damage or death. Common causes are premature separation of the placenta, prolapse of the umbilical cord, difficult labor (dystocia), depression of the respiratory center due to excessive anesthesia, and obstruction of the respiratory airway (Chamberlin, 1975).

PHYSICAL TRAUMA

Physical trauma during the birth process can result in intracranial vascular injury. While it has been greatly reduced by modern obstetric procedures, it still occurs, particularly in connection with prematurity or difficult labor. Massive brain hemorrhage is usually fatal, but small intracerebral hemorrhages can lead to motor abnormalities, seizures, and mental retardation (Chamberlin, 1975).

Herpes Infections

This is a viral infection of the genitals that is occurring with increasing frequency in pregnant women (Sells & Bennett, 1977). Following initial infection, the virus is generally quiescent within the maternal tissue until reactivated by a variety of stimuli and resulting in renewed infection. The herpes virus is extremely contagious. It is transmitted from mother to infant during childbirth with about half of the newborns affected (Nahmias et al., 1971). When the maternal infection is recognized close to the time of birth, delivery may be by cesarean section. Because of the neonate's immature immunological system, spread of the infection is common, and results in death or serious sequelae in about 80 percent of cases (Nahmias et al., 1975). Common sequelae are retardation and blindness (Nahmias & Tomeh, 1977).

POSTNATAL HAZARDS

Postnatal biological factors causing mental retardation consist of infectious diseases which affect the brain, cerebrovascular accidents (most often from head injury), brain tumors, poisons, environmental toxins, and severe dietary protein deficiency.

Infectious Diseases

There are two kinds of infections that can result in permanent neurological sequelae and mental retardation—encephalitis and meningitis. Encephalitis is inflammation of the brain, and meningitis is inflammation of the three membranes[4] that line the brain, the meninges. The diseases of particular interest here are usually of either viral or bacterial origin and occur mainly in infancy.

ENCEPHALITIS

Inflammation of the brain leads to injury to nerve cells (neurons). This may result from an initial invasion of the brain by an infectious agent (primary encephalities) or following the infection of another organ (secondary encephalitis). The major sources of primary encephalitis are the viruses of mumps, herpes simplex, and infectious mononucleosis. Mumps virus is the most common and can produce death or such permanent neurological deficits as retardation, cerebral palsy, and seizures. Among the secondary encephalitides, the most common is measles encephalitis, but it can also be associated with whooping cough (pertussis encephalitis). Measles encephalitis is a very rare complication of ordinary measles, occurring in about one in 1200 cases and usually only after severe attacks. The course of the disease is unpredictable, with about 20 percent suffering permanent damage (Hodes, 1977).

MENINGITIS

In meningitis, there is infection of the meninges with consequent inflammation and symptoms of increased intracranial pressure (fever, bulging of the fontanelles, projectile vomiting, alternating periods of drowsiness and irritability). In serious infections associated with high fever, one sees convulsions, stupor, or coma (Einhorn, 1977). With the development of antibiotics and other drugs, there has been a major reduction in mortality rate in the most serious of the meningitides, bacterial meningitis, but a sizable proportion of children affected in the first year of life are still left with crippling neuromuscular problems, hearing and visual impairments, seizures, and cognitive deficits (Sell, Merrill, Dayne, Zimsky, 1972; Sells & Bennett, 1977).

Cerebral Trauma

Among children, accidental injuries are the greatest threat to life. More than half of child deaths are due to motor vehicle accidents and, typically, with the child remaining *inside* the car. About 40 percent of all trauma cases in children involve head injuries, and some of these must also be attributable to such "nonaccidents" as child abuse. Most injuries to the head are simple concussions or mild contusions, and there is usually complete recovery without complications. The head injuries that are more serious are those that involve intracranial bleeding. Bleeding between the outermost membrane covering the brain (and spinal cord), the dura mater, and the brain itself, *subdural hematoma*, can result in cerebral atrophy and neurological deficit. Fortunately, neither organic dementia nor intellectual deficit, as such, is a common outcome of cerebral trauma. In the adult, following head injury, one may see the "posttraumatic syndrome"; its symptoms are headache,

---

[4]The outermost membrane is the dura mater, next comes the arachnoid, and then the pia mater.

irritability, and postural vertigo (dizziness). The condition is seen less often in children, and it manifests itself differently. The main symptoms are enuresis, disturbance of sleep patterns, episodically aggressive behavior, and decline in school achievement (Hammill, 1977).

Cerebrovascular Accidents

In addition to possible sequelae of intracranial bleeding due to trauma, one may also see cerebrovascular accidents. Though these are most common in older people, they are not infrequent in children. While congenital heart defects are a predisposing factor, trauma leading to subarachnoid bleeding is the most common cause of intracranial hemorrhage. Bleeding may also result from the rupture of a blood vessel malformation, an aneurysm (a pathological blood-filled swollen blood vessel), or from infections, toxins, metabolic disorders, and tumors (Gold, Hammill, & Carter, 1977).

Brain Tumors

Brain tumors are the second most common form of cancer in children, leukemia being first. The clinical picture is of increased intracranial pressure, and there may be focal neurological signs (Chatorian, 1977). In children under 2 years of age, brain tumors may go unrecognized because the visual and motor problems associated with them (e.g., visual loss and staggering gait) are erroneously attributed to developmental delay (Fessard, 1968).

Poisons and Environmental Toxins

In the earlier section on prenatal factors, reference was made to the potentially adverse environment to which a fetus might be exposed through maternal use of drugs. There are also some postnatal dangers to the brain associated with drug use. Glue sniffing has been linked to brain damage, and barbiturate abuse has been related to impairment in cognitive functioning (Casarett, 1975). The most important of the toxic dangers, however, are lead and mercury.

LEAD POISONING

Lead encephalitis is a complication of lead poisoning. It usually results from prolonged ingestion by the infant or young child of flaking leaded paint, the kind found in dilapidated housing (Lin-Fu, 1972). Daily consumption of only a few small chips for 3 months can produce lead poisoning (Challop, 1971). Most cases of acute lead encephalitis occur in children ages 1–3 years, of whom about 5 percent die and 50 percent sustain permanent brain damage (Chisolm, 1977). Federal legislation (the Lead-Based Paint Poisoning Act of 1971) has set new standards for the amount of lead allowable in toys and paints. There have also been a large number of screening programs in high-risk areas, and these show elevated blood lead levels in about 8 percent of the children. Almost two-thirds of the dwellings in these areas still have lead-paint hazards. It is also thought that automobile lead exhaust emissions may now be the largest contributor to the lead to which children are exposed (Chow & Earl, 1970).

The problem of lead exposure is not limited to the amount that results in encephalitis. Earlier workers had reported some intellectual impairment at levels considered undesirable but below that necessary to produce symptoms, so-called asymptomatic lead exposure (Gibson, Lam, & McRae, 1967; Moncrieff, Koumides, & Clayton, 1964). Subsequent studies have examined this lesser level of lead exposure, especially in children who live near lead-battery dumps or lead smelters or who are exposed to lead paint in their homes. These are children with blood lead levels of 40–80 μg/100 ml (Gregory, Lehman, & Mohan, 1976; Gregory & Mohan, 1977).

A review of this research by Milar and Schroeder (1983) indicates that where IQ effects are found they usually do not exceed six points. Nor do moderate levels of exposure produce hyperactivity (Rummo, Routh, Rummo, & Brown, 1979), a symptom seen at higher lead level exposure.

It has also been suggested that effects might be found on attention span and personality (Burde & Choat, 1975). With regard to attention span, a striking relationship was reported between lead level in *teeth* and distractibility (Needleman et al., 1979). Some researchers have begun to question the usefulness of *blood* lead level as a measure of toxicity (Chisolm, personal communication; Needleman et al., 1979).

MERCURY POISONING

Dramatic evidence of the toxic effects of some metals has also been shown for mercury. Although exposure to mercury compounds has long been known to be an occupational hazard ("mad as a hatter") (Robinson & Robinson, 1976), more recently an entire community in Japan was affected by the eating of shellfish contaminated by mercury waste products that had been dumped by a new plant into a local stream. Serious neurological problems followed involving memory, skin sensation, vision, gait, and emotional stability. In the younger children were found cerebral palsy and intellectual impairment (Miller, 1967). In addition to these effects, mercury consumption by pregnant women has been tied to prenatal brain damage (Beliles, 1975; Koos & Longo, 1976).

Malnutrition

One of the most perplexing questions in retardation has been the role of malnutrition on mental development. In our own country it has been suggested that the poorer intellectual functioning and school achievement of disadvantaged children is attributable to malnutrition, although the degree of dietary deficiency observed is not regarded as of sufficient severity to affect brain growth and mental development.

Malnutrition is humankind's most pervasive health problem. It is estimated that at least half of the children in developing countries are moderately or severely undernourished—with basic *caloric* deprivation as the primary problem.

DEGREES OF MALNUTRITION

About 5 percent of the world's children know severe malnutrition. It has two clinical manifestations—*kwashiorkor*, or protein deficiency, and *marasmus*, or overall food (calorie) deficit. Marasmus results in a wasting away of tissues and extreme growth retardation. Kwashiorkor usually occurs after weaning, when milk, which is high in protein, is replaced by high-starch but low protein food. The clinical picture in kwashiorkor is usually of stunted growth, edema (accumulation of water), skin sores, and reduced hair pigmentation. *Moderate malnutrition* is usually related to general food deprivation and results in some growth retardation. There are also specific vitamin or mineral deficits that can produce such diseases as rickets or pellagra. In the United States, marasmus and kwashiorkor are quite rare, but about 20 percent of our children are undernourished; that is, they consume less than the recommended daily calorie minimum. This condition affects nearly one-third of our low-income families. Fortunately, however, virtually all these children are getting a sufficient amount of protein, and it is this foodstuff that is most closely linked to brain growth and mental development (National Institute of Child Health and Human Development, 1976).

BRAIN DEVELOPMENT

There are two growth spurts in the development of the human brain. The first occurs in the second trimester of pregnancy and is associated with an increase in the number of neurons. The second spurt begins in the third trimester and continues on through about age 6 months. During this period the supporting cells of the nervous system (glia) multiply, and branches (dendrites) from the neurons grow to form connections with other neurons (synapses). Animal studies are commonly cited as illustrating how nutritional deprivation retards brain growth and can cause retardation. But in the rat, for example, a degree of nutritional deprivation equivalent to a 40 percent reduction in weight gain is necessary before permanent neurological deficits occur. Such growth curtailment in man is rarely seen except in marasmus or kwashiorkor or in low–birth weight babies who fail to grow adequately after birth.

Research efforts to relate malnutrition specifically to intellectual impairment have been continually confounded by the fact that malnutrition usually does not occur alone but rather in combination with other biological and psychological hazards to normal mental development. For example, infectious diseases may be the most important cause of malnutrition (Das & Pivato, 1976). The malnourished child has limited resistance to infection, and the infection itself aggravates nutritional stress by elevating calorie requirements (Birch & Cravioto, 1966). In the psychological realm, there is some indication that the amount of home stimulation of the infant may affect nutritional state (Cravioto & Delicardie, 1972).

Two studies of children with *severe* malnutrition in the first 2 years of life have noted intellectual deficits relative to sibs (Birch, Pinuro, Atchalde, Toca, & Cravioto; 1971; Hertzig, Birch, Richardson, & Tizard, 1972). In the first of these, it was severe malnutrition during the first 6 months that was regarded as particularly damaging, although in the Hertzig study, no differential age effect was noted. It would appear that survivors of kwashiorkor or marasmus *in infancy* do show some adverse effects on cognitive functioning in later childhood. Whether such differences are irreversible is another matter. In a study of nondisadvantaged children whose nutritional problems were related to the digestive disease cystic fibrosis, cognitive differences between them and their unaffected sibs were found in the preschool years only; they were no longer present in adolescence or adulthood (Lloyd-Hill, Hurwitz, Wolf, & Shwachman, 1974). Although this study is cited as illuminating the role of early malnutrition on mental development without the confounding influence of family factors, the degree and type of nutritional deficiency associated with it are not comparable to those in kwashiorkor or marasmus.

In summary, while severe malnutrition in infancy does have at least temporary effects on mental development, the long-range consequences are yet to be determined. At lesser levels of malnutrition (e.g., chronic undernourishment), there is as yet no evidence of specific damage to brain function and general intelligence. What continues to be clear is that the environment that fails to meet minimum nutritional requirements is also often lacking in the kind of conditions that more broadly foster mental development and school achievement. This is addressed in the following chapter.

MAJOR NEUROLOGICAL DISORDERS OFTEN ASSOCIATED WITH MENTAL RETARDATION: CEREBRAL PALSY AND EPILEPSY

Cerebral Palsy

DEFINITION
Cerebral palsy refers to a group of disorders of movement and posture caused by a nonprogressive brain lesion (Box, 1964). Together with the motor disability, there are commonly found mental retardation, epilepsy, and sensory disorder. Cortical, subcortical (basal ganglia), or cerebellar pathways may be involved and determine the kinds of motor symptoms seen. The incidence is about 1–2 per 1000 births (Molnar & Taft, 1973).

ETIOLOGY
Cerebral palsy is most often associated with perinatal brain injury, but it may also originate in prenatal or postnatal events. During the prenatal period, the kinds of fetal stresses described earlier can cause permanent motor impairment—infections, trauma, toxemias, radiation, and blood incompatibilities. The syndrome can also result from faulty implantation of the ovum or from maternal disease. In the perinatal period, asphyxia and cerebral hemorrhage are the major determiners. The former is considered to be the most common cause of brain injury. In either case, the premature newborn is particularly vulnerable; even full-term but small-for-gestational-age babies are especially susceptible. In the neonatal period, excessive levels of bilirubin (kernicterus) are one of the causes of the athetoid form of the disorder. Kernicterus-caused cerebral palsy is associated with hearing loss and eye-muscle weakness as well as with retardation. Finally, in the postnatal years, infections such as meningitis and encephalitis can cause cerebral palsy as will arterial blockages (Low, 1977).

FORMS OF CEREBRAL PALSY

There are a variety of motor problems in cerebral palsy—weakness, paralysis, incoordination, involuntary movements, and imbalance. The variation in motor symptoms is the basis for three broad categories of relatively "pure" forms—spastic, dyskinetic (athetoid), and ataxic—and a fourth "mixed forms."

Spastic Cerebral Palsy

This is the predominant variant (Low, 1977, Molnar & Taft, 1973, Peterson, 1972), accounting for about two-thirds of all cases. The clinical picture is of muscular stiffness in the limbs (high muscle tone); movement is slow, made with much effort, and its range is limited. Occasionally, movements are jerky and explosive (Fleming, 1973; Peterson, 1972). The cause of the extreme muscle rigidity is that muscle flexors and extensors do not work reciprocally. Instead of extensors relaxing when flexors are contracting and vice versa, they are both in constant flexion. The brain lesion that causes spasticity is in the *pyramidal tract*, the motor pathways that descend from the cortex and control voluntary movement. Within the spastic form there are a number of subvarieties distinguished by the number and laterality of the limbs affected. In *hemiplegia* there is involvement of the limbs on one side and with the arm usually more affected than the leg, in *tetraplegia* (or quadriplegia) there is involvement of all limbs to the same degree, in *diplegia* there is involvement of all four limbs but with greater impairment of the legs than the arms, in *paraplegia* both legs are affected but without involvement of the arms, and *monoplegia* and *triplegia* are rare subforms involving one and three limbs, respectively. In the latter, one arm is usually unaffected (Low, 1977).

Dyskinetic Cerebral Palsies

In this group there is impairment of motion caused by uncontrolled and purposeless movements. They disappear during sleep. Muscle tone varies from tense to flaccid. The lesion is in the basal ganglia, affects the extrapyramidal motor tract, and accounts for about a third of the cerebral palsies. The most common type of movement is *athetosis*. This a relatively slow, wormlike, writhing movement which usually involves all four limbs, as well as the face and neck to a lesser degree. When these movements have a jerky element they are dubbed choreic, and the term *choreoathetosis* is applied. In addition to these two main forms, lesser variants are dystonia (above-average muscle tonus), tremors, and rigidity. The dyskinesias usually involve all four limbs, and the involuntary movements tend to be exaggerated during volitional activity.

Ataxic Cerebral Palsy

This is the rarest of the three major forms and accounts for about one-tenth of all cases. Its cause is a lesion of the cerebellum or its pathways. The motor picture is of poor balance while standing and walking. Gait is wide based, and there is difficulty in turning rapidly. There are also difficulties in performing fast, repetitive finger movements. This form has the best prognosis for functional improvement (Low, 1977).

Mixed Forms

Symptoms of more than one type are found. The most common combination is spasticity and athetosis; less frequent is that of ataxia and athetosis.

ASSOCIATED CONDITIONS

Speech

The most common abnormality associated with cerebral palsy is speech. About 75 percent have some impairment with the highest rates, about 90 percent, in those with the athetoid and ataxic forms. Speech problems are manifest in articulation, voice quality, and rhythm. There is special difficulty in pronouncing the sounds of *s, z, th, ch,* and *r*; the voice has a hoarse, harsh, or breathy quality, and speech is rendered in a monotone (Lundeen, 1972). For those whose speech is unintelligible, there is now use of "communication boards" on which are shown words, pictures, or symbols that the "speaker" can denote by pointing (e.g., Bliss symbols).

Intelligence

The assessment of intelligence in persons with cerebral palsy has always been a problem because of the impairment in expressive language and in general motor ability. The capacity to respond at either the verbal or motor level is simply more restricted. Within these limitations, studies have typically found retardation in about half of the population (Stephen & Hawks, 1974), with the remainder equally distributed among those with borderline and normal intelligence (Taylor, 1959). With reference to the long-term stability (reliability) of IQs in cerebral palsy, a 14-year follow-up study indicated good reliability for scores in the normal and severely/profoundly retarded ranges. More variability was found for IQs in the intermediate ranges of borderline and mild retardation (Klapper & Birch, 1967). Within the various forms, those with ataxia and dyskinesis (athetoid) are the least impaired; a higher frequency of retardation is found in spastics, and the greatest impairment is seen in mixed forms. Although all combinations of physical and mental ability are found, it is suggested that the combination of severity of motor deficit *and* seizures seems most predictive of the degree of retardation (Molnar & Taft, 1973).

Other

Following speech and intellectual impairment, *seizures* are the third most frequently associated condition. They are found in about one-third of cases. Seizures are more common in the postnatally acquired forms and are especially prominent in those with spastic hemiplegia. They are less common in other spastic variants and in the dyskinetic and ataxic forms (Low, 1977). *Visual* problems are seen in about a quarter of the cases; these consist of strabismus, refractive errors, and defects of the visual field. *Deafness* due to auditory nerve damage is found in athetosis caused by kernicteris, and impairment of *tactile* perception is seen in spastic hemiplegics who also have some involvement of the parietal lobes. They have difficulty in recognizing the size and shape of an object by touch (stereognosis) and in identifying stimulated areas on the skin when it is simultaneously touched at two different points (Molnar & Taft, 1973).

TREATMENT

The treatment of cerebral palsy involves procedures designed to reduce the degree of motor disability. They comprise straightforward exercises, the use of reflex therapies (e.g., Bobath method of inhibiting and activating postural reflexes), training in functional activities, and surgery for contractures. (For more details see Chap. 7). Early treatment, especially before age 1 year, is considered vital. Since the commencement of treatment depends on recognition of the disease within a context of delayed motor development, it is important to distinguish between motor delay due to cerebral palsy and that which may relate only to mental retardation. The distinguishing feature of cerebral palsy is the persistence and predominance of reflexes that are normal in early infancy but which generally disappear by about age 6 months, especially the *tonic neck* and *tonic labyrinthine* reflexes. Their persistence is seen as a cause of motor impairment, because they interfere with the appearance of the automatic postural reactions of righting and balance which are necessary to controlled motor activities.

Where motor symptoms are only minimal, persistence of primitive reflexes may not be found. Instead there may be a delay in the acquisition of the automatic postural reactions (Molnar, 1978).

THE CEREBRAL PALSIED ADULT

In spite of the multiplicity of disabilities, from a third to a half of those with spastic hemplegia achieve independence as adults (Crothers & Paine, 1959). Many who do not attain independence are capable of employment, though primarily in sheltered work settings. The regularly employed individual tends to differ from those in sheltered employment by having better speech, gait, hand function, and general mobility (Garrett, 1966; Moed & Litwin, 1963). One of the greatest aids to maximizing the adaptive potential of these individuals is to avoid overprotecting them. Rather, they should be exposed to as wide a variety of experiences as possible. And if you take the time, you discover that inside the outer shell of motor abnormality is a person who has the same needs for intimacy, success, and autonomy as you and I.[5]

Epilepsy

DEFINITION

Epilepsy refers to recurrent paroxysmal attacks associated with altered states of consciousness and, usually, a succession of *tonic* (stiffness) or *clonic* (jerking) muscular spasms. In addition, these attacks (seizures, fits, convulsions) may also

---

[5]The British documentary film *Like Other People* is highly recommended as a way of discovering what persons with cerebral palsy are "really like."

include abnormal sensory experiences and disturbances of intellectual, behavioral, and vegetative functions. Seizures have the quality of sudden onset and spontaneous cessation. They may be found as isolated episodes in infants with high fever (hyperthermia) and never recur. It is only the *recurrence* of seizures that is termed epilepsy.

AGE

Epilepsy is primarily a disorder of childhood, its peak onset being in the age range of 4–10 years. It tends to disappear by the end of adolescence. This age range is particularly true of epilepsy that is apparently of genetic (idiopathic) origin as distinguished from that caused by some metabolic disorder or underlying brain lesion (symptomatic). In the latter, seizures may occur *before* age 2 years. In the young adult with no prior history of convulsions, seizures are seldom seen except when caused by trauma, drug abuse (particularly alcohol), or infection. After age 35 years their onset may be due to vascular disease or brain tumor.

PHYSIOLOGICAL NATURE

The seizure itself results from abnormal electrical neuron discharge in the brain. This activity, normal as well as abnormal, can be recorded on the electroencephalogram (EEG), and the resultant electrical wave pattern in epilepsy has been shown to correlate with the types of seizures seen. Both the EEG and pneumoencephalography (brain air study) are used as diagnostic procedures in epilepsy (Chao, Carter, & Gold, 1977).

CAUSATION

We have already noted the distinction between idiopathic and symptomatic epilepsies. In the former, there is a small but significant pattern of familial occurrence and an absence of demonstrable structural lesion in the brain. The risk in first-degree relatives, parents and sibs, of persons with the idiopathic form is about 2–4 percent (Neel & Schull, 1954; Reed, 1955) as contrasted with a general prevalence in the population of less than 1 percent. Twin data, too, show high frequencies of similarly affected persons in identical twin pairs (concordance of about 67–85%) whereas among fraternal twin pairs, the concordance rates are much lower, varying from 3 to 24 percent (Falek & Glanville, 1962). The difference in concordance rates is consistent with a genetic determinant. In the symptomatic group, seizures are associated with specific metabolic errors or organic brain pathology (Chao, Carter, & Gold, 1977). In the production of a seizure the structural or metabolic lesion in the brain serves as a focus for the initiation of abnormal electrical activity. The neuronal discharge and its behavioral effects may be localized and involve only isolated organ systems or may spread and involve the entire body. Interestingly, there is even some indication that vulnerability to symptomatic epilepsy has a genetic basis. It appears that heredity affects susceptibility to seizure at the level of our basic EEG pattern (Lennox, Gibbs, & Gibbs, 1945). A given biological stress will have different probabilities for resulting in seizure depending on that underlying pattern. This is the same kind of heredity-environment interaction that will be described in terms of intelligence in the next chapter.

TYPES OF SEIZURES

Seizures vary from virtually imperceptible, brief lapses of consciousness to violent, generalized convulsions lasting several minutes.

Generalized Convulsions

The most common form of seizures is the generalized convulsion or grand mal attack. The classic grand mal seizure is sudden in onset, although some are typically preceded by an *aura*—a subjective sensation, olfactory or visual, which the person learns to recognize as a warning that the attack is imminent. With the attack there is an immediate loss of consciousness and a stiffening of the body. There may be a sharp loud cry caused by the muscles of the larynx which, like the rest of the body, go into sudden contraction (tonic phase). If standing, the person falls forcibly to the ground—hence the name given to the condition by Hippocrates, "the falling sickness." The pupils dilate, eyes roll up to one side, and the face becomes pale or flushed. The change in skin color is due to tonic interference with breathing. Spastic contraction of the respiratory muscles produces a brief period of oxygen deprivation. After some 10–30 seconds the tonic phase is replaced by spasmodic rhythmical jerking of the entire muscular system (clonic phase). This can last for from 1 to 5 minutes or longer. Breathing resumes but is labored, and there may be profuse perspiration and salivation. The tongue may be bitten, and in severe attacks there is sometimes involuntary bladder and bowel evacuation. Gradually the attack diminishes; the muscle contractions become less violent and finally cease. If the episode is of short duration there may be a quick recovery of conciousness with little or no aftereffect. More usually, there is a stuporous state which is followed by sleep for at least an hour. After awakening there may be headache, fatigue, and restlessness. One also may see transient neurologic abnormalities. These can be helpful in the localizing of a focal lesion.

Grand mal seizures vary greatly in frequency, duration, and intensity. Occasionally they occur so frequently that one attack is barely ended before another begins. This condition of continuous grand mal seizure is called *status epilepticus* and, if not treated promptly and effectively, may persist for hours or even days. It can produce exhaustion, severe anoxia, or brain hemorrhage; there may be serious sequelae or even death. It is regarded as a medical emergency.

A grand mal variant in which there is unconsciousness and body stiffness but no jerking is called the *tonic seizure*. Unlike the classic grand mal, there is no clonic phase.

Focal Seizures

Here the initial symptoms of a seizure indicate a specific point of origin in the brain. The abnormal electrical discharge may originate anywhere in the brain; it may remain confined to the hemisphere of origin (and stay localized) or it may spread across the midline of the brain to the opposite hemisphere and become generalized. The symptoms of these seizures may be either motor or sensory.

Focal motor seizures either involve muscles on one entire side of the body (hemiconvulsive) or are limited to an extremity and/or the face. The best known of these, Jacksonian epilepsy, originates in one part of the motor cortex and then spreads to the rest of the cortical motor region. The usual points of origin are the thumb, face, and toe—structures having relatively large areas of cortical representation. In *focal sensory seizures*, there are numbness and tingling. The sensation originates in the sensory cortex but may spread to the motor cortex and result in motor seizures. In *focal adversive seizures*, there are loss of consciousness and a turning of the head, eyes, and trunk away from the side of the cerebral lesion from which it originates. *Occipital seizures* produce simple visual impressions, such as dimness, shadows or clouds in front of the eyes, or a temporary blindness. *Inhibitory seizures* result in paralysis rather than in motor activity.

Psychomotor seizures are the most common type of focal seizures in childhood. They usually originate in the temporal lobe (temporal lobe epilepsy) and manifest as a drawing and jerking of mouth and face. This form of epilepsy is notable for some extraordinary behavioral effects. The eyes may stare in a searching manner, there may be a tonic posturing (as in catatonic psychosis), or there may be a desire to urinate. Most remarkable, they can produce what may appear to be complex voluntary movements. These pseudopurposeful movements (automatisms) are performed in a repetitive and stereotyped manner—clutching, fumbling, kicking, walking or running in circles, swallowing, smacking, chewing, licking, spitting. Pill rolling, athetoid, or flinging movements are less commonly observed. Affective behavior such as laughing or crying are not unusual, and one may also see outbursts of aggression. The onset of psychomotor epilepsy is highest in the 3- to 6-year age range.

Petit Mal

These seizures consist of abrupt and momentary lapses of consciousness accompanied by a cessation of voluntary activity. The child shows a blank expression and stares into space. These episodes rarely exceed 5–15 seconds and end as abruptly as they begin. The child recovers his senses and resumes activities as if nothing had occurred. Petit mal seizures are often referred to by those involved with the child as "staring attacks," "little absences," or "little blackouts." There is usually no aura or any postseizure difficulty. In from 60 to 70 percent some myoclonic movement is seen, the most common being a slow rhythmical blinking of the eyes and rhythmical jerking of the head, arms, or trunk. The child rarely falls or loses bladder control. Some petit mal episodes include automatisms such as snapping of fingers, patting movements, or walking around or in circles.

The frequency of these attacks varies tremendously, from an occasional one to hundreds per day. Keeping the child interested in activities appears to reduce their frequency. The age of peak onset is 4–10 years, and there is a slightly higher prevalence in girls. They tend to decrease with time and, in about half the cases, completely disappear in the late teens. From one-third to one-half of children with petit mal also have grand mal seizures, with the former usually appearing first. Ordinarily there are no long-term mental or physical consequences of petit mal epilepsy.

Minor Motor Seizures

In akinetic seizures (drop fits), there is a sudden loss of muscle tone. It may be limited to the neck muscles and result in bobbing of the head; more usually, the entire body is affected, and the child simply collapses. These attacks are so abrupt and unexpected that there is no warning, and, with frequencies that can reach hundreds per day, serious physical injury is a constant threat. These seizures usually occur in symptomatic epilepsy, and their onset is much earlier than in the idiopathic form. The cause is commonly unknown, but the history often suggests a diffuse brain disease (e.g., measles encephalitis) or other viral diseases and toxins. It is also seen in tuberous sclerosis (see Chap. 3). As a rule, the course of the condition is protracted, and some intellectual impairment usually exists.

Myoclonic epilepsies are clonic spasms of an isolated muscle or group of muscles. They may occur in the genetic epilepsies, in association with either petit mal or grand mal seizures. More severe myoclonic seizures are frequent in symptomatic epilepsies incident to either progressive or nonprogressive brain disease. In the latter, they are seen in the age range of 2–6 years, and residual neurologic deficit is common.

Infantile spasms (massive myoclonic spasms) are seizures peculiar to infants. They consist of sudden flexion or extension, following a cry, and are also referred to as "lightning" or "jackknife" seizures. They may occur in apparently normally developing infants or in those with obvious abnormality since birth. In the latter, one may find a history of prenatal, natal, or postnatal cerebral insult. These seizures usually arise in the first 3–6 months of life; onset after 2 years is uncommon. The course of the condition is protracted, with a gradual reduction in spasms over a period of months to years. Occasionally, they are replaced by focal, grand mal, or other minor motor seizures. Coincident with their onset, there is either an arrest or regression in development and, as they persist, both mental and motor functions deteriorate. About 10–15 percent succumb, and of the remainder, about 90 percent are mentally retarded (Pincus & Tucker, 1974).

Autonomic epilepsy (seizure equivalent syndrome) consists in sudden episodes of autonomic disturbance, most commonly headache and abdominal pain, which generally last for minutes and which may or may not be associated with other types of seizures. Their peak occurrence is at 6–7 years. In about half the cases there is a history of organic insult (Chao, Carter, & Gold, 1977).

Management

The standard treatment for epilepsy is drug therapy, and about 60 percent of seizures can be controlled. Grand mal seizures in idiopathic epilepsy generally respond to drugs, and the seizures themselves tend to disappear after age 20. Among the symptomatic epilepsies, posttraumatic and focal seizures have a favorable prognosis; psychomotor and minor motor seizures are more difficult to control. In addition to drug therapy, a special "ketogenic" diet (high fat, low carbohydrate) is used with akinetic seizures, and surgery is utilized for certain types of focal epilepsy such as temporal lobe (Chao, Carter, & Gold, 1977).

Epilepsy and Intelligence

From the aforegoing it is apparent that intellectual functioning is more likely to be impaired when the epilepsy is associated with some organic brain dysfunction. Here the retardation is likely to be simply another manifestation of an injured brain. In fact, in persons with from moderate to profound retardation, a degree of impairment where some organicity is assumed, the frequency of seizures is about 20 percent as contrasted with about 5 percent in those who are mildly retarded (Corbett, Harris, & Robinson, 1975). Other studies report frequencies of epilepsy in retardation of from 16 to 24 percent (Richardson, Koller, Katz, & McLaren, 1981; Rutter, Tizard, & Whitmore, 1970).

It has been noted that mental retardation is most often associated with seizures occurring in early infancy and that, of these, infantile spasms carry the greatest risk (Jeavons, Bower, & Dimitrihoudi, 1973). Within the population of children with infantile spasms, the prognosis is particularly poor for the 50–60 percent in whom there is some evidence of brain pathology. Interestingly, the children who present a later picture of mental retardation are said to show a highly characteristic behavioral picture and one that resembles that of early infantile autism. Their motor development is relatively normal, but they all have severe language deficits and show stereotyped movements. Also carrying fairly grave consequences are seizures that occur in the first 4 days of life. These tend to be found in small-for-date newborns with hypoglycemia. Nearly half of these neonates either die or suffer some serious handicap. In contrast, seizures beginning the fifth to seventh days and associated with a too-low blood calcium level (hypocalcemia) have a good prognosis.

Although retardation has been seen as generally another consequence of the basic seizure-causing abnormality, there is some indication that seizures themselves can impair mental functioning. This is particularly true in status epilepticus and is also a rare complication of the earlier cited fever (febrile) convulsions. The latter are seen in about 2 percent of infants. Febrile seizures can progress into status epilepticus and cause secondary brain damage. Prolonged febrile seizures are also commonly found in persons who later manifest temporal lobe epilepsy.

The prevention of febrile convulsions is regarded as an important means of diminishing risks of retardation as well as of other organic brain sequelae (e.g., hemiplegia and hyperkinetic behavior). A special drug treatment, phenobarbitone, is recommended for "high-risk" children—those who are less than 13 months old, who have a family history of febrile convulsions, or who have had at least two such episodes (Corbett et al., 1975).

In idiopathic epilepsy, intellectual functioning seems to be grossly normal. Seizures do not appear to generally produce adverse cognitive effects, though there is probably a somewhat higher proportion of at least mildly impaired persons in this population. Within the group of epileptic children of normal intelligence, there is a particular link between behavior disorders and temporal lobe (psychomotor) epilepsy (Corbett et al., 1975), and in one study of persons who become psychotic after a long history of seizures, evidence of temporal lobe abnormality was predominant (Slater, Beard, & Glithero, 1963).

Psychological Factors in Mental Retardation

OVERVIEW

The causes of mental retardation are to be sought in the psychological as well as biological realm. Though the precise role of psychological factors is generally less explicit than that of the biological ones, that they do affect mental development seems undeniable. In this chapter, three aspects of the psychological dimension are considered: (a) research supporting the conclusion that intelligence is affected by environmental factors; (b) the implications of this research for the prevention of mental retardation through early environmental intervention; and (c) the nature of "effective parenting" and the quality of that experience in the child who is at high risk for nonorganic retardation.

PSYCHOLOGICAL EXPERIENCE AND GENERAL INTELLIGENCE

In this initial section of the chapter research is cited that reveals *general* relationships between certain kinds of experiences and intellectual development. The term "general relationships" is intended to convey the fact that although developmental research has been able to successfully define "normative" behavior throughout the age span, it has been unable to explain the *process* by which a child reached, maintained, or diverged from such behavior. We cannot yet explain why children who have experienced apparently similar qualities of care have different outcomes or how children can emerge from either the most supportive or the most brutalizing of environments as equally able and competent (Escalona, 1968; Sameroff & Chandler, 1978). The complexity of this process is most clearly seen in the few cases of children who were reared in the seemingly most depriving of environments until age 6–7 years but who were able to recover from the experience and move ahead developmentally (Davis, 1947; Koluchova, 1972; Mason, 1942). These case studies as well as findings in Guatemalan children by Kagan (1972), where retardation in infancy did not preclude normal adulthood, have called into question the relative immutability of experiences of infancy and early childhood and *suggest a much longer period of growth potential than has been hitherto assumed.*[1] Given this "disclaimer," we now want to look at four types of studies that indicate the general relationship between experience and intelligence. They are (a) children raised in grossly unfavorable environments, (b) children reared by retarded parents, (c) children of parents with retarded or borderline intelligence adopted by normal parents, and (c) studies of twins, with particular emphasis on identical twin pairs reared in different homes.

Children Reared in Grossly Unfavorable Environments

CONDITIONS OF DEPRIVATION

We begin to address the complex nature of the impact of experience on intelligence by asking what it is that constitutes an "unfavorable" (or favorable) environment. First let us see two examples of extraordinary deprivation, albeit associated with remarkable recovery.

Koluchova (1972) describes a pair of identical twin boys who were reared by a hostile stepmother under conditions of extreme isolation. Their plight was not discovered until they were 6 years old, after which they were removed from the home and placed in group and then foster care. The stepmother was imprisoned, and both she and the father lost parental rights.

> For more that 5 years the twins lived under most abnormal conditions. Some neighbors were unaware of their very existence! The father was once seen beating them with a rubber hose, but neighbors did not interfere because they feared conflict with the twins' stepmother.
>
> The twins grew up in almost total isolation. They lived in a small unheated closet and were not allowed in the rest of the house.
>
> Following their discovery they were admitted to a hospital at age 7. In the hospital kindergarten they were timid and mistrustful, and did not join in activities. They had to be brought to the kindergarten in a wheelchair, as they could barely walk! Their long-term virtual imprisonment and limited opportunity for using their legs in normal child activities had apparently affected their motor development.
>
> The extraordinary degree of deprivation of normal childhood experiences was evident in their reaction to objects and activities that are familiar to most children. They showed surprise and horror at such things as moving mechanical toys, TV, children doing physical exer-

[1]Hunt (1979) in a major review article on "early experience" states, "A major share of early losses can be made up if the develop-fostering quality of experience improves, and a great deal of early gain can be lost if the quality of experience depreciates."

cises, and street traffic. These reactions gradually disappeared, and they began to explore their environment. Their shyness also diminished, and they began to respond positively to adults but in the kind of indiscriminate fashion seen in affection-deprived children.

Their speech was very poor, and they communicated with others through gestures. They tried to imitate adult speech but could only repeat fragments of sentences, and words were poorly articulated.

Their spontaneous play was very primitive; initially it consisted only of manipulating objects, but soon imitative play appeared. They did not join in the play of other children.

A remarkable finding was their lack of understanding of the meaning of pictures. To help them learn that pictures were representations of real objects, pictures were initially used that were identical in size and color to the objects portrayed. After repeated comparisons, the twins began to understand the relationship. At the time of their rescue they were functioning developmentally at about the 3-year mental age level. Though this was comparable to at least a moderate level of retardation, it was assumed that their basic abilities were much higher and that, indeed, they were not really retarded.

Following hospitalization they were placed in a home for preschoolers, and there they made good progress. They began to interact with other youngsters, and this was aided by the fact that the other residents were younger. In effect, the twins' social immaturity made it easier to interact with younger children. Their motor skills improved, and they learned to walk, run, jump, and ride a scooter. Comparable progress was also seen in fine motor skills.

At age 7-7, their progress was evaluated again. Their mental age score had increased to 4 years, and there was less variability in their range of successes and failures. Though their mental development had exceeded expectations, their ultimate educability was still in question. It was not until age 9 that they were deemed ready for school, but continued impairment in speech and in fine motor skills led to their initial placement in one for retarded children. About this time they were moved from the children's home to a foster home. Their new "parents" were two unmarried, middle-aged sisters, intelligent, having wide interests and demonstrably capable of forming good relationships with children. One of the sisters had earlier adopted a baby girl who was now an intelligent and well-educated 13-year-old. The second sister became the twins' foster mother.

The twins have memories of their original home, though their foster mother tries to avoid talking to them about it. It was not until age 9 that they had enough language to even describe in outline their earlier life. They refer to their stepmother as "that unkind lady," an apparent understatement. They recalled how they were hungry and thirsty and beaten on their heads. Their scalps are badly scarred!

For a long time they dreaded the darkness. They appreciated the physical warmth of their new house, the good food, and refuge from being beaten. They early had to be reassured that they would not be taken away from their foster mother.

In a school with retarded children, the twin excelled. Their abilities to write, draw, and concentrate improved remarkably, and at age 10 they were transferred to a second-grade class in a regular school. Their progress there indicated that they could successfully complete their country's "basic 9-year school course" though at age 18 rather than the normal one of 15.

A summary of psychological test results shows that in the 25-month period from ages 7–9 to 9–10, their mental age scores increased by 3 years! Apparently, a dramatic change in living conditions was able to effect major mental growth even in children as old as 7 years. Beginning at age 8–4, they were tested with the Wechsler Intelligence Scale for Children (WISC), and these scores are shown in Table 9. Over the period from 8 to 11 their Full Scale IQs increased from 80 and 72 to 95 and 93. By age 11, then, their mental abilities were in the average range of intelligence. Some 5 years earlier they had been functioning in the range of moderate retardation! The greatest change is seen on the Verbal Scale, where scores increased from IQs of 80 and 69 at 8–4 to 97 and 96 at 11.

We have here a picture of remarkable growth in mental and social development which transformed two children who were functioning in the moderately retarded range into apparently grossly normal youngsters. And all of this occurred beginning at age 7 and appears to have continued through at least age 11.

A similar picture of deprivation and recovery is seen in a girl who, because of her illegitimacy, was locked with her deaf and aphasic mother in a room with drawn shades for $6\frac{1}{2}$ years! When both escaped, the child was extremely malnourished and also suffering from rickets which had so bowed her legs that the soles of her shoes nearly came together. When discovered she was functioning at about a 3-year developmental level, although her cognitive abilities were only at about 19 months. As in the case of the twins just described, language was especially impaired, but here, too, we see acquisition of a human capacity long after its normal age of appearance. A description of her rapid development of language over a 5-month period is given by her speech therapist (Mason, 1942):

11-16-38: Admittance to Children's Hospital, Columbus, Ohio

11-17-38: Cried almost continuously; would not partake of food except milk and crackers; showed recoil, disinterest, or fear of everyone with whom she came in contact.

11-20-38 My second visit. Isabelle showed interest in the watch, ring and doll which I brought here. Partook of some food when seated at a small table.

TABLE 9   Wechsler Intelligence Test Scores (WISC)

IQ			
Twin P.		Twin J.	
8 years 4 months			
Verbal	80	Verbal	69
Performance	83	Performance	80
Full Scale	80	Full Scale	72
9 years			
Verbal	84	Verbal	75
Performance	83	Performance	76
Full Scale	82	Full Scale	73
10 years			
Verbal	97	Verbal	94
Performance	85	Performance	86
Full Scale	91	Full Scale	89
11 years			
Verbal	97	Verbal	96
Performance	93	Performance	90
Full Scale	95	Full Scale	93

11-25-28: First vocalization. Attempt to say the words "ball" and "car" and "bye" (good-bye).

11-26-38: Repeated the words "baby" and "dirty" in imitation of words spoken to her in the form of play. "Baby" was the most distinct articulation to date.

11-30-38: Said "flower," "one," "two." Jabbered succession of nonsense syllables in imitation of my rather lengthy explanation to Jane that she should not appropriate Isabelle's toys.

12-03-38: Isabelle began to associate the word with its object; does not associate individuals with their names, but recognizes her own name when spoken.

12-08-38: Said: "watch, ring, blue, car, ball, lady, bell, bow-wow, hot, cold, warm, one, two, three, red, dirty, pretty, baby."

1-13-39: Distinguished yellow from the other colors and said "yellow" voluntarily.

2-08-39: Says the following sentences voluntarily: "That's my baby; I love my baby; open your eyes; close your eyes; I don't know; I don't want; that's funny; 'top it—'at's mine (when another child attempted to take one of her toys)."

2-11-39: She now associates people with names.

3-09-39: Isabelle said, "Say please," when I asked her to hand me something. Later said, "I'm sorry," when she accidentally hurt another child's finger.

3-04-39: Isabelle said "I love you, Miss Mason."

3-09-39: Identified printed form of the words "blue" and "yellow," and matched the word with the color.

By age 8 she had learned the meaning of a great many words, and her number concepts were equivalent to those of a normal 6-year old. By age 14 her intellectual function was said to be average (Sauer, 1947).

We have presented two examples of extraordinary deprivation. They reveal the remarkable resiliency of at least some children and the enigmatic nature of the environment-organism impact. But even the staunchest advocate of a lengthier period of growth potential than hitherto assumed would not minimize the importance of the early years or that the capacity for change diminishes with time.

Another but somewhat less dramatic example of the effect of deprivation is the growth retardation in infants with the *failure-to-thrive* syndrome (English, 1978). These are children who, though full-term and normal weight at birth, come to show poor weight gain, slow motor development, and both irritability and lethargy (Glaser, Heagarty, Bullard, & Pivchick, 1968). This symptom picture is most often found in the first year of life, usually by age 6 months. It is typically associated with difficulties in feeding, with the syndrome referring to infants whose weight falls below the third percentile. The distinction is drawn between organic and nonorganic causes. In one study, 62 percent were attributed to organic factors, the most common of which were either gastrointestinal or neurological in nature. With reference to the latter, failure to thrive was frequently associated with retardation, cerebral palsy, neurofibromatosis, microcephaly, and asphyxia (English, 1978). In the nonorganic cases it is presumed that the cause lies in a disturbed mother-child relationship.

Irrespective of origin, the clinical picture is remarkably similar. The children are described as fussy eaters who do such things as spit, vomit, turn away, and even fall asleep during feedings. Their mothers characterize feeding as a time of conflict, and even experienced nurses regard the feeding of these children as requiring particular patience and skill. But their mothers are perceived as lacking the nurturing skills necessary to overcome their babies' feeding peculiarities, and the resultant conflict leaves the mothers feeling anxious, guilty, and angry. The clearest evidence of a psychological basis is in those infants who, following hospitalization, show weight gain with nothing more than food and lots of attention. Follow-up studies of nonorganic failure-to-thrive infants reveal that a substantial minority continue to be below the third percentile in weight (Glaser et al., 1968; Elmer, Gregg, & Ellison, 1969). They tend to be skimpier eaters and actually consume about 300 calories per day less than normal age mates—1400 as against 1700 (Pollitt & Eichler, 1976).

Two sets of investigators have reported intellectual status at follow-up; their data suggest increased rates of at least mild retardation. In one study of 40 children, three (8%) were in the 50–70 range (Glaser et al., 1968), and, although a much larger proportion of at least mild to borderline retardation is noted in the second study, overall family impairment obscures the role of earlier failure to thrive. One worker (Kearsley, 1979) has coined the term *iatrogenic* retardation to refer to developmental delay in nonorganic failure-to-thrive children who are functioning normally on experimental cognitive measures for infants. He suggests that, in some instances, an early developmental lag is interpreted to the parents as retardation, and this leads them to have low expectations and to understimulate the child. Whether these cognitive measures will correlate with general indices of intelligence remains to be seen, but there is no doubt that understimulation would be a common outcome in an *organically based* failure-to-thrive child. Thus, to whatever developmental lag is attributable to neurological deficit, there might be added an additional overlay that is really psychological. Hence the importance of early stimulation of the handicapped infant, an issue addressed in the next chapter.

DEFINING A "FAVORABLE" ENVIRONMENT

Our own shock at the earlier-reported brutalizing of children provides at least an emotional cue as to the kinds of experience to which neither children nor adults should be exposed. But let us try to move beyond a purely affective response and seek to define the elements of a favorable developmental environment.

As a result of our own experience, each of us has his own idea as to what a child should be exposed to. There would be no difference of opinion as to the child's need for adequate nutrition and health care, so sadly lacking in these three children, but there would probably be some disagreement as to the nature of a good parent-child relationship. Perhaps the use of a single frame of reference, here the "need reduction" personality model presented in Chapter 2, can unify our individual views. We recognize that a child needs love (intimacy), but in certain degrees it can be smothering. The child need guidance, limits, and direction (structure) but also freedom (autonomy). The child needs to feel competent (success) but also challenged if adaptive skills are to broaden. Our assessment of the favorableness of the child's environment will be in terms of the psychological needs for structure, self-esteem, and self-expression and on the effect of that environment on the resources (abilities) through which needs are at least partly met. Our particular focus will be on self-esteem and the degree to which the child is offered experiences that foster intimacy, success, and autonomy. Given the needs here posited, we can quickly recognize why certain kinds of early experiences have been regarded as important to healthy mental and emotional development, though the deprivation recovery cited here suggests an important organismic contribution to developmental outcome.

The "Responsive" Parent

Perhaps the most general characteristic of a healthy child-rearing experience is to be raised by a "responsive" parent (Harriet Rheingold, personal communication). By this is meant a parent who is both sensitive to a child's needs and willing to make the effort to respond to them. Such a parent loves the child, is concerned about its development, and tries to provide the kind of "personalized" experiences that make the child happy and foster growth. How utterly removed from these motivations were the people who controlled the destinies of our deprived children.

Ainsworth and Wittig (1969) define a healthy environment as one that encourages competence (success) and normal social responsiveness (intimacy). It is one in which (a) the mother is sensitive to her baby's signals and willing to time her interventions to his rhythms; (b) there is frequent and sustained physical contact, especially during the first year, and baby's discomfort is soothed through physical contact; (c) there is mutual delight in the mother-infant interplay; and (d) the infant feels some control over what happens to him. The last mentioned has been referred to as the baby's need for "contingent" stimulation (Bronfenbrenner, 1972)—that is, that the baby's actions produce some meaningful effect on its environment. The absence of such experience is seen as creating attitudes of "learned helplessness" and generally diminished motivation (Martin, 1977). In terms of the personality model, the first three elements clearly relate to intimacy, and the last pertains to success and autonomy.

Intelligence

Regarding intelligence, developmental theorists stress the importance of *stimulation*, particularly of the contingent kind (Casler, 1961; Thompson, 1960). In addition to stimulation, another extremely important parental function in encouraging mental development is that of "verbal mediator" between the child and his experience. Here the parent interprets or explains the world to the child, helping him to understand his experiences (Feuerstein & Krassilowsky, 1972; Miller, 1970). Still another parental behavior seen as affecting cognitive development is the style of parental control. The distinction has been drawn between control through "authority" and control through "reason" (Hess & Shipman, 1965). In control through authority, rules are established, but there is little attention to the unique characteristics of a given situation. Unlike control through reason, there is no attempt to *teach* the child about the why's of his behavior. This also constitutes a deficiency in the "verbal mediator" parental role. The author has referred to this as the "teacher" facet of parenthood, and we shall return to it in the last section of the chapter.

CHILD REARING IN GROUP-CARE SETTINGS

One of the most widely studied of child-rearing environments has been the orphanage. The very word "orphan" has an alien ring to contemporary adult ears because of the dramatic change in our own lifetime in the rearing of orphaned children as well as those who have parents but are unable to live with them. Prior to World War II, such youngsters were placed in orphanages where they remained until adulthood unless adopted or placed in a foster home. As a result of psychological studies of the effects on mental and emotional development of being raised in a large group-care setting, such practice is now avoided, and early placement is sought in either adoptive or foster homes. The problem with large group-care settings is that they fail to provide the kind of individualized, intimate, one-to-one experience that is the very essence of "responsive parenting." The same problem exists in large group-care settings, "institutions," serving mentally handicapped children and adults, and is seen as encouraging the kinds of negligence and personal abuse that have led to national efforts to depopulate them—the so-called deinstitutionalization movement. The intent is to substitute for them smaller and more intimate, community-based residential settings—for example, group homes (see Chap. 9). Let us now consider the relevant research.

Skeels and Dye Study

An important early study on the effects of institutional care on mental development was that of Skeels and Dye (1939). Their attention was called to two infant girls who had been reared in an orphanage and whose lagging development at 13 and 16 months led to placement in an institution for the mentally retarded. "The youngsters were pitiful little creatures . . . they were emaciated, undersized, and lacked muscle tone or responsiveness. Sad and inactive, the two spent their days rocking (stereotypy) and whining" (Skeels, 1966). Their developmental levels were less than half of average for their age though neither child had any apparent organic abnormality. The 13-month-old was not attempting to stand, she was producing little vocalization, and her IQ on the Kuhlman-Binet intelligence test was 46. The older infant was even further delayed: at 16 months she neither walked, vocalized, nor showed interest in play. Her IQ was 35. The institution to which the children were admitted had no program for infants, and each was placed on a ward housing mildly retarded adolescent girls. The children came to be ward "pets," as each received a great deal of mothering from the older girls. Six months after admission, striking changes were noted in their behavior. They were retested, and both showed tremendous gains—from 46 to 87 and from 35 to 77. At their subsequent adoption 27 months after admission, both children had IQs in the 90–100 range.

After learning of the dramatic developmental changes in these two little girls, Skeels and Dye decided to try to repeat this "natural" experiment with other young children in the orphanage who were also functioning at a retarded level. Thirteen infants, average age 19 months and mean IQ 64 (range 35–89), were transferred to the institution for the retarded. They, too, were free of organic abnormality. At the institution they received the same kind of intense mothering as the first two had, and 19 months later their average developmental score had risen to IQ 92. All of the children gained in mental ability, the range being 7–58 points, with a mean gain of 28 points. Other studies to be mentioned later also show apparent environmental effects of from 20 to 30 IQ points. No control group was ever established, but children who remained in the institution showed a decline in IQ; their retardation appears to have been organic in origin. A follow-up study of the early-placed children in adulthood found them to be functioning normally (Skeels, 1966).

What was the nature of the orphanage experience that seemed to retard development in infancy—a retardation that could be erased through intensive mothering? Up to age 2, children in the orphanage lived in a special hospital nursery wing where they were given good physical and medical care but *little personal attention.* Contacts with staff were largely limited to meeting basic self-care needs. The children were attended by nurses and by young girls who served as nurses' assistants. The latter viewed their duties as a necessary evil and took little interest in the children. There were few play materials and little desire to teach the children how to use them. How stark the contrast with their later experiences where they were lavished with attention and their achievements were a source of pride to the girls who were mothering them. It is said that there was competition between wards to see which would have its baby walking or talking first, and much time was spend in "teaching" these activities. In terms of our personality model we can see how intimacy and success experiences were provided to the children through an intensive period of *cognitive* and *social stimulation.* At least in the early childhood period, and under the supervision of normal adults, mildly retarded young women were capable of meeting crucial psychological needs.

The reader should not interpret the thriving of these children as typifying the effects of early placement in institutions for the retarded. The combination of circumstances that made possible the meeting of affectional needs and the fostering of development is not likely to be found in large group-care settings—hence the encouragement of family rather than institutional placement by child-care agencies. The most important findings of the study were that (a) lack of personal attention and general stimulation appears capable of delaying normal developmental stages,[2] and (b) such developmental lag can be reversed by intensive mothering and stimulation, at least before age 2.

Other Studies

The Skeels and Dye study was the forerunner of a large number of investigations on the effects of institutional residence on young children. While some researchers reported particularly adverse ones on mental and/or emotional development (Bowlby, 1940; Goldfarb, 1955; Kirk, 1958; Provence & Lipton, 1962; Spitz, 1945), the latter particularly referring to difficulties in establishing deep emotional ties, others have found no such effects (Dennis, 1960; Dennis & Najarian, 1957; Rheingold, 1960, 1961). One of the most prominent of the investigators, Bowlby (1952), had concluded in a World Health Organization report that deprivation of maternal care would almost always lead to retardation. Following a later study, Bowlby and his collaborators (Bowlby, Ainsworth, Boston, & Rosenbluth, 1956) indicated that the case for maternal deprivation had been overstated. In a major review article, Thompson and Grusec (1970) deduce that since not all children raised in institutions show adverse effects, in spite of the fact that all have suffered maternal deprivation, that is, *have been separated from their*

---

[2]In his highly influential book, *Intelligence and Experience,* Hunt (1961) notes other research indicating that "deprivation" delays the onset of normally seen developmental behaviors. Kagan, Kearsley, and Zelazo (1978) observed maturational delays in Guatemalan infants they attributed to a diminished *variety* of stimulation.

parent,[3] other causes for these effects must be sought. They conclude that children in institutions are more likely to suffer "perceptual deprivation and restriction of learning opportunities." The author would characterize the institutional environment as one in which the necessity of caring for large numbers of children decreases the likelihood of experiences of *contingent stimulation* and of receiving *individualized* or *responsive* care from a *loving* adult who also serves as a "verbal mediator."

POSITIVE EFFECTS
OF OUT–OF–HOME PLACEMENT

Though few have claimed benefits for out-of-home placement (Freud & Burlingham, 1944), gains in IQ have been seen in mildly retarded adolescents and adults *following* institutional placement (Clarke & Clarke, 1954). Apparently, many came from poverty backgrounds, and the amount of gain in IQ was inversely related to the quality of their home. Those coming from "very bad homes" gained an average of 10 IQ points, an increase not attributable to the institutional program itself. Although this degree of gain is "modest" and potentially explicable in terms of motivational factors, it does suggest a freeing of capacity. While we would hesitate to suggest that these youths were necessarily "happier" in the institution than in their own homes, the quality of life in some of their homes must have been similar to that described in the next section and would imply that one's own home is not necessarily to be preferred to residence elsewhere. Until recently this had to be an "institution," but now a wider range of options exist.

Children Reared by Retarded Parents

Another group of children whose childhood experiences may hinder mental development are those reared by parents who are themselves retarded. In spite of the apparent benefits of at least short-term mothering by retarded women, as shown in the Skeels and Dye study, the majority of children of retarded parents are not of normal intelligence. This is not to suggest that the higher frequency of retardation in the children of retarded parents is necessarily environmental in origin, since in these families the role of environment is confounded by the possible influence of heredity. To the degree that genetic factors affect intelligence, a larger proportion of the children of retarded parents would also be retarded. Let us now look at the intelligence of children of retarded parents when reared in their own homes. Later we will look at similar children reared in adoptive ones.

CHILDREN OF TWO RETARDED PARENTS

Studies of children of two retarded parents have found frequencies of retardation in the children from 39 to 61 percent (Birch, Richardson, Baird, Horobin, & Illslcy, 1970; Halperin, 1945; Penrose, 1938; Reed & Reed, 1965; Scally, 1968). For purposes of rough estimate, approximately half of the children of

---

[3]A curious definition of maternal deprivation—perhaps intended to show the inadequacy of earlier uses of the term.

retarded parents, *if reared in the parental home*, will be retarded. The next-largest cluster, about one-third, will function in the borderline range (IQ 70–90), and the remaining one-sixth will show normal intelligence. The IQ distribution in the children, though not clearly attributable to environmental factors because of the confounding effects of heredity, does indicate that intelligence is not wholly a function of environment, since this would not explain the normal children who emerge from such families. When we look later, however, at the intellectual status of foster and adopted children of retarded parents, the powerful role of environment becomes apparent.

CHILDREN IN FAMILIES
WITH ONLY ONE RETARDED PARENT

Some evidence for an environmental effect is seen in the children of families where only one parent is retarded (Reed & Reed, 1965). Where it was the mother who was retarded, the proportion of retarded children was more than twice as great as in those where it was the father who was retarded, 19 to 8 percent. Since there is no evidence for a differential genetic contribution of either sex to the intelligence of the child, this maternal effect is presumed to be psychological in nature and due to her likely greater contact with the child than is ordinarily true of the father. Admittedly, however, this effect could also be biological in that the retarded mother would be less likely to provide adequate health care to her children (and to herself). A differential parental effect on intelligence was also found in a study in which children of mothers of either very high or very low intelligence more closely resembled their mothers than their fathers (Willerman & Stafford, 1972).

With regard to the children of retarded parents, we can inquire as to the nature of the potentially adverse environment to which they may be exposed. At least a partial answer is found in a description of the family settings from which children emerge who were earlier classified as having "cultural-familial" retardation.

CULTURAL-FAMILIAL
(PSYCHOSOCIAL) MENTAL RETARDATION

Although this term has been abandoned in the current AAMD nomenclature,[4] it is included here because it does accurately depict the two central features in families which are at high risk for children with mild retardation in the absence of organicity—similarly affected parents and/or siblings and the probability of a less-than-ideal child-rearing experience. The sometimes frightful conditions of life in these families have been graphically depicted in earlier studies (e.g., Bice, 1947; Goddard, 1912; Town, 1939), and there has been some specific focus on the child care practices of the retarded mother (Mickelson, 1947; Scally, 1973). Spec-

---

[4]The 1973 revision of the AAMD classification substituted "psychosocial disadvantage" for "cultural-familial," presumably because the latter included the possibility of a genetic contribution (Robinson & Robinson, 1976). Since the 1961 AAMD definition specifically disavowed any etiological implications for the term, its removal without explanation is questioned.

ulation regarding presumed child care limitations of the retarded mother refer to diminished responsiveness and possible indifference, inconsistency, and lack of stimulation (Sarason, 1959). Undoubtedly, within these families can be found wide variations in basic child care practices. At their best, such families can at least minimally meet the child's basic needs for physical care (survival) and love (intimacy). The author was much impressed by a retarded couple who were seeking assistance for health problems in their children. The father was employed as a bookbinder, they owned their own home, and both seemed to be responsible individuals.

At their worst, such families can rear children under conditions that are shocking. The children may be ill clothed and ill fed, routine preventive health care is unknown, and medical treatment is limited to emergencies. Even emergency care may be uncertain, especially in rural areas, because of the lack of a telephone or a dependable vehicle. Although the children do poorly in school, the retarded ones prior to "mainstreaming" were commonly found in classes for "educable" pupils, the parents seem unconcerned. Their children's performance is little different from their own. Even if it is acknowledged that doing well in school is a means of getting a decent job and moving up economically, the parents are unlikely to provide the kind of encouragement and stimulation necessary to translate the wish into reality. Rather, such families unwittingly teach maladaptive ways of thinking and behaving. The experience has been characterized as fostering absolute and concrete modes of thought rather than relative and abstract ones, of teaching the expectation of failure, and of inculcating low self-worth (McCandless, 1952). In the Baroff model, this refers to diminished self-esteem arising, in part, from the prominence of failure rather than success. Moreover, this failure is attributed to an environment that does not enhance the child's intellectual resources. The effect is to assure the generational continuity of poverty and of socially maladaptive behavior.

Some sense of life in these families is dramatically depicted in the following descriptions of two families in which at least one parent is retarded and in which there are also retarded siblings. In addition to giving a picture of the family as seen from outside, letters are included that document the experience as seen by those who live it.

The "J." Family

The "J." family epitomizes the impoverished, multiproblem family in which retardation in parents and children is but one of a number of seriously disabling conditions. There are four children in the family, three girls and a boy, and all are mentally retarded as are the mother and probably the father. A brief description is given of each member of the family and of the home conditions as seen by the local social services department.

Edith, age 27, IQ 60, was admitted to an institution for the retarded at age 7. She had twice been excluded from first grade because of extremely aggressive behavior toward other children. She was described as overactive, noisy, destructive, having a short attention span, and tending to wander from home. There was a very poor relationship between Edith and her parents, particularly with her father. The parents were said to not understand her and to be very hard on her. When the father, an alcoholic, was drunk, he would be severely punitive while the mother was always screaming at her. The poor relationship with the father is seen in a letter from Edith to her mother when she was 13:

> august 22, 1965
>
> Dear Mother,
>   I got your letter & sure was glad to here from you but I was not pleased with what Daddy said. Mother Daddy said he doesn't under stand me but I don't understand him either. Mother I was not mad at you and I dident mean to get you upset, but I did mean every word I said about not coming home unless Daddy wants me home enough to behave himself. Mother I love you all very much and I would like to come home and I would if Daddy would behave himself. Daddy makes me very unhappy when I am at home and I don't want to come home for a while. Mother I would like to see you if you could come down here. well I had better close up for now

The letter reveals a young woman who has the capacity to appraise a situation and to make a decision that is probably painful to her. At the institution she was described as one of the few girls in her group who was able to look at and understand some of the nuances of her own behavior. Additionally, the letter indicates relatively good academic skills; her reading and number abilities are at the fifth-grade level. After 11 years at the institution, Edith was returned to the community. She shortly became pregnant and was encouraged to have an abortion to which she consented providing she was not also sterilized. One of her concerns regarding the abortion was its cost. Seemingly illustrating the reasoning impairment of a retarded individual was

Edith's comment that if the operation was expensive she would just as soon skip it and have the baby. Edith is now married, has two children, and appears to be the only child who has avoided chronic difficulty.

John, age 25, IQ 65 (IQ 70 on Beta), is serving a life term in prison for forcible rape. He had always been the favorite child, although he is said to have disobeyed his father and struck his mother. He was seen as much pampered by his parents, who were unable to provide any controls for him. He had poor school adjustment; he repeated the first grade, and there was much absence. Although recognized as eligible for special class placement by the third grade, this was not done, and there was continued truancy which ultimately led to court referral at age 10. At that time the mother was in a psychiatric hospital, and he was seen by the court as a "neglected" rather than "delinquent" child. For a short time John lived in a foster home, but he soon returned to that of his parents where the pattern of truancy resumed. At ages 12 and 14 he was again referred to the court, but "malicious mischief" was now added to truancy. He was seen as beyond control and was sent to a juvenile correction institution, where he remained for 1 year. On returning home he was placed in junior high school in a special education class, but he again left school and then went to work as a "helper." Although for a brief period of time he appeared to have made an adequate adjustment, at age 17 he was again in trouble and was convicted of "breaking and entering" and auto theft. He was placed on 3 years' probation. During the next 3 years he worked as either a laborer or truck driver and is said to have had a stable work record. Nevertheless he began to drink, and at age 20 he was arrested and convicted of driving without a license, driving under the influence of alcohol, and conspiring to commit armed robbery. Presumably, before sentencing he committed the act of rape, which led to his present imprisonment. He is said to be getting along well in prison and is active in an inmate Alcoholics Anonymous group. His general achievement level is at fourth to fifth grade.

Doris, age 24, IQ 54–61, is currently a patient in a psychiatric hospital. She has been hospitalized for about 1 year and is under treatment for "unsocialized aggressive behavior." Owing to psychiatric depressions of the mother, Doris had spent much of her childhood in foster care. Until puberty she had made an adequate adjustment in the foster home and in a special class, but, thereafter, there were behavior problems in both settings. In the classroom she was usually cooperative though excessively demanding of the teacher's attention. Illness in the foster parents caused her to have to leave the foster home, and she was admitted to the same institution for the retarded as her sister Edith. Doris was at the institution for 4 years and was then placed in a family-care group home in the community. She had difficulty in adjusting there and elsewhere, as frequent temper tantrums led to continual changes in residence. She worked in a sheltered workshop, where she was described as demonstrating extremely variable behavior. She could either engage in immature attention-getting behavior or show unusual maturity. Her central problem was extreme temper tantrums, the last of which went on for many hours, included self-hitting and smearing of the face with food and, ultimately, intervention by the police. She was bodily carried by them to the psychiatric hospital where she now resides. She is on tranquilizing medication and is said to be getting along adequately. It is soon planned to place her in a group home in another community. She functions academically at about a fourth-grade level.

Susan, age 19, IQ 58, was admitted to a mental retardation center at the same time as her sister Doris. She continues in residence at this time, though some possibility of community return is entertained. Susan was institutionalized at age 10 and was described as a highly distractible and active youngster who did not get into difficulty if she was kept occupied. Like Doris, Susan was eager for adult attention, and she would often ask her foster parents to do things for her that she could do herself. Susan, too, was in special education, and in the classroom she had difficulty remaining in her seat and following class routine. When upset she had tantrums that were only quelled by allowing her to sit on the floor either next to or under the teacher's desk. In the early teen years she was seen as a friendly and rather outgoing youngster who still had some difficulty in accepting class routine. In recent years she has shown the same pattern of emotional instability as her sister. She has numerous physical complaints related to the vagina, exhibits public masturbation, and has frequent episodes of aggression when frustrated. She has been on tranquilizing medication for at least 2 years. On interview, she appears to be very immature and shows extremes of emotional behavior. She appears to be much more immature than Doris. Academically, she functions at about a first-grade level.

Mr. J. is 53 years old, attended school to only third grade, lacks functional reading skills, and is employed as a laborer. He has a long history of alcoholism and has had at least one psychiatric hospitalization in connection with his drinking. At age 44, drunk and enraged at criticism of his drinking by a family acquaintance, he threatened this man by cursing him and firing his shotgun in the air. His aquaintance was less obliging; he returned the fire and shot Mr. J. in the leg. Some 8 months later Mr. J. resumed employment, and he is currently a maintenance worker for the city. He is described by a social worker as a likable and sentimental person who cried when he saw his daughter Susan on a Christmas vacation at home. To the social worker he seemed more like a real person than Mrs. J.

Mrs. J., age 50, completed sixth grade. She has a long history of depressions which required psychiatric hospitalization, and during one of these she was found to be retarded. Mrs. J., though fond of her son John, has shown little interest in her three daughters, especially Doris and Susan. The mother made no effort to see the girls when they were in foster care because she said they were "nerve-racking." She has always been easily upset and unable to tolerate stress. On one occasion she disappeared for a year but was later found in another state and returned to the family home. On a recent visit, she was described as extremely nervous, and her conversation centered around her nervousness, her husband's drinking, fighting with her husband, and fears of returning to the hospital. She is said to have functional reading and writing skills.

This family epitomizes the multiproblem nature of such impoverished settings—problems of alcoholism, psychiatric disorder, mental retardation, and criminality. The children grew up in a home that often lacked basic necessities, they were frequently without adequate clothing and food. The parents were unable to exercise control, the mother was openly rejecting of her daughters, and on at least one occasion, she simply abandoned the family. Except for Edith, all of the children are currently in institutional settings, and, with their shared failure in dealing with feelings of anger, the future for Doris and Susan is not bright.

The "R." Family

Here we see another example of the multiproblem home and one in which there is cultural-familial retardation. But here we also encounter a mother who, in spite of her limitations, is devoted to her children. While there is a question of her ability to meet their needs, there is no doubt about her sustained interest and concern for them. There are three children, two girls and a boy. Both girls are retarded as appear to be the parents and the father's mother and siblings. Amid mental subnormality, rural isolation, and deprivation, one child, the boy, has managed to achieve normal ability and a successful adult adjustment.

Troy, age 27, is married to a schoolteacher and is employed as a lab technician. He is making a good adjustment. Apparently of normal intelligence, he recognized the problems of his parents and sibs and has served a liaison role between his family and the social agencies with which they have been involved.

Emma, age 24, with tested IQs ranging from 46 to 66, was initially placed in an institution for the retarded at age 11. She repeated first grade in a rural school where she was described as restless, unable to concentrate, excessively demanding of teacher attention, and interacting poorly with classmates. Various kinds of nonsexual aggressive behavior were displayed toward the boys in her class, and as a teenager she was seen as immature, having a childlike self-image, and very demanding of adult attention. She did not do well in the institutional program that prepares residents for community return, but both she and her mother wanted her home. At about 19 she returned to the family home and for a while lived with her mother who had since divorced the father. For a time she attended an adult day activity program and there met a retarded man whom she married. During the period before and after her marriage she was in continuous difficulty in the community and was in and out of psychiatric hospitals. She lived with her husband for 3 months and said that they fought all the time. Asked what they fought about, she said that he wanted her to wash clothes and do dishes and that she did not want to do that. In the community she was sexually exhibitionistic both alone and with her husband! She also continued the pattern of aggressive behavior of her childhood years and would destroy property in fits of anger. She is seen by a social worker as "mean." She has had no children, as she was sterilized when she returned home. She is now in a psychiatric hospital, declared incompetent, and in the legal custody of her father. In the hospital, she continues to be sexually active and has been treated for gonorrhea. The hospital does not see itself as doing anything more than providing a residence for her, because the community will not tolerate her behavior.

Teresa, age 22, with tested IQ ranging from 35 to 45, was institutionalized with Emma when Teresa was 11 years old. She also had much difficulty in school—her behavior was very much like her sister's. At the institution for the retarded she was seen as a fairly attractive and shy girl who got along well with others. She was discharged from the institution to a group home where she lived while working in a sheltered workshop. Without explanation she was returned to the maternal home, where she has continued to reside. She became pregnant, but the child was removed from both her custody and that of her mother and was placed in foster care. Neither she nor her mother was seen as able to provide adequate supervision for the child. At placement, the child was seen as slightly delayed in development but grossly normal. Like her sister, Teresa attends a local adult day activity program, but she has functioned well in it and is soon expected to be placed in regular employment. Unlike her sister, Teresa is stable and, apparently, able to function in the community. She has never married and continues to live with her mother.

Mr. R., age 49, attended school to the third grade and works in unskilled jobs. His mother and his siblings are retarded, and a younger brother was in a correctional facility. Mr. R. is said to have whipped his children excessively and to have regularly beaten his first wife, who has since divorced him. He has since remarried, apparently to another retarded woman, and they are now expecting a child.

Mrs. R. (first wife and mother of Troy, Emma, and Teresa), age 43, had only a fourth-grade education, was married at age 15, is described as "very erratic," and has had at least one psychiatric hospitalization. In spite of her limitations, Mrs. R. seems to represent the kind of socially impoverished parent who cares about her children. All the time that Emma and Teresa were institutionalized, the mother was regarded as genuinely interested in them but unable to provide the needed guidance. During their years in the institution for the retarded, she maintained continuous contact with them as shown in frequent correspondence and in a direct wish to have the girls back with her. The letter (pp. 202–203) gives a picture of her maternal concern and of her willingness to expose herself to continued physical abuse from Mr. R. if this was necessary to her not losing custody of them. Mrs. R. now lives with Teresa and is perceived by the social service agency as continuing to make only a very marginal community adjustment.

The experience of these children and their parents has been one of cultural isolation and deprivation. They were always very poor and lived in a remote rural area. They often lacked the barest necessities and were long know to social agencies. Both parents are seen as "very limited"; the father is said to have squandered his meager earnings and frequently left the family without food or adequate clothing. Some sense of the family's cultural isolation is that prior to the institutionalization of the girls, not only was the home without television, a not necessarily fatal flaw, but the children had never seen a movie.

Two families have been depicted in which parents and children are retarded. It is improbable that these life-styles are typical of such families, as the selection of people with institutional histories biases the population to those from less stable homes. These families are presented as illustrating adverse child-rearing environments. In them it was probably difficult to maintain a state of good health, to have a sense of stability, to be assured of parental love and protection, and to be encouraged in the development of one's interests and aptitudes. They were homes that taught brutality, neglect, fear—a way of life seemingly far removed from the comfortable America that is the experience of so many of us.

Foster Children, Adopted Children

It is the view here that the most convincing evidence for the impact of environment on mental development is to be found in studies of children of retarded parents who were early placed in foster or adoptive homes and in studies of twins. The latter, in particular, appear to indicate that *both* environmental and genetic factors influence intelligence.

There are a large number of studies that show that the children of mothers with borderline or retarded intelligence will consistently show average to near-average mental development when reared in foster or adoptive homes of normal parents (Freeman, Holzinger, & Mitchell, 1928; Illingworth, 1971; Skeels & Harms, 1948; Skodak & Skeels, 1949; Snygg, 1938; Stippich, 1940). Moreover,

Dear Mr.

I thought I would Drop you a few lines concerning [redacted] an [redacted]. that is in school. As I suppose you know that their Daddy and I Do not live together. We have been separated since October the 4th. Althae we were separated once before I went back to him gave him a chance to be good to me. All he would Do is knock me Around an curse me. thae I know that you Can not help the Cause thae I want to ask you a few Questions. I would Come Down there and talk to you thae I Don't have a dolar at

and I cannot hire any way dust now. thae someone told me when we signed for the girls To Come Down there that we signed our nights away from the girls and if I Did not live with their Daddy. that I Could never get them on a vacation. Also they told me That if I Did not go back To him. the welfaris would have the right to adopt the girls out to him. I would like for you to write me And Tell me if this be so. if so. I will try to live with him for the sake of the Chilluns Althae That he knocks me Around And Kurse me Aching until I am not Able to take Care of the girls, when they are at home. an I feel much better away from him for when Im not living in the home with him he cannot trust me around. An I am much more able to look after the girls away from him then with him. And also I take the girls to church when they are with me And Im sure nothing would happen to them while I am at. Otther you know I love the girls, I may not be able to get them out for christmas due to finacally problems short of money. But I will try to come an see them an get them for a vacation just as soon as I can be sure an write an tell me if I love to live with him an be abused by him So I me freedom with the girls

And also he may try to get the girls out for christmas If he dais I would rather that They were not let out with him unless I was with him for he will not have any one to look after them for they stayed with me for a week when they were out for thanksgiven they are sweet girls that is bad to get in things. And Im can anything happens or if you more am let me know at ████ ██ Mrs ████

Answer real soon

PS
I Am ████ and
M the

the earlier the placement, preferably before age 2 years, the better the child is likely to do (Dennis, 1967; Freeman et al., 1928; Speer, 1940). The impact of these findings on at least one set of investigators is seen in the following quote:

> Perusal of the child's social history . . . and comparison [of it] with the field agent's pre-placement evaluation of the adoptive home was disheartening. It did not seem possible that children with such meager possibilities as projected from the intellectual, academic, and occupational attainments of their parents could measure up to the demands of cultured, educated parents. Yet careful examination of one child after another showed none of the retardation or misplacement (in terms of adoptive home) which might have been anticipated. (Skodak & Skeels, 1949)

This finding is all the more remarkable considering that the main factors in matching child to adoptive parents were religion, sex, and hair color!

The Skodak and Skeels study merits description because of its scope and the representativeness of its findings with regard to the intelligence of the adopted children, and because it appears to illustrate the influence of heredity as well as environment. One hundred children were studied, 60 boys and 40 girls, each of whom had been placed in an adoptive home by age 6 months. The intelligence of the children was assessed four times between ages 2 and 13 with the mean IQ usually falling in the bright-normal range (100–120). For purposes of comparing the intelligence of the children with that of their biological mothers, their mean IQ at age 13 is used. At that age the children were tested on both the 1916 and 1937 versions of the Stanford-Binet intelligence test with mean IQs being 107 and 117, respectively. Since the IQs of the biological mothers are based on the 1916 test, it is this version of the Binet that is used for comparative purposes. At age 13 the mean IQ of the adoptive children was 107, exceeding that of the general population by at least seven IQ points and that of their biological mothers by 21 points. The average IQ of 63 biological mothers for whom test scores were available was 86. The range of IQs in the children was 65–144, with two-thirds of them functioning in the average to bright-normal range. On the basis of the information available, the precise magnitude of the influence of the adoptive home is not ascertainable, but, had the children been reared by their own mother, and assuming some regression to the mean, an average IQ of 95 is more probable than one of 107. It is reasonable to propose that early placement in homes of adoptive parents of above-average educational and socioeconomic status increased the IQ of the children by at least 12 IQ points. This figure probably underestimates the environmental impact of the adoptive homes and certainly does for the children of the biological mothers who were retarded. There were 11 such mothers with IQs below 70; their average IQ was 63. The mean IQ of their children was 96, exceeding the maternal mean by 33 points. In spite of having retarded mothers, within advantaged adoptive homes the majority of these children achieved at least average intelligence.

Analogous findings are reported in several more recent studies. In one (Willerman, 1979), the adoptive children of a group of biological mothers with mean IQ 89 (n = 27), tested an average 14 points higher ($\overline{X}$ IQ 103). In an interesting French study (Schiff et al., 1978), lower socioeconomic biological mothers gave up a child for adoption but also reared a full or half sibling themselves. The adoptees were all reared in more advantaged homes, and their average IQ was 111. Their nonadopted sibs had an average IQ of 95. Finally, Scarr and Weinberg (1967) studied black children adopted by advantaged white families in Minnesota. The mean IQ of the black children (n = 130) was 106; it exceeded by 16 points the average IQ of black children in that geographical area. Moreover, the earlier the adoption the greater the effect. For even late adoptees, those adopted after age 1 year, the gain was at least 10 points, and this was doubled to as much as 20 points for early-placed children.

HEREDITY—ENVIRONMENT INTERACTION

But the Skodak and Skeels study discloses more than just an environmental effect on intelligence. Though the IQs of the children typically surpassed those of their biological mothers, the children themselves differed from each other in intelligence. Recall that their IQs ranged all the way from 65 to 144, a spread that is very similar to that of the general population (the standard deviation was 14 points). Thus, in spite of being reared in similar kinds of adoptive homes, the children were no more alike in their measured intelligence than a random population of children reared in the homes of their biological parents. Recognizing that the adoptive homes were clearly much more homogeneous in their sociocultural makeup than would be true of a random sample of family settings, what could account for such IQ diversity? The answer cannot be the environment but rather is to be sought in the meaning of a statistical relationship observed between the adopted child and the biological mother.

A correlation of .44 was found between the intelligence of the biological mother and the child from whom she had been separated since early infancy. The size of this correlation is only slightly less than that found when the child is reared by his own mother (or father), .50, and means that parent and child tended to occupy relatively similar positions in their respective IQ distributions. Biological mothers whose IQs were above their group mean of 86 had children whose IQs tended to be above their group mean of 107. Similarly, biological mothers whose IQs fell below their group mean of 86 had children whose IQs tended to be below their group mean of 107. This relationship is illustrated in Figure 24, where the upper line shows the mean IQs of the total group of adopted children (M') and of subgroups of eight children of bright biological mothers (A') and 11 children of retarded biological mothers (B'). The corresponding mean IQs of the biological mothers, shown on the lower line, are M, A, and B. The mean IQs at A and A' are 111 and 118; at B and B', 63 and 96; and at M and M', 86 and 107.

How can we explain the existence of a very significant relationship between the intelligence of mothers and children who have been separated since infancy?

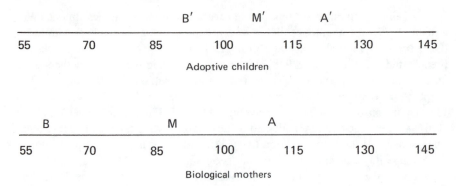

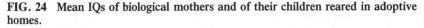

FIG. 24   Mean IQs of biological mothers and of their children reared in adoptive homes.

Surely the parents and children did not share a similar child-rearing experience, although some selective adoptive placement is said to have occurred with children of mothers who were at the extremes of the IQ distribution. What the mothers and children did share was not environment but heredity. Through heredity, through the genes, the biological mother and father are seen as determining their child's capacity to use or benefit from the adoptive home. Parental influence was exercised through the kind of nervous system or biological equipment that their genes enabled the child to develop. Although an enriched environment led to essentially normal mental ability in the children of retarded mothers, it is heredity that still left these children well below the means of the children of the brighter mothers. The effect of environmental enrichment was to elevate the mental ability of the adopted children well above what might have been expected if they had been reared by their own mothers, but this enhancement did not eliminate all differences between them. The differences persisted, though at a higher IQ level, and it is heredity that is seen as maintaining the differences. Heredity acted to regulate the adopted child's capacity to benefit from the enriched child-rearing experience.

A very similar finding is noted in the earlier-cited Willerman (1979) study of adopted children. As a part of that study Willerman looked at the children whose mothers represented the extremes of IQ in the maternal IQ distribution. The lower IQ group had a mean of 89 ($n = 27$), and the higher a mean of 122 ($n = 34$). As in the case of the Skodak and Skeels study, the children of the least bright mothers functioned in the normal range. Their average IQ was 103; the maternal mean was exceeded by 14 points. But as in the former study, the children of the least bright group did not function at the same level as those of the brightest group of mothers. The children of the latter averaged 118, a difference between the two groups of adoptees of 15 points. There was a four-point difference between the means of the adoptive parents in favor of the brighter adoptees (115 to 111), but this is not presumed to be a primary cause of the 15-point difference.

Another major difference between the two groups is in the proportion of each functioning at the extremes of their distribution. Of the children of the brighter biological mothers, 44 percent had IQs of 120+. None (0%) of the other group had such scores. And 15 percent of the children of the least bright mothers had IQs of 95 or less, in contrast to 0 percent of the children from the other group of mothers. Willerman sees these data as also reflecting a heredity and environment interaction wherein the environment produced a significant effect but where the *magnitude* of that effect was influenced by heredity.

Separated Identical Twins

Perhaps the most convincing evidence for the role of environment on intelligence, and for a heredity-environment interaction as well, is found in studies of twins, particularly identical twins separated early in childhood and reared in different homes. Twins occur with a frequency of about one in 86 births (Neel & Schull, 1954), and their usefulness in research is based on the existence of two types—identical (monozygotic) and fraternal (dizygotic). One-third of all twins are identical, with the remaining two-thirds equally divided between same-sex and opposite-sex fraternals.

IDENTICAL TWINS

Identical twins or identical triplets, quadruplets, quintuplets, and so on are the product of a single fertilized egg which, either prior to or shortly after placental implantation, divides by fission and creates two or more separate embryos that are genetically identical because they are derived from the same sperm and egg cell. Identical twins are unique in the human species, being the only examples of persons sharing the same heredity. It will be recalled that ordinary siblings generally share about half of the parental chromosomes (and genes) in common. In a sense, identical twins and their other multiple birth counterparts can be regarded as "pseudoclones." It is, of course, their genetic identicalness which accounts for their striking physical similarities; it is often difficult to tell them apart. Since sex, too, is determined by the genes (on the sex chromosomes), identical twins are always of the same sex.

FRATERNAL TWINS

Fraternal twins, and their multiple birth counterparts, are the result of the simultaneous fertilization of two (or more) different ova by two (or more) different sperm cells. They have the same degree of genetic relationship as single-born siblings and may be either of the same sex or opposite sex.

IMPLICATIONS

The implications that follow from these two types of twinning are twofold. First, since identical twins are genetically alike, all differences between them must be of nongenetic or environmental origin. Furthermore, the degree of difference indicates the range of variation the environment can effect on a given genotype. This is the dimension *reaction range*, which was discussed in the prior chapter. Second, since fraternal twins are no more alike genetically than ordinary siblings, differences between them may be of either genetic and/or environmental origin. Twin studies typically compare identical and fraternal twins on some trait whose heritability is in question. If the identical twin pairs are significantly more similar, it is concluded that the trait *may* have a genetic basis. Qualification is necessary because of an assumption underlying the twin comparisons—that the environment of the identical twins was no more similar than that of the fraternal ones. Unless this can be shown, the observed greater similarity between identical twins could be attributed to environment rather than to heredity, the physical similarities of the twins themselves evoking more similar treatment.

The use in twin research of a special group of identical twins, those reared apart, helps to obviate this difficulty. They are assumed to have experienced less similar environments than identical twins reared together. Since differences between them are necessarily environmental in origin, should they be less similar than identical twins reared together, this would support an environmental effect. Thus, of particular interest will be a comparison of the degree of intellectual similarity between identical twins reared together and those reared apart, though our analysis will also include same-sex fraternal twins reared together.

TWIN STUDY FINDINGS

In addition to a number of studies of IQ differences among identical and fraternal twins reared together, there have been four of identical twins reared apart. The accuracy of the data in at least one of them (Burt, 1966) has been called into serious question (Kamin, 1974) and is not included here. In Table 10 are presented the relevant twin findings.

Comparing the two types of identical twins, we find that those reared apart are less similar than those reared together. This is evidence for an environmental effect. Moreover, differences of as much as 24 points have been found in twins who were reared in very different homes (Newman, Freeman, & Holzinger, 1937). This IQ effect is very similar in magnitude to that found in the earlier-noted studies on the adoptive placement of children of mothers with borderline or retarded intelligence. We would agree with Scarr-Salapatek (1975) that "a reasonable reaction range model for most genotypes (not severely retarded or extremely gifted) would include phenotypes in a 25 point IQ range."

Still further evidence of an environmental effect is found in the one study reported on retarded twins and, specifically, in those without organic impairment. Although all of the identical twins were both affected (100% concordance), a

TABLE 10   IQ Differences Among Twins [a]

Types of twins	Number of studies	Median intrapair correlation	Median intrapair difference[b]
Identical twins reared together	11	+.87	5
Identical twins reared apart[c]	3	+.68	7
Fraternal twins reared together	13	+.53	11

[a]*Source:* Erlenmeyer-Kimling & Jarvik (1963).
[b]*Source:* Jensen (1971).
[c]Represents 69 pairs.

concordance rate of 88 percent was also found for fraternal twins. Although the perfect concordance in identical twins is consistent with a genetic etiology, such a high rate in fraternal twins would not be expected on a purely genetic basis, and is attributed to an environmental influence (Allen, Kallmann, Baroff, & Sank, 1962).

But the combined twin data do not only show an environmental effect. If environment alone affected IQ, then fraternal twins reared in the same home should be more similar than identical twins reared in different ones. But this is not the case. In Table 10 we see that in spite of being raised in different homes identical twins are still more similar than fraternal ones. This argues strongly for a genetic as well as environmental component in intelligence. Fuller (1973) has indicated that the earlier-cited Reeds' data on the frequency of retardation in children of retarded parents is consistent with a polygenic model. They estimate that between 22 and 100 genes control intelligence and that about 70 percent of the variation in IQ is of genetic origin.

The research on foster and adopted children and on twins indicates that intelligence is not exclusively a function of heredity or environment. It is clear that the environment can either enhance or depress intellectual development and, most importantly, to a degree that makes the difference between essentially normal mental functioning and mental retardation. But the organism is not infinitely malleable. Even within a shared environment, be it home or institution, variation rather than sameness is the rule, and this is seen as reflecting differences in the biological (genetic) capacities of each individual to respond to that environment. This interdependence or "coaction" is the essence of Fuller's (1954) conception of heredity as *the capacity to use an environment in a particular way.*

PREVENTION OF MENTAL RETARDATION THROUGH EARLY ENVIRONMENTAL INTERVENTION

Head Start

The material cited thus far strongly suggests that it is possible to prevent the kind of mild mental retardation found in physically normal children who come from disadvantaged family backgrounds. Another of the potential sources of enlightenment on this question is Head Start. This is the federally funded national preschool program that began in 1965 and is intended to enhance school achievement in disadvantaged children. While Head Start has not been specifically directed toward the prevention of retardation, the children it has served include those coming from high-risk backgrounds. This is reflected in disproportionate numbers of disadvantaged ethnic and racial minorities in special classes and is the source of the "labeling" controversy discussed in the first two chapters. The intent of Head Start is to provide to disadvantaged children the kinds of preschool experiences that are thought to underlie school achievement and that are often not available in their homes. The theoretical rationale for early intervention lies in animal and human research (Caldwell, 1970; Uzgiris & Hunt, 1975) and its educational implications (Hunt, 1961). Bloom (1964) sees the intellect as particularly trainable during the preschool years, with marked environmental changes in the early years producing greater effects on intelligence than equally marked changes later on. Within this context a national preschool effort was begun in the 1960s and continues to the present. The most comprehensive evaluation of its effectiveness was presented by Bronfenbrenner (1974) in his monograph *Is Early Intervention Effective?* From more than 20 major studies he selected seven that met three criteria—2 years of follow-up information, a control group, and data that could be compared across studies. The seven projects were of two kinds, five primarily preschool (Beller, 1972; Gray & Klaus, 1970; Herzog, Newcomb, & Cisin, 1972; Hodges, McChandless, & Spicker, 1967; Weikart et al., 1970) and two focused on home-based intervention—working with the child's parent in the home (Levenstein, 1970; Schaeffer, 1968; Schaeffer & Aaronson, 1972).

PRESCHOOL EFFECTS

The preschool programs varied in length from a full summer combined with year-long home visits to 1- and 2-year preschool attendance. The earliest began at age 3. Preschool programs have been commonly evaluated in terms of IQ effects, and the general finding is that children attending them usually show a gain of about 10 points relative to controls. These gains are typically found at the end of the first year of participation, and continued attendance does not increase them. There is some indication that these gains may be primarily *motivational* rather than cognitive, as Zigler and Butterfield (1968) were able to demonstrate comparable IQ changes in Head Start children *prior* to the preschool experience by testing the children so as to maximize success and avoid extended periods of failure.

IQ differences between preschool and control children tend to disappear following entry into school. The controls commonly show a spurt in IQ which is presumed to be due to the new stimulation offered by school attendance, whereas the former preschoolers manifest a slight decline. The disappearance of the earlier IQ advantage of the preschoolers also has a school achievement counterpart. By the end of fourth grade there is only slight academic advantage seen for them. Not only were IQ effects temporary, but, surprisingly, there was no indication that the length of the program influenced their magnitude or permanence. Children starting earlier did no better than those starting later. And in one 5-year program (Deutsch, 1971), there was no significant difference between preschoolers and controls, their respective IQs being 97 and 93. At age 9 years, the mean IQ of the children who were in the various preschool programs is about 90.

The content of preschool programs can be categorized as either highly structured and cognitively-academically oriented or as relatively unstructured and "discovery" or free play in thrust. The latter was characteristic of pre–Head Start nursery school programs, those typically serving more affluent youngsters. It is clear that the more structured programs produce greater gains in disadvantaged children. But the "discovery" approach appears to lead to more "active" kinds of problem solving and to more positive attitudes toward learning. Bronfenbrenner (1974) suggests that an optimal mix would begin with structure but gradually invite discovery in increasing measure.

HOME-BASED INTERVENTION

Two kinds of home-based programs were reviewed by Bronfenbrenner. The first involved extensive work in the home with children, ages 1–3 years, but did not systematically involve the mother (Schaefer, 1968). Little effect was found relative to a control group, but the children who did gain were those whose mothers showed interest in the child's development and demonstrated some degree of "verbal expressiveness." As a result, Schaefer (1970) called for a "family-centered" rather than child-centered intervention approach. Precisely this kind of model is illustrated in the second study (Levenstein, 1970. Here the intent was to stimulate a mother-child interaction in 2- and 3-year-olds by providing toys that had educational potential. Especially noteworthy was the finding that there were not only significant IQ effects relative to controls, and of a much greater magnitude than usually found, 18 to 20 points, but that these differences persisted for from 3 to 4 years *after* cessation of the program. Analysis of maternal behaviors associated with IQ gains indicated the importance of "verbal interaction" as reflected in *responsiveness* to the child, *clarity* of verbal expression, expressed *approval*, and the use of *reason*. While this study supports the importance of a family- rather than child-centered intervention approach, there do not seem to have been any subsequent related academic advantages. For the most part experimental children differed little from controls and, like them, were tending to fall behind achievementwise by the end of the first grade!

At least two studies that combined home-based intervention with preschool did not show any IQ advantages for the experimental children. In one of them (Karnes, Hodgins, & Teska, 1969), the absence of a maternal effect was attributed to the simultaneous access of the children to a preschool. It is presumed that the mothers regarded their role as less important. In the second study (Gilmer, Miller, & Gray, 1970), children who had had the combined intervention showed less IQ decline after its termination. Bronfenbrenner likens parent involvement to a "fixative" in chemistry. It stabilizes gains produced in other ways. Home-based programs are perceived as effective, at least IQ-wise, to the degree that the target of intervention is neither the parent nor the child exclusively but rather the "parent-child system." Another benefit of parent involvement is that its effects can be transmitted to other children. Thus gains are found in younger sibs as well, so-called "vertical diffusion."

In summary, family-centered intervention before age 3 involving the mother in verbal activity of an educational nature with her child appears to produce several effects. First, it results in IQ gains that are as great as or greater than those of preschools alone or of even home-based child tutoring, but not by the mother. More importantly, even when parent intervention commences *after* 3 years of age, the gains achieved are more resistant to erosion when intervention has ceased. Finally, parental involvement can be expected to benefit later-born children.

In reviewing the experiences that seem to underlie the advantages of family-centered intervention, Bronfenbrenner concludes, "The psychological development of the young child is enhanced through his involvement in progressively more complex, enduring patterns of *reciprocal contingent* interaction with persons with whom he has established a mutual and enduring emotional attachment. . . .

Any force or circumstance which interferes with the formation, maintenance, status or continued development of the parent-child system in turn jeopardizes the development of the child." Since even preschool programs can unwittingly diminish the mother's perception of her importance in the development of her child, Bronfenbrenner recommends a phased sequence of parent and preschool intervention. The involvement of the mother should begin at 1 or 2, with preschool experiences not introduced until later.

An examples of such phased intervention is one in which there were weekly home visits during the first and/or second years of life followed at age 3 by a preschool (Gordon, 1971). There were three main findings: (1) the earlier the onset of parent intervention, the more lasting the effect; preferably, it should commence during the first year; (2) when parent intervention *precedes* preschool, the effects will endure until at least school age (e.g., IQ 96 vs. IQ 89); and (3) the participation in a preschool *following* parent intervention does not lead to further IQ gains and, paradoxically, may result in some loss relative to children who have parental intervention and no preschool. This is thought to be another instance of the possible undermining of the earlier-established importance of the maternal influence.

Another example of the significance of parental involvement is seen in the response of children to a preschool follow-up supplemental kindergarten program as a function of whether or not there had earlier been maternal intervention (Radin, 1969). Interestingly, it was the children who had earlier experienced parent intervention who benefited most. Furthermore, additional IQ gains associated with the supplementary kindergarten program were limited to children whose mothers were also receiving home counseling. It appears that parent involvement in the preschool years increases the impact of a subsequent school experience, especially when the mother continues to be involved. This hypothesis was subsequently tested (Radin, 1972) by looking at the intellectual status of children of school age who earlier had a preschool experience but who differed with regard to parent intervention. At kindergarten age, it was again children who had experienced both maternal and preschool intervention who continued to make IQ gains. Bronfenbrenner sees the special significance of Radin's work as demonstrating that parent intervention not only provides a "fixative" but that it also is a "catalyst" which enhances the impact of educational experiences that may accompany or follow parent intervention.

Finally, where maternal intervention programs that stress an active mother-child interaction are compared with maternal interventions limited to courses or information dissemination, it is only the former that have shown promise (Amidon & Brim, 1972).

IMPLICATIONS FOR MENTAL RETARDATION

Given the apparently extraordinary importance of the mother in determining the effectiveness of preschool programs, and of later ones as well, what are its implications for mental retardation? More specifically, can the mentally retarded mother be an effective agent in the "parent-child" system? In the last major section of this chapter we consider again, and in some detail, the specific ingredients, both affective and cognitive, of a growth-enhancing child-rearing experience and the probable limitations of the mentally retarded mother.

Follow-Through

This is an ongoing major national education effort to provide supplemental education in the early elementary grades to disadvantaged children and assistance to their parents. Follow-Through is intended to be a continuation of Head Start— an effort to preserve any earlier gains associated with a preschool experience. Evaluation of its effectiveness has been complicated by its dual focus—some programs being primarily educational and child-oriented while others have taken a parent/social services thrust. Only the educational impact has been comprehensively studied (Stanford Research Institute 1971a, 1971b; Stebbins, St. Pierre, Proper, Anderson, & Cerva, 1977), and the findings are controversial (House, Glass, McLean, Walker, & Hutchins, 1977). The effect of Follow-Through on the educational achievement of disadvantaged children through third grade has been disappointing, and Stebbins et al. (1977) concluded that it is genuinely hard to raise achievement scores by the compensatory methods applied. The extent of academic difficulty in these children is such that by spring of third grade, even with Follow-Through, about a third are already 1 year behind in grade level. Within the basic skill subjects of the early grades, their area of greatest weakness is "language" (punctuation, capitalization, word usage, and sentence "sense"— recognizing affirmative, interrogative, and incomplete sentences). But despite this picture of academic difficulty, there are some bright spots, and they are consistent with earlier findings in Head Start. Follow-Through comprised a number of educational models, but those that produced the highest levels of achievement combined *high structure* with an emphasis on teaching basic *academic skills*. Interestingly, the single most effective program, the (DISTAR) curriculum, also places a strong emphasis on the home environment. Recent follow-up studies of DISTAR-instructed children at fifth and sixth grades show continued benefits relative to non-Follow-Through children, particularly in reading, word recognition, math problem solving, and spelling (Becker & Gersten, 1982). But in relation to standard achievement expectations, even these children show major declines. The loss of ground after leaving Follow-Through is reflected in failure to master long division and complex multiplication and in difficulties with vocabulary and reading comprehension. The conclusion is drawn that the DISTAR method of instruction needs to be continued into the intermediate grades.

Follow-Through has also sought to evaluate its impact on self-concept, an area of particular interest in light of our earlier stress on self-esteem as one of the major dimensions of personality. It was found that children who were exposed to teaching models that stressed basic skill acquisition also had better self-concepts. Contrary to the view that self-esteem is a prerequisite to learning, it is learning itself or experiences of success that foster self-esteem.

Preschool Experience
and Prevention of Mental Retardation

Head Start and Follow-Through give no direct answer to the question of the prevention of retardation, but they point to the importance of the role of the family in mental development. Moreover, Head Start and Follow-Through have focused on the "average" disadvantaged child while the high-risk child represents a special subgroup of that population, those whose mothers are themselves retarded (Heber, Dever, & Conry, 1968). We now look at several studies that have examined the impact of a preschool experience on children who are either already functioning as mentally retarded or who, because of retardation in the mother, are at risk. These studies have largely dealt with physically normal children who came from the kind of social milieu earlier depicted with regard to cultural-familial or psychosocial retardation.

Early Studies of Retarded
or High-Risk Children

The first effort in this realm involved a 2-year preschool program for 15 mildly retarded, institutionalized children. In comparison with a control group of 12 children who did not attend preschool, the former showed a mean IQ gain of 12 points, from 61 to 73, while the latter declined—from 57 to 50 (Kirk, 1958). The gain in the preschool group is comparable to that found in Head Start children.

An attempt to replicate the Kirk study by Fouracre et al. (1962) was unsuccessful because their population came to consist largely of retarded children with organic impairment. Over a 2-year period their sample of 54 children showed a nonsignificant IQ gain of from 59 to 65. But this finding parallels one of Kirk's (1958) with a subgroup of retarded children with organicity. It was the nonorganic retarded child and the youngster from a disadvantaged background who were most likely to profit IQ-wise from a preschool experience. These IQ gains can be understood as a response to increased stimulation in children who have earlier experienced little of what we have called a "mother-teacher." Since organically impaired children come from all social class backgrounds, they are much less likely, as a group, to have experienced parental understimulation. Presumably, the child who is *both* organically impaired *and* understimulated would show benefits from a preschool experience.

Another illustration of the quality of life in high-risk families is found in a study by Kugel and Parsons (1967). They examined the intellectual, health, and social needs of disadvantaged families where mothers had IQs in the range of 70–84. Though this research effort was focused on the prevention of retardation in high-risk children, it has received little attention, undoubtedly because of methodological limitations and data incompleteness.

A vivid picture is given of home conditions in families where crisis is frequent, sometimes catastrophic, but where there is a stoic acceptance of disaster. The mothers, though loving of their children, were ineffective in discipline, gradually losing control of them, until as adolescents they were responded to more as peers than as children. The families were socially isolated, and the adults were lonely people with few friends or community contacts. Physical conditions in the homes were dismal. They were meagerly furnished and very crowded. Often regular dishes were not available, and meals were eaten from kitchen pans or makeshift dishes. Half of the families had no sheets on their beds; people slept directly on mattresses and in their clothing. Blankets were usually dirty and smelly, towels were frequently just pieces of torn clothing, and closet and drawer space was negligible. In these crowded homes there was little privacy, and the possessions of the children were communal. The children were poorly dressed and were said to look and to feel like misfits. They were not well accepted by more advantaged children and adults; discrimination against them started in their early life and left its mark.

These families included 35 children who attended a preschool daily on a year-round basis. It is not clear how long the program continued, but it would appear that the younger children had at least 2 years in it. The program itself is described as the "usual nursery school curriculum," as no modification was deemed necessary for these children. In light of Head Start and Follow-Through, it is clear that maximal gains are related to programs with high structure and a cognitive-instructional emphasis. At entry into the preschool the average IQ of the children was 75 (range 55–105), and reevaluation at intervals of from 2 to 4 years showed a mean gain of 16 points and a group average of 91 (range 63–116). The amount of gain was related to age, with the younger children, ages 2–4, showing greater gains than the older ones.

Of particular interest was the fate of 12 children whose initial IQs were in the retarded range, 55–69. With the exception of one child whose IQ was 55, the rest were in the 60s. None of them had gross signs of organicity, although one had borderline microcephaly. At reevaluation all were functioning above the retarded range except the child with IQ 55. Their mean IQ increased from 64 to 87 (range 72–113), a gain of 23 points. Though there was no control group, the magnitude of the change observed is certainly consistent with earlier-cited studies on the potential impact of the environment on young children who are free of gross organic abnormality. This investigation also points to the multiproblem nature of the poverty family and to the need for comprehensive family assistance in health, child rearing, housing, and employment. With reference to the children, stress is placed on the importance of *early* preschool intervention, preferably before age 4. While the age effects on IQ gain predicted by the Bloom hypothesis (Bloom, 1964) have not been found in Head Start, Bronfenbrenner would still start preschools no later than age 3.

THE MILWAUKEE PROJECT

Of all of the early-intervention programs directed toward the prevention of retardation in high-risk families, none has created greater interest and controversy that the Milwaukee Project. Its focus was on children of mothers with IQs of less than 75, women whose children comprise a disproportionate segment of the Milwaukee inner-city retarded population. On the basis of an earlier prevalence study it was concluded that it is not slum residence itself that is associated with retardation but rather the presence in the family of a mother who is retarded (Heber et al., 1968). Intervention consisted of working with 20 children from such families beginning at age 3 months, first in the home, and then continuing throughout the remainder of infancy and the preschool years with a day-long preschool program. Some attention was also given to the mothers but mostly in vocational, reading, and home management skills. There was a control group of a like number of children.

The interest created by this relatively massive intervention stems from its purported effect on IQ. The experimental children not only consistently scored 20–30 points higher than the controls, but, on the Stanford-Binet test, the experimentals hovered around IQ 120. While a 20- to 30-point "environmental" effect is perfectly consistent with earlier reported studies, it is the absolute level of IQ attainment that is unexpected. It should be noted that after the preschool years the children were tested with the two Wechsler children's scales—the Wechsler Preschool and Primary Scale of Intelligence (WPPSI) and the Wechsler Intelligence Scale for Children (WISC). On these tests lower scores have been obtained, for controls as well as experimentals, a common phenomenon when comparing Binet and WISC or WPPSI findings (Sattler, 1974). At age 8 their respective WISC IQs were 104 and 81. Questions have been raised about the reliability of the Binet IQs, the precise nature of the preschool program, and the research methodology (Page, 1973). Doubts about the Binet IQs led to acknowledgment that there had been some training on test items through their fortuitous inclusion in the preschool curriculum (Page, 1973). The published data are extraordinarily incomplete; for example, we are not given the means and standard deviations for maternal IQs, nor are statistical tests of significance offered to support apparent effects.

Uncertainties about the test scores have not been eased by what is sketchily known about the children's school achievement, at least through third grade. In the first edition of this book, agreement was expressed with the Milwaukee investigators' view that "any ultimate evaluation, of course, must be based on the performance of these children as they move through the education system" (Heber, Garber, Harrington, & Hoffman, 1972). Although IQ scores are reported for both groups to age 9, no comparable grade achievement data are presented. In an unpublished paper given by Garber,[5] the experimental children are said to have exceeded the achievement level of the controls throughout at least second grade, but that in third grade there had been a major decline in their reading level. This was attributed to a combination of poor communication between parent and school and to unstable and conflict-ridden family situations. Given the extremely meager information on the educational status of the children, we can judge neither the degree of reported decline nor the factors accounting for it. We certainly do not doubt the existence of home environments that fail to meet the child's need for a "mother-teacher" and are not surprised at Heber's assertion that intervention and support for children reared by intellectually inadequate parents and living in dis-

---

[5]Paper presented by Howard Garber at Gatlinburg Research meeting on mental retardation, Gatlinburg, Tennessee, 1978.

rupted family environments must continue through the school as well as preschool years (Heber, 1976). This, of course, is what much of Follow-Through is all about.

Given the paucity of current information, it is extremely difficult to evaluate the effectiveness of a program whose massive intervention and reported IQ effects have promised so much. One can only hope that the following statement in a letter to the author from the Milwaukee public schools understates its impact: " 'Project pupils' are probably equal to or better than a control group in terms of measured ability, academic achievement, and personal adjustment." If this is the *best* that can be said at this time, then the effectiveness of the Project is seriously called into question by the investigators' own criteria.

THE ABECEDARIAN PROJECT

This project[6] mirrors the Milwaukee one in intent and extensiveness, although, in the specificity of its curriculum, it aspires to a greater degree of replicability. Its target is also disadvantaged children, but where the Milwaukee Project focused on children of mothers with IQs of less than 75, the mean IQ of the mothers of the Abecedarian children is in the low 80s. The risk for these children would not be expected to be as high, and, indeed, the mean IQ of the older siblings of the project populations ("educationally treated" and control) is also in the low 80s, comparable to the IQs of their mothers and well above the usual range of retardation. The "educationally treated" group consists of children who have attended a day nursery and preschool since 3 months of age. Data on their intellectual functioning are available up to age 4 years, and one additional IQ evaluation is intended at age $6\frac{1}{2}$. There are 27 children in this group, the first two of four cohorts, and 23 in the control group. The mean WAIS IQs of the mothers of the educationally treated and control children were 83 (SD 12) and 81 (SD 12), respectively. There was no specific "parent intervention" component, although all families were offered basic health care and social services. The control children also received a diet supplement up to age 15 months. This was to assure the adequacy of their diet during the period of rapid brain growth and to maintain comparability to the day care children who were receiving meals at the center.

Given a curriculum that focused on cognitive, linguistic, and social development, significant differences in IQ between the two groups have been found from ages 2 to 5. Although both groups were at 106 at 1 year, day care children have consistently scored in the mid-90 range, whereas the controls have functioned in the 80s. The smallest difference between them is found on the latest test, at 5 years, when their respective means were 98 (SD 12) and 91 (SD 14). The associated IQ ranges were 71–119 and 68–123. The narrowed difference at 5 years may reflect the "climbing control group" phenomenon noted in the Head Start research. Whether the control group IQ will begin to decline back into the 80s, as was true of the older sibs, remains to be seen. In any case, the level of functioning

[6]Taking its name from the sound of the first four letters of the alphabet, "abecedarian" refers to one who teaches or studies the alphabet.

in the day care children is very similar to that seen in the better Head Start programs, and, since these did not usually begin until age 4, we have additional support for the absence of an age effect on IQ elevation. The range of scores found in the control group also confirms the expectation that these children are not really at risk for retardation. Only the very tail end of their distribution falls into the below-70 range, and, in fact, the two ranges are extremely similar. But the day care program has not only apparently elevated IQ, it has also reduced some of the variability in the children's functioning. They are more homogeneous (note the smaller standard deviation).

Another interesting finding is the absence of a significant mother-child IQ correlation in the educationally treated children. In contrast to a correlation of .43 between mother and child in the control group, recall that .50 is the usual parent-child correlation, that correlation was −.05 in the experimentals. These correlations were computed for IQs obtained at age 3. The lack of any significant relationship between mother and child IQ in the educationally treated group is regarded as evidence of an environmental effect, one that has eliminated the usual predictability of maternal IQ. But the day care program did not erase all family influences, and several factors that did positively affect IQ in the children related directly to the "parenting" function. They were (a) the emotional and verbal responsiveness of the mother, (b) the quality of playthings available to the child, and (c) the predictability and regularity of the child's home environment. These parenting behaviors recall earlier references to "responsiveness," "verbal mediator," and the general need for "structure." A second major study is under way, and this will involve "parent intervention," working with the mother beginning at age 3 months. This is clearly the message of all of the early intervention research.

Is Cultural-Familial (Psychosocial) Mental Retardation Preventable?

We have reviewed research on the effects of varying kinds and degrees of early intervention on the mental development of physically normal children who are at risk for either retardation or for a lesser but still significant intellectual impairment–IQ 70–85. Is intellectual functioning in these ranges preventable in biologically intact children? The answer seems to be an unequivocal "yes"! Intervention studies that involve the most radical form of environmental modification, adoption, regularly report IQs in the 100+ range. A "reaction range" of 25 points attendant on such drastic intervention seems evident, but even the lesser intrusiveness of the combination of parent intervention and preschool seems capable of elevating IQ at least 10 points. Of course, only the latter form of intervention is widely possible in our society, the implication being that we must maximize our effort to reach the high-risk mother during the infancy of her firstborn and involve her as a "teacher" to her child, offer comprehensive day care to her children beginning about age 3, and continue to offer support to the mother into at least the elementary school years.

ON THE NATURE OF "APPROPRIATE" INTERVENTION

Given the presumption that the mental development and related academic and vocational potential of economically disadvantaged children can be materially altered, attention is again directed toward the nature of the child-rearing experience that can produce this effect. We shall also consider how the disadvantaged parent, usually the mother, may be unable to provide these experiences. The oft-cited disproportionate contribution of our most economically impoverished social class to the population of nonorganically impaired persons with mild retardation is not confined to the United States. It is also seen in Scottish data shown in Figure 25.

Basic Health Care

A major goal of early intervention is to assure that every child, *irrespective of all other considerations*, receives basic health care. The disadvantaged child is "at risk" biologically as well as psychologically; recall that basic health care is offered in the Abecedarian preschool project. Social class appears to affect our perception of health and illness (Bergner & Yerby, 1968). Poor people have less accurate health knowledge, tend to place little stress on prevention, and delay longer in seeking medical care. Moreover, desires to take advantage of available services can be blunted by demeaning encounters with health professionals and the inconvenience of long waits in unpleasant surroundings. The consequences of these "health attitudes" are higher rates of inadequate (or no) prenatal care, pre-

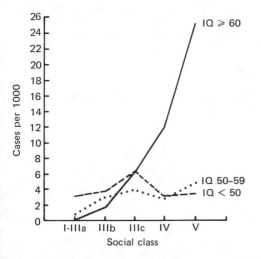

FIG. 25 The prevalence of different levels of IQ in mentally subnormal children from different social classes. From Birch et al. (1970). Copyright © 1970 by Williams and Wilkins Co., Baltimore. Reprinted by permission.

maturity, infant mortality,[7] and underimmunization. In Chapter 4 we discussed the significance of prematurity or low birth weight in neonatal death and in neurological abnormality and its association with the quality of prenatal care. Both prematurity and prenatal care are much influenced by social variables—maternal education and parental occupation, for example. Since the mid-1960s, tremendous progress has been made in reducing the frequency of inadequate prenatal care in poor pregnant women, the proportions declining from nearly 40 percent in the 1960s (Bergner & Yerby, 1968) to about 15 percent in 1975 (Gortmaker, 1979). In view of the relationship of maternal education to prenatal care, it can be assumed that it is the prospective retarded mother who probably constitutes a disproportionate contributor to that 15 percent. While statistical tables do not, ordinarily, make for interesting reading, the health statistics of poverty tell a powerful and sad story. Some from the early 1960s are shown in Tables 11 and 12. Above all, they reveal the utter vulnerability of the child born into the poorest of families.

Table 12 starkly reveals the vulnerability of the poverty child. Only half had received the "standard" immunizations of infancy, less than half against smallpox, and less than a quarter against polio. In the decade of the 1970s, smallpox has been totally eliminated throughout the world, but, imagine, at least 4 years after polio vaccination was a standard part of well-child care,[8] three-quarters of the children

[7]Death of a baby born alive in the first year of life.
[8]Personal communication from Bergner.

TABLE 11   The Relation of Health Problems to Poverty in New York City, 1961–1963

Problem	Total	In 16 poverty areas	In rest of city	Percentage excess in poverty over nonpoverty areas
Percentage infant deaths per 1000 live births	26	35	22	59
Percentage live births weighing 2500 g or less	10	13	8	63
Percentage of maternal mortality per 1000 live births	7	12	5	140
Percentage of mothers with late or no prenatal care	22	38	14	171
Cases of infectious syphilis per 100,000	96	207	52	298
Percentage of out-of-wedlock births	11	20	5	300
Crude death rate per 100,000				
Diabetes	23	23	22	4
Home accidents	12	14	12	16
Pneumonia and influenza	45	54	41	31
Tuberculosis	9	15	7	114

Source: Adapted and modified from Bergner & Yerby (1968), by permission of *The New England Journal of Medicine* (278, 541-546, 1968).

TABLE 12   Immunization of Children Ages 1–4 Years According to
Family Income (New York City, 1964)

Family income ($)	Percentage fully immunized		
	Diphtheria, pertussis, and tetanus	Polio	Smallpox
0–1,999	51	24	45
2,000–3,999	65	40	69
4,000–5,999	78	55	85
6,000–7,999	83	63	88

Source: Adapted and modified from Bergner & Yerby (1968), by permission of *The New England Journal of Medicine* (278, 541-546, 1968).

were still not immunized. The health data, like those of Head Start, illustrate the extraordinary importance of reaching the parents of these children.

Growth-Enhancing Psychological Experiences

A favorable developmental environment was earlier defined as one that would provide experiences to meet our basic psychological needs for structure, self-esteem, and self-expression. Such experiences would also enhance our "resources," the abilities or capacities we employ to meet our needs. The most important agent in that environment was termed a "responsive parent." "Responsive" or "effective" parenting can be conceptualized in at least two dimensions— emotional (affective) and cognitive. Examples of each are shown in Table 13

TABLE 13   Effective Parenting

Emotional (affective)	Cognitive
Loving one's child: providing tactile stimulation to the infant; relieving stress; providing acceptance, approval and praise more than criticism	Providing socially adaptive goals
	Using appropriate reward-and-punishment systems (contingencies) to encourage motivation to achieve adaptive goals and to apply these in a reasonably consistent manner
Accepting unpleasant as well as pleasant feelings in one's child (e.g., anger, fear)	Fostering skills that will enable goals to be achieved: curiosity, self-reliance, persistence
Managing one's own feelings of anger without brutalizing one's child	Functioning as a "verbal mediator"—explaining to the child the why's and wherefore's of behavior; utilizing reason as well as authority
Accepting one's child's sexuality	Encouraging a sense of competence—of "can do"—by providing developmentally appropriate experiences (e.g., play, chores, part-time employment)
	Proving enrichment experiences
	Encouraging the transition from dependence to independence

where the "cognitive" dimension is equated with the role of parent as "teacher."
It is true, however, that how parents deal with emotions also "teaches" the child.
In any case, it is useful to think of the child's parents as his first "teachers" and of
home as the child's first classroom. In Table 14 these same behaviors are organized in terms of basic needs.

Effective Parenting

MEETING THE "EMOTIONAL" NEEDS OF THE CHILD

Of the two components of parenting, the high-risk parent is more likely to
function adequately in the emotional domain. There is no reason to believe that
socioeconomic status or IQ affects the capacity to love, although the stresses to
which at least some of these families are daily confronted can block its expression.
The retarded mother, in particular, appears to be vulnerable to stress and to suffer
more quickly in the maternal role as family size increases. As her own children
reach adolescence she is also more prone to abandon a true parental role and to
assume one that is more siblike. A survey of the children of retarded parents in
Northern Ireland (Scally, 1973) indicated that only 30 percent were considered to
be adequately cared for, the remainder apparently being placed outside the family
home. The reasons for placement are not given.

TABLE 14   "Effective Parenting" and the Meeting of Biological
and Psychological Needs

Biological	Structure	Self-esteem	Self-expression
Meeting "survival" needs: food, cloth- ing, shelter Maintaining a state of health Accepting sexual ex- pression	Adaptive goals Appropriate reward systems— "understanding the contingencies" Access to a "verbal mediator"	*Intimacy* Loving one's child: tactile stimulation; reliev- ing distress; accept- ing, approving, and praising more than criticizing *Success* Encouraging a sense of compe- tence; fostering curiosity and per- sistence; explaining the why's and wherefore's of be- havior; using rea- son as well as au- thority *Autonomy* Encouraging independence and a sense of personal control over one's life	Providing experiences of enrichment (gen- eral stimulation)

MEETING THE "COGNITIVE" NEEDS OF THE CHILD

Whatever the limitations of the high-risk parent in the emotional domain, there is no question that it is in the cognitive sphere that the greater difficulty is likely to arise. The area of greatest cognitive impairment in the disadvantaged child, in general, and, presumably, of the retarded and disadvantaged parent in particular, is in "language" (Miller, 1970). Low-income children are said to spend less time interacting with adults (Keller, 1963), and, when speaking to them, their verbalizations are shorter (Deutsch, 1964). Language deficits relative to more advantaged children are found in word knowledge, verbal categorization, and grammatical syntax, and these deficits are cumulative, increasing in the elementary grades (Deutsch, 1967).

We have earlier referred to the language impairment of the disadvantaged child in connection with Follow-Through. It has been suggested that the language difficulties of the disadvantaged child are due to an impoverishment of the mother-child communication system (Hess & Shipman, 1965). An analysis of maternal teaching behavior in these families showed reduced verbal output, inadequate levels of conceptualization, and fewer attempts to teach the child about the relationship between events. The last mentioned epitomizes what is meant by the parent as "teacher." In contrast, middle- or upper-class mothers tend to verbalize more with the child, to use more complex syntax and longer sentences, and to be generally more effective as teachers (Martin, 1975). Gray and Klaus (1965) note that when information is given by the poverty mother it is likely to be vague and too general—"You're a bad boy"—rather than specifying the nature of the problem.

Another worker, John (1963), regards the greater concreteness of the disadvantaged child as due to reduced exposure to a mother who serves as a tutor. One of the common reading problems of these children is in phonics, analysis of words by their sounds, and it is considered that this is due to diminished "word game" experiences with adults, such as rhyming and being read to (Wallach & Wallach, 1977).

Two conversations are now offered that illustrate parental differences in readiness to assume a teaching role. They are drawn from Bernstein's (1967) analysis of social-class language differences in Britain but also seem applicable to our own society. They take place on a bus, where a mother has a child seated on her lap.

Mother: Hold on tight.
Child: Why?
Mother: Hold on tight.
Child: Why?
Mother: You'll fall.
Child: Why?
Mother: I told you to hold on tight, didn't I?
Mother: Hold on tight.

Child: Why?
Mother: If you don't you'll be thrown forward and fall.
Child: Why?
Mother: Because if the bus stops suddenly, you'll jerk forward.
Child: Why?
Mother: I told you to hold on tight, didn't I?

In the first exchange, the mother short-circuits the opportunity for teaching the child something about motion and safety by limiting herself to control through authority. The natural curiosity of the child is blunted. In the second exchange, the child is exposed to cause and effect. This mother is no less protective and, in the end, also resorts to control through authority, but she also wants her child to understand *why* he must hold on tight.

OTHER CONSEQUENCES

Not only is the high-risk child adversely affected by reduced access to a "teaching" parent, but this condition unwittingly encourages the child's emotional investment in behavior that can be maladaptive. The educationally unprepared child will come to devalue school achievement as a source of self-esteem because the experience there is one of failure, ridicule, and diminished self-worth. To maintain self-esteem the child will, necessarily, look to other kinds of experiences and may find that mastery through aggression becomes a means of winning positive recognition, at least from peers. It is "masculinity" (macho), in the male, that becomes the chief prop on which self-esteem depends. This is not to say that the educationally prepared youth is indifferent to gaining approval through physical means but rather that that youth has a wider range of behaviors (resources) on which to draw. To the degree that one is not dependent on any one resource for maintaining a sense of worth, there is greater acceptance of limitations and less need to constantly prove oneself.

THE MENTALLY RETARDED PARENT

If, as presumed here and elsewhere (Robinson & Robinson, 1976), the mentally retarded parent is inevitably going to be impaired in the cognitive-teacher domain of parenting, what are the implications? We deal now with one of our most fundamental rights, the right to be a parent. Although society has earlier sought to interfere with the procreative potential of retarded persons through institutional segregation and involuntary sterilization, the abuses attendant on these measures have produced strong counterreactions, and any infringement on the rights of retarded persons is now the subject of careful scrutiny. But all "rights" carry with them corresponding "responsibilities." In our view, this calls for communicating to retarded adolescents and young adults the needs of children and the responsibilities of parenthood. It calls for extensive sex education, for separating marriage from parenthood, and for encouraging the use of health and family services for those who want children. To do less or to pretend that the problem does not exist is to do a disservice to retarded persons, to the children they will bear, and to that society of which we are all a part. (This topic is again addressed in the section on sexuality in Chap. 9.)

An Overview of Services to Retarded Individuals and Their Families

OVERVIEW

Through the first five chapters of the book our focus has been on the nature of mental retardation and its causes. In this chapter and in the remainder of the book, the emphasis shifts to its management. In its most general sense, management refers to how society responds to the retarded person and to the adaptive difficulties the condition engenders. This chapter introduces the management aspect by considering four major dimensions: (a) the "right" of retarded people to receive appropriate services; (b) "normalization"—a philosophy of management that seeks to accord retarded persons opportunities and experiences that most nearly parallel those of the rest of us; (c) the "continuum of care"—the array of services needed by retarded persons and their families and, in this chapter, with special emphasis on diagnostic ones; and (d) the creating of an array of services with particular attention to scope (prevalence), coordination, and administrative organization. In the chapters that follow each of the major services is treated in depth.

THE RIGHT TO SERVICES

Until very recently, the most visible signs of society's response to the needs of retarded persons were special education classes in the public schools and large residential institutions. Special education typically served children and youths with mild or moderate retardation, roughly equivalent to the school designations of "educable" and "trainable." Though initiated in the United States in the 1890s, as late as the early 1970s only about 40 percent of these children were receiving a public education (President's Committee on Mental Retardation, 1969). In the 1970s, sparked by judicial decisions and federal legislation, there was an explosion of educational services, and, by the end of the decade, at least 90 percent of the total retarded population was receiving some kind of educational program (Kirk & Gallagher, 1979).

The large state institutions have also been a focus of tremendous concern. As early as 1963, President Kennedy was calling on Congress to reduce the number of mentally ill and mentally retarded persons in institutions (Scheerenberger, 1976). Together with media exposés of abominable institutional conditions and such pictorial essays as *Christmas in Purgatory* (Blatt & Kaplan, 1966), a picture emerged of generally inadequate care that, coupled with numerous instances of outright resident physical abuse, fueled the "normalization" and deinstitutionalization movements. The latter involved an attempt both to improve institutions and, more importantly, to reduce the number of persons served in them by creating residential programs at the community level.

In a sense, the recent thrust for the development of services for retarded people is part of a broader social movement toward improving the quality of life for all disabled persons, a movement that reached one pinnacle with the enactment and implementation of the Rehabilitation Act of 1973. Apart from provisions that prohibit various forms of discrimination in programs receiving federal dollars, the intent of this and related legislation was to change the status of handicapped persons from one of separateness and exclusion to one of integration and inclusion. But such change does not come easily. The conditions that produced absent or inadequate services reflect our basic attitudes toward handicapped individuals. In one view (Goffman, 1963), all forms of physical and mental disability have the power to disturb us; we come to expect that others will be like ourselves, generally whole and unblemished. When we encounter persons who are "different" in some significant way, there is the tendency to perceive them as not quite "human," as a kind of alien. In these encounters we may experience discomfort, anxiety, and fear (Bartel & Guskin, 1971). Where there is physical deformity, shock and repugnance are common. Even when handicapped individuals demonstrate capacities that evoke our admiration or even awe, as in the ability of some blind people to "read" their physical environment, they are still largely perceived in terms of characteristics we would not want for ourselves. Our culture has tended to regard handicapped persons as objects of scorn and ridicule, and even our positive feelings are often fringed with pity. Given this traditional attitude, it is hardly surprising that we have either ignored their existence or placed those with mental and emotional disabilities out of sight and mind in custodial-like institutions and hospitals.

Basic Rights

Undoubtedly, the civil rights movements of the 1950s and 1960s created the kind of climate for the redress of grievances which led to assertions of the "rights" of retarded persons by national and international organizations (Scheerenberger, 1976). In 1968 the International League of Societies for the Mentally Handicapped proclaimed rights of retarded persons pertaining to education and training, work, place of residence, guardianship, and legal safeguards. Their "Declaration of General and Special Rights of the Mentally Retarded" was adopted by the United Nations in 1971. In 1973 the American Association on Mental Deficiency (AAMD) issued its own "rights" statement and later developed a series of "position papers" elaborating on the rights already mentioned and dealing with such issues as sterilization, habilitation, and aversive treatment procedures. As a backdrop for later discussion of the infringement or denial of rights and its associated litigation, the following statement of "basic rights" promulgated by AAMD is quoted:[1]

> I. The basic rights that a retarded person shares with his or her nonretarded peers include . . . those implied in "life, liberty, and the pursuit of happiness" . . .
>
> A. *The right to freedom of choice within the individual's capacity to make decisions and within the limitations imposed on all persons.*
>
> B. *The right to live in the least restrictive individually appropriate environment.* (Nonretarded adults have considerable latitude to control their own lives, particularly in terms of choosing place of employment and place of residence. Insofar as he or she is able to make these choices, a retarded adult should have the same freedom of choice. A classification of mental retardation is not, of itself, sufficient cause to restrict an individual's freedom of movement.)
>
> C. *The right to gainful employment, and to a fair day's pay for a fair day's labor.* (A retarded individual should be allowed to work at whatever job he or she is capable of performing and should be paid at a level reflecting his or her productivity. If a retarded person cannot work in the community at large and is to be appropriately employed in the maintenance of the public or private institution at which he resides, then he also should be paid according to his level of productivity . . . [possible use of residents as unpaid employees, protection against *peonage*]. In no event should a retarded individual be retained at any facility solely because his or her presence enables the institution to maintain itself.)
>
> D. *The right to be part of a family.* (A retarded individual should not be summarily excised from his family, and should be permitted and encouraged to be with them whenever his developmental needs can be satisfactorily met in this manner. If . . . an institutional resident, family visits should be encouraged . . . .)
>
> E. *The right to marry and have a family* . . . (Any retarded citizen who can be effectively self-supporting, and who can be reasonably expected to discharge effectively the obligations of marriage and parenthood, should be permitted to marry and to raise a family; in no event, once . . . married, should the marriage be annulled on the basis of the exclusive circumstance of mental retardation, nor should that

---

[1]Position Papers of the American Association on Mental Deficiency, approved by AAMD Council 1973–1975.

person's right to bear and rear children be abridged. [The author's concerns re retarded persons as parents were presented in the preceding chapter] . . . If it should become evident that a retarded individual has become incapable of rearing his or her children, as may also occur with nonretarded parents, the same legal and professional procedures concerning parenthood that are applicable to families of nonretarded citizens should be applied . . . .)

F. *The right to freedom of movement, hence not to be interned without just cause and due process of law, including the right not to be permanently deprived of liberty by institutionalization in lieu of improvement.* (If . . . brought to trial and ruled incompetent to defend himself, legal counsel must be approved, at public expense if necessary. A retarded person must not be remanded to any public institution interminably. When . . . judged to be incompetent to stand trial [unable to participate in own defense and, presumably, remanded to an institution] . . . must be provided an integrated, individualized, and comprehensive habilitative program. Regular judicial and programmatic review of an individual's program must be maintained.)

Specific Extensions (of Basic Rights)

A. *The right to a publicly supported and administered comprehensive and integrated set of habilitative programs and services designed to minimize handicap or handicaps.* [The retarded individual may reasonably expect a program of habilitation geared to . . . individual needs at public expense. The program of habilitation should recognize the individual's handicap(s), but should be geared to allowing that individual to function in a way as nearly as possible approximating the functioning of nonretarded citizens. Each individual, however severe his handicaps, should be helped to realize his maximum potential through an individualized habilitative program that takes maximum advantage of all relevant services, . . . social welfare . . . , medical . . . , housing . . . , vocational . . . , transportation . . . , legal . . . , and financial assistance. . . . The program should be subject to regular reevaluation and open review, and should be adapted to reflect the growth and learning of the retarded individual. For those severely handicapped individuals who may never be able to function independently, it is the responsibility of the larger society to provide effective and humane supervised care using the full spectrum of resources essential to the person's optimal development in the least restrictive setting consistent with . . . capacities and needs.]

B. *The right to a publicly supported and administered program of training and education including, but not restricted to, basic academic and interpersonal skills.* (The society must make every effort to enable its retarded citizens, from childhood, to learn and use the skills that are necessary to function in the least restrictive setting possible and to function in the community . . . with the least supervision that is appropriate. Among the skills that retarded persons should be afforded the opportunity to learn are self-help skills, money handling, use of transportation services, adaptive interpersonal behavior, reading, writing, the ability to take advantage of other services and sources of assistance in the community and rewarding use of leisure time.)

Rights of Special Concern in Mental Retardation

LEGAL IMPLICATION OF LABEL "RETARDED"

The rights retarded persons seek to exercise are identical to those you and I take for granted but which may be denied to them in "casual" fashion. One legal scholar (Wald, 1976) has grouped them into two categories: *personal* rights—to marry, to have sexual relationships, to bear and raise children, and *civil* and *commercial* rights to contract, work, sue, vote, hold office, and serve on a jury. These rights are viewed as fundamental to the human condition and the very essence of citizenship. It is contended that we had created a dual legal system based on "labels" or classifications under which all members of a class were equally affected but that recent Supreme Court decisions have called for more individualized rather than class-determined methods of restricting or denying these rights when such action is deemed necessary. Wald argues that laws that restrict rights for an entire group are inevitably overdrawn. For example, while society should have minimum child care qualifications, it is inappropriate to deny in a blanket manner the right of retarded persons to rear their own children. To establish that a given parent, retarded or not, is unfit to raise his or her children, an individualized determination should be required.

THE RIGHT TO LIBERTY

Attention has been called to the denial of liberty itself (Friedman, 1976). Confinement to an institution necessarily involves restriction of the fundamental right to liberty and other rights that depend on liberty—the rights to travel, to free association, and to privacy. Once institutionalized, other rights that may be affected are those of habilitation, sexual expression, and even protection from harm.

The most blatant infringement on liberty has been the practice of indefinite commitment to an institution of a person charged with a crime but found incompetent to stand trial and defend himself. The law does not proceed against a defendant who is deemed unable to understand the nature and object of the proceedings against him or to make a rational defense. When mentally handicapped persons are found incompetent to stand trial, they are often committed to psychiatric hospitals or institutions for the retarded with the understanding that a trial will ensue if they ultimately become competent.

For persons with mental illness, recovery of a state of competence is at least a reasonable presumption, but in the case of incompetency associated with retardation, such a change is less probable, and the commitment may be permanent. This issue was addressed by the Supreme Court in the decision *Jackson v. Indiana.*[2] Jackson was a 27-year-old deaf-mute with a mental age of about 4 years and no ability to communicate apart from limited sign language. He had been charged with two counts of larceny—purse snatching and stealing property worth nine dollars. Found incompetent to stand trail, he was committed to a mental hospital until he should become competent. Although the maximum sentence for these misdemeanors, had he been convicted, was 6 months, he had already been confined for 3 years and might well have remained there for life had the Supreme Court not heard his case. The Court ruled:

> A person charged by the state with a criminal offense who is committed solely on account of his incapacity to proceed to trial cannot be held more than the reasonable period of time necessary to determine whether there is a substantial probability that he will attain the capacity in the foreseeable future. If it is determined that this is not the case, then the State must either institute the customary civil commitment procedure that would be required to commit indefinitely any other citizen, or release the defendant.

Since Jackson's prior adjustment had show that he was able to live independently and, at least on that ground, was not committable to an institution for the retarded, nor was he proven to be a danger to others (in court), he was released.

THE RIGHT TO HABILITATION

But does civil commitment even when appropriate to the person's condition negate his rights? This important issue relates to the often undesirable conditions in institutions to which retarded persons were committed. A landmark Alabama case[3] addressed this concern. Begun on behalf of state mental hospital patients, the plaintiffs were broadened to include retarded residents of its sister facility and the federal court held as follows:

> The evidence . . . has vividly and undisputedly portrayed Partlow State Hospital and School as a warehousing institution which, because of its atmosphere of psychological and physical deprivation, is wholly incapable of furnishing habilitation to the mentally retarded and is conducive only to the deterioration and the debilitation of the residents. . . . The evidence has reflected further that safety and sanitary conditions . . . are substandard to the point of endangering the health and lives of those residing there, that the wards are grossly understaffed, rendering even simple custodial care impossible, and that overcrowding remains a dangerous problem often leading to serious accidents, some of which have resulted in deaths of residents.

[2] 406 U.S. 715 (1972).

[3] *Wyatt v. Stickney,* supra, Unpublished Interim Emergency Order, March 2, 1972.

The nature of this case is landmark because, for the first time, a federal court held that retarded persons committed to a state institution had a constitutional right to habilitation. This right involved (1) a humane psychological and physical environment, (2) an individualized habilitation and training plan for each resident, and (3) qualified professional and paraprofessional staff in sufficient numbers to deliver individualized habilitation and training. These guidelines were subsequently incorporated in national standards for services to retarded persons[4] and in related federal legislation.[5] In the years following the Alabama decision, improvements were noted, but some residents were perceived as still not receiving suitable programs. These appear to have been primarily severely and profoundly retarded individuals. The state asked the court to modify its original standard and to substitute for these residents an "enriched environment" rather than regular programs of training and education. The basis for this request was the contention that some retarded persons were not capable of continued significant growth.

The court rejected this appeal[6] but does not appear to have addressed the question as to whether *permanent growth* in abilities is to be expected for severely and profoundly retarded persons or, indeed, for all persons. There do seem to be limits set on our growth potential—witness the frustration of attempting to teach functional academic skills to most "trainable" pupils. Assuming the reality of growth limitations, workers will have to distinguish between *skill development* and *skill maintenance* phases. The latter would allow for continued "horizontal" if not "vertical" growth in the sense that the individual is provided new experiences at a level of complexity that is within rather than beyond his apparent highest level. An example of this in the academic sphere would be "graded" readers. While one may not be able to read beyond the first-grade level, there are an infinite number of reading experiences that could be generated at that level. It is also probably true that the provision of such "maintenance" experiences might themselves have the effect of causing some further skill growth. In any case, this is an issue that workers in the field will have to address.

In 1982 the Supreme Court spoke to the right to treatment in the case of an institutionalized retarded adult in Pennsylvania who alleged physical abuse and repeated physical confinement with arm restraints. The Court declined to uphold a right to habilitation as such. Rather it held that institutions must provide "minimally adequate or reasonable training *when* training could significantly reduce the need for restraints or the likelihood of violence." With regard to the broader question of right to treatment per se, the Court stated, "This case does not present the difficult question whether a mentally retarded person, involuntarily committed to a state institution, has some *general constitutional right* to training, per se . . ." (*Youngberg v. Romeo*; emphasis added).

---

[4]Standards for Services for Developmentally Disabled Individuals. Joint Commission on Accreditation of Hospitals, 1977.

[5]Developmental Disabilities Act of 1970 (Ph 94-517) and Education for All Handicapped Children Act of 1975 (Ph 94-142).

[6]*APA Monitor, 11*, 1 (1980).

LEAST RESTRICTIVE ENVIRONMENT
AND FREEDOM FROM HARM

Earlier assertions of a right to habilitation had come to include the right to receive it in the setting that is least restrictive of individual liberty and where one is protected from harm. The former means living as normally as possible and receiving appropriate services in the least separate or most integrated setting. The case that brought these elements into play involved Forest Haven, an institution for the retarded operated by the District of Columbia (*Evans v. Washington*, 1978). The decision in this case called for depopulation of the institution and the creation of alternative living arrangements and other appropriate programs in the community. A similar decision was rendered in a suit brought against the Pennhurst state institution in Pennsylvania. In the judge's view, "minimal habilitation cannot be provided in an institution such as Pennhurst. . . . Pennhurst does not provide an atmosphere conducive to normalization which is so vital to the retarded if they are to be given the opportunity to acquire, maintain, and improve their life skills (*Halderman v. Pennhurst State School and Hospital*, 1978). It was later ordered that all school-age residents be moved from the institution and provided with residential and educational services at the community level. The concept of "the least restrictive alternative" has become a guideline in all kinds of services to retarded individuals and is most often encountered in its application to school programs as in "mainstreaming." In the just-cited Supreme Court decision, the Court did uphold the right of a behaviorally disturbed, institutionalized, retarded individual to at least that level of training or care that would reduce the need for physical restraints.

A right to be kept "free from harm" was first enunciated in the Willowbrook case (*New York State Association for Retarded Children v. Carey, 1975*). The conditions at Willowbrook State School, an institution for the retarded in New York City, were regarded as so deplorable as to cause its residents physical, mental, and emotional deterioration. This was interpreted as a violation of right to be protected from harm, a right inferred from the Eighth Amendment to the Constitution, which prohibits "cruel and unusual punishment." Though traditionally applied to persons in prison, it is now deemed applicable to any person for whom the state accepts residential care (Friedman, 1976).

RIGHT TO EDUCATION

The "right" of retarded persons that has had the widest impact is that of "education." The Education for All Handicapped Children Act (PL 94-142) enacted by Congress in 1975 requires that all states receiving federal dollars for their schools must provide an appropriate education for all the handicapped children in the state. The law refers to all handicaps—mental retardation, physical disability, visual or hearing impairment, learning disability, and emotional disturbance. The law applies to both handicapped children who are not in school and receiving educational services and to those who are in school but not receiving an appropriate education. The law stipulates that (a) the schools develop an individualized educational plan (IEP) for each child, (b) the child be placed in classes with normal youngsters to the degree possible ("mainstreamed" or placed in the "least restrictive alternative"), (c) the procedures used to evaluate children with learning difficulties not be culturally or racially biased, and (d) parents have access to "due process" administrative procedure whereby educational decisions of the schools regarding their child become subject to challenge.

Although the Supreme Court in the historic civil rights decision *Brown v. Board of Education* held that "education is perhaps the most important function of state and local governments," the Constitution does not specifically *guarantee* citizens a right to education. But it does guarantee "equal protection" and "due process." The "equal protection" provision prohibits the government from unfairly discriminating against either an individual or a group. Given (a) the importance of education to the individual citizen and to his society and (b) judicial agreement with the assertion that all retarded individuals are capable of benefiting from some kind of education and training,[7] where state or local government provides education under compulsory education laws, they cannot withhold these opportunities from retarded children. However, "due process" requires that governmental actions that exclude such children from the same educational opportunities offered others must be of such nature as to accord with fundamental concepts of fairness. The PARC decision was the first to acknowledge the special learning needs of retarded children, and, as a result, Pennsylvania agreed to assure a free, appropriate, and public education for each retarded child (Herr, 1976). With regard to "equal protection," the court concluded that there was no rational basis for denying public education to one group while providing it to others. Regarding "due process," the court relied heavily on the stigma that comes from misplacement or exclusion. The stigma is presumed to arise from the process through which children are classified (or "labeled") and is seen as requiring due process procedural safeguards (e.g., parents or guardians participating in the development of the educational plan for their child and the right to challenge the school's decision before an impartial hearing officer).

In the second "fairness" case on the right to education (*Mills v. D.C. Board of Education*), it was held that denial to retarded persons of educational opportunities offered others and arbitrary suspension and exclusion procedures violated due process. As noted, it is in the area of education that judicial and legislative actions have had their greatest impact in mental retardation. In the decade of the 1970s, the proportion of retarded children receiving at least some public education more than doubled. In spite of acknowledged pressures placed on schools and teachers, the nation appears to be finally facing up to its educational responsibilities to its handicapped children.

GUARDIANSHIP

The concept of guardianship pertains to the rights of retarded individuals because it gives to one person the legal authority to make decisions for another. It

[7]From landmark decision in *Pennsylvania Association for Retarded Children (PARC) v. Pennsylvania*.

brings into potential conflict two important social goals for retarded persons—the necessity *to protect them against injury and exploitation* and the obligation to *encourage maximum personal freedom and independence* (Friedman, 1976). The principle of "the least restrictive alternative" offers a means of reconciling this conflict. It requires that when a compelling public or societal interest justifies invasion of one's *personal* interest, the public interest should be no more intrusive than is absolutely necessary.

"General" and "Limited" Guardianship

Traditionally, guardianship has been an all-or-none affair. Distinctions were not made as to either the extent or kind of guardianship needed; guardianship meant only total care (Lippman, 1976). Further, its intent was chiefly financial—to protect the property of the ward. It took no account of the ward's capacity for prudent decision making in nonfinancial concerns such as employment, socializing, marriage, and childbearing. Usually the parent has served as guardian, but if the person was institutionalized it was common to automatically designate the institutional superintendent as guardian. The effect was to grant to an unrelated public official total control of both the life and property of the person, an administrative arrangement that is regarded as failing to represent the ward's interests if they were in conflict with those of the institution.

If the least restrictive alternative is applied to guardianship, it calls for tailoring it to the prospective ward's pattern of competencies. *General* guardianship would be appropriate for retarded adults who lack the capacity for any complex decision making. This would apply to profoundly retarded individuals and to severely retarded individuals who function at the lower end of their range. At lesser levels of retardation, however, limited or partial guardians may be feasible. This itself has two forms: guardianship of the *estate* (the right to make financial decisions) and guardianship of the *person*. The latter gives the guardian "custody" of the ward and the right to make a wide range of decisions (e.g., residential and educational but *not* financial).

But the concept of limited guardianship is not restricted to simply separating estate and personal interests. It also calls for the limiting of powers within each domain. A Wisconsin state statute stipulates:

> Any finding of limited incompetency shall specifically state which legal rights the person is incompetent to exercise. Guardianship of the person shall be limited in accordance with the order of the court accompanying the finding of incompetence. No person shall be deprived of any legal rights, including the right to vote, to marry, to obtain a motor vehicle operator's license, to testify in any judicial or administrative proceedings, to make a will, to hold or convey property, and to contract except upon specific findings of the court. Such findings must be based on clear and convincing evidence of the need for such limitations. (Wisconsin State Statutes, S 880.33, 1974)

Protectorship

The exercise of limited guardianship has also been described as "protectorship"—an apparent formalizing of the "benefactor" role mentioned in Chapter 1. It involves making available to retarded persons such counseling, guidance, and general assistance as may be needed with or without court action. Such assistance might be offered through the kind of local "care management" center to be described in the last section of this chapter.

While access to protectorship clearly meets an important need for retarded persons who are attempting to function as independently as possible, its provision through state or county agencies has some inherent limitations. Protectors (caseworkers) employed by public agenices will feel pressures to respond to the needs of their employing agency if these should come into conflict with those of the retarded client. Other potential limitations are the inherent lack of flexibility associated with employment in public agencies and the possible lack of opportunity for a sustained relationship between worker and client. It is suggested that publicly operated protective services will have difficulty in being responsive to individual needs (Wolfensberger, 1972).

Advocacy

One response to the limitations of publicly employed protectors is the concept of the *citizen advocate*. These are persons who as *volunteers* participate in one-to-one relationships with retarded persons (protégés) for the purpose of protecting their rights and/or meeting their needs for a social relationship. The former has been termed "instrumental advocacy," and the latter "expressive advocacy" (Wolfensberger, 1972, 1976). *Instrumental* advocacy involves helping the retarded protégé to solve significant problems including the securing of appropriate services from relevant agencies. In its instrumental aspect the *volunteer* advocate is free of the potential conflicts of interest implicit in protectors who are employed by the same governmental agency responsible for delivering those services.

Expressive advocacy is primarily a "friend" or, perhaps, someone fulfilling a big-brother or big-sister relationship who seeks to meet some of the social or interpersonal needs of retarded individuals, principally adolescents and adults.

Another very important kind of advocacy is *legal* or *case* advocacy. It is this form of advocacy that has formally challenged the denial of rights to retarded and other handicapped persons and won for them new forms of judicial and legislative protection. Legal advocacy has involved both individual representation (case advocacy) and representation of groups of individuals with a common concern (class advocacy). While case advocacy has largely been the responsibility of lawyers, nonlawyer "paralegals" have also been trained to represent retarded persons in the kind of "due process" administrative hearings to which we have earlier referred and, in fact, in court cases too, when appointed by a judge to be *ad litem* guardians (Cohen, 1976). Every state now has a protection and advocacy agency whose role is to support and defend the rights of retarded citizens and to train both lawyers and concerned citizens to function as advocates. It is particularly important that these agencies, though publicly supported, operate independently of the service delivery system. To the extent that this is true, they can more fully serve the needs of the client when these come into conflict with those of the service system. While judicial and legislative actions have been the most visible evidence of "legal" advocacy, its more frequent application has been in the school procedures related to the development of educational plans.

Consent

In this section on guardianship reference has been made to the dual concerns of social policy for retarded persons—the need to protect and the need to maximize personal freedom. The legal process of "consent" is germane to both. "Consent" applies when our approval is sought for some procedure or action that will have a significant effect on us (e.g., an operation for the retarded person, institutional placement, or a sterilization procedure). Valid legal consent depends on three conditions associated with the giving of consent: (1) the provision of *information* on the nature and consequences of the choices under consideration, (2) the capacity to understand the information and to weigh choices, and (3) the opportunity to exercise choice free of *coercion*, expressed or implied. It is presumed that much of the legal consent given by retarded individuals in the past was pro forma, and the effect of recent concerns is to assure that the consent given by a retarded person or by a surrogate really meets these criteria. In the case of the retarded person, at least, this means taking the steps necessary to help that person fully understand the situation for which consent is sought.

Normalization

Much of the legal and legislative activity on behalf of retarded persons is an outgrowth of the philosophy of "normalization," a "treatment" concept first advanced in Scandinavia (Bank-Mikkelson, 1969) and elaborated in the United States and Canada by Wolfensberger and his colleagues (Perske, 1972; Wolfensberger, 1972; Wolfensberger & Glenn, 1973, 1975). As initially defined by Nirje (1969), normalization means "making available to the mentally retarded patterns and conditions of everyday life which are as close as possible to the norms and patterns of the mainstream of society." Wolfensberger has broadened its application to make it relevant to *all* human services and has defined it as the "utilization of *means* which are culturally normative as possible, to establish and/or maintain personal *behaviors* and *characteristics* which are as culturally normative as possible."

Normalization places stress on the *means* through which services are provided. It seeks to reduce the degree of deviancy inherent in retardation and in other disabilities by encouraging the provision of experiences and development of skills that will help the person to most closely approximate normality within his or her culture. Its primary mechanism for accomplishing this goal is "integration"—that is, the *inclusion* of handicapped persons within the general society, a condition that should encourage positive "modeling." Integration should also reduce the likelihood of subjecting retarded persons to the kind of dehumanizing experiences that are encouraged by providing services in apartheid settings—out of sight, out of mind.

One of the concerns raised about normalization is its emphasis on the *milieu* within which services are offered rather than on the clients themselves (Mesibov, 1976). Its proponents had *assumed* that its application would produce positive behavioral outcomes, and research appears to have borne out their expectations (Eyman, Silverstein, McLain, & Miller 1977; Eyman, Demaine, & Lei, 1979, MacEachron, 1983). The related findings are presented in the section on residential services in Chapter 9.

In our view there are two extremely important benefits to be derived from its application to human services. First, by seeking to place the retarded individual in settings that most nearly approximate those of nonhandicapped persons, it automatically assures exposure to the *most complex* environment to which the person can adapt, thus maximizing behavioral potential. Second, integration will mean *our* more frequent exposure to persons who are different and devalued; it is only through such exposure that our fears and avoidance tendencies can be eased as we come to recognize that behind the outer manifestations of intellectual and/or physical difference there is a *person*—one who shares with us the same physical and psychological needs.

THE CONTINUUM OF CARE: AN ARRAY OF SERVICES

The "continuum of care" refers to an array of services designed either to prevent mental retardation or to help retarded individuals achieve their highest level of adaptation. These services meet our most elementary needs—a place to live, something meaningful to do, and access to social experiences. The continuum has both *horizontal* and *vertical* dimensions. At the horizontal level, the focus is on possible needs at any single moment in time for a multiplicity of services. Thus a retarded preschooler might be living in a foster home, attending a preschool developmental center, and receiving medical care for epilepsy and physical therapy for cerebral palsy. The vertical dimension reflects a time continuum, the need for services at each stage from infancy to adulthood. When this preschooler reaches school age, there will be service needs appropriate to that developmental level—educational, social, recreational, and vocational. As an adult there will be need for employment or the opportunity to engage in some other meaningful activity, for social, sexual, and recreational outlets, and, where there is at least moderate retardation, access to a community residential setting when the family home is no longer available.

Continuum of care also implies a *continuity* of services. It suggests a rational progression of experiences appropriate to one's age and abilities. Nor does the provision of these services constitute special or preferential treatment. Most can be provided by the agencies that serve all segments of the population—health, mental health, the schools, social services, vocational rehabilitiation, and recreation.

Let us now consider the array of services. They will be described briefly here and then treated in depth in the remainder of the book. Table 15 presents them arranged according to developmental periods from prenatal status to adulthood. At each stage there are identified (a) the required services, (b) the service agencies that deliver them, and (c) the professions with which they are associated. The table makes clear the extraordinary number of agencies and disciplines involved in serving retarded persons and their families. It is this diversity that has led to chronic problems of service coordination—an issue dealt with in depth later.

TABLE 15   Array of Services

Services	Service agents	Service disciplines
Prenatal		
Prevention Genetic counseling, prenatal care, amniocentesis, therapeutic abortion	Health Agents Primary physician, local health department, hospital clinic, fetology service	Physician, public-health nurse, genetic counselor
Infancy and preschool		
Prevention (medical) Metabolic screening (e.g., PKU), adequate diet, immunization, avoid toxic substances, follow-up of high-risk neonates, routine medical care	Health agents Primary physician, well-baby clinic at local health department, hospital	Physician, public-health nurse, nutritionist
Prevention (psychological) Stimulation	Child care agents Home, foster care (social service), infant stimulation, developmental day care	Parents or parent surrogate, teacher, aide, social worker, volunteer
Identification Screening, diagnosis, parent counseling, medical treatment, early intervention: sensory stimulation, physical therapy, encouraging motor, language, and cognitive development	Health agents Well-baby clinic (health department, hospital), physician (general practitioner or specialist, e.g., pediatrician or neurologist), special diagnostic clinic	Public-health nurse, pediatrician, psychologist, social worker, audiologist, physical therapist, occupational therapist, speech therapist, speech therapist, educator, dentist
Training and education Self-help (feeding, dressing, toileting), gross motor and fine motor, language, cognitive, social-emotional skills	Early childhood workers Infant stimulation in the home, child development center (generic and specialized)	Teacher, teacher aide, physical therapist, occupational therapist, speech therapist, social worker, psychologist
Residential	Care givers Home, adoptive home, foster home, small group home, respite care, "medical support" home	Parent, foster parent, group home parent

TABLE 15 Array of Services (*Continued*)

Services	Service agents	Service disciplines
Parental Training in child development, emotional support, respite care, parent organizations, social services	Early childhood workers, social service agencies, parent associations (local and regional)	Parent trainers, social workers
Coordination and advocacy Coordination of multiagency services (as needed), helping parents become "advocates" for their child	Case managers and advocates Case management agency; advocacy agency	Case managers (social workers, etc.), volunteers, lawyers, paralegals
School age		
Training and education As in preschool plus academic, prevocational and vocational preparation; sex and family life education; stress on acquisition of skills in activities of daily living	Education, vocational rehabilitation, health, and special therapies Public school, special school, homebound program, institution; vocational rehabilitation agency and health department; physical, occupational, and speech therapy	Teacher, aide, school psychologist, guidance counselor, rehabilitation counselor, sex educator, physical therapist, occupational therapist, speech therapist
Residential As in preschool but adding programs for special populations	As in preschool years plus special facilities for youthful offenders and behaviorally disabled	As in preschool years plus behavior management specialists
Recreational	Community parks and recreational programs Generic and special recreational resources; day programs, camping—day and overnight, summer, year-round; scouting, Special Olympics	Recreator, group worker, volunteer (e.g., student)
Coordination and advocacy As in preschool years but with special emphasis on assuring that schools fulfill their responsibilities under Education for Handicapped Children Act (PL 94-142)	As in preschool years	As in preschool years but with paralegal advocates assisting in school hearings
Adulthood		
Vocational Prevocational, vocational (as appropriate), and on-the-job training; competitive employment, sheltered employ-	Semiskilled and unskilled jobs in industry, services, and government; sheltered workshop, vocational rehabilitation agency	Employer, personnel manager, rehabilitation counselor, staff of sheltered workshop (administrator, work evaluator, work supervisor, personal

TABLE 15   Array of Services (*Continued*)

Services	Service agents	Service disciplines
ment		adjustment counselor, instructor)
Day "activity" program Primarily for severely and profoundly retarded adults and providing continued training in basic self-care skills and activities of daily living, recreation, and prevocational activities	Day "activity" center	Teacher, aide
Educational Courses on money management, human relations, music appreciation, health, sexuality, cooking, camping, etc.	Community colleges For example, Metropolitan State, Denver; College of Staten Island, New York; Northern Virginia Community College, Annandale, VA; Mesa Community College, Mesa, AZ	Educators
Residential From semiindependent living to specialized residential facilities for profoundly retarded and medically involved	Care givers and counselors Supervised/supported boarding placements, apartment clusters, and coresidential living; subsidized family living placement; minimum-supervision group home, intensive training group home, health care facility (ICF-MR), specialized facility for persons with chronic medical problems	As in earlier years plus health workers
"Support" services Home	Respite resources, homemaker, personal care, and chore services	"Respite" care givers, homemakers, personal-care attendants
Health	Medical and dental	Health professionals
Transportation	Community agencies	
Social and recreational	Organizations and community recreation resources	As in earlier years
Advocacy	Advocacy agency	As in earlier years
Coordination	Case management agency	As in earlier years

Preventive Services

BIOLOGICAL

This form of prevention refers to those services that enhance the likelihood of the conception and birth of a healthy infant. It refers to the planning of pregnancies, to the knowledge of genetic risk if it exists, to obtaining prenatal care, and to availing oneself of amniocentesis where risk is increased either because of chronological age, as in Down syndrome, or because of known genetic metabolic disorders detectable through this procedure. At birth, prevention entails the identification of high-risk babies (e.g., small for gestation age), screening for metabolic abnormalities, and commencement of appropriate dietary and medical procedures. Postnatal prevention, therefore, involves "routine" health measures: immunization, adequate diet, avoidance of toxic substances, and periodic examinations.

PSYCHOLOGICAL

Although we can be quite specific about the kinds of health measures that minimize the probability of retardation, in the psychological realm we are on somewhat fuzzier ground. The research cited in Chapter 5 leaves little doubt of the importance of the environment on cognitive development, but its specific nature is yet to be defined. It is clear that early stimulation is important, but the time span during which stimulation can be impactful may be broader than once thought. There is growing evidence that the involvement of the mother (or father) as "teacher" or "verbal mediator" is crucial to maintaining whatever benefits are achieved through programs of early stimulation, and this has enormous implications for workers in early childhood education and social welfare. The means through which psychological prevention can be achieved is "educational" in nature. It does or will incorporate family life education in our schools, health education for prospective parents, child access to early childhood education, and a "teaching" parent. With the rapid increase of women in the work force, there is a special challenge to social policy to make it possible for young children to have access to "teaching" parents, at least during their first 2 years of life.

Diagnosis and Intervention

In spite of our best efforts at medical and psychological prevention, there will continue to be children with congenital (present at birth) and postnatally acquired forms of retardation. We now consider the procedures, disciplines, and agencies involved in diagnosis and intervention. In this section, the diagnostic process is presented in some detail and is followed by an overview of the full array of services that ought to be available to retarded persons and their families in preschool, school, and adult years. In the chapters that follow, these "postdiagnostic" services are described in detail.

PREDICTING FUTURE RETARDATION
IN THE YOUNG CHILD

In some forms of retardation, (e.g., Down syndrome), the physical signs are commonly recognizable at birth and with them future expectations of intellectual impairment. It is standard pediatric practice to inform parents immediately of the child's condition and to try to provide the emotional support that will be needed. But here, as elsewhere, the physician should be cautious with regard to predicting the ultimate degree of cognitive deficit, since programs of early stimulation may result in somewhat higher levels of functioning than are usually found (see Chap. 3). But many if not most children who are eventually found to be retarded do not show a characteristic clinical picture at birth, and the nature of their abnormality only becomes detectable over time as the child's development lags relative to normative developmental milestones. *But developmental lag itself calls for extreme caution in interpretation.* At 8 months of age, for example, developmental delays of as much as 4 months are still compatible with future normality (Holsen, 1972). Apart from infants who at age 8 months are functioning at less than half of their chronological age, it is not until at least 2 years of age that developmental scores become reasonably predictive of future mental status, and even this is only true for children already functioning in the retarded range (Hatcher, 1976) and in whom the retardation is associated with biological abnormality (DuBose, 1976; Fishler, Graliker, & Koch, 1965; VanderVeer & Schweid, 1974). IQs in infants whose physical development is grossly normal are notoriously poor predictors of later intellectual functioning (Bayley, 1970).

CASE FINDING: A ROLE FOR THE SOCIAL SERVICE AGENCY

Though periodic examination of the infant and young child by physician or public-health nurse is the best means of identifying children with significant developmental delay, it cannot help the children whose parents use such services only in emergency. Many of these children are found in families receiving public assistance, and the "eligibility" worker who visits the home can also "screen" the children and inquire about those whose development is clearly deviant for their age. This will require training of eligibility workers in "growth and development," but it will bring to light infants and young children who are in need of medical and educational services.

The Diagnostic Process

MULTIDISCIPLINARY

The determination of mental retardation in the infant and young child is a complex procedure involving the assessment of sensory, motor, language, cognitive, and personality resources. Such a comprehensive evaluation is best accomplished in a multidisciplinary setting and one in which *evaluation is tied to intervention.* The clinical and behavioral picture presented by the child will dictate the range of assessments necessary; the most commonly involved are pediatrics, psychology, social work, physical therapy, occupational therapy, speech and hearing, education, public-health nursing, and child psychiatry. Of these, all except social work have the child as their main focus. The social worker will be primarily concerned with the family. The diagnostic process in the school-age child will generally not require the same breadth of assessments; ordinarily, associated health, sensory, or motor problems will have been recognized earlier.

SENSORY AND MOTOR PROBLEMS SIMULATING MENTAL RETARDATION

The need for caution in interpreting developmental delays stems not only from the kind of individual changes in developmental level already noted (Holden,

1972; VanderVeer & Schweid, 1974) but also from lags in development that may be due to sensory and/or motor problems unrelated to mental retardation. For example, lack of responsiveness to environmental sounds and the failure to develop speech may be caused by deafness (Telford & Sawrey, 1967). Similarly, diminished curiosity, prolonged mouthing of objects, and poor motor development may be associated with blindness (Lowenfeld, 1971). Slow motor development is not seen only in retardation; it is also found in hypotonia, a non-retardation-producing neuromuscular disorder, and, more frequently, in cerebral palsy. Of course, the latter commonly includes retardation.

BEHAVIOR DISORDERS IN THE YOUNG CHILD

In addition to the sensory and motor impairments that can simulate retardation, the behavioral picture can include severe personality disorder. In particular, developmental lag and behavior disorder will often be found in the child with infantile autism; the overlap between these two conditions was discussed in Chapter 2. The frequent presence of at least some degree of personality disorder, though not necessarily of the severity seen in autism, indicates the need for mental health skills in the assessment team. This may be provided by the psychologist or by a child psychiatrist. The importance of mental health skills in the diagnostic staff not only pertains to the child but can also be important in helping parents deal with the emotional consequences of a finding of retardation.

FAMILY ASSESSMENT: SOCIAL WORK AND NURSING

Evaluation of the emotional climate of the retarded child's family is the domain of the social worker. The focus of this discipline is on the family's capacity to cope with stress—here induced by the presence of a handicapped child (Schild, 1971). The social worker in the diagnostic team is concerned with (a) support of the family under stress, (b) optimizing growth opportunities for its retarded member and, preferably, within rather than outside the family setting, and (c) maintaining decision-making responsibilities with the family rather than with the professionals; it is only the family that must live with the consequences of those decisions!

Although the focus of the nurse is on the developmental status of the child, her attention is also directed to the family, especially in relation to its meeting of the child's health, nutritional, and training needs (Krajicek & Roberts, 1976). The nurse is often the first professional to evaluate the child—either in the home as an "advance" member of the diagnostic team or in health department well-baby clinics. She brings to the team knowledge of "growth and development" and skill in using such developmental screening procedures as the Denver Developmental Screening Test (DDST) (Frankenburg, Dodds, & Fandaz, 1973; Frankenburg, Goldstein, & Camp, 1971) and the Functional Screening Tool (Paulus, 1966).

ROLE OF THE PHYSICIAN

Recommendations on the nature of the pediatric evaluation as well as on the general role of the physician in mental retardation are found in several sources:

Mental Retardation: A Handbook for the Primary Physician (American Medical Association, 1965), the "Pediatrics" chapter in Wortis's series *Mental Retardation* (Drayer & Guzman-Neuhaus, 1971), and the chapter "Mental Retardation" in *Pediatric Neurology* (Chamberlin, 1975). The basic elements in the diagnostic examination are (a) a full family and personal history stressing pregnancy, birth, the neonatal period, and the child's subsequent development, (b) a careful physical and neurological examination, and (c) a determination of developmental status relative to chronological age. The importance of a comprehensive assessment has been noted by Illingworth (1966), who attributes the limited predictiveness of the infant examination to inadequate performance of these procedures, and an excessive reliance on sensorimotor tests. The latter concern is shown by other pediatricians as well and is reflected in the broadening range of procedures, described in the next section.

At the therapeutic level, the physician is reminded that no drugs or medical procedures can reverse intellectual impairment but that early detection of metabolic disease (i.e., PKU and galactosemia), can either prevent retardation or minimize its effects (Drayer & Guzman-Neuhaus, 1971). If the question of the possible placement of the infant outside the home is raised, the physician should avoid "prescribing" but rather stress the kinds of services that are increasingly available to help the parent rear the child at home—home-based infant training and specialized day care. The handicapped child is entitled to no less parental love and devotion than the normal child, and, without it, the already considerable burden is much intensified. The physician needs to recognize the right and the responsibility of the parent in making decisions as to the child's placement. Most importantly, the physician should educate himself to the general developmental expectations for retarded persons and to the range of services through which these expectations are achieved. This will provide the physician the kind of perspective necessary if the diagnosis is to be regarded as something other than ultimate catastrophe.

Neonatal Neurological Assessment

The desirability of the earliest possible detection of children at risk for retardation highlights the limitations of the standard pediatric and neurological examination in the newborn. Some neurological abnormalities present at birth are only *transient* perinatal effects (Illingworth, 1966; Parmelee & Michaelis, 1971). For example, drugs given to the mother just prior to delivery can reach the fetus and produce temporary abnormalities of color, respiration, muscle tone, and ability to respond to life-threatening mucus in the airway. These newborns need constant nursing during this transient period of depressed functioning (Tronick & Brazelton, 1975). On the other hand, Illingworth (1966) suggests that it is possible to recognize in early infancy the *mildest* form of cerebral palsy.

The traditional neurological examination of the neonate focuses on reflexive behavior associated with the midbrain (e.g., pupillary response to light) rather than on such complex behavior or integrated responses as visual tracking. Although this is an effective way of detecting gross abnormality, it is insensitive to mild central nervous system dysfunction. It also has the undesirable effect of classifying as neurologically suspect infants who later prove to be normal (Tronick & Brazelton, 1975). More recent neurological diagnostic procedures do not view the neonate as functioning at only a midbrain level. Infants who have only a midbrain and no cortex (e.g., anencephalics) do not show the habituation or grading of responses to stimulation seen in normal neonates (Prechtl & Beintema, 1964). Moreover, it is suggested that, apart from gross CNS abnormality, injury to the infant brain is more likely to be manifest in impairment of (a) more complex behavior, (b) states of arousal, and (c) total body tone than in the elimination of specific tendon or skin reflexes (Parmalee & Michaelis, 1971). An examination that incorporates both behavioral and reflex elements is Brazelton's Neonatal Behavioral Assessment Scale (Brazelton, 1973). In comparison with standard neonatal neurological assessment, it is as sensitive in identifying infants who will show permanent CNS abnormalities, but it is much less likely to misclassify as neurologically suspect infants who will later prove to be normal (Tronick & Brazelton, 1975). The more complex and integrated behaviors measured on this scale are infant regulation of their states of consciousness, habituation, attention to stimuli and control of tone and activity while so doing, and performing integrated motor acts.

Experimental Measures of Cognition in Infancy

The current interest in the evaluation of more complex behaviors in newborns is also related to earlier-cited research on identifying measures of cognitive functioning in infants that do not depend on intact motor skills (Kearsley & Sigel, 1979). Such measures would be particularly valuable in the assessment of infants with cerebral palsy, those in whom the capacity to communicate may be severely limited (Zelazo, 1979). They are also seen as a means of revealing normal mental capacities in the nonorganic failure-to-thrive children described in the previous chapter (Kearsley, 1979). The kinds of responses studied are smiling, vocalizing, visual attention, and changes in heart rate. Smiling is thought to be one response to the sudden understanding of some event and is accompanied by a release in tension (Sroufe & Waters, 1976; Zelazo, 1972). Vocalization appears to be more ambiguous in meaning. In infants under 1 year, it may reflect boredom with redundant events, but toward the end of the first year, like smiling, it appears to follow sudden understanding (Kagan, 1971; Zelazo, Kagan, & Hartman, 1975).

There is much research that reveals the sensitivity of the infant to change in its visual environment. Infants will show longer-sustained looking at stimuli that are moderately discrepant from what they already know—"variety" (e.g., Kinney & Kagan, 1976; Zelazo, Hopkins, Jacobson, & Kagan, 1974). Finally, change in heart rate seems to accompany activity of psychological significance. A slowing of heart rate often accompanies orientation and initial attention to a new event (Lewis & Goldberg, 1969), and an increase is found following the presentation of moderate novelty (McCall & Melson, 1969) and to situations evoking active thought or fear (Campos, 1976; Kagan, 1972; Kahneman, Tursky, Shapiro, & Crider, 1969;

Lacey, 1967). There is preliminary indication that normal and retarded infants can be distinguished by their attention-cardiac response to an auditory stimulus (Bradley-Johnson & Travers, 1979).

ROLE OF THE PSYCHOLOGIST

The psychologist has an extremely important function in the evaluation and management of problems of retardation. At the level of evaluation, the psychologist is responsible for assessment of intellectual and personality functioning; at the level of management, or intervention, he contributes through procedures that involve behavioral and psychodynamic methods.[8]

Intellectual Assessment in Infancy

Three of the most widely used infant measures have been the Gesell Developmental Schedules, the Cattell Infant Intelligence Scale, and the Bayley Scales of Infant Development.[9]

The Gesell Developmental Schedules (Gesell et al., 1940) permit evaluation of children from birth to 6 years in four developmental areas—motor, adaptive, language, and personal-social. In each, the child's level of functioning is compared with developmental norms and is reported in terms of a *developmental age* and *developmental quotient*. A major limitation is a relatively heavy emphasis on motor and physical skills. If these are not very deviant, the overall score will have little predictive value. The Schedules were described by their chief developer, Gesell and Amatruda (1947), as "in no sense a formal examination but a selective screening device which will serve to indicate those cases which do need a formal developmental examination. . . ." As a "screening" device, the Gesell is probably being replaced by the later developed Denver Developmental Screening Test (Frankenburg, Goldstein, & Camp, 1971).

Until the advent of the Bayley Scales, the Cattell Infant Scale (Cattell, 1947) was the most widely used infant test. It was designed as a lower extension of the Stanford-Binet and covers the age range of 2–30 months. Although its items closely resemble those of the Gesell, the intent was to minimize tasks that were primarily of a sensorimotor nature. It measures language development, perceptual functions, and manipulatory skills and is well regarded in spite of deficiencies in the standardization population relative to size and representativeness (Anastasi, 1961). Because of its continuity with the Binet, it is often used with older retarded persons who are functioning at less than the 2-year mental age level (Magrab, 1976).

The Bayley Scales (Bayley, 1969) cover the same age range as the Cattell, 2–30 months, and are by far the best standardized of the infant tests. The Scales have three separate components—Mental Scale, Motor Scale, and Infant Behavior Re-

---

[8]Chapters 1 and 2 contain reviews of the main intelligence test and personality findings in mental retardation.

[9]For a review of these tests in the evaluation of handicapped infants and young children, see Hosking and Ulrey (1982).

cord. The Mental Scale assesses sensorimotor skills, response to novel situations, social behavior, problem solving, and language. The Motor Scale measures body control, large-muscle coordination, and hand and finger manipulation. The Infant Behavior Record is a personality measure. The Bayley is considered to be particularly useful in the evaluation of motor-impaired infants because it separates the motor and cognitive domains (Magrab, 1976). It is also helpful in planning stimulation activities for the child.

With growing interest in the intellectual assessment of children with the most severe degrees of handicap, the Uzgiris-Hunt Ordinal Scales of Psychological Development (Uzgiris & Hunt, 1975) offer the possibility of in-depth Piagetian evaluation of six dimensions of cognitive development seen in the first years of life. The Piagetian constructs are object permanence, achieving desired environmental events, vocal and gestural limitation, operational causality, object relations in space, and schema for relating to objects. Unlike other infant tests, the items are organized by cognitive dimension rather than by age, permitting simultaneous determination of both where the child is developmentally and a "curriculum" for where he needs to go. A limitation, however, is that age norms for the steps in each sequence are not available.[10]

In spite of the popularity of the Bayley Scales, it shares with other infant tests the earlier-noted limited predictiveness for future mental ability. Of some reassurance, however, is the indication that IQs in the retarded range in children with clear biological abnormality are the most predictive of all infant intelligence measures (e.g., DuBose, 1977).

Intellectual Assessment After Infancy

After infancy, the most often used tests are the Stanford-Binet (Terman & Merrill, 1960) and the Wechsler scales—the revised Wechsler Intelligence Scale for Children [WISC-R] (Wechsler, 1974), the Wechsler Preschool and Primary Scale of Intelligence [WPPSI] (Wechsler, 1967), and the Wechsler Adult Intelligence Scale [WAIS] (Wechsler, 1955). The usefulness of these in the evaluation of children and adults with possible retardation has been reviewed by Sattler (1974). The Stanford-Binet appears to be the most preferred test in the years from 2 to 8. Although the WPPSI was introduced as a downward revision of the WISC, $4-6\frac{1}{2}$ years, and like the other Wechsler Scales has the advantage of separately assessing verbal and performance abilities, the Binet appears preferable, at least in the evaluation of disadvantaged children. In at least two studies, disadvantaged children performed better on the Binet than on the WPPSI (Barclay & Yater, 1969; Fagan, Broughton, Allen, Clark, & Emerson, 1969). Apart from disadvantaged youngsters, the WPPSI would be most appropriate for less severely handicapped children—those with relatively good language skills and on-task behavior. After age 8, the WISC-R tends to be preferred over the Binet, as does the WAIS in adulthood. Regarding level of intelligence, none of the Wechsler Scales are useful with children who appear to be

---

[10]Ulrey (1982) has discussed the usefulness of this test, also called the Infant Psychological Development Scale (IPDS), and offers cognitive training activities based on it.

severely or profoundly retarded, as the minimum IQ obtainable on them is 40. Here one would turn again to the Binet or to its downward revision, the Cattell.

One of the problems confronting psychologists is the comparability of scores between tests. Different tests of the same individual do not produce the same scores, a phenomenon that is disconcerting to persons who perceive IQ as some intrinsic aspect of the person rather than a function of the test itself. Fortunately, there is less of a problem in retardation because it is precisely in the below-normal ranges that the WISC and Binet are most comparable. Contrariwise, in the superior range, IQ 120+, WISC scores are commonly below Binet scores by from 16 to 18 points (Sattler, 1974). But comparability diminishes when either WISC or Binet scores are compared with the WAIS. The WAIS yields IQs that are from 8 to 15 points higher than those of the WISC or Binet (Fisher, 1962a, 1962b; Sattler, 1974), and only differences of more than 15 points are interpretable as reflecting significant change in intellectual status.

Psychological Assessment in Nonmultidisciplinary Settings

Though evaluation of the infant and preschool-age child may well occur in a multidisciplinary setting, this is less likely to be true with school-age youth and adults. The older groups may be seen in the setting of the school, mental health center, social service agency, mental hospital, institution, or in private practice. Here the psychologist will need to obtain his own developmental history or secure it through a social worker. Under this condition, it will be useful to complement intelligence testing with such a measure of general behavioral functioning as the Vineland Social Maturity Scale (Doll, 1964) or the test specially developed for assessing adaptive behavior in retarded persons, the AAMD Adaptive Behavior Scales (Nihira, Foster, Shellmaas, & Leland, 1969). Both Scales provide scores based on information obtained through interview of a person who is knowledgeable about the testee's general level of functioning. A variant of the Vineland, the Cain-Levine Social Competency Scale (Cain, Levine, & Elzey, 1963), is designed for children between the ages of 5 and 14 years who are at least moderately retarded. For those with severe or profound retardation the psychologist can look to the Balthazar Scales of Adaptive Behavior (Balthazar, 1971).

Assessment of the Multihandicapped Child

The intelligence measures specified thus far are appropriate when there are no major sensory and/or motor disabilities. But children with delayed development often have disabilities that can seriously limit the usefulness of the standard tests. The psychologist must be prepared to assess mental ability in children with deafness, blindness, deafness *and* blindness, lack of speech, and motor dysfunction. For a good review of test procedures with multihandicapped infants and young children, the reader is referred to Ulrey and Rogers (1982) and to DuBose et al. (1982).

1. Deafness: Intellectual evaluation of the deaf child requires the use of non-language tests, and the Nebraska-Hiskey Test of Learning Aptitude is useful (Hiskey, 1966). It is administered through pantomime and includes measures of memory,

pictorial analogies and associations, and spatial relations. It is appropriate for deaf children ages 4–10, and its validity is based on a correlation of .83 with the 1937 Stanford-Binet on a group of hearing children (Hiskey, 1955). For evaluating deaf youth over age 10, one can try the Performance Scale of the WISC-R or WAIS or the Arthur Performance Scale (Arthur, 1947). The Arthur consists of form boards, mazes, and tests of visual memory, block design, and picture completion. There is also the Arthur Adaptation of the Leiter International Performance Scale (Arthur, 1950), a test that can be administered through pantomime.

2. Blindness: Testing of blind children ordinarily requires verbal items, but many legally blind children (corrected vision of 20/200) do have some functional vision. The WISC Verbal Scale has been utilized in general studies of blind children (Cohen, 1966; Tillman & Osborne, 1969) as well as a modified version of the Binet, the Hayes-Binet (Hayes, 1950). Two more recent scales are those of Newland (1969) and Reynell and Zinkin (1975). Newland's Blind Learning Aptitude Test uses bas-relief for sampling discrimination, generalization sequencing, analogies, and matrix completion. It is considered to be a useful measure (Ramey et al., 1982; Salvia & Ysseldyke, 1978).

In their review of the evaluation of the visually impaired child, Hensen et al. (1982) indicate that many clinicians merely pick items from existing tests (e.g., Bayley, Binet, McCarthy, WPPSI) and combine these with observational data. There is also a Vineland-type scale that was developed for blind children, though its range is limited to the preschool years. It is the Maxfield-Buchholz Social Maturity Scale (Maxfield & Buchholz, 1957) and it measures self-help, communication, socialization, and motor skills.

3. Deaf-blind condition: The term "multihandicapped" is a euphemism when one is confronted with a child who is both deaf and blind. This combination of sensory deficit, and sometimes also including motor impairment, is seen in some rubella children. The sensory modality through which these children can be reached is "touch" (Wolf & Anderson, 1969), but, as yet, formal intelligence measures using this modality do not exist. Form boards are one means of evaluation, and the writer has also contrived simple learning tasks involving differential reinforcement. The speed with which the child learns the reinforced response gives at least an intuitive impression of general intelligence.

There is now available a "developmental" measure for deaf-blind children, the Callier-Azusa Scale (Stillman, 1975). It evaluates motor, perceptual, and language domains, and daily living and socialization skills. Scores are given in terms of "developmental ages" (Hosking & Ulrey, 1982).

Another recent measure for deaf-bind children is the Peabody Intellectual Performance Scale (Kiernan & DuBose, 1974). It consists of selected items adapted from infant scales. In at least one study, children scored significantly higher on it than on the Cattell Infant Scale (DuBose, 1981).

4. Speech and/or motor impairment: This combination of disabilities is often found in cerebral palsy, and, where there is a lack of intelligible speech, picture vocabulary tests such as the Peabody (Dunn, 1959) or the French (French, 1964) are necessary. The latter, the French Pictorial Tests of Intelligence, may be prefer-

red because they sample a wider range of abilities (e.g., memory and concepts of size and number). For infants with cerebral palsy or older children functioning at less than the 2-year-old level, an adaptation has been made of the earlier-cited Uzgiris-Hunt Scales (Robinson, 1976).

Rogers (1982) provides suggestions for overcoming problems of responding in the severely motor involved child. She points out the importance of proper "positioning" so as to minimize the effects of "primitive reflexes" (see "Physical Therapist") and the need to take advantage of whatever movements the child can make. For a comprehensive treatment of the evaluation of the cerebral palsied child, the reader is referred to Taylor (1959).

Personality Assessment

Chapter 2 dealt at length with personality in mental retardation. Here we want to limit ourselves to indicating some of the procedures found helpful in its evaluation. Certainly *observation* of the child in his interactions with others and with play materials offers important impressions and, apart from parental reports, will be the basic source of information on the very young child. For older children, the Children's Apperception Test (CAT) and the Thematic Apperception Test (TAT) may be useful. The former requires at least a mental age of 3 years, and the latter requires about an 8-year mental age level (Magrab, 1976). Other recommended procedures are figure drawings and self-concept measures, such as the Piers-Harris Self-Concept Scale (Piers & Harris, 1966) and the Self-Concept Scale for Children (Lipsitt, 1958; Simpson & Meaney, 1979).

Intervention

Though much attention has been devoted to the assessment role of the psychologist, involvement at the therapeutic or habilitative level has come to be at least as important if not more so. This has stemmed from the extraordinary impact of learning theory on behavior management as reflected in the treatment modality "behavior modification." Reference to behavior modification was made in Chapter 2, and its basic principles will be presented in the introductory section of the next chapter. The chapter is devoted to habilitative programs for infants and preschoolers, and knowledge of behavior principles is as important to the teacher as to the psychologist. It suffices here to state only that behavorial principles have provided a strategy for looking at how experience can affect behavior and a powerful tool for systematic intervention.[11]

Counseling will be helpful in working with parents, especially those in whom chronic states of emotional arousal indicate stress and conflict. We have touched earlier on the stresses associated with parenting a child who is "different," and where parental feelings interfere with the child's basic need for intimacy or impede the implementation of appropriate programs, counseling is necessary. Other disciplines that may as-

---

[11]Chapter 10 is devoted to the application of behavior principles to problem behaviors seen in those with severe and profound retardation.

sume this responsibility are social work and psychiatry. In addition to individual counseling or family therapy, group counseling of parents and/or siblings has long been recognized as an important therapeutic tool in helping family members cope with retardation-related family stresses (e.g., Grossman, 1972; Ross, 1964).

ROLES OF THE AUDIOLOGIST AND SPEECH PATHOLOGIST

Speech problems have been touched on in connection with intellectual assessment of the child by the psychologist. Here are addressed the roles of two other and related disciplines, audiology and speech pathology.

Audiologist

The audiologist evaluates hearing. Since intact hearing is essential to normal language development, the language delays characteristic of retardation require the ruling out of hearing loss (Smith, 1976). (Rogers and Soper [1982] also point out the importance of ruling out hearing loss in the psychological assessment of young children with language delay.) Of course, as we have just seen, hearing loss and retardation are not an uncommon combination as, for example, in rubella or in kernicteris.

Speech Pathologist

Assuming normal hearing acuity, the role of the speech pathologist is to characterize the child's level of receptive and expressive language relative to other areas of development, and to inaugurate appropriate intervention. For treatment purposes, Knobeloch (1976) distinguishes between children whose language levels are consistent or inconsistent with their general level of development. The term "language disorder" is reserved for children in whom there is a significant disparity between language and nonlanguage abilities. In these children, specific remediation procedures are intended to elevate language to the level of the more intact areas. For children whose language development is congruent with their general level of development, "language stimulation" rather than remediation would be the recommended procedure. Significant language gains beyond the child's mental age would not be anticipated.

Evaluation

Language evaluation measures recommended by Knobeloch (1976) are (a) The Receptive-Expressive Emergent Language Scale (Bzoch & League, 1971); its items are grouped as either receptive or expressive and are scored as typical, emergent, or absent; (b) The Test for Auditory Comprehension of Language (Carrow, 1973), like the Peabody Picture Vocabulary Test (Dunn, 1959), which is also recommended, it does not require a verbal response but it is weak in items pertaining to the understanding of syntax; and (c) Assessment of Children's Language Comprehension (Foster, Giddon, & Stark, 1973)—also a picture test that does not require language. Other evaluation procedures relate to articulation and oral-motor skills, areas of particular concern in cerebral palsy.

Remediation

Recommended for remediation is the Kent Language Acquisition Program for the Retarded (Kent, Klein, Falk, & Guenther, 1972). This consists of a number of preverbal and beginning verbal activities. The preverbal ones are "attending" and motor and vocal imitation; the verbal ones are initial receptive and expressive language. Other training models suggested are Programmed Conditioning for Language (Gray & Ryan, 1973) and "GOAL," Game-Oriented Activities for Learning (Karnes, 1972). The latter is based on the language model of the Illinois Test of Psycholinguistic Abilities (ITPA) and is appropriate to children with mental ages of from 3 to 5 years.

ROLES OF THE PHYSICAL THERAPIST AND OCCUPATIONAL THERAPIST

These two disciplines have come to be very important in the treatment of motor-related disabilities.

Physical Therapist

The physical therapist is concerned with posture and locomotion and the specific motor functions on which they depend (Harryman, 1976). The physical therapist looks for problems of muscle tone (hypertonus or hypotonus), movement, strength, balance, and coordination. These are the disorders seen in cerebral palsy and in other conditions associated with motor impairment. The physical therapist attempts to establish the child's "motor age" and to determine whether motor delays are in part attributable to persistence of primitive reflexes. The latter are normal reflexes present in infancy but which disappear as the infant matures (Molnar, 1978). The earliest reflexes are called tonic reflexes (e.g., tonic, asymmetrical tonic, symmetrical tonic, tonic labyrinth, and positive supporting reaction), and their disappearance permits the development of the kind of "righting" reactions that enable us to maintain balance or cushion our falls.

The abnormal persistence of the tonic reflexes literally prevent the infant from assuming or maintaining normal posture and locomotion. For example, one of the earliest-appearing motor skills is the ability to raise one's head, a task usually accomplished by age 1 month. Head control is fundamental to achieving an upright position. In the neonate, prior to 1 month of age, one sees the influence of the tonic labyrinth reflex when the infant is lying prone. It creates a predominant posture of *flexion*—of arms, legs, and neck. It is the flexion of the neck, as well as of arms and legs, that inhibits the raising of the head. Head raising involves "extension," the muscular opposite of flexion, and the persistence of this reflex will interfere with head raising and with ultimate attainment of upright position.

From a treatment standpoint, the physical therapist, like the speech therapist, distinguishes between a motor lag that is consistent with the general level of development and that which reflects specific motor dysfunction, the latter being due to a particular brain abnormality. Where there is overall developmental delay, the adequacy of the child's posture and locomotion is judged by comparing it with the degree of maturity of the automatic postural reactions—righting, tilting and protective extension. If the automatic postural reactions are at a higher level, then a program is undertaken to improve posture and locomotion. If the motor lag is due to brain injury, as in cerebral palsy, muscle tone will be increased, and treatment is designed to reduce it and the related spasticity as well as to encourage normal postural reactions while inhibiting the primitive ones.

Occupational Therapist

Where the focus of the physical therapist is on basic muscle function, the occupational therapist is concerned with the impact of motor impairment on the performance of daily activities (Gorga, 1976). In the case of children, particular attention is directed toward motor problems that impede self-feeding, dressing, and toileting. In school-age youths the stress tends to be on the gross and fine motor skills that underlie academic tasks.

One of the very important areas in the young child is feeding, and here the occupational therapist will be evaluating the basic motor skills that underlie it— grasping, holding, moving from plate to mouth, and oral movements (e.g., lip closure, jaw and tongue control). Like the physical therapist, the occupational therapist is concerned with the problems created by the persistence of primitive reflexes. Prolongation of neonate sucking, rooting, and biting reflexes can interfere with later eating behavior. An interesting example of this is seen with the asymmetric tonic reflex. This reflex causes the infant to assume the "fencing" posture. When the head is turned to either side, the arm on that side tends to be extended (in "extension"). The persistence of this early reflex posture interferes with attempts at self-feeding because it prevents the child from bringing his hand to his mouth while facing the hand that holds the food! To accomplish this requires flexion of the arm rather than extension, but the early reflex promotes extension. Treatment procedures for this and related problems involve identifying special postures that will permit performance of the function and modifying objects to make them usable ("adapted" equipment—e.g., a wide handle on a fork for a child with an inadequate grasp).

The Nature
of the Diagnostic Formulation

The interpretation of diagnostic findings requires much care and sensitivity. We have repeatedly stressed the need for caution with regard to the predictiveness of IQ scores obtained in infancy; it is not until age 2 years that the combination of retardation and organicity allows for some presumptions regarding future status. In the case of children who are less than a year old and whose rate of development is at least one-half of normal, it is prudent to avoid offering any diagnostic label except, of course, if a syndrome is present that is regularly associated with retardation. We have already noted that it is the practice to immediately convey to new parents the diagnosis of Down syndrome, but even this catastrophic experience can be softened by the knowledge that programs of infant stimulation and preschool experiences appear capable of reducing, at least to some degree, the extent of intellectual impairment. In the absence of a recognizable mental retardation syndrome, the diagnostic statement should be confined to a characterization of the child's state of health and developmental level and the offering of suggestions on appropriate forms of stimulation. The formulation of early diagnoses must be for the purpose of early treatment (Johnston & Magrab, 1976). If the parents raise the issue of retardation, it should be acknowledged as a possibility, but within the context of the limited predictability of infant measures. It can be pointed out to parents that only time and the child's response to early intervention measures will determine the significance of the current developmental delay. Where, however, by at least age 8 months the rate of development is less than half of normal or where the child has been seen until at least 2 years, the diagnostic formulation can be less tentative and should avoid encouraging parental hopes for any major change.

INTERPRETATION AS
A STAGEWISE PROCESS
The intellectual and emotional assimilation of an unwanted event requires *time*. In Chapter 1, we described both the immediate and long-term impact of a diagnosis of mental retardation on parents. These reactions will vary from resigned acquiescence to hysterical denial, and parental emotional state will determine how much is "heard." Interpretation should be viewed as a stagewise process (Ross, 1964) with gradual emotional acceptance, over time, making it possible for parents to hear and assimilate more and more of what is being said. Initially, their main need is *emotional support*, and this is rendered through the provision of future appointments during which they are encouraged to express their feelings and to raise questions about the child's current and future needs.

THE SUPPORTIVE ROLE
OF THE SOCIAL WORKER
The role of the social worker in the mental retardation diagnostic process was seen as focusing on the child's parents, with the goals of providing support under stress, assisting in the securing of services, and maintaining parental decision-making responsibility as regards the child. It is after diagnosis that the social worker becomes the most common source of support. Adams (1971) has identified three kinds of assistance the social worker can offer: (a) assistance during the "acute reactive phase"; (b) assistance in stabilizing the family as it begins to assimilate the child and exercise parental functions; and (c) long-term availability on a kind of "retainer" basis.

Each type of assistance involves three essential elements of the "helping process"—reality, empathy, and support. It is the social worker's focus on the *reality* of child and family needs that helps the family gradually to come to grips with the nature of the child's difficulties and to begin to meet its needs as well as theirs. *Empathy* enables the social worker to recognize and communicate to the parents an understanding of the feelings they experience and, thereby, free them to express what may be bottled up or a source of conflict. And it is through helping child and/or parents to secure needed services that the social worker performs what is often the most powerful form of *support* (Apthekar, 1957).

Postdiagnostic Services

The most constructive thing to be done for child and parents following a finding of significant developmental delay is to recommend therapeutic activities in the areas of deficit and to assist and support the parents in their implementation (Abramson, Gravink, Abramson, & Sommers, 1977; Stone, 1975). In one large study the average age when retardation was first suspected was 6 months, but it was not until 2 years that services were generally begun (Abramson et al., 1977). The effect of this delay is to potentially deprive that child who is most in need of stimulation of the kinds of cognitive, motor, and language experiences that can only encourage its development.

INFANT AND PRESCHOOL-AGE SERVICES[12]

Programs for children who are less than 2 years of age (infants) are typically conducted in the *home* (e.g., Portage Project) (Shearer & Shearer, 1976), where "early intervention workers" instruct parents in appropriate activities for the child. In one such program neonates at risk for significant difficulties are so identified when discharged from a postnatal intensive care unit and then followed for 1 year by a worker who comes into the home[13] (*Mental Retardation: The Leading Edge*, 1978). In addition to the provision of stimulation and training to the infant, the involvement of the parent in this activity encourages parent-child "affectional bonding," a potential problem area in children whose possible lack of responsiveness can interfere with the development of normal parental attachment (Stone, 1975). At about 2 years, retarded children can begin to attend day care (child development) centers. These will provide peer (social) experiences for the child and will focus on continued growth of self-help, motor, language, and cognitive skills. They also can offer special programs for parents and sibs. It is the combination of early home-based training and a later preschool experience that is presumed to account for above-average developmental rates in Down children exposed to such a program (Hayden & Dmitriev, 1978). These preschool experiences are usually offered in special centers serving handicapped children, but these youngsters can also be integrated in day care programs serving nonhandicapped children (Guralnick, 1978). For the handicapped child this offers exposure to normal peer models and preparation for varying degrees of integration in the school years and beyond. For the nonhandicapped child this means encounters with children who are "different" early in life and before stereotyping can occur. With teacher leadership and pleasurable interactions, more positive attitudes about them can be fostered.

Another important service to families is *respite care*. This provides a temporary substitute care giver for the child and offers relief to parents from the sometimes exhausting burdens of caring for handicapped children. The states of Wash-

---

[12]See Chapter 7 for an in-depth treatment of these services.

[13]Follow-up Intervention for Normal Development (FIND), San Bernardino, CA. See also Cohen (1979).

ington[14] and California (Apolloni & Triest, 1983) have developed programs that provide a pool of respite-care providers from which parents may choose. Washington also enables families to purchase therapeutic services not available through their regular local community programs—for example, physical therapy and special equipment for families in low-population areas.

With reference to residential services (see Chap. 9), there has been a strong trend toward the rearing of the retarded child in his own home. The earlier, not uncommon recommendation of immediate institutional placement has been softened by the much publicized limitations of institutional care and the growing array of community-based services. If we think in terms of the personality model presented in Chapter 2, it would appear that it is within the child's own home that resources are most likely to be fully developed and needs met. It is parental love (attachment) that most nearly assures that needs for *survival* (health), *structure, self-esteem,* and *self-expression* will be met. But all children, handicapped or not, do not have access to a parental home. Here child care agencies ordinarily choose between adoptive and foster homes. The range of retarded children who are adoptable is narrower than those served in foster care (Gallagher, 1968), though the adoptive potential of handicapped children has clearly been underestimated (Franklin, 1969; Wolfensberger, 1972). Foster care is temporary care purchased from families who offer their homes to children (Garrett, 1970; Paige, 1971) or adults (Justice, Bradley, & O'Connor, 1971). It may even be combined with institutional services for children who must leave their own homes to obtain services not available in their own communities.

SCHOOL–AGE SERVICES

The school years are vital to the later adult adjustment of retarded persons (see Chaps. 8 and 9). It is then, if not before, that the retarded child is brought into contact with the wider community and is given the opportunity to acquire the skills necessary to an optimal adult adjustment. Both the range and quality of these coping skills will depend heavily on the nature of that educational experience, and it is here that the effect of the Education for All Handicapped Children Act will be felt. Virtually all retarded children are now receiving some kind of education, and, within these schools, mildly retarded (educable) children are increasingly served in classes with nonhandicapped ones (mainstreaming). Although children who are at least moderately retarded (trainable and below) are still housed in separate (self-contained) classes, these classes are now expected to be at least physically located in schools serving normal children. The physical and psychological separation of the retarded child is diminishing, and both normal and retarded children can expect to benefit. In the past, children with severe and profound retardation were usually completely excluded from the public schools and instead attended such day center programs as were available. But this, too, is changing, and the schools are beginning to open their doors to these youngsters as well.

Although the setting in which retarded children are served is changing, their

---

[14]Bureau of Developmental Disabilities, Olympia, WA.

educational goals have not. Whether "mainstreamed" or not, and irrespective of cultural background, the child whose IQ on a standard intelligence test falls below 70 is going to have major academic problems and require special attention. In this regard, one of the concerns about "mainstreaming" is the degree to which traditional objectives of special education can be maintained (Childs, 1979). Mildly retarded youths can be expected to acquire some functional academic skills, although their average achievement level in reading and arithmetic is only about third grade (Bilsky, 1970). In spite of this, the majority are expected to operate independently as adults,[15] and their education should be focused on the kinds of *functional* academic, social, and vocational skills necessary to achieve and sustain independence. On the other hand, youths with at least moderate retardation are not expected to achieve complete independence and will always require at least some degree of supervision. Their education will have a lesser degree of academic emphasis, although within this population are found children who can acquire at least a low level of functional academic skills (Kirk & Gallagher, 1979). One task of the educator is to recognize the existence of such a subgroup and to encourage its full development while not pressing other trainable children for similar gains.

It is probable that the rate of gain per unit of time will be the ultimate criterion for determining when to continue to press for higher grade-level achievement and when to take whatever level has been achieved and make it as functional as possible. Apart from academic considerations, trainable pupils will benefit from activities focused on self-help, social, motor, language, recreational, and work skills (Kirk & Gallagher, 1979). With reference to work skills, though the trainable student will not ordinarily move into regular competitive employment, he can be very productively employed in the sheltered workshop. Success in the sheltered workshop, as in any other work setting, depends on good work habits, and these can be fostered in school through experiences that simulate work—presenting a *specific task* that is to be completed within a *specific time period* and meets a *specific standard of quality*. For children with severe and profound retardation, the public schools are only beginning to assume educational responsibility, and the curriculum focus is on self-care, language, recreational, motor, and some vocational preparation (Wehman, 1979). Regarding vocational potential, researchers have demonstrated that these individuals can learn to perform complex motor assembly tasks (Gold, 1973, 1976; Hunter & Bellamy, 1976). These are usually performed in sheltered settings (Bellamy, 1976; Gold, 1976; Karan, 1979; Wehman, Schutz, Renzaglia, & Karan, 1977), though some possibility of competitive potential has been suggested (Wehman, Hill, & Koehler, 1979).

During the school years the family home will continue to be the primary residential resource. If out-of-home care is necessary, it may be in a family setting with several children or in a group home, thus affording the retarded child opportunities for peer experiences and normalizing models.

Another need that becomes apparent in the school years, especially in adolescence, is for social outlets and recreational skills. It is in adolescence, if not

[15]See Chapter 1 re adaptive potential of retarded persons.

before, that the retarded youngster begins to experience some neighborhood peer isolation, and the local recreation department can be a vehicle for creating activities that provide both fun and social experiences.

ADULT SERVICES

The postschool years present challenges to the retarded person and his family that differ somewhat from earlier ones. Largely they focus around the *need for finding meaningful ways to "bind time"* once the time-binding experiences of the school years end. For the mildly retarded person the problem is less severe because of the capacity to seek out vocational, social, and recreational activities independently. Even here, however, as indicated in Chapter 1, there is greater occupational vulnerability and proneness to some degree of isolation. For individuals with more than mild retardation there will be a greater dependence on resources outside oneself to meet these needs.

At the *vocational* level, there will have to be access to sheltered workshops and adult day activity centers. While the former is, essentially, a place of employment, the latter, typically serving persons with severe and profound retardation, commonly includes educational and recreational activities as well as vocational ones. Educational services are also beginning to be available to retarded adults at community colleges (see Table 15). Apart from the use of adult day care centers for social and recreational experiences, the main resource for such programs will be community recreation departments, often working in concert with mental retardation agencies and parent organizations.

The adult years are also the period during which the need for residential services other than those provided by parents may be a reality. While aging and the death of parents will require residential change in the older dependent retarded adult, even the younger person may benefit from movement out of the family home. Family care and group homes can provide the opportunity for growth in independence and access to long-term peer social relationships. From the standpoint of increasing personal autonomy, both can also be stepping stones to a still higher level of independence (e.g., sharing a "sheltered apartment" with another retarded adult). Such apartments are usually clustered within a regular apartment complex and include access to a counselor who also resides there. For the aged retarded adult, the community-based options to institutional placement are family care, foster care, and rest homes (homes for the aged). Though there is general national concern over the quality of life in facilities serving the aged, small rest homes that allow for resident privacy and some autonomy and which provide some meaningful activity can meet needs satisfactorily. We are just beginning to look at the needs of this population (Segal, 1977; Tymchuk, 1979).

CREATING AN ARRAY OF SERVICES

To this point there has been described the array of services necessary (a) to prevent mental retardation, (b) to identify it in the young child, and (c) to optimize the adaptive potential of affected persons. Historically, these services were largely educational and institutional. Although for at least a decade our rhetoric has called for the deinstitutionalizing of retarded persons and the creation of community-based services, the development of these services has lagged. Paradoxically, during a period of continuing deinstitutionalization, e.g., 1977-1985, the federal government has increased its level of funding support to state institutions from 26 percent to 46 percent (Braddock, Hemp, & Howes, 1986). As a nation we have not yet really confronted the economic, social, educational, and residential implications of trying to serve *all* of our handicapped citizens, retarded and otherwise, and the effect is a picture of extraordinary diversity in the nature, quality, and quantity of services currently available to retarded persons in their home communities. Given the effect of recent court decisions, it can be expected that the immediate future will be a period of attempting to respond to court-determined rights by finding means for the creation and orderly delivery of such services. In this section our intent is to assist the planner of services in determining the scope of service needs in his own planning or "catchment" area.

Predicting Prevalence in a Service Area

As society increasingly seeks to serve retarded persons in the community, it is important for mental retardation planners to be able to estimate the scope of services that will be required within their own service (catchment) areas. To make such projections, one needs to be able to estimate the numbers of persons within a catchment area who will require them. The author has offered a basis for projecting prevalence within a catchment area and one that incorporates the "adaptive behavior" aspect of our mental retardation definition (Baroff, 1982). Planners have traditionally relied on the 3 percent prevalence[16] rate—a rate that refers only to IQ and that ignores "adaptive behavior," a central part of the AAMD definition of retardation since 1959 (Heber, 1959). When the criterion for classification as "retarded" includes both IQ and adaptive behavior, the rate is estimated at only about 1 percent (Mercer, 1973; Tarjan et al., 1973). Even the usual 3 percent rate is only a population *average*, as much variation is found as a function of chronological age, sex, race, ethnic group, social class, and urban or rural status (Conley, 1973, 1976; Reschly & Jipson, 1976).

SOCIAL CLASS AND RACE

Of the various elements affecting prevalence, social class is clearly the most predictive. In one of the major studies on prevalence, one that incorporated measures of social class (based on parental occupation and education), children from the lowest of the five social classes were almost 13 times as likely to be retarded as those from the upper three (Lemkau & Imre, 1966), and this socioeconomic effect cut across all racial groups. It is the relationship between socioeconomic status and

---

[16]"Prevalence" is an epidemiologic term that refers to the number of individuals classifiable according to a given trait at any one moment in time. "Incidence," a term often used synonymously with "prevalence," refers to the number of *new* cases per unit of time (Morton & Hebel, 1978).

retardation that is thought to largely account for the higher rates of retardation among economically disadvantaged racial and ethnic minorities (Maloney & Ward, 1979). This disproportionate representation is almost entirely limited to mild retardation, typically of the "sociocultural" variety, though there is also a slightly greater risk for more severe degrees of impairment (Conley, 1973).

AGE

An age effect is well established, as the prevalence of retardation is significantly elevated in the school-age population, especially in the 10–14 age range. Conley (1973) notes that, in virtually every prevalence study, the frequency of retardation increases with age until the middle teens and then it begins to decline. This variation in prevalence is particularly pronounced with regard to individuals identified as retarded by agencies *other* than the school and certainly reflects the distinction drawn by Mercer (1973) between school and nonschool criteria for the labeling of a person as retarded.

URBAN OR RURAL STATUS

There is a consistent finding of increased rates of retardation among rural as against urban populations (Conley, 1973). This is especially true of economically disadvantaged minorities and is also reflected in diminished educational attainment (U.S. Census, 1970).

DEGREE OF RETARDATION

Mild

Another limiting aspect of the 3 percent rate is that it is unrelated to the "adaptive behavior" criterion of the AAMD mental retardation definition (Heber, 1959; Mercer, 1973). This element particularly affects those in the 55–69 range who will be classifiable as retarded. While IQs in the 55–69 range are certain to severely limit academic progress, IQ tests being best understood as measures of scholastic aptitude, these adaptive behavior deficits during the school years do not preclude age-appropriate levels of independence either before or after that period. Certainly, in the adult years, the majority of such individuals achieve independence and self-sufficiency (Edgerton & Bercovici, 1976; Richardson, 1978), and this will probably be most characteristic of the 80 percent who are free of an obvious organic basis for their intellectual limitation. About 20 percent of persons in the 55–69 IQ range can be expected to have some organic impairment (Tarjan, 1970), and it is only this segment that is likely to show adaptive deficit throughout life and, potentially, to warrant continuous classification as "retarded."

The effect of "adaptive behavior" is to reduce the level of mild retardation of from about 2.3 percent (Kauffman & Payne, 1975; Maloney & Ward, 1979) to not more than 0.5 percent. Since those with IQ 55–69 represent almost 90 percent of all persons with IQs of less than 70, this fivefold reduction has a tremendous impact on the overall retardation rate. Two recent Scandinavian studies found similar rates in the IQ 50+ population, 0.55 percent (Rantakallio & Von Wendt, 1986), and 0.56 percent (Hagberg, B., Hagberg, G., Lewerth, & Lindberg, 1981), though this was based on IQ alone.

The greatest impact on the 3 percent rate was the 1978 federal legislation pertaining to "developmental disabilities" (PL 95-602; Rehabilitation, Comprehensive Services, and the Developmental Disabilities Amendments of 1978). Under it the term *developmental disability* was redefined from a categorical (mental retardation, cerebral palsy, epilepsy, and autism) to a functional basis. Of particular significance was the narrowing of its application to persons with a "severe" disability—one that would require services of a "lifelong" or "extended duration" nature. Among the rationales for the redefinition of the client group was the need to focus scarce resources on that segment of the developmentally disabled population most in need of services. In light of the current fiscal difficulties of community-based mental retardation services, that rationale was painfully prophetic. In any case, the 1978 "DD" amendments gave legislative legitimacy to the adaptive behavior dimension; individuals with mild retardation, IQ-wise, are no longer eligible for services unless they have other handicaps that substantially limit their ability to function. The effect of this is to concentrate services to those with from moderate to profound retardation.

Moderate to Profound

The projection of prevalence rates for the current client target group is relatively straightforward. Individuals with IQs in the below-55 range will generally not meet age-appropriate standards for personal independence and will require services, at least sporadically, throughout life. Acknowledging the limitation of this generalization, as of most others, the mental retardation planner can consider all members of this group as at least *potential* clients.

Apart from behavioral considerations, the rates of retardation in the moderate to profound range are not subject to the same degree of variation seen in the mild range (Conley, 1973). Using the pre-AAMD tripartite classification of mental retardation which sets the upper limit of the moderate range as 49, Conley projects a school-age rate of 0.40 percent (4/1000) for those with IQs of 0–49 (0.12% with IQ 0–24 and 0.28% with IQ 25–49). His overall rate in the 20–64 age range, adjusted for a higher mortality, is 0.32 percent. Our own estimates are slightly higher, as they represent a broadening of the upper limit of the IQ range to 54. They are 0.50 percent at school age and 0.40 percent in the 20–64 age range. The overall rate for the entire population is estimated at 0.41 percent, or about four persons per thousand. This is also the estimate derived by Abramowicz and Richardson (1975) from a review of a large number of population studies. Recent studies of the retarded population in British Columbia found a rate of about 2/1000 for the moderate to profound group though approximately equal rates for the severe and profound suggests some underreporting of the "severe" category. (Baird, 1983; Baird & Sadovnick, 1985). Much higher rates are reported in the Scandinavian studies; 0.74 percent in northern Finland (Rantakallio & Von Wendt, 1986) and 0.63 percent in Gothenburg, Sweden (Hagberg et al., 1981).

DETERMINING PREVALENCE
FOR INDIVIDUAL CATCHMENT AREAS

Table 16 offers the planner a means of estimating the number of "developmentally disabled" mentally retarded persons within a catchment area. It is limited to individuals with from moderate to profound retardation, the population for whom prevalence estimates appear most reliable. Since services are often developed on the basis of chronological age and degree of retardation, the table is so organized. Within this population, the ratio of moderate to severe to profound is about 60 percent moderate, 30 percent severe, and 10 percent profound (e.g., NARC 1963 projection of 6.0%, 3.5% and 1.5% [Maloney & Ward, 1979]). For predicting between age groups, the proportions are 0–4 years 7.1 percent, 5–19 years 27.2 percent, 20–64 years 55.0 percent, and 65+ years 10.7 percent. Table 16 illustrates the use of these prevalence estimates for a hypothetical catchment area of 100,000 persons. The numbers have been rounded off to avoid decimals.

Table 16 projects a grand total of 413 individuals who would be eligible for mental retardation services. Thus the mental retardation planner can estimate the number of persons with from moderate to profound retardation as about 4/1000 of general population. If the mildly retarded subgroup of 0.5 percent or 5/1000 is added to this, then the maximum number of potential clients is estimated at 0.9 percent, or 9/1000.

PREVALENCE OF MULTIPLE
DISABILITIES

As attention has shifted to persons with greater degrees of impairment, the population of multihandicapped individuals becomes more visible. To assist the planner of services, Table 17 projects the numbers of retarded children per one thousand of population who will also have other disabilities commonly seen in retardation.

TABLE 16   Projected Prevalence of Persons with Moderate to Profound Retardation in a Hypothetical Catchment Area of 100,000

| | Age range | | | |
	0–4	5–19	20–64	65+
Total population	7100	27,200	55,000	10,700
Total of moderate	(7100 × 0.5%)	(27,200 × 0.5%)	(55,000 × 0.4%)	(10,700 × 0.2%)
to profound retardation	36	136	220	21
Moderate	(36 × 60%)	(136 × 60%)	(220 × 60%)	(21 × 60%)
	22	82	133	13
Severe	(36 × 30%)	(136 × 30%)	(220 × 30%)	(21 × 30%)
	11	41	67	7
Profound	(36 × 10%)	(136 × 10%)	(220 × 10%)	(21 × 10%)
	3	13	20	1

TABLE 17   Multihandicapped Retarded Children

	Estimated frequency per 1000[a]	
Disability	In general population	In retarded children
Cerebral palsy	2–3	90
Epilepsy	5–9	80
Blindness	1	30
Deafness	1	20

[a]Estimates are based on Conen, 1979; Conley, 1973; Conroy and Derr, 1971; Payne, 1968; Reynolds and Reynolds, 1979.

Service Delivery Systems

There is no single model for the delivery of services to retarded persons. In part, this stems from the fact that except for traditional state control of institutions, no single agency, state or local, has exclusive responsibility for all services to retarded persons within a catchment area. The services that do exist represent a mix of state and local, public and private, and generic and specialized agencies. This variety was illustrated in Table 15. Other sources of diversity are changing definitions of the client population in federal legislation, multiple sources of funding, multiple planning bodies, and multiple service delivery models—medical, educational, vocational, custodial, and developmental (Magrab & Elder, 1979). The effect has been to create a fragmentary "nonsystem" of services with chronic problems of absent or inadequate services, service duplication, interagency bickering, and a general lack of coordination.

In an early paper, Begab (1963) questioned whether a single pattern of service delivery could fit all catchment areas. He pointed out that communities differ in their prevailing social philosophy, size, economic conditions, and manpower resources and that these differences would dictate different problems of service delivery. Although these factors are all important influences on how individual catchment areas respond to major social problems, the effect of recent federal legislation (e.g., Education of All Handicapped Children Act [PL 94-142]) is to require equivalent services irrespective of catchment area preferences. The challenge of the 1970s was ensuring the "rights" of handicapped citizens to services that were traditionally available to the nonhandicapped. The challenge of the 1980s and beyond is to see that legislative and judicial intent is translated into concrete services that meet some minimal standards of quality and that are offered in a coordinated and expeditious manner.

SERVICES AND COMMUNITY VALUES

Apart from the cost of services, perhaps the most crucial element in the creation of an effective system is the attitude toward the prospective client group held by those who make the political and administrative decisions that affect services (Pollard, Hall, & Keeran, 1979). The scale and quality of services that our society provides to any group are a reflection of how that group is perceived or *valued*. The current quality of services to the aged is a case in point, although, as the aged proportion of the population and corresponding influence grows, we can anticipate that some of the current horrors will be eliminated.

In this respect retarded people are at a disadvantage in several ways. Not only does society have a very negative attitude toward their disability, but, apart from school programs, society's traditional involvement has been limited to creating large residential institutions. What we have had is a "custodial" service model in which minimal care, even if in a setting that also offered a variety of other services, came to be the primary function. Although the deinstitutionalization thrust has resulted in the exodus of less impaired persons from the institutions, the custodial model can expect to persist if only because the residual institutional population is largely made up of persons with severe and profound retardation. About 70 percent of the institutional population is composed of individuals with the severest forms of retardation (Scheerenberger, 1982).

In any case, it was the abuses of the custodial model that sparked the normalization movement and the effort to serve retarded people in environments that most nearly resembled those of nonhandicapped individuals. But the translation of normalizing goals and the development of a community-based rather than institutional model will require an attitudinal re-educative process. This will take time and, in a sense, be a bootstrap operation, because it will be the creation of some community programs themselves and the opportunities they provide for "experiencing" retarded people that will constitute the re-educative process.

FACILITATIVE VALUES

There are at least four values whose promulgation will hasten the development of community-based services: (a) the recognition that retarded individuals are like us, *persons* and *citizens*, and as such are protected by the same rights and entitled to the same opportunities as we are; (b) that retarded persons can grow in their adaptive capacities given appropriate educational experiences (the "developmental" model); (c) that maximum growth in adaptive potential for *all* persons occurs in environments that demand from each of us the highest level of complexity with which we can cope (the "least restrictive alternative") and, for the retarded person, this means experiencing environments that most nearly approximate those of nonhandicapped individuals; and (d) that to the degree that we deal with less advantaged fellow human beings in a sensitive and compassionate manner, a milieu is created that will be responsive to *our* own needs when we, too, are in need of assistance, *as one day we will be!*

STRUCTURAL ELEMENTS
OF A COORDINATED SYSTEM OF SERVICES

Though "values" provide the motivational support for any system of services, an effective, coordinated, community-based system will also have some "structural" prerequisites. In his review of our national effort toward deinstitutionalization, Scheerenberger (1976) identified five such prerequisites—local authority, an independent standard setting and monitoring agency, backup services, advocacy, and adequate financial support.

Local Authority

The development of an effective "system" of services within a catchment area requires the creation of a single agency or board with *statutory* authority to plan, implement, and coordinate mental retardation services and to be legally accountable for their quality. Sixteen such services are specified in the federal developmental disabilities legislation: evaluation, diagnosis, treatment, day programs, training, education, sheltered employment, recreation, personal care, domiciliary care, special living arrangements, counseling, information and referral, follow-up, protective and other sociolegal services, and transportation (Scheerenberger, 1976). Of particular importance is that all state funds for mental retardation services except for the public schools and, perhaps, the institutions, are channeled through this local authority. Under the impact of other federal legislation pertaining to comprehensive mental health planning, such statutory responsibility is now commonly vested in a catchment area mental health and/or mental retardation authority. It is this authority that operates the local mental retardation services program.

In the performance of its comprehensive role as planner, implementer, and coordinator, the local mental retardation program is increasingly looking to persons who function as "case managers" or expediters of services (Hansell, Wodarczyk, & Visotsky, 1968). It is especially with regard to the "coordinator" role that case management is seen as a necessary function. As noted earlier, there are a host of agencies involved in providing mental retardation services, and many of them are administratively independent of each other as well as of the agency that has the statutory authority and accountability for the services. Their own traditions and need to protect "turf" are also major bars to coordination (Elder, 1979). Under these conditions a mechanism must be found for locating in one place a person or persons who can follow the client through the service maze. The case manager is seen as the link between the retarded person and his family and the various service providers in that catchment area. In this respect, the case manager's activities are akin to some of those of the social worker. From a catchment area standpoint, the case manager should be regarded as *the* locus for the initial referral of retarded persons into the service system (Pollard, Hall, & Keeran, 1979), as multiple portals of entry defeat coordinative functions.

In the planning of appropriate client services, the case manager typically functions in collaboration with a service planning team. The latter are professionals from the key provider agencies, and it is they who have the ultimate responsibility for developing the final service plan for each client. The case manager operates as "staff" to the planning team. He collects preliminary data on each client, presents a tentative service plan to the team, assures that the client enters the service system, monitors the services that are rendered, and provides ongoing follow-up.

Of the case manager's various responsibilities it is that of "monitoring"' that will perhaps be the most difficult to pursue. It literally requires that the case manager determine how effectively other service agencies are performing their responsibilities to the client. Since these services are often provided by agencies that are not administratively responsible to that of the case manager (e.g., social services, sheltered workshop, group home, etc.), the power of the case manager is likely to be limited. Another factor that can undercut monitoring is that there is often little choice in the selection of service providers. Where the option is limited to using inadequate services or none at all, it is essential that the case manager assume a "consultant" role and assist the service provider to perform more satisfactorily.

In large metropolitan areas where resources may be more plentiful, case managers can exercise the option of *choosing* among agencies to which their clients are referred. Such choices give to the case manager his most powerful option—the "power of the purse." Goldman (1975) has suggested not only that case managers should, like vocational rehabilitation counselors, have control over client service expenditures but that this control should include the state institutions that serve that catchment area! He has pointed out how service systems tend to fund *agencies* rather than *services*, thus assuring the existence of the service agency apart from the quality of services it provides. Goldman suggests that service funds should be tied to the *client* wherever he is, thus following the client from one service to another. Whether such flexibility is feasible is another matter, since any service agency has to have sufficient funding to assure that there is the capacity to provide the service when called on to do so.

An Independent Standard Setting and Monitoring Agency

The setting of standards is a means of assuring that the scope and quality of services will meet some minimum level of adequacy. Since the funds appropriated for services are both federal and state in nature, both will have standards applied to the service provider agencies that receive them. When services are provided under a local (nonstate) catchment area authority, the state has a dual role to perform. It not only monitors agency performance relative to standards but, in its consultative role, helps agencies to meet them. Where the state is also a provider of services, as in the case of state institutions, its capacity for monitoring is compromised. Self-monitoring constitutes the epitome of conflict of interest. Ultimately, standards review must be made by an agency that is administratively independent of the one actually providing the service.

One protection against conflict of interest, at all levels, is the giving of responsibility for evaluation to *independent* organizations whose only purpose is to provide such review and accreditation. In the 1970s such review was provided by a division of the Joint Commission of Accreditation of Hospitals. Originally it offered only review of institutional (residential) programs, but it later added standards for community agencies.[17] In the 1980s the responsibility of accreditation

---

[17]Standards for Community Agencies (Serving Persons with Mental Retardation and other Developmental Disabilities). JCAH, 875 North Michigan Avenue, Suite 2201, Chicago, IL 60611.

shifted, as the meeting of federal standards assured eligibility for federal funds. These apply only to residential services, but the *Standards for Community Agencies* as published by the Joint Commission in 1973 are still useful, since one aspect of accreditation involved an initial self-survey with the standards.

A particularly helpful, if rigorous, form of assessment is through Wolfensberger and Glenn's (1975) normalization rating scale—Program Analysis of Service Systems (PASS). This is a 50-item scale which measures the degree to which mental retardation and other human services programs meet normalization goals in such areas as integration, age appropriateness of activities, appropriateness of program model, growth orientation, and quality of setting. The writer has participated in PASS training and can state unequivocally that it is an extremely effective way of learning what normalization is all about and how we can use PASS to improve programs.

One final comment about standard setting and monitoring: the monitoring of standards cannot take place in a consequence-free milieu. Somehow programs need to be rewarded for meeting standards and penalized for failing to meet them. In the absence of such consequences change is unlikely to occur. As noted in the earlier discussion of the case manager's monitoring role, the application of consequences also requires the availability of sufficient resources to make choices—that is, to move funds from one potential provider to another so as to create new services when viable alternatives do not exist. Where there is no freedom to exercise choice, one can anticipate that change will only come about through litigation, a tortuous procedure which takes its toll on the retarded client and family as well as on the service provider.

Backup Services

The concern here is with assuring that community service providers have access to whatever mental retardation expertise exists in their area. In the past, persons most experienced in mental retardation, apart from special education teachers, were associated with institutions. The creation of community services, especially for persons with severe and/or multiple handicaps, will call for both the training of new workers in the field and the use of selected personnel from institutional and university programs as resource people in that endeavor.

The personnel problem, per se, is one in which the author has had continuing interest. For the most part, our states and local communities have gone about developing programs with only minimal concerns for the people who will operate them. Although state institutional programs have been much maligned, at the very least they commonly include some kind of in-service training for their workers. In part, this stems from the relatively large number of typically untrained persons recruited to work in them as "attendants." But even the professional staff often lack prior education and experience in mental retardation. Although the university-affiliated mental retardation centers around the country do offer varying degrees of exposure to students, the bulk of professionals currently in the field at either the institutional or community level are without specific preparation in mental retardation. In some respects one must regard the continued absence of concern about a trained manpower pool as another reflection of our society's negative attitude toward retarded persons. Our general goal in retardation should be to "professionalize" the field by creating greater in-service educational opportunities and by tying career growth in the field to both education and experience.

Advocacy

Early in the chapter we discussed various forms of advocacy on behalf of retarded persons. There now exists in all states a federally supported "Protection and Advocacy" agency which is expected to protect the rights of retarded individuals and to assure their access to appropriate services. Local advocacy groups are necessary as a means of monitoring the local service delivery system. The key to such monitoring is the administrative independence of the advocacy group from the service provider agencies. Advocacy is also an appropriate role for case managers and can be most readily pursued when the case manager is outside the service delivery system. One attempt to achieve this is by placing the case manager in an office associated with the government of the catchment area, for example in the mayor's or the county commissioner's office.

Some states (e.g., Ohio and New Jersey) have created "protectorship" agencies whose duties include client advocacy. Protectorship was also referred to earlier in connection with forms of guardianship. The responsibilities of the protector agencies are comprehensive and include counseling, needs assessment, referral to service agencies, monitoring, guardianship, and advocacy. The limitations of such publicly employed "protectors" were also indicated previously. As state employees the caseworkers as guardians have an implicit conflict of interest where clients are being served by state agencies. State protection and advocacy agencies, even if independent of the service delivery system, are still part of the state government. Moreover, an employee of the governmental system will probably have more difficulty in negotiating its bureaucracy that one who is outside it.

Adequate Financial Support

The scope and quality of services within a catchment are will depend mainly on its fiscal base. The importance of local control of service funds has been noted, but the funding base itself must be adequate to client needs. Whether one likes it or not, "dollars" determine which client group will receive which service and, since these dollars are finite, competition for them is inevitable, and the general health of the economy will determine the fierceness of the competition. Apart from struggles for tax dollars *between* disability groups (e.g., mental retardation vs mental health), *within* retardation there is the potential competition between institutional and community programs. In spite of the acknowledged inadequacies of many large institutions, their long histories, well-established roles, and organized constituencies (e.g., parents of residents and employee unions) suggest that in the competition for funds the newer community programs are at a severe disadvantage (Rothman, 1979). One way in which institutions can help in the development of community services is by directing funds earned by institutions through federal medical accreditation to the communities. But the spin-off of federal institutional dollars can only be a small contributor to the overall need. In the final analysis the development of new services will depend on our readiness to be taxed for their creation and operation.

A Specific Service Model

Figure 26 illustrates the array of services along a continuum that varies from "most restrictive" to "least restrictive."[18] "Restrictiveness" refers to the degree to which the setting encourages maximum personal responsibility, decision making, and independence. At least some of the variables that appear to contribute to this are number of clients served, ratio of staff to clients, and management model. The demarcation of each program is a purely subjective estimate which tries to take each of these elements into account.

To flesh out the picture of a service system that seeks to serve retarded persons in the least restrictive setting, a model is offered of how such services might be administratively organized (see Fig. 27). Though some models are organized wholly on a functional basis and ignore age distinctions (Lensink, 1976), the proposed scheme divides services according to two dimensions—the age of the population and the types of services offered. It consciously seeks to separate child and adult services as *the* major organizational distinction. This is particularly important in mental retardation because of our tendency to think of the retarded adult in terms of "the eternal child." The administrative separation should increase the likelihood that the retarded adult receives more age-appropriate kinds of services. Another important reason is that it should facilitate coordination among workers providing different services to the same individual. The preschool child who requires some kind of out-of-home residential placement will also need a developmental day care program. Similarly, residential resources for an adult must be tied to some kind of meaningful activity, preferably of a vocational nature. The proposed model does not seek to divide all services according to age group, however, and includes a division that would be responsible for more occasional kinds of service (e.g., advocacy) as well as those designed primarily for the family.

[18]The figure largely represents the work of Tony Dalton, Senior Staff Trainer, Developmental Disabilities Training Institute, University of North Carolina at Chapel Hill.

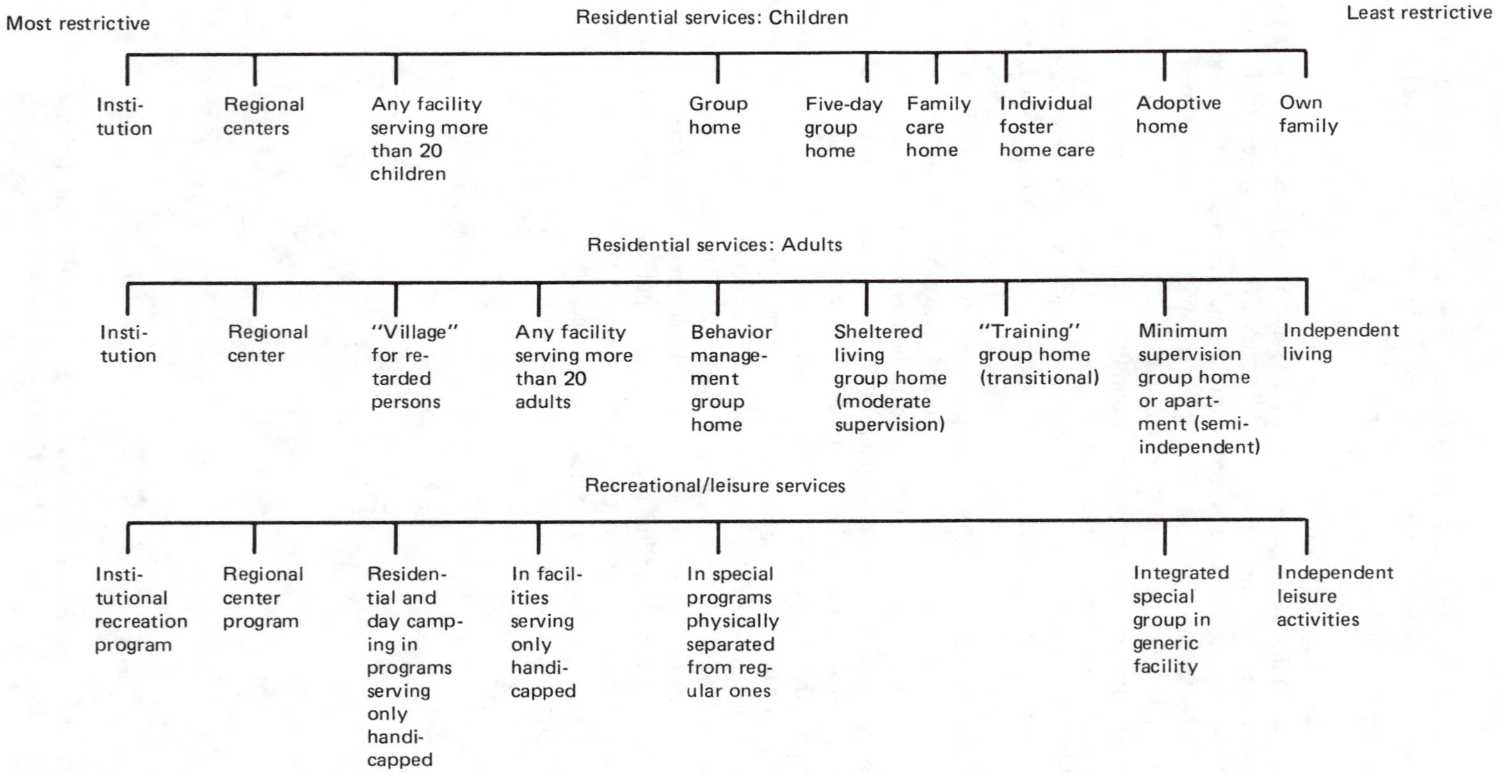

FIG. 26 Continuum of services by degree of "restrictiveness."

Most restrictive   Least restrictive

Residential services: Children

| Insti-tution | Regional centers | Any facility serving more than 20 children | Group home | Five-day group home | Family care home | Individual foster home care | Adoptive home | Own family |

Residential services: Adults

| Insti-tution | Regional center | "Village" for re-tarded persons | Any facility serving more than 20 adults | Behavior manage-ment group home | Sheltered living group home (moderate supervision) | "Training" group home (transitional) | Minimum supervision group home or apart-ment (semi-independent) | Independent living |

Recreational/leisure services

| Insti-tutional recreation program | Regional center program | Residen-tial and day camp-ing in programs serving only handi-capped | In facil-ities serving only handi-capped | In special programs physically separated from reg-ular ones | Integrated special group in generic facility | Independent leisure activities |

270

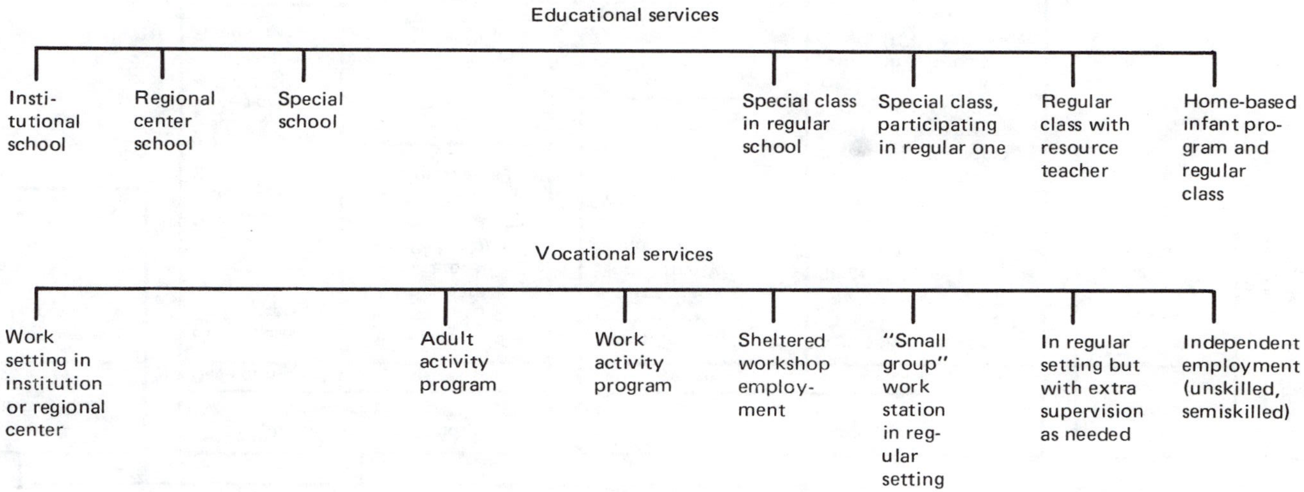

FIG. 26 Continuum of services by degree of "restrictiveness." *(Continued)*

Educational services

Institutional school — Regional center school — Special school — Special class in regular school — Special class, participating in regular one — Regular class with resource teacher — Home-based infant program and regular class

Vocational services

Work setting in institution or regional center — Adult activity program — Work activity program — Sheltered workshop employment — "Small group" work station in regular setting — In regular setting but with extra supervision as needed — Independent employment (unskilled, semiskilled)

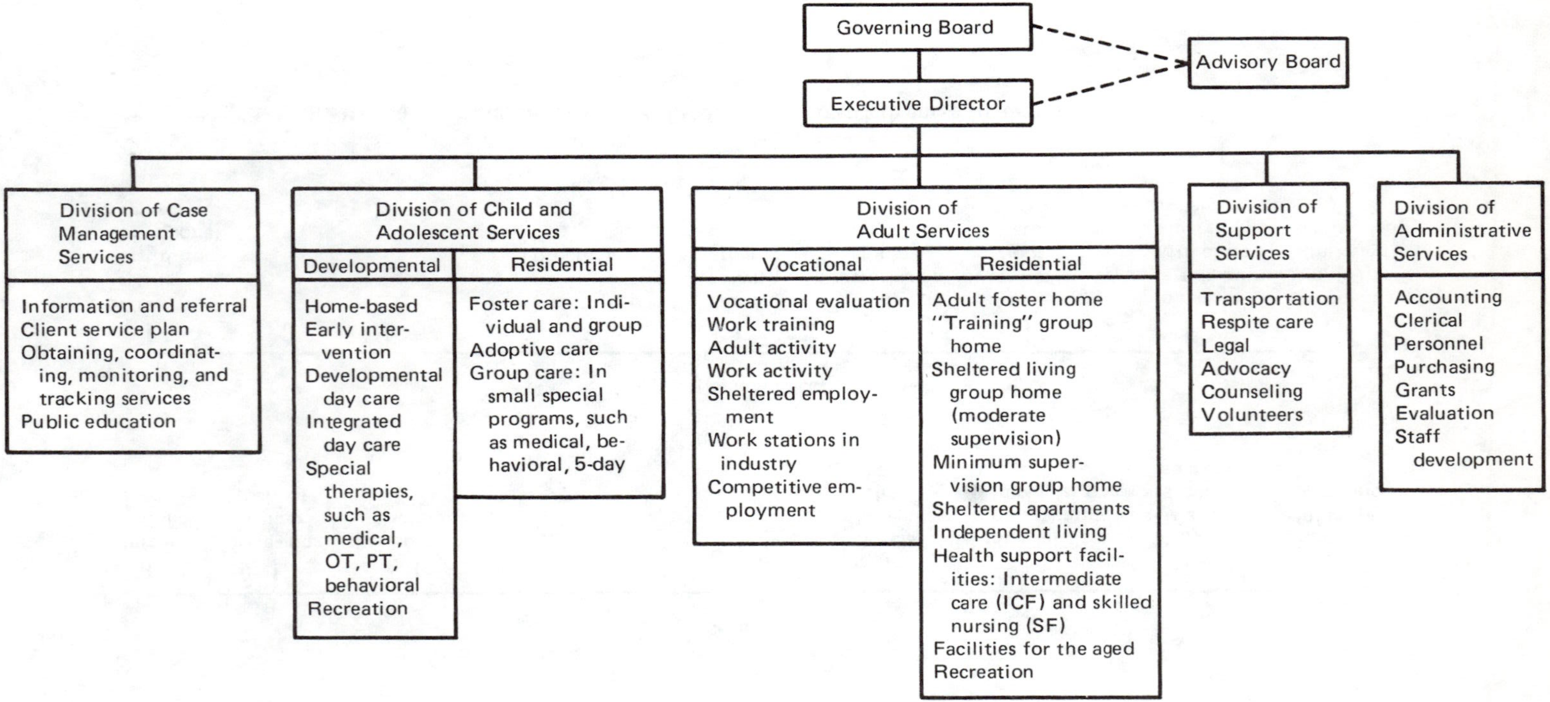

FIG. 27 An administrative model for an area MH/MR/SA mental retardation service system.

Infant and Preschool Programs

OVERVIEW

We now begin the in-depth review of educational and treatment programs for retarded persons. The review begins with an examination of programs for the retarded infant (age 0–2) and preschooler (age 2–6). The topics addressed are (a) general objectives of infant and preschool programs; (b) behavior modification; (c) the instructional process; (d) the nature and effects of infant training programs; (e) the nature and effects of preschool (early childhood) programs; (f) the preschool curriculum: self-help, cognition, language, motor, and social-emotional development; and (g) the role of parents, sibs, and other family members.

GENERAL OBJECTIVES OF INFANT AND PRESCHOOL PROGRAMS

The objectives of infant and preschool programs are at least threefold: (a) to maximize cognitive, communicative, motor, and personality resources as these are applied to age-related developmental tasks; (b) to assist the child's family, parents *and* sibs, in the understanding and rearing of their handicapped member; and (c) to prepare the child to function as fully as possible in a world of nonhandicapped persons.

Developmental Tasks of Infancy and Early Childhood

The age-related developmental tasks of the preschool years focus on the acquisition of *self-help skills* (feeding, dressing, and toileting), *cognitive development* (through "preoperational" thought in Piagetian terms), *functional communication*, gross and fine *motor skill*, and *social skills*.

Parents and Sibs

Infant and preschool programs not only serve the child; they also help the family through direct assistance in child training and by offering to parents and sibs the opportunity to meet others who are facing similar challenges.

Preparing for Life in a Nonhandicapped World

Though the preschool years may involve only limited contact with nonfamily normal children and adults, the effect of seeking to provide services within the least restrictive setting will ensure that by school age, if not earlier, the handicapped child will be interacting with normal children and adults. Under appropriate conditions these encounters can, through modeling, enhance the handicapped child's resources while simultaneously offering to normal children the possibility of developing more positive attitudes toward children who are "different."

Attainment of Training Objectives

The child's capacity to benefit from infancy and preschool programs depends on many things—the child's abilities, teacher skills, appropriateness of the teaching objectives, the physical setting, and, most importantly, the attitudes of family and teachers toward the child's "teachability." If little is expected or required *because* of the disability, then little will be forthcoming. Coversely, if the child is expected to accomplish at least those developmental tasks commensurate with his abilities, this too will be realized. Appropriate expectancies can be fostered by helping teachers and parents to understand their training objectives and the methods through which those objectives can be attained. In the section that follows is presented one methodology that teachers and parents will find useful. The remainder of the chapter offers the specific training content or "curriculum" of infant and preschool programs.

BEHAVIOR MODIFICATION

Behavior modification is a therapeutic approach that has been widely applied to the education, training, and behavioral management of retarded children. Its fundamental rationale is that *behavior is governed by its consequences.* Consequences may be "positive" or rewarding (positive reinforcers), "negative" or punishing (negative reinforcers), or absent altogether. The basic premise of behavior modification is in accord with the "first-order" need posited in the personality model presented in Chapter 2—that we are ultimately governed by the need to obtain pleasurable consequences and to avoid painful ones. The popularity of this educational and behavioral approach stems from its appeal to common sense, as we are all familiar with the use of rewards and penalties as motivators. Although its underlying principles are easily understood, their implementation is not. As applied to educational or behavioral objectives they involve (a) the specifying of the target behaviors in an objective and measurable manner, (b) determining the method of measuring changes in the target behavior,[1] (c) choosing potential reinforcers, (d) specifying the conditions (contingencies) under which the desired behavior will be rewarded and the undesired behavior punished (providing "structure"), (e) ensuring that procedures are carried out, and (f) monitoring the effectiveness of the contingencies in terms of measurable behavior change, and (g) modifying contingencies of reward and punishment as needed. For a comprehensive treatment of the application of these principles in mental retardation, the reader is referred to Thompson and Grabowski (1977) and Matson and McCartney (1981). The discussion here is limited to the behavioral consequences. It is these contingencies, either positive and/or negative, that are the main tools of the behavior modifier. In Chapter 10, there is again a focus on behavior modification with regard to the management of behavior problems in severely and profoundly retarded individuals.

Behavioral Consequences

Rewards (Positive Consequences)

In behavior modification particular stress is placed on the use of rewards (positive reinforcers) as a means of encouraging desired behavior. The actual administration of rewards is called "positive reinforcement." In choosing potential positive reinforcers, one considers what will be rewarding to a particular child—what does he like, what will he work for. Four types of rewards are recognized—social, symbolic, material, or activities.

Social

Social reinforcers are the most common and the easiest to provide. They consist of forms of positive teacher attention to desired behavior, typically verbal praise—the omnipresent "good boy" or "good girl."

Symbolic

Symbolic rewards are those that stand for or signify approval; tokens or stars are common examples. They represent concrete forms of positive recognition and have the important virtue of a much longer "half-life" than social ones. Not only do they constitute a continuing evidence of adult approval, but they can also be accumulated and used to obtain other rewards.

Material

Material reinforcers typically consist of edibles—food and candy, and, of course, require that the child be in some state of "need" if they are to be effective. The reinforcing of that need must also be done with care so as to avoid reducing it through "satiation."

---

[1]Some believe that the observing and recording of behavior is itself the most important contributor to behavior change (Hall, 1971; Sherman & Bushell, 1975). It clearly has the effect of sensitizing the observer to what the child is actually doing, an especially important consideration with respect to the antecedents and consequences of undesirable behavior.

Activities

Access to desired activities as a reward for appropriate behavior is a widely used incentive. For the child it can take the form of additional free play time, the opportunity to play with a particularly desired toy, or even additional teacher attention.

Universality of Reward Systems

In the use of rewards to encourage the achievement of behavioral and educational objectives, behavior modification does not represent some new and exotic approach. All of us who attempt to influence the behavior of others recognize that incentives are a powerful ally. It is only that behavior modification is much more explicit and systematic in their dispensation. Some workers may initially resist the use of rewards because they are perceived as "bribes." If *we* were expected to meet parental and teacher expectancies without the inducement of specific rewards, why should others be treated differently? But even cursory reflection on our own childhood experience and consideration of the personality model presented earlier reveal that our response to parents and teachers was not made in an incentive-free vacuum. The incentives *were* and *are* there, though not necessarily explicitly stated. The need for intimacy was both nurtured and fulfilled through parental love. Throughout our lives we continue to need experiences of intimacy as approval is sought from persons whose esteem we value—teachers, peers, employers, persons in authority, and always our parents. Together with intimacy, experiences that meet needs for success and autonomy all feed our extraordinary need for self-esteem. For the child, doing well in school can be a powerful means of obtaining parental and teacher approval (intimacy) as well as affirming some sense of personal effectiveness (success). Later in life, possibilities of job promotion and accompanying wage increases and greater prestige create strong incentives. We too, then, are also locked into a reward system.

But even the use of the term "bribe" in this context is inappropriate. A bribe is an incentive to do something that we ought *not* to do. It is an inducement to violate accepted behavioral standards. But the use of rewards in behavior modification is intended to provide an incentive to do what we *ought* to do. Furthermore, the conscious and conspicuous dispensing of rewards cannot be a permanent basis for maintaining desired behavior. Rather it is an encouragement to move in the desired direction. Whether the reinforced behavior "takes" will, ultimately, depend on whether the behavior itself becomes rewarding.

PENALTIES (PUNISHMENT)

Just as rewards are used as incentives to do something desirable, so are penalties (negative reinforcers) employed to discourage that which is undesirable. Although we would wish that all of our interactions with others were pleasant and rewarding, this is clearly not possible. Each of us, child and adult, learns through pleasure *and* pain. Effective adaptation requires awareness of the possibility of unpleasant consequences as well as pleasant ones. Our preferences for the use of positive rather than negative consequences rests on many factors. One of these is the wish to avoid control that is primarily coercive since control based only on fear of punishment is going to diminish once the threat of punishment is absent. We also want the child to perceive persons in authority as sources of positive reinforcement rather than pain, since this will induce "approach" rather than "avoidance" tendencies. In principle, an ideal series of consequences will involve the use of rewards and penalties (this is discussed in Chap. 10). Indeed, it has been suggested that a program that limits itself to punishment, especially if it is particularly aversive (e.g., brief electric shock) and does not simultaneously offer the opportunity for positive reinforcement, cannot be justified (Richmond & Martin, 1977). A review of ethical and legal issues pertaining to the use of punishment with institutionalized retarded persons calls attention to principles referred to in the prior chapter. Though preschool children are less likely than older ones to engage in the kind of disruptive behavior that calls for severe consequences, we need to be sensitive to the desirability of selecting "the least restrictive consequences," of avoiding "cruel and unusual punishment," and of obtaining parental consent (Thompson & Grabowski, 1977).[2]

One method of punishment is called *aversive stimulation*. It is the most controversial of all forms of punishment since it involves the direct imposition of very painful though physically noninjurious stimulation. Various types of corporal punishment would be examples of aversive stimulation, though the form is most commonly equated with the use of electric shock. Such procedures have absolutely no place in the management of children, and even with adults their use must be minimal and carefully monitored. We will return, in Chapter 10, to the use of aversive stimulation in the management of self-injurious behavior.

Overcorrection is a consequence wherein the child is literally required to engage in behavior that restores the desired state, such as cleaning up an area that the child has soiled. The distinction is drawn between *restitutional overcorrection*, the restoration of the former state, and *positive practice overcorrection*, in which restoration is supplemented by additional related activities (e.g., after cleaning up the soiled area, the child would also be required to clean other areas that he has not soiled).[3] While such procedures are thought to have an "education" component (Foxx & Azrin, 1973b), their performance under conditions of coercion suggests that negative attitudes toward ordinarily appropriate behavior might also be engendered. One would want to avoid incorporating in restitutional overcorrection activities or chores that are normally expected of the child.

Exercising Restraint

The right to punish carries with it the responsibility of restraint. The legal issues to which we have just referred are explicit guidelines in this regard. Punishment that involves the direct infliction of pain, as in spanking, should be avoided

---

[2]Modified guidelines for the use of aversive and deprivation procedures as developed by Minnesota are found in *Behavior Modification of the Mentally Retarded* (Thompson & Grabowski, 1977). See also Nolley et al. (1980).

[3]Overcorrection is dealt with in depth in Chapter 10.

(Ross, 1981). The recognition that behavior is governed by its consequences can lead to serious difficulties when mild punishments are ineffective. Reason will direct us to seek increasingly more aversive consequences, a condition that can gradually lead us to ever more abusive behavior. It is then that we should welcome the legal and ethical restraints on our freedom to punish. We protect the child from possible cruelty and ourselves from brutalization.

Ignoring Behavior (Extinction)

In the use of rewards and penalties, we *react* to behavior we want to influence; we do something. But another option open to us in trying to eliminate undesirable behavior is to do nothing at all. If behavior is governed by its consequences and a particular behavior evokes no response at all, it can be expected to disappear. The deliberate ignoring of behavior is called *extinction*. This procedure will be particularly appropriate to behavior that is perceived as "attention-getting" in intent and is dangerous to neither the child nor others. Attention-getting reflects the need for intimacy, but when it seems excessive or occurs at inopportune times, its gratification is undesirable. Bedtime disturbances are a common example of attention-getting behavior. Although the child has been put to sleep and parents have retired to their own interests, the child does not immediately accept separation, and crying ensues. The crying brings the parents, who then spend additional time with the child. In effect, the child's crying has been reinforced or rewarded by renewed parental attention. The child's "need" system now begins to encroach on those of its parents and is experienced by them as a "demand."

But if parents decide to adhere to a bedtime schedule and not return to the child once goodnights have been said, the crying will eventually cease. Not immediately, because if prolonged goodnights have been encouraged (reinforced) in the past, the failure to produce the parents with crying will lead to its intensification. But if parents stick by their guns and refrain from responding to the crying, it will gradually cease. It is through such experiences that the child gradually becomes "socialized"—that is, he learns that his own needs cannot be gratified whenever and wherever he desires.

This is particularly important for the handicapped child, who often evokes overly permissive parental behavior. But children can and do learn that others have needs too and that the satisfaction of their own needs depends on some degree of responsiveness to the needs of others. But this technique is only appropriate if the child is generally receiving adequate attention; it cannot be expected to work with children who are in periodic states of real attention deprivation, such as children who come from economically disadvantaged backgrounds. The ignoring of undesirable behavior is an effort to reverse the usual condition in which "the squeaky wheel gets the grease" and rather reminds us to be attentive to the child when he is behaving properly.

Negative Reinforcement

This behavioral contingency, paradoxically, refers to a positive state resulting from the cessation of an unpleasant one. The choice of this term was unfortunate because it is easily confused with negative reinforcers, events associated with punishment. Examples of negative reinforcement would be the cessation of a time-out period that was aversive to the child (Ross, 1981) or a feeling of relief following the taking of a medication. Negative reinforcement usually occurs in unplanned situations and so has a minor role in child management. Perhaps it is most often used at mealtime, when food may be offered that the child initially resists. The author often saw retarded children who were very resistive to new foods—for example, the child who would drink only Coke and rejected milk and all other liquids. Apart from attempts to wean the child gradually from Coke to milk by mixing one with the other, presentation of milk only while preventing access to other fluids will eventually produce the desired effect: thirst must be quenched!

Behavior Modification and the Teaching Process

The principles of behavior modification have had an enormous impact on the training and education of handicapped learners. Their understanding is regarded as one of the most important competencies in working with severely impaired children (Fredericks, Anderson, & Baldwin, 1979).[4] Two other important skills identified by these researchers are *maximizing instructional time* and *task analysis*. Where children are particularly limited in abilities to attend and persist, the judicious use of incentives (reinforcers) can help them to be more responsive to teacher objectives. The guide to teacher objectives lies in the child's level of development and in another major feature of the behavioral approach, the principle of *successive approximation*. This principle calls attention to the fact that new behaviors or skills are usually acquired in stages and that the degrees of skill mastery need to be rewarded as well as the end product itself. The concept of stepwise learning requires the instructor to break down the learning objective into its component parts (task analysis), teach them individually, and then gradually chain them together into the desired whole. The process is shortly illustrated in the teaching of self-care skills in dressing.

Finally, behavior modification lends itself particularly to an individual approach, though it can also be used with groups (Sherman & Bushell, 1975), and it is the former that is especially appropriate to the young handicapped child. Within a preschool group there are likely to be wide differences in ability and in developmental levels, and much of the instruction, of necessity, will be individual in nature. It is, of course, this very "individualization" that permits the teacher to be most responsive to the child's learning needs.

THE INSTRUCTIONAL PROCESS

Core Teacher Knowledge

Although one of the teacher skills important to effective instruction is knowledge of behavioral principles, these principles are merely the method through which one seeks to alter the child's developmental level. It is the child's development that is the focus of our educational effort, and, in preschool programs, this

---

[4]The use of behavioral principles in education is also illustrated in Chapter 8 in connection with educational programs for severely and profoundly retarded adults.

will relate to the areas of self-help, cognition, language, motor skills, and socialization. It is the *scope* and *sequence* of development in infancy and early childhood along with the learning characteristics of young children that constitute the fundamental body of knowledge pertaining to preschool education.

Teacher Attitudes

Together with skills, the effective teacher will reflect certain attitudes. These will include acceptance of where the child is developmentally, optimism regarding the child's capacity to develop, and awareness of the importance of providing experiences of success. As a corollary to the belief that some growth is possible in virtually all children, there is acceptance of the fact that the responsibility for the attainment of instructional goals lies with the teacher rather than with the child. This is a reverse of the usual way of perceiving the teacher-child relationship. Ordinarily, it is the child who must adapt to the teacher's methodology, and if the child fails to learn, the fault is his. Our newer vision relates the child's progress to the *conditions of learning* rather than to the child per se. If the child fails to learn, the teachers asks herself in what way did the lesson plan *prevent* the child from achieving the instructional objective. She then seeks to modify the learning situation as appropriate.[5]

The Teaching Process

Let us now examine the teaching process itself. It is divisible into five major steps: (a) evaluating the child's current level of functioning; (b) selecting, on the basis of that evaluation, learning objectives that either strengthen existing skills or teach next higher level ones; (c) translating learning objectives into concrete lesson plans; (d) supporting the lesson plan through appropriate teaching methods, including the use of reinforcers; and (e) determining whether goals have been met and modifying lesson plans and reinforcers accordingly.

EVALUATION

The evaluation process serves two functions—establishing the appropriateness of a child for a given program and the identification of specific teaching objectives. Evaluation itself may have two phases—an initial "screening" assessment which indicates the general level of functioning in developmental areas and a subsequent more in-depth assessment on a measure which also provides specific training goals.

SELECTING LEARNING OBJECTIVES

Screening Assessment

A common screening battery for handicapped preschoolers consists of the Denver Developmental Screening Test (Frankenburg, Dodds, & Fandal, 1967,

---

[5]For a series of articles on preschool education for handicapped children, see "Managing the Preschool Environment," *Topics in Early Childhood Special Education*, 2, 1 (1982).

1970; Frankenburg, Goldstein, & Camp, 1971), the Receptive-Expressive Emergent Language Scale (Bzoch & League, 1970), and the Oseretsky Tests of Motor Proficiency (Doll, 1946). For a single assessment tool specifically developed for the handicapped infant and young preschooler, see also the *Early Learning Accomplishment Profile for Developmentally Young Children Birth to 36 Months* (Early LAP) (Glover, Preminger, & Sanford, 1978). In conjunction with *Competency-Based Training: A Manual for Staff Servicing Developmentally Disabled Children* (Fullagar & Glover, 1977), they provide an integrated evaluation and teaching combination. The manual incorporates assessment, programming, error-free teaching, organizing and scheduling a teaching day, and clear description of how the teacher can use behavioral principles. Its only limitation pertains to ill-defined success criteria.[6]

All of these scales will be limited in their usefulness if serious sensory and/or motor handicaps exist. DuBose (1981) has discussed the special problems of evaluating the severely impaired young child. She points out the effects of hearing loss on language and visual loss on both motor and cognitive skills. Physical impairments, of course, affect motor skills, and behavior problems and attentional disorders create their own barriers. Of particular interest are guidelines for the informal assessment of such children in the basic developmental areas.

Another important, potentially contaminating influence is medication. Drugs are commonly used for the control of seizures and for the management of behavior problems—typically hyperactivity in the young child. Although appropriate drug levels can facilitate evaluation, very high levels may reduce the child's capacity to respond.[7]

Prescriptive Assessment

A screening assessment period of about 6 weeks enables the teacher to become familiar with the child and the child to become adapted to a new setting. At its conclusion the teacher is ready for a second evaluation, but this time using one or more scales that are particularly helpful in selecting teaching objectives. A battery of scales may be in order to capitalize on the particular strengths of each. A combination might include the Vulpe Assessment Battery (Vulpe, 1977), because of its focus on motor-impaired children; the Early LAP or CAO (Sanford, 1973) for the older preschooler; and the Uzgiris-Hunt Ordinal Scales of Psychological Development (Uzgiris & Hunt, 1975). The LAP is seen as strong in the cognitive area, and the Uzgiris-Hunt is wholly focused on the kinds of cognitive processes found in normal infants or in retarded children who are functioning at mental age levels of less than 2 years.

[6]For a reference to early childhood materials see *Early Childhood Curriculum Materials: An Annotated Bibliography* (Technical Assistance Development System, 1975).

[7]For a brief review of medication effects in handicapped preschoolers, see Simeonsson and Simeonsson (1981).

TRANSLATING OBJECTIVES
INTO LESSON PLANS

Task Analysis

Even the simplest of skills consists of a series of subskills. Teaching a child to put on a pair of pants involves the mastery of a number of individual steps of which the practiced performer is no longer aware—finding leg holes, lifting and inserting legs, grasping a waistband, pulling up the pants, buttoning, zipping, and tying a belt. It is the mastery of each element that brings the total task within the child's capacity, no small achievement for the motor-impaired child. Task analysis involves not only identifying task subskills but also determining the sequence with which they will be taught (Espech & Williams, 1967)—"We learn to walk before we run." Later in the chapter a model sequence is offered that is particularly appropriate to cognitive and academic objectives.

Maximizing Success

In the teaching of children with learning difficulties there is special need for minimizing failure. So-called error-free learning seeks to accomplish this through task analysis and by using such teaching methods as modeling, prompting, cuing, and reinforcement (Findlay et al., 1974).

APPROPRIATE TEACHING METHODS:
TEACHING IN SMALL STEPS

Three elements are involved in teaching in small steps—shaping, chaining, and fading (Bigelow, 1977). *Shaping* refers to the reinforcement of behaviors that gradually approximate the final teaching objective. For example, if we are interested in teaching a normally nonverbal child to imitate a particular sound correctly, we may initially reinforce *any* sound and then follow this by gradually reinforcing only those sounds that increasingly approximate the desired one.

Chaining refers to the uniting of the individual subskills that underlie a particular task. Thus, in teaching a child to put on his pants, chaining involves a gradual combining of individually taught subskills into larger and larger segments. Curiously, it is "backward" rather than forward chaining that is most often appropriate. Here the child is taught the *last* step in the chain first and then worked backward through it. The intent of this reversal of the usual method of instruction is to enable the child to have an experience of success and reward in the learning of relatively difficult tasks, though at first only one step in the chain is mastered. If, as in usual practice, we commence training at the beginning step rather than at the last, as, for example, in putting on pants, each of the several intermediate steps increases the likelihood of some error and frustration for child and teacher. In starting with the last step, however, the child is guided by the instructor through each of the preceding steps, and it is only the last one in which training actually takes place. Reinforcement would then follow that mastery of the last step. The instructor then moves successively to each preceding step while always reserving the largest reinforcement for the completion of an ever lengthening chain. This form of instruction seems best suited to self-help skills, but it is also appropriate to such a stepwise activity as assembling puzzles (Bigelow, 1977). Table 18 illustrates both task analysis and a training sequence.

Fading, the third element in small-step instruction, refers to the gradual reduction in the level of assistance provided by the teacher as task mastery increases. In teaching the putting on of pants, the instructor may, initially, fully assist the child in all but the last step, the one being trained. As each preceding step is mastered, the degree of instructor assistance inevitably diminishes or is "faded." Fading also refers to the degree of assistance provided in teaching any subskill. Common forms of assistance are *modeling* (demonstrating the desired response), *prompting* (physically guiding the learner through the correct response), and *cuing* (giving hints to the desired response). With reference to modeling, demonstration is clearly superior to only verbal instructions as a teaching method (Rosenthal & Kellogg, 1973). The retarded learner, like you and me, learns best by "doing" but appears to have particular difficulty in utilizing the verbal medium. The nature of this "verbal" limitation was discussed in the first chapter. Teachers should avoid lengthy verbal explanations in the introduction of tasks. As mastery is achieved it *is* appropriate to provide their verbal representation, but *language represents the formulation of the completed act* rather than greatly assisting in task mastery itself.

In a study of a population of severely handicapped children who differed in educational gains, it was found that the most significant factor was the amount of teacher time spent in actual instruction (Fredericks, Anderson, & Baldwin, 1979). Teachers whose children made the greater gains provided an average of 40 minutes

TABLE 18   Teaching a Child to Put on His Pants

Goal or Step (student behavior)	Method (teacher behavior)
6. Picks up pants, grasping both sides of waist-band	6. With child seated, give command, "_____, put on your pants." Have child grasp both sides of waistband and pick up pants
5. Puts right foot through waist and into leg hole	5. Have child pull up his right leg (bending it at knee) while spreading open the pants waist. Insert right foot into the correct leg hole
4. Puts left foot through waist and into left leg hole	4. Same as step 5 but for left foot
3. Pulls pants to knees	3. While child is seated, have him pull waistband to knees
2. Pull pants to midthigh	2. Have child stand and continue pulling pants to midthigh
1. Pulls pants to waist	1. Have child pull until pants are completely on (some straightening of waistband may be necessary)

Note. These individual training steps and methodology are taken from the Murdoch Center C & Y Program Library: A Collection of Step-by-Step Programs for the Developmentally Disabled. Distributed by Murdoch Center at Butner, NC, the Library consists of over 350 task-analyzed training programs in the areas of self-help, residential skills, gross motor skills, fine motor skills, preacademic, academic, and social skills.

more instruction per day ($4\frac{1}{3}$ hours vs. $3\frac{3}{4}$). In such programs the majority of teacher time tends to be spent in "caretaking"—toileting, diapering, feeding, and dressing (McCormick & Goldman, 1979)—but training can be incorporated with caretaking (McCormick, Cooper, & Goldman, 1979). This involves the caretaker's requirement of some relevant behavior from the child.

INFANCY: THE FIRST TWO YEARS OF LIFE

In recent years there has been much stress on the earliest possible identification of children who are at high risk for mental retardation. The first 2 years of life not only may afford this opportunity for children who are chronologically infants, but they also have educational implications for clearly retarded persons of all ages who are functioning cognitively at not more than this developmental level.

Development in Infancy

The first 2 years of life are marked by tremendous growth in all aspects of development (see Table 19). *Motorically*, there is change from an initial state of very limited mobility, in part due to the early predominance of reflexive activity (Johnston, 1976), to one in which there is ease of movement and relatively good hand-eye coordination. *Languagewise*, we see development from an initial cooing and babbling to one in which there is a rapid expansion of single-word vocabulary and a common stringing of words together in little two-word utterances. *Cognitively*, it is a period during which one learns that things exist independent of our perception of them, there is understanding of simple cause-and-effect relationships, and there develops a capacity to innovate solutions to accomplish goals (Uzgiris & Hunt, 1975). In the *social-emotional* sphere, the infant shows very early the nature of humans as social animals. By 6 months there is inviting of attention and a beginning distinction between parents and "strangers." Attachment grows, and separation from caretakers becomes more difficult. There is recognition of different emotional states in others and a reaction to them. The parent dominates the child's social life, but during the second year there is a growing interest in other children. In the self-help domain there is a considerable movement, from one of total dependency, tied in part to limited motor capacities, to one in which there is partial ability to feed oneself with cup and spoon and to participate in undressing. Toiletwise, the 2-year-old is dry at night if taken up and has begun to signal toilet needs.

Infant Training Programs

The content of infant programs will consist of varying combinations of basic sensory stimulation (Johnson & Werner, 1975) and of specific training in each of the aforementioned areas. The teaching is intended either to accelerate potentially delayed development or to maximize its level where significant delay already exists. Of the training areas, the motor sphere will be of special concern because abnormalities here will generally be evident fairly early. In Chapter 4 there was

TABLE 19 Normal Development in the First Two Years of Life[a]

Months	Gross and fine motor	Language	Activity-cognition	Social-emotional	Self-help
3	Prone—can raise head and chest, some head sag when held in sitting; rolls from back to side and returns, on either side; hands usually clenched; held standing, lifts foot	Looks at face and eyes of person talking to him; babbles or coos when talked to	Growing interest in world but primarily centered on parents, looks longer at human face than at objects, becoming more active	In response to smile, may smile, coo, and blow bubbles; crying tends to sharply decrease at sound of person approaching	
6	Rolls from prone to supine and from supine to prone; prone—pushes up on hands and can raise chest and abdomen off surface; sits erect when supported; bears almost all weight when standing supported; approaches and grasps with one hand; movement is not smooth; uses raking motion in picking up, fingers against palm	"Talks" to mirror image, responds to voices by turning head toward source, usually stops crying when spoken to	Discriminates strangers, smiles and vocalizes to mirror image, looks at objects while handling, mouths toys, resists removal of toys; moves toward objects; may repeat chance occurrences to reproduce a desired effect	Holds arms out to be picked up, shows displeasure when person tries to take toy, first evidence of separation anxiety	

285

TABLE 19 Normal Development in the First Two Years of Life[a] (*Continued*)

Months	Gross and fine motor	Language	Activity–cognition	Social–emotional	Self-help
9	Pulls self to sitting and sits without support for 10 minutes; pushes up on hands and knees and creeps; stands holding on for 5 minutes, while standing—makes stepping movements; can now oppose thumb and forefinger in "pincer" grasp	Imitates sounds made by himself, recognizes own name, appropriate head shaking for "No"	Becoming interested in putting objects together; enjoys dropping things into a cup and then removing them; reaches out to people playfully; can recognize object when only part is visible; acts begin to become clearly intentional and can use one activity to accomplish another (e.g., pulling a string to get a ring)	Is reserved with strangers but enjoys social play such as pat-a-cake and bye-bye	Takes solids well, finger-feeds; holds, bites, and chews cracker
12	Rapidly creeps on hands and knees, rises from hands and knees to standing without assistance, begins to walk; deft pincer grasp, can put cube in cup and release, can throw with a pushing motion	Says two words besides "Mama" and "Dada"; jabbers expressively (beginning of "jargon" stage); recognizes some familiar objects and body parts by name; may repeat familiar words	Can search for object seen hidden (has concept of "object permanence"); can follow simple directions; at nighttime has difficulty in settling down for sleep and wakes easily; some rocking, head rolling, and head banging may be seen; enjoys simple tricks and games, especially being chased while creeping at top speed; can respond to	Increased dependence on caretaker, and any separation is difficult; tries to attract attention by squealing or crying; capable of recognizing anger, jealousy, and fear in others, and may react to these emotions	Finger-feeds self part of meal, inhibits drooling; cooperates in dressing; can take off hat and shoes; bowel movements are regularized

15	An active walker— walks with feet wide apart and with short steps, may be able to walk down stairs holding your hand and may be able to crawl up stairs by himself; can place one block on another, but voluntary release is exaggerated; can turn pages, usually several at a time	Vocalizes and gestures to indicate wants; uses jargon; mimicks sounds	music and enjoys single repetitive rhythmical sounds; beginning understanding of form. Very active, "gets into things"; enjoys picture books, filling boxes; can make simple drawing stroke; remembers objects that are out of sight; may be puzzled when can't find something in its usual place	As he becomes more independent, he is a little less compliant; temper is easily aroused and loudly expressed though it may be short-lived	Feeding: chews most foods well, holds glass with two hands but is apt to spill; can grasp spoon and insert in dish but fills spoon poorly and is apt to turn upside down when it enters mouth; dressing: pulls off socks; toileting: shows wet or soiled pants
18	Runs; may walk down stairs aided only by rail or wall; can seat self in small chair and climb into an adult one; pushes and pulls objects; can throw a ball over- hand and doesn't fall; scribbles spontane- ously with pencil; voluntary release is still exaggerated	Vocabulary is increas- ing, and child is bet- ter able to make wants understood; words are beginning to accompany and even replace ges- tures; "baby talk" is being abandoned; two-word combina- tions may appear	Knows where things belong, can follow simple two-step di- rections, still explor- ing and able to move things to extend reach; can point to named pictures; likes to imitate the activi- ties of older children and adults; solitary onlooker play	Behavior varies from independence at one moment to clinging dependency in the next; calls adult to admire constructions; sudden changes pro- duce negativistic behavior; may seem defiant	Feeding: growing inde- pendence leads to prolongation of eat- ing and a messy op- eration, handles cup quite well, fills spoon but apt to turn it in mouth, places in mouth; dressing: unzips, can take off mittens, hat, and socks, tries to put on shoes; toileting: reg- ulated for both bowel and bladder control, may awaken at night and ask to be changed

TABLE 19 Normal Development in the First Two Years of Life[a] (*Continued*)

Months	Gross and fine motor	Language	Activity-cognition	Social-emotional	Self-help
21	Runs stiffly and with fewer falls, alternates quickly between standing, squatting, and sitting; assumes squatting position in play; walks up stairs using rail and placing two feet on each step; creeps backward down stairs	Has vocabulary of at least 20 words, uses words in simple requests, speaks in two-word combinations	Loves rough-and-tumble play, usually plays near other children but not with them; boys and girls tend to imitate their mother more and more; possessive attitude toward toys—refers to "me" and "mine" and with little sharing; can look at pictures alone; enjoys rhythmical sound patterns; good immediate memory, but attention span is short, and child is easily distractible; recognizes names of several body parts; refers to self by name rather than as "I" and "me"	May be showing some interest in other children, may quickly show affection, attempts to delay bedtime in order to remain with family	Feeding: lifts, drinks, and replaces cup well; uses spoon with moderate spilling, no longer turns spoon in mouth, dawdles and plays with food, refuses foods; toileting: asks for toilet and uses same word for both functions, increased frequency of urinating

288

Runs well, walks down stairs placing both feet on each step, jumps from bottom step, one food leading, and usually lands on all fours or in squat; picks up object from floor without falling, kicks large ball, jumps in place, attempts to imitate folding of paper, builds tower of 6–7 blocks, imitates vertical and circular stroke, turns pages singly

Verbalizes immediate experiences, "talks" about activities while ongoing (soliloquies); jargon has disappeared, speaking vocabulary has sharply increased and may consist of 200–300 words; pronouns are beginning to be used, also negative and interrogatory phrases; average "sentence" length is still about 2 words

Increasing attention span, understands such concepts as "another," "same," and simple spatial ones such as "on" and "under"; can identify objects by their name and has mastered the cognitive skills associated with what Piaget refers to as the "sensorimotor" period—the child understands simple causality and has the capacity to modify situations and mentally innovate solutions to accomplish desired ends

Still playing beside other children rather than with them (parallel play); apt to snatch, push, and kick rather than social give and take; does not ask for help in play, and adult must be watchful

Feeding: holds small glass with one hand while drinking, uses spoon with moderate spilling but is able to insert spoon in mouth without turning, still needs help in feeding—dawdles and plays with food, refuses foods; dressing: pulls on simple articles of clothing, pulls up pants, can remove shoes but needs help with laces; takes off clothes with help on buttons, hooks and unhooks, cooperates well in dressing; toileting: dry at night if taken up; squats, holds self or verbalizes toilet need

Sources: Gesell et al., 1940; Glover, Preminger, and Sanford, 1978; Wabash Center for the Mentally Retarded, 1977.

reference to the importance of the early recognition and treatment of the motor problems associated with cerebral palsy. Physical and occupational therapy and the management of feeding problems caused by motor impairment are some of the most prominent treatment activities of this period (Finnie, 1975). The cognitive and language areas will also receive much attention, the Uzgiris-Hunt scale providing a basis for cognitive training, itself a prerequisite to language development (Kahn, 1971; Uzgiris & Hunt, 1975).

Another very important dimension is assistance to the family. Since the child's development is viewed as at least partially tied to the quality of the mother-infant interaction, intervention also focuses on fostering a strong mutually gratifying mother-infant relationship. It is particularly in high-risk infants that this relationship is often disturbed (recall Kearsley's conjecture about "iatrogenic" retardation [Kearsley & Sigel, 1979]), but it is the mother (and/or the father) who is the most continuous source of potential stimulation during infancy. Although infants do not have to be induced to develop, the experiences that facilitate growth are totally dependent on what the parents provide (Lambie, Band, & Weikart, 1974). And especially where the child's natural responsiveness is diminished, parents may be less inclined to provide the kind of stimulation that can help the child grow.

HOME-BASED PROGRAMS

An important vehicle for encouraging maternal intimacy as well as providing direct support to parents is to bring the training program directly into the home. Such efforts are also necessary where place of residence does not permit access to day centers. This will be particularly true in sparsely populated rural areas. Perhaps the best known of the home-based programs is the Portage Project (Shearer & Shearer, 1976). Developed in rural Wisconsin, it serves all preschool-age children. A regular teacher is assigned to each child and his family and visits weekly.

CENTER-BASED PROGRAMS

Here parents and infant may visit a day center on a weekly basis with the parents sharing in the instructional activities. The parents will be encouraged and assisted in continuing these activities in the home. After infancy, center-based programs become the primary means of serving preschoolers (examples of them are found in Tjossem, 1976).

Effects of Intervention on Handicapped Infants

Current research suggests that programs of stimulation to the handicapped infant can accelerate the rate of development. This is particularly true of gross motor skills (Connally & Russell, 1976), but it is also reported for sensorimotor cognitive processes (Brassell, 1977; Dunst, 1974; Henry, 1977; Kahn, 1978). The research literature indicates, however, that the rate of speech development, in preschoolers as well as infants, may be the most difficult to alter. This is especially true in Down syndrome (e.g., Hayden & Dmitriev, 1975; Rynders & Horrobin,

1975, 1980), where a special speech deficit is well established (see Chapter 3). It is presumed that *problems of accelerating language acquisition relate to its apparent dependence on the level of cognitive development* (Bloom, 1975; Kahn, 1979). Significant growth in even single-word vocabulary usually does not occur until about 18 months of age in the normally developing infant, a time that heralds the onset of the final phase of cognitive development in the sensorimotor period. Moerk (1975), in particular, has described the order and specific sensorimotor stage within which appear the cognitive skills that are prerequisite to speech. Significant gains in language *can* be expected when the infant's language development is well below its cognitive level (Nielsen et al., 1975) except, of course, where speech-related problems exist, as in cerebral palsy or Down syndrome.

To what degree accelerated rates of development can be maintained remains to be seen. There are some relevant findings in the cognitive domain, but these are conflicting. Dunst (1976) found neither long-term retention nor generalization of earlier gains, but some later studies report both effects (Henry, 1977; Kahn, 1979). In the section that follows, the effects of intervention programs carried through to school age are presented. This will afford at least some inkling of the possible benefits of prolonged stimulation in children whose developmental lag is traceable to organic brain pathology.

EARLY CHILDHOOD: AGES TWO TO SIX

The same broad curriculum objectives of the infant programs exist in those for preschoolers and are typically pursued in day centers. For a description of some of the major ones the reader is again referred to Tjossem (1976). These day centers have tended to serve only handicapped children, though the "mainstreaming" thrust in educational services to school-age youth now includes the preschool population as well. We earlier touched on the importance of encouraging interaction between handicapped and nonhandicapped children as a means of providing more normalizing models for the handicapped youngsters and creating more accepting attitudes in normal ones. Models of such integrated preschool settings are described in Guralnick (1978), and specified aspects of it are discussed later in the chapter in the section dealing with social-emotional development in retarded preschoolers.

Effects of Preschool Programs

Attempts to evaluate the effects of intervention have been beset by extraordinary methodological problems (Bricker, 1978), chief of which pertain to the common absence of adequate control populations against which treatment children can be compared. Most often, effects are defined in terms of changes in the child's skills following intervention, irrespective of possible gains attributable to "maturation" per se. A somewhat more defensible method has been described that relates intervention effects to changes in the child's *rate* of development following intervention (Summers, McGregory, Lesch, & Reed, 1980). The method requires repeated assessment of the child over time following intervention and the assumption that the child's status at entrance into the program was a valid reflection of the prior developmental rate. Given the limitations of the current data, they still do point to the possibility of significant developmental benefits—again, most prominently in the realm of gross motor skills (Edgar et al., 1969; Maloney, Ball, & Edgar, 1970; Moore et al., 1979).

One of the major studies provides follow-up data on 13 Down syndrome children who were then 9 years old (Hayden & Haring, 1976). The total group is depicted as near normal on the Denver Developmental Screening Test at both 1 year and 6 years of age. This is in striking contrast to the usual developmental picture in Down syndrome (see Chap. 3) and is attributed to the influence of the preschool program. At age 9, the subgroup of 13 children is still reported to be functioning at 95 percent of normal; this in contrast to a nonpreschool control group, which was at 61 percent of normal. These developmental percentiles are based on a special scale developed by the researchers, the Down's Syndrome Performance Inventory. What is unclear is the relationship between the Down's Inventory and standard measures of intelligence because the average Stanford-Binet IQ of these children was 52.[8] Thus, though depicted as essentially normal on the Down's Inventory, their measured intelligence is in the retarded range, albeit at a higher level than is typical for this disorder.

A very similar picture of relatively advanced development in Down children is found in a series of 35 who were in a preschool program from ages 6 months to 5 years (Rynders, Spiker, & Horrobin, 1978). Of these, four (11%) had IQs on the Binet beyond the retarded range. Of the remainder, two-thirds tested in the mildly retarded range, with the rest showing at least moderate retardation. We are left with the impression that early intervention can positively affect overall development, though it would appear that the effects of biological abnormality cannot be fully eliminated. Whether both groups of children will continue to maintain these relatively high levels remains to be determined.

Self-Help Skills

See Table 20 for developmental norms from age 2 to 6 in all preschool domains.

EATING

In teaching appropriate eating behaviors, social as well as manual, snacks and mealtimes in the preschool become one of the important "natural" training activities. If only one meal a day is served at the center, sandwiches should be discouraged, and the child should eat at a table in the company of others. The child learns to share in setting and clearing the table and is taught table manners. At least in its early stages, the acquisition of appropriate eating behavior should be publicly recognized (rewarded); grossly inappropriate behavior should not be accepted and, when it occurs, should lead to prompt removal from the table for at least short periods (punished). Children's appetites vary, and they should not be

[8]Reported by Alice Hayden at a meeting of the American Association on Mental Deficiency.

forced to eat, nor should they have to eat everything served, though all foods should be at least tasted before getting dessert. Dessert should not be served with other foods, as its appearance signals the end of the meal except for beverage.

Teaching the Use of the Spoon

Teaching the use of the spoon typically follows finger feeding and, once begun, attempts to finger feed should be discouraged by temporarily halting the meal.[9] Food is withheld until it is accepted on the spoon. To help the child begin to master the spoon, food to be "spooned" is more easily picked up from a bowl than a dish.

Specific steps are now offered in teaching spoon use. Similar instructions will be offered for other self-help skills and in the other curriculum areas. In depicting these teaching procedures in fairly specific terms, they assume a highly mechanistic quality. *This is not the intent.* The training should be conducted in a warm and informal manner, and these procedures should not be regarded as inviolate. They are intended to serve only as guides toward achieving teaching objectives. Teaching methodology should be viewed as a means, not an end!

1. Place the spoon in the child's hand and hold your hand over his. Guide (prompt) the child in filling the spoon and in bringing it to the mouth. At first it is necessary to guide the spoon all the way to the mouth to prevent complete spilling. You will find that the child will at first tend to eat from the side of the spoon. This is a developmental phenomenon related to limited capacity to rotate the wrist. As this motor skill matures, the front of the spoon becomes accessible.
2. With the child accepting the spoon and being rewarded for it both by teacher approval and the food that it brings into the mouth, training consists of gradually reducing spilling. After step 1 has been practiced for several meals, the instructor begins to release the child's hand as it gets close to his mouth. The proper distance is governed by the degree of spillage. Remember that some spillage is to be expected, especially in the younger retarded child. After all, this is a learning process that goes on over many months in the normally developing infant.
3. The instructor begins to require the child to fill the spoon by himself.
4. The instructor discontinues any physical assistance. The child has a spoon and is expected to use it.
5. Once the child can handle a spoon fairly easily, the normal serving plate is substituted for the bowl.

Teaching the Use of the Fork

The child is developmentally ready to learn to use a fork when he is able to eat off the front of a spoon with little spilling. By that time, he will have developed

[9]Unusual prolongation of finger feeding increases the likelihood of pica (see Chap. 10).

TABLE 20   Normal Development 2–5

Age	Gross motor skills	Fine motor skills	Understanding of language	Spoken language
24–36 Months	Runs forward well. Jumps in place, two feet together. Stands on one foot, with aid. Walks on tiptoe. Kicks ball forward.	Strings 4 large beads. Turns pages singly. Snips with scissors. Holds crayon with thumb and fingers, not fist. Uses one hand consistently in most activities. Imitates circular, vertical, horizontal strokes. Paints with some wrist action. Makes dots, lines, circular strokes. Rolls, pounds, squeezes, and pulls clay.	Points to pictures of common objects when they are named. Can identify objects when told their use. Understands questions of what and where. Understands negatives no, not, can't, and don't. Enjoys listening to simple storybooks and requests them again.	Joins vocabulary w together in two phrases. Gives first and las name. Asks what and wh questions. Makes negative sta ments (for exam Can't open it). Shows frustration not being under stood.
36–48 Months	Runs around obstacles. Walks on a line. Balances on one foot for 5 to 10 seconds. Hops on one foot. Pushes, pulls, steers wheeled toys. Rides (that is, steers and pedals) tricycle. Uses slide without assistance. Jumps over 15 cm. (6″) high object, landing on both feet together. Throws ball overhead. Catches ball bounced to him or her.	Builds tower of 9 small blocks. Drives nails and pegs. Copies circle. Imitates cross. Manipulates clay materials (for example, rolls balls, snakes, cookies).	Begins to understand sentences involving time concepts (for example, We are going to the zoo tomorrow). Understands size comparatives such as big and bigger. Understands relationships expressed by if . . . then or because sentences. Carries out a series of 2 to 4 related directions. Understands when told, Let's pretend.	Talks in sentences three or more words, which ta the form agent-action-object (I the ball) or age action-location (Daddy sit on c Tells about past ex ences. Uses "s" on noun indicate plural. Uses "ed" on ver indicate past ter Refers to self usin pronouns I or n Repeats at least on nursery rhyme can sing a song Speech is understa able to stranger but there are sti some sound err
48–60 Months	Walks backward toe-heel. Jumps forward 10 times, without fall-	Cuts on line continuously. Copies cross. Copies square.	Follows three unrelated commands in proper order. Understands compara-	Asks when, how, why questions. Uses models like will, shall, shou

Cognitive Skills	Cognitive Skills	Self-help skills	Social skills
Responds to simple directions (for example: Give me the ball and the block. Get your shoes and socks). Selects and looks at picture books, names pictured objects, and identifies several objects within one picture. Matches and uses associated objects meaningfully (for example, given cup, saucer, and bead, puts cup and saucer together). Stacks rings on peg in order of size. Recognizes self in mirror, saying, baby, or own name.	Can talk briefly about what he or she is doing. Imitates adult actions (for example, housekeeping play). Has limited attention span. Learning is through exploration and adult direction (as in reading of picture stories). Is beginning to understand functional concepts of familiar objects (for example, that a spoon is used for eating) and part/whole concepts (for example, parts of the body).	Uses spoon, spilling little. Gets drink from fountain or faucet unassisted. Opens door by turning handle. Takes off coat. Puts on coat with assistance. Washes and dries hands with assistance.	Plays near other children. Watches other children, joins briefly in their play. Defends own possessions. Begins to play house. Symbolically uses objects, self in play. Participates in simple group activity (for example, sings, claps, dances). Knows gender identity.
Recognizes and matches six colors. Intentionally stacks blocks or rings in order of size. Draws somewhat recognizable picture that is meaningful to child, if not to adult. Names and briefly explains picture. Asks questions for information (why and how questions requiring simple answers). Knows own age. Knows own last name.	Has short attention span. Learns through observing and imitating adults, and by adult instruction and explanation. Is very easily distracted. Has increased understanding of concepts of the functions and groupings of objects (for example, can put doll house furniture in correct rooms) part/whole (for example, can identify pictures of hand and foot as parts of body). Begins to be aware of past and present (for example: Yesterday we went to the park. Today we go to the library).	Pours well from small pitcher. Spreads soft butter with knife. Buttons and unbuttons large buttons. Washes hands unassisted. Blows nose when reminded. Uses toilet independently.	Joins in play with other children. Begins to interact. Shares toys. Takes turns with assistance. Begins dramatic play, acting out whole scenes (for example, traveling, playing house, pretending to be animals).
Plays with words (creates own rhyming words; says or makes up words	Knows own street and town. Has more extended attention span.	Cuts easy foods with a knife (for example, hamburger patty, tomato slice).	Plays and interacts with other children. Dramatic play is closer to reality, with atten-

TABLE 20   Normal Development 2–5 (*Continued*)

Age	Gross motor skills	Fine motor skills	Understanding of language	Spoken language
	ing. Walks up and down stairs alone, alternating feet. Turns somersault.	Prints a few capital letters.	tives like pretty, prettier, and prettiest. Listens to long stories but often misinterprets the facts. Incorporates verbal directions into play activities. Understands sequencing of events when told them (for example, First we have to go to the store, then we can make the cake, and tomorrow we will eat it).	and might. Joins sentences together (for example I like chocolate chi cookies and milk). Talks about causality by using because and so. Tells the content of a story but may confuse facts.

Source: Lynch et al. (1978).

the wrist rotation necessary to the use of a fork. Initial fork use will be limited to picking up food.

Teaching Drinking from a Glass

The same principle of successive approximation applied in teaching spoon use applies to the use of a glass. The instructor initially places the child's hands on the glass and then her hands over them. The child is guided in bringing the glass to the mouth, and assistance is gradually faded as control increases.

Special Feeding Problems

The acquisition of eating skills is seriously complicated in children with motor problems. The infant or young child with cerebral palsy, for example, will be commonly delayed in learning how to suck, swallow, and chew. Sucking can be taught with a straw, while swallowing is aided by gently stroking downward from just below the chin to the chest. *It is difficulty in swallowing that is associated with drooling.* Swallowing is also encouraged by placing food toward the back of the tongue.

Tongue control is itself a problem. It can be strengthened by placing food at either side of the mouth and on the lips and encouraging the child to reach the food with the tongue. Chewing may be delayed and further complicated by poor tooth

Cognitive Skills	Cognitive Skills	Self-help skills	Social skills
having similar sounds). Points to and names 4 to 6 colors. Matches pictures of familiar objects (for example, shoe, sock, foot; apple, orange, banana). Draws a person with 2 to 6 recognizable parts, such as head, arms, legs. Can name or match drawn parts to own body. Draws, names, and describes recognizable picture. Rote counts to 5, imitating adults.	Learns through observing and listening to adults as well as through exploration. Is easily distracted. Has increased understanding of concepts of function, time, part/whole relationships. Function or use of objects may be stated in addition to names of objects. Time concepts are expanding. The child can talk about yesterday or last week (a long time ago), about today, and about what will happen tomorrow.	Laces shoes.	tion paid to detail, time, and space. Plays dress-up. Shows interest in exploring sex differences.

alignment. Start with mashed or strained foods, those requiring little chewing, and gradually increase solid foods. Chewing is also helped by placing one's hand on the child's jaw and moving it up and down while simultaneously making chewing movements of your own that can be seen and imitated.

One of the most important elements in feeding of the motor-impaired child is proper *body positioning*. The child may be unable to sit up and assume the normal eating position. Some do best when propped up or semi-inclined, and others prefer to eat in a doubled over jackknife manner. When beginning to eat solids, some may prefer to keep their jaw down on the table while being fed from below. Finnie (1975), in particular, has described how the motor problems of the cerebral palsied child interfere with normal eating and offers excellent illustrations of appropriate kinds of positioning. She also notes how eating utensils can be altered when the child's disabilities prevent their being held in the usual manner (e.g., modifying handles) (see Fig. 28) (U.S. Department of Health, Education, and Welfare, 1973.)

Banerdt and Bricker (1978) illustrate some of these procedures in a training program for a $2\frac{1}{2}$-year-old spastic, cerebral palsied child who was functioning at the 6-month level. The child was initially unable even to finger-feed himself. He could not bring his hands to midline without assistance, and his only attempts at self-feeding involved a raking motion to pick up small bits of food. Adaptations were made to a high chair to inhibit extension reflexes and to facilitate normal

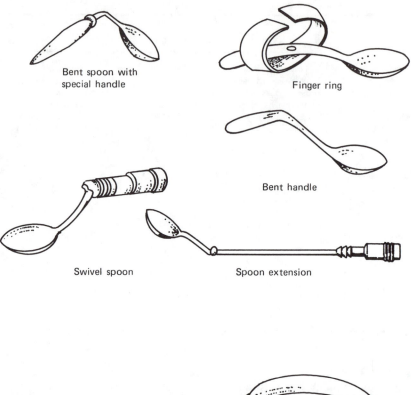

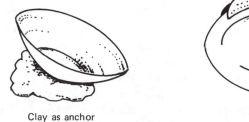

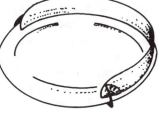

FIG. 28   Adapted utensils and plates.

eating movements. Over a period of 3 months he learned to pick up pieces of food placed at midline and to bring it to his mouth within 10 seconds.

Dressing and Grooming

The acquisition of dressing and grooming skills will be affected by the child's general level of cognitive development and motor coordination. In general, girls learn to dress themselves earlier than boys because of greater wrist flexibility and, at least in early childhood, better fine motor skill (Hurlock, 1964).

In the teaching of dressing and grooming skills, we utilize behavioral principles and the method of backward chaining. Table 18 illustrates backward chaining in the teaching of the putting on of pants. In the next chapter the reader will find additional dressing and grooming programs. Though focused on severely and profoundly retarded youth and adults, the methods employed will also be appropriate to young handicapped children.

Dressing the motor-impaired child may also require the modification of usual procedures. For example, infants with either the spastic or athetoid form of cerebral palsy and who have strong extensor movements might be more easily dressed or undressed while lying across one's knee or on their side. Children who are unable to maintain balance while sitting need support from behind. As with eating, Finnie (1975) provides excellent illustrations of managing dressing problems.

Toileting

Of all the self-help areas, none is so emotion-laden as toilet training. Parents and child-care workers both show this concern, which is likely to be heightened in retardation because of the general delay in self-help skills. The mother of a Down youth, recalling his early years, saw toilet training as an *ordeal*. She felt that it was necessary to be more patient and that she should have waited until he had more understanding of what was expected (Kramm, 1963). This observation deserves comment. She is speaking to the importance of the child coming to understand the connection between elimination and the toilet. In a very real sense, the intent of a systematic approach to toilet training is to speed up the making of that connection, seen most dramatically in a regimen that is reported to achieve training in less than a week (Foxx & Azrin, 1973a). This program was specifically designed for older severely and profoundly retarded persons who, after many years, had failed to achieve bladder and bowel control. Its appropriateness for preschoolers would depend on the readiness of staff to carry out the stringency of its procedures. These are described in Chapter 8.

The Nature of the Task

Gaining control of elimination begins with day training and is only later extended to the night. It is appropriate to start when the child is periodically dry; evidence of sufficient bladder control to exercise some retention of urine. Though urine retention is a signal for undertaking training, bowel and bladder training go on simultaneously. Toileting involves other skills as well—getting to the toilet (mobility), undressing, sitting on the commode for a period of time (typically not more than 10 minutes for preschoolers), and cleaning and dressing oneself.

Teaching "Sitting on the Toilet"

Children vary in their readiness to accept placement on the toilet. Some will cooperate without undue urging or restraint, and others will resist. The latter includes children who are disturbed by anything new or different and/or who have had previous unpleasant experiences around toileting, often reflecting struggles between child and adult. Adults can become very frustrated when children fail to use the toilet and, shortly thereafter, soil themselves. The instructions that follow are directed toward the resistive child but are also appropriate to compliant ones.

Step 1: Encourage the child to sit on the toilet (or potty) without physical restraint or verbal threats. The resisting child should be rewarded as soon as he has sat for only a few seconds. Once seated, it may be necessary to restrain the child if he tries to get up. The child should be released from restraint as soon as struggling ceases but should not be allowed to get off the toilet. The child may fuss, squirm, and cry, but this should be ignored. Eventually the fussing will cease, and, as soon as the child remains seated without restraint, he should be rewarded again. One procedure used with older adults and severely retarded youths was to feed them while on the toilet. If the individual attempted to get up, feeding was temporarily interrupted (Giles & Wolf, 1966).

Step 2: Getting the child to sit quietly on the toilet. Once the child accepts sitting without restraint, the next goal is to remain there without fussing. The child is no longer rewarded only for sitting without restraint; reward is now given only when crying ceases or the degree of upset is much diminished.

Step 3: Getting the child to sit long enough to use the toilet. With the child now sitting quietly on the toilet, our next goal is to extend the time of sitting so as to increase the likelihood that the toilet will actually be used. Our goal for preschoolers is at least 10 minutes, and this can be encouraged, as necessary, by periodic rewards during the interim. The Foxx-Azrin program recommends a 20-minute period, but this would generally be excessive for preschool-age children.

Reward Considerations

The amount and kind of reward to be used are chiefly determined by the frequency with which the reward is offered. When reward intervals are short, small amounts are given to avoid satiation. Appropriate rewards are small bits of preferred food, dried cereal, cookies, candy, and/or sips of juice. When the reward comes at longer intervals, either its amount is increased or its nature is changed. Instead of an edible reinforcer for sitting quietly for several minutes, the child could be offered a preferred activity.

Once the child has accepted sitting quietly on the toilet for at least 10 minutes or until toilet use, rewards are discontinued for only "sitting" and are now reserved for actual use. Foxx and Azrin (1973a) recommend the use of relatively stronger rewards for actual toilet use since this is *the* behavior we are actually trying to teach.

Scheduling Daily Training Times

The mastery of the prior steps is prerequisite to toilet training, and now it can begin. It typically consists of toileting the child at regular intervals and observing the *pattern* of response. Children are generally initially toileted on an hourly basis, and this gradually provides an indication of when it is most likely to be used. In programs with multiple toilets, up to five children can be supervised in hourly toileting by one worker. As toilet use increases, hourly visits are reduced, especially during period when toilet use is rare. "Accidents" are to be expected during the early months of training, but unless there is a persistent pattern of them, they should be dealt with a minimum of fuss. Where they persist, the child may be required to participate in clean-up activities and be denied potential rewards. Both of these responses are intended to be unpleasant consequences and ones that can lead to a rapid reduction of persistent accidents. This phase of training ends when the child is using the toilet on his own and without being rewarded for it. Ultimately, the child comes to prefer the state of being dry and clean; this is the reward. At this point the child is considered "day" trained. Occasional lapses will still occur, and these should be followed by immediate reinstatement of training procedures. Prolonged lapses may be early signs of a urinary or intestinal disorder.

Nighttime Toilet Training

Nighttime training should not commence until day training has been achieved. The latter is usually accomplished well before equivalent nighttime control (Foxx & Azrin, 1973a). In older retarded children nighttime control usually quickly follows day training, but this is less true of the preschooler. Though during the day the toilet is easily accessible, the physiological demands of urine or bowel retention over an entire night may be beyond the child's muscular capacities. This problem is generally solved by awakening the child once or twice during the night.

As with day training, the initial approach is to determine the *timing* of nighttime accidents. They usually occur just after retiring or just before awakening in the morning, and placement on the toilet at these times should be adequate. If there is prolonged failure to achieve urine control, the use of mechanical alerting devices should be considered. They are relatively inexpensive and easy to use. They typically consist of a water-sensitive pad that is placed under the sheet. When urine touches the pad, an alarm sounds and the child awakes. The effect of this procedure is to gradually increase the child's sensitivity to muscular contractions of the bladder while still sleeping. (In Chap. 8 there is a description of the Foxx-Azrin nighttime training regimen.)

Cognitive Skills

DEVELOPMENTAL SEQUENCE

We earlier touched briefly on cognitive development during infancy. This is the so-called sensorimotor period (Piagetian designation)—one in which there is a gradual linking or integration of sensory and motor behaviors, a recognition that objects exists apart from our ability to see them (object permanence), a beginning understanding of causality, and simple but creative problem solving. The last quarter of this period, beginning at about age 18 months, is one of rapid language development. In fact, as noted earlier, it is often the failure of the child to speak at age 2 that indicates to parents that development is abnormal. The postinfancy preschool period incorporates the next two Piagetian developmental stages—preconceptual thought (ages 2–4) and intuitive thought (ages 4–7). Beyond the preschool level in normal children there are two additional periods—concrete operations (ages 7–11) and formal operations (age 11 plus). (All stages were described in Chap. 1.).

These developmental stages are also seen in retarded children, and the extent to which they are present in preschoolers will depend on their degree of retardation. Since the majority of retarded preschoolers are likely to have mental ages of 4 years or less, it can be expected that we will primarily see children who are functioning at the sensorimotor and preconceptual stages.

SPECIFIC OBJECTIVES

The learning content of the preconceptual stage will pertain to understanding and labeling body parts and common objects in the child's environment; acquiring concepts of size, shape, space, weight, texture, color, and number; and academic "readiness" activities. A method of teaching this material now follows.

A Sample Teaching Procedure

The integration of these cognitive objectives is achieved in teaching lessons directed toward learning the names of common objects and then becoming familiar with such attributes as their function, major parts, shape, color, size, smell, and texture. The lesson that follows proceeds from the concrete (actual object) to the representative (e.g., picture of object) and from the whole to parts. The intent here is to offer the teacher a systematic way of approaching educational objectives—one that recognizes the learning difficulties of the child and the need for careful stepwise teaching. Its most general characteristic is a clear identification of the learning objective and a teaching methodology that will minimize error. The method is illustrated in teaching "apple."

Step 1: Recognizing it by name. Teacher holds an apple in front of a child (or several children) and says, "This is an apple, touch apple." (Encourage and reward as necessary.)

Step 2: Distinguishing between apple and nonapple in a two-choice situation. Teacher holds an apple in one hand and a dissimilar object in the other and says, "Touch apple." At this level the child can make an error. If the child shows uncertainty, the teacher will promptly cue the correct response. If the child touches the nonapple, the teachers says, "No, this is the apple. Touch apple." It is undesirable to identify the nonapple, because many alternatives will be used and this will only divert the focus from "apple." *By teaching only one thing at a time, we reduce confusion for the child with learning difficulties* (Roberts, 1976).

Step 3: Discriminating apple from a larger number of nonapples. With an apple and several nonapples presented simultaneously, say "Touch apple."

Step 4: Recognizing a picture of an apple. We move now from the concrete to the representational. In addition to a slight increase in complexity, we also have much more flexibility in teaching about objects. This is particularly true for objects whose size makes them physically unmanageable. Hold up a picture that shows only an apple and say, "This is a *picture* of an apple. Touch apple."

Step 5: Distinguishing between a picture of an apple and pictures of other objects. Hold a picture of an apple in one hand and the picture of a nonapple in the other and say, "Touch apple."

Step 6: Discriminating the picture of an apple from several pictures of other objects. Present several pictures and say, "Find apple."

Step 7: Identifying a major function. Present the child with a picture of an apple and a picture of a nonapple and say, "We eat an apple. Touch the one we eat."

Step 8: Identifying related attributes, such as color and shape. In the course of teaching "apple" there is the opportunity to introduce related cognitive content. Developmentally, at the same time as the child is learning the names of things, he is also learning their functions (e.g., eating an apple), he is beginning to discriminate between simple shapes and colors, and he is developing initial number concepts. It is important to remember, however, that each new element is added only after the prior one has been mastered.

Step 9: Identifying major parts. As appropriate, present the major parts of an object (e.g., the skin of an apple). If the child has been taught that an apple is red, he can now see that it is the skin of the apple that is red.

Step 10: Verbalizing the name of the object and its related attributes. This step represents a very large jump, because here, for the first time, we ask the child to use words to indicate his understanding. While the normally developing child is rapidly expanding his vocabulary at the same time as his understanding grows, there will commonly be a significant lag in the speech development of the retarded child. In a later section, the special language problems of retarded children are described, and methods for developing speech are presented. Here it is necessary only to recognize that the normal difference between what a child understands and what he can express (receptive vs. expressive vocabulary) is commonly much greater in retarded children. Their understanding is likely to far exceed their speech. Thus cognitive training should not be equated with speech acquisition per se. While attempting to elicit language, cognitive training can use *any* expressive modality available to the child—for example, pointing.

Returning to our example, the teacher variously says, "What is this? What do we do with this? What color is this? What shape is this?", and so forth.

Summary

The ten steps are now listed for easy reference.

Step 1. Object being taught is labeled by teacher.

Step 2. Discriminating actual object in two-choice situation.

Step 3. Discriminating actual object among a group.
Step 4. Recognizing picture of the object.
Step 5. Discriminating picture of object in two-picture choice situation.
Step 6. Discriminating picture of object among pictures of other objects.
Step 7. Recognizing major functions.
Step 8. Recognizing major attributes.
Step 9. Recognizing major parts.
Step 10. Verbalizing name and related content.

Language Skills

DEVELOPMENTAL SEQUENCE

It is during the latter half of the second year that speech, in its usual sense, really begins to emerge. Such preverbal communication forms as gestures are beginning to be accompanied and then replaced by words. "Baby talk" is disappearing; words are used to convey labels ("naming"), negatives, and questions are frequently strung together in two-word combinations.

Interestingly, one of the oldest but still useful measures of the level of speech development is the average length of the child's utterances (mean length of utterance—MLU). Steady growth in length is found between 24 and 42 months. The average at 24 months is about 1.5 words and then expands to an average of about four words at 42 months. Thereafter the rate of growth is much slower, increasing only to about 4.5 words per utterance at 60 months (Belugi, 1972; McCarthy, 1930).

During the third year, pronouns are first used though not always correctly. Speech is commonly employed as an "accompaniment" to action and for play itself, but it is also increasingly used for purposes of communication. As the normal child reaches age 3, we see increasing integration of speech and action, longer utterances, and use of plurals and past tense. By this age the mechanics of speech are largely in place, though traces of infantile pronunciations will persist and can be heard in children up to school age. In comparison to the 3-year-old, the child at 4 is a chatterbox. He talks about everything, plays with words, questions continuously, stretches simple answers into lengthy narratives, and comments on his own behavior as well as that of others. The language of the 4-year-old is often rambling. An answer to a question may lead to a "flight of ideas" that are tied to each other only by associations, not by the question itself. At 5, this free-flowing quality is gradually replaced by a greater control and appropriateness (Gesell et al., 1940).

SPEECH TRAINING

Of the various preschool educational domains, none has received greater attention than language. Language development is delayed in retardation (Miller & Yoder, 1974; Yoder & Miller, 1972), but it is assumed that the differences between retarded and nonretarded children are essentially quantitative—of degree rather than kind. It is this assumption that underlies virtually all speech training strategies with this population.

Speech and Mental Development

The central premise of language scholars is that speech is tied to cognition; the child's language at any moment in time being viewed as the outcome of interaction between *experience* and *level of cognitive development* (Kahn, 1979; Miller & Yoder, 1974). More specifically, "comprehension," a cognitive function, precedes and "paces" speech production (Horton, 1974). It is this inextricable tie between language and cognition that affects remedial efforts.

Speech and Social Development

Together with its cognitive component, speech is seen as a "social" act whose purpose is to achieve communication with others (Mahoney, 1980; Vigotsky, 1962). In normal development speech appears only after a relatively sophisticated nonverbal communication system has been established. These prespeech modes include crying, eye contact, facial expression, babbling, and gestures. In this sense, speech represents a refinement of earlier means of communication (Mahoney, 1980). Even speech development itself reflects this principle. The change in speech complexity between the single-word utterances at 18 months and the two-word utterances of the 2-year-old are really more changes in *form* than in *substance* (Miller & Yoder, 1974). "Mommy" as a one-word utterance may mean "I want Mommy," which at the 2-year level is expressed as "want Mommy." The meaning has not changed; it is only that the speaker is learning how to communicate with greater precision.

Both the cognitive and social aspects of language have relevance for profoundly retarded children. It is this population that is least developed cognitively and socially. Their attainment of speech will ultimately depend on both the acquisition of a level of mental development comparable to that of the 18-month-old child (Kahn, 1979) and a desire to communicate. The latter requires the creation of social dependencies in the child which will provide a motive for communication. This is seen most clearly in autistic children. Their total speaking vocabulary may be limited to just a few words, but each of them carries much significance for the child in the communication of wants—"cookie," "ice cream," "no!"

LANGUAGE TRAINING MODELS

Two types of language training models can be distinguished—developmental and remedial. The developmental model takes the course of language development in the normal child as its rationale, the language of the retarded child being regarded as merely reflecting a slowing of this process (Miller & Yoder, 1974). Others have challenged the normal developmental sequence as the basis for language remediation (Gray & Ryan, 1973; Guess, Sailor, & Baer, 1974, 1976). In their view there are not yet sufficient empirical data to enable us to know whether a particular set of language behaviors is prerequisite to the learning of others. As a consequence, they introduce some elements earlier than would be expected, for example, teaching the asking of questions. This approach also appears to place less stress on comprehension as a prerequisite to language. It is also an approach that seems to have been designed primarily for the older nonverbal retarded person rather than for the child (Guess et al., 1974). In a review of this and other issues in language training, Ruder and Smith (1974) conclude that there are sufficient observational data on the sequence of language development (Bloom, 1970; Brown, 1973) to justify the use of the developmental model.

ASSESSMENT

Language assessment involves establishing where the child is cognitively, speechwise, and socially. At the cognitive level our interest is in the child's understanding of what is heard. Our everyday interactions provide this information, as do more formal assessment procedures such as the Peabody Picture Vocabulary Test (Dunn, 1959). At the speech level, we have the child's spontaneous utterances and/or speech elicited specifically for remedial analysis (e.g., Lee & Canter, 1971). At the social level, our focus is on the degree to which there is interest in others, eye contact with them, and some responsiveness to verbal requests.

TRAINING CONTENT, SEQUENCE, AND FORMAT

A number of speech programs have been developed that can serve as models for workers with young handicapped children. For the child who has no speech at all, the language acquisition programs of Kent (1972), Bricker (1972), and Guess, Sailor, and Baer (1976) are appropriate. The latter two also seek to move the child beyond the one-word utterance level. For children who are already using single-word or single-sound utterances, the training programs of MacDonald et al. (1974) and Miller and Yoder (1974) should be considered.

Content and Sequence

The verbal content of one of the beginning programs (Guess et al., 1976) consists of six categories of words: words for persons and things, words for actions with persons and things, and words for possession, color, size, and location. Initial studies indicate that words that depict actions are the most readily learned and that those that convey possession are much more difficult to master.

Since comprehension precedes verbalization, words to be trained should be understood and should occur frequently in the child's experience (Miller & Yoder, 1974). They should also, as noted earlier, be words whose expression "makes a difference" (Guess et al., 1976). In keeping with the normal developmental sequence, initial language training will be in the form of single-word utterances.

Language training also involves the expansion of single-word utterances into longer and longer chains. For example, teaching the child to express the idea that daddy is hitting a ball might consist of a sequence of first "Daddy," then "hit ball," and then "Daddy hit ball." Though all of the training programs to which we have referred are intended to carry through to multiword utterances (phrases or sentences), that of MacDonald et al. (1974) appears to offer a particularly promising way of expanding single-word utterances. Working with Down syndrome children, though admittedly with a small sample, and using parents as well as professionals as trainers, they were able over a period of several weeks to increase the frequency of spontaneous two-word utterances from a pretraining rate of 15 percent to a posttraining rate of 50 percent. They chose to focus on word combinations expressing action/agent (e.g., throw ball) and object or action/location (e.g., ball chair) relationships. These are two of the earliest developing types of word combinations (Brown, 1973).

Format

A typical model of systematic speech instruction for retarded children is shown in Tables 21–23. It has three components, which are presented in a single 45-minute period: *imitation, conversation,* and *play,* each for 15 minutes. The method essentially involves the pairing of a specific object or event with its speech

TABLE 21   Training Model for Imitation

Speech stimulus	Correctness of child's response	Instructor's reaction	Examples
This consists of a pair of nonlanguage and language cues designed to elicit verbal imitation of a particular utterance length	Correct (complete repetition of language cue)	Acknowledgment of correct response and repetition of language cue as feedback model	"Good. Say, 'throw ball.' "
		Social praise	"Good talking."
		Token	Plastic chip leading to tangible reward
Nonlanguage cue: throwing a ball in the air		Proceed to next word	
Language cue: Say, "Throw ball" (the form of the utterance is also appropriate to the child's developmental stage)	Partially correct (closer to correct than any previous response)	Repetition of language cues	"Throw ball."
		Social praise	"Good try."
		Token	Token
	Incorrect (shorter utterance length than in cue or response unrelated to cue)	Pause: no attention for 3 seconds	—
		Repetition of nonlanguage and language cues	Trainer says, "Say, 'throw ball,' " as he throws ball in the air

Source: MacDonald et al. (1974).

TABLE 22   Training Model for Conversation

Speech stimulus	Correctness of child's response	Instructor's reaction	Examples
Designed to elicit conversationlike response reflecting a particular grammatical rule	Correct (response reflects the action/ object rule)	Acknowledgement of correct response and repetition of it for modeling purposes	"Good! Say, 'throw ball.' "
		Social praise	"Good talking."
The language cue is either a question or a command		Token	Token
		Proceed to next words	
Nonlanguage cue: throwing a ball into the air	Partially correct (closer than previous attempt or correct in either utterance length or rule)	Imitative cue	"Say, 'throw ball.' "
		Social praise	"Good try."
Language cue: "What am I doing?"		Token	Token
		Repetition of conversation stimulus set once	"What am I doing?" as ball is thrown into air
	Incorrect (briefer than utterance length being trained and not using grammatical rule)	Pause for 3 seconds with no attention given	Pause
		Imitation cue	"Say, 'throw ball.' "
		Repetition of conversational stimulus set once	"What am I doing?" as ball is thrown in air
	No response (no verbal response within 5 seconds)	Pause for 3 seconds with no attention given	Pause
		Imitation cue	"Say, 'throw ball.' "
		Repetition of conversational stimulus set	"What am I doing?" as ball is thrown in air

Source: MacDonald et al. (1974).

equivalent and eliciting speech through the three modalities of imitation, conversation, and play.

The first modality, imitation, is central to all initial teaching in these language programs. For the nonverbal child, the first words and even lengthier utterances are taught through imitating the adult model. Imitation requires the gaining of the child's attention and the reinforcement of verbal utterances that gradually approximate those of the model. Some workers suggest that imitation of motor behavior (e.g., pointing or sitting) should precede attempts to achieve vocal imitation. Gross body movements are easier to demonstrate and to prompt and guide than vocalizations (Brocker & Bricker, 1970). It is not clear, however, that such motor imitation actually speeds the onset of vocal imitation. On the other hand, it certainly should be considered if initial efforts to elicit verbal imitation are unsuccessful. The basic model of imitation training involves first teaching the prerequisite "attending" behaviors—sitting still and looking at the teacher—and then eliciting motor and/or verbal responses that increasingly mirror those of the model.

With reference to all three of the teaching modalities, *instructions should be stated in language that is generally just one word beyond the child's stage of utterance* (Miller & Yoder, 1974). In other words, adult speech should be expressed at the child's level. This speech model also illustrates the use of two behavior modification contingencies. Correct responses are rewarded with praise, and incorrect ones are ignored.

Apart from such reinforcers as praise and tokens, the technique called "reciprocal change" seems useful as a motivator (Murray, 1972; Ruder & Smith, 1974). Here access to a desired object(s) depends on the correctness of the verbalization. There is an immediate and meaningful consequence which is directly tied to speech. The method is probably best employed to encourage relatively small changes in children who already have speech but who use the correct verbalization only sporadically. It should not be used to taunt children.

COMMON PROBLEMS

Problems of speech clarity due to poor articulation are common in retarded children. Attention has earlier been called to the speech of children with Down

TABLE 23   Training Model for Structured Play

Speech stimulus	Correctness of child's response	Instructor's reaction	Examples
Designed to incorporate words being trained in play For example, father might hold ball and pretend to throw it while asking child, "What do you want me to do?" Designed to help "expand" correct response	Correct (as in conversation)	Compliance with child's request	Throw ball
		Repetition of response and expansion if appropriate	Say, "Daddy throw ball."
	Partially correct (as in conversation)[a]	Social praise	"Good try."
		Expansion to correct response	Say, "Daddy throw ball."
		Compliance with child's verbal request	Throw ball
	Incorrect (as in conversation)[a]	No compliance with child	Do not throw ball
		Pause, followed by modeling of correct response	After pause, say, "Daddy throw ball."

Source: MacDonald et al. (1974).
[a]See Table 22.

syndrome and with cerebral palsy. Pronunciation problems are also found in the speech of normally developing children, and it is not until after age 3 that rapid improvement in intelligibility occurs (McCarthy, 1954).

Apart from the absence of speech itself in children with severe and profound degrees of retardation, there may be little use of newly learned words in non-speech-training settings (Guess et al., 1976). This is why it is important for parents to try to provide conditions that are intended to elicit such words. The MacDonald et al. (1974) program is one of many that specifically seek to encourage transfer of learning (generalization) by involvement of parents.

THE CEREBRAL PALSIED CHILD

Except for hearing-impaired children or those with profound retardation, the most serious speech problems are seen in cerebral palsy. The difficulties here result from neurological interference with the organs that enable us to produce sounds—lips, tongue, and larynx. The nature of these difficulties and remedial procedures are described by Finnie (1975). The child with either the spastic or ataxic form of cerebral palsy will be slow in producing a sound, and the athetoid child will show extremes of pitch and loudness as well as grimacing. Speech training consists of various activities intended to strengthen control of tongue and lips, encourage articulation, build sentences, and reduce drooling. Drooling is common, because the child tends to keep his mouth open and has difficulty in swallowing.

AUXILIARY COMMUNICATION MODES

While a primary goal in language training is the development of speech, this is not always achieved. Persistent teacher pressure for intelligible language may prove very frustrating and weaken the desire to communicate. It is for these motor-impaired children as well as for either those with uncorrected cleft palates or those who have simply not responded to speech stimulation that auxiliary communication modes are increasingly in vogue (Nietupski & Hamre-Nietupski, 1979). Interestingly, these *nonspeech* communication modes are not only used as substitutes for speech but can also be employed in conjunction with or to augment speech training itself. Fears that the teaching of nonspeech modalities might inhibit speech development, an old concern in the education of deaf children, appear unwarranted. To the contrary, they may actually increase or improve vocalizations (Grinnel, Detamore, & Lippki, 1976; Vanderheiden, 1975).

There are three types of nonspeech methods—*manual, communication aids,* and *communication codes.* Manual forms for retarded children commonly involve the use of generally understood gestures. Communication aids ("communication boards") are display devices that may consist of objects, pictures of objects or actions, symbols, and even printed words. These boards permit the child to circumvent speech by pointing to what he wishes to convey. Boards are usually homemade, though there are two commercial versions—Blissymbolics (Bliss, 1965) and the Non-Speech Language Initiation Program (Non-SLIP) (Carrier, 1976; Carrier & Peak, 1975). Bliss symbols represent objects, relationships, feelings, and ideas, and they tend to be abstract rather than direct representations of what they symbolize. Four of the symbols are shown as well as how they are used to complement each other, the symbol for "school" being made up of three other symbols.

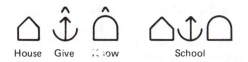

House   Give   Know   School

Non-SLIP is based on animal language training (Premack, 1971) and consists of masonite symbols of various geometric shapes and colors. They are used to teach how words are sequenced in a grammatical communication. Non-SLIP is intended to provide a strategy for acquiring language rather than offering a set of functional communication responses as such (Nietupski & Hamre-Nietupski, 1979). Figure 29 shows the most common kind of communication board. It provides a realistic pictorial representation of the elements to be expressed. Communication codes involve simple actions, which essentially serve as yes/no answers to questions. They might be only an eye blink or a foot tap.

Choosing Appropriate Auxiliary Modes

Guidelines for the selection of the appropriate modes are offered by Nietupski and Hamre-Nietupski (1979). The *manual* modes should be considered

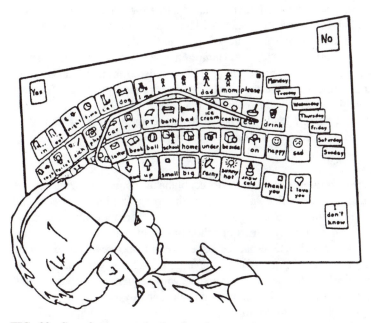

FIG. 29 Sample communication board.

where there are no motor impediments, the child is able to attend to and imitate others' actions (e.g., see Topper, 1975), and workers are willing to learn the system. A comprehensive list of "signs" used in manual training is found in Fristoe and Lloyd (1979), though many would be beyond the comprehension of preschool-age retarded children. *Communication boards* are appropriate where there are motor impairments, where the child tends to be inattentive to the actions of others, and where workers are less ready to learn a manual system (e.g. see Vanderheiden, 1975). Communication boards are particularly useful with nonambulatory children, but ambulatory ones can carry their board with them or use such a variant as a picture card apron. Anderson (1980) has called attention to the need for determining both the child's visual functioning and range of arm movement in the placement of visual materials on the boards. *Communication codes* are clearly the least functional and should only be used when motor limitations prevent all but the simplest of movements.

Choosing the Initial Vocabulary

Apart from the issue of utility, one will try to initially teach signs, gestures, and symbols that are different from each other and that also resemble their referent. In one program using the Bliss symbols, the first taught were yes/no, hello/goodbye, more, teacher, toilet, want, eat, and drink. All of these were already a part of the child's receptive vocabulary and were related to daily experiences (Vanderheiden et al., 1975).

Teaching Procedures

Physical assistance, imitation, and prompting are the main methods of teaching these nonverbal communication modes. The sign or symbol is shown, the worker models the sign or points to the symbol, and the child is encouraged to imitate the worker's action (Nietupski & Hamre-Nietupski, 1979; Vanderheiden et al., 1975). Specific procedures for teaching signs are also offered by Guess et al. (1976) as an added feature of their general language training program. Teachers will want to combine speech with nonverbal modes as a means of facilitating speech itself (Kopchick & Lloyd, 1976) and to encourage the use of nonverbal modes in the home as well as in the school.

ECHOLALIA

In Chapter 2, reference was made to echolalia in connection with speech problems in autistic children. Echolalia refers to the rote parroting of speech, and it is also observed in children variously labeled as retarded, emotionally disturbed, and brain-injured. There are two forms of echolalia—immediate and delayed. Immediate echolalia occurs when a verbal request evokes a response that is expressed in the same form as the request—for example, Q: "What's your name?" A: "What's your name?" In the delayed variant, a word sequence is produced that reflects something heard earlier but that has no relevance to ongoing activities.

Interestingly, echolalialike vocalization is heard in the prespeech behavior of normal infants of about 9–10 months of age. It consists of the apparent imitation of sounds. Though soon followed by the initiation of first words, some echolalia may persist in normal children, though not beyond $2\frac{1}{2}$ years (Rutter & Box, 1972).

Causes of Echolalia

All workers stress that an echolalic response indicates that the child does not understand the meaning of what is echoed (Garber & David, 1975). It is most likely to occur around questions that seek information from the child ("What is your name?") and is less frequent around requests that have immediate behavioral consequences ("Do you want a cookie?") (Matheney, 1968). The latter type of request is also more concrete, since it refers to something the child can know through the senses—hearing, touch and vision.

Treatment of Echolalia

Given the association between echolalia and lack of comprehension, the most obvious strategy is to simplify the verbal request. Apart from this "cognitive" approach, behavior modification procedures have been commonly employed. They involve the attempt to capitalize on the echoic response by facilitating the echoing of the *correct* one (Ausman & Gaddy, 1974; Freeman, Ritvo, & Miller, 1975; Garber & David, 1975; Risley & Wolf, 1967; Palyo et al., 1979). The limitation of this procedure is that its effects are specific to the situation in which it is used (in fact, this is the basic rationale of behavior modification) and generalization to other settings will require comparable programming (Cooke, Cooke, & Apolloni, 1976; Garcia & DeHaven, 1974; Palyo et al., 1979). Although the cognitive approach may be the most effective in the long run (Garber & David, 1975), a combination of it and behavior modification might produce at least some immediate reduction in its frequency. The behavioral method is illustrated in Figure 30; as presented here it involves an instructor and an aide as well as the child.

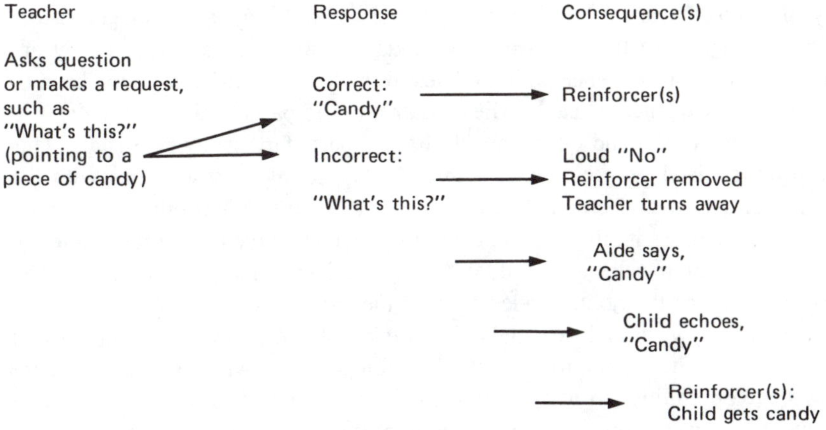

Teacher	Response	Consequence(s)
Asks question or makes a request, such as "What's this?" (pointing to a piece of candy)	Correct: "Candy" ⟶	Reinforcer(s)
	Incorrect: "What's this?" ⟶	Loud "No" Reinforcer removed Teacher turns away
	⟶	Aide says, "Candy"
	⟶	Child echoes, "Candy"
	⟶	Reinforcer(s): Child gets candy

FIG. 30   A method for the direct reduction of echolalia. Modified from Palyo et al. (1979).

The teacher will want to begin with questions that can be simply put, refer to something visible, and provide an immediate and natural consequence.

Motor Function

Disorders of motor development are prominent in retarded children, especially those with some organic brain impairment. These disorders consist of abnormalities of movement, posture, and balance.

NORMAL MOTOR DEVELOPMENT

The first year of life is characterized by a growing control by the infant of the movement of its body. One can think of this process as a gradual *liberation* from the influence of involuntary movements and postures caused by so-called "primitive" reflexes (Bobath, 1971). As the child learns to inhibit these reflexes or as they actually disappear, the body comes increasingly under its own control. Another important development in the first year is the appearance of so-called "automatic" or protective reflexes. These are "righting" responses, which enable the infant to maintain normal body positions and balance. It is this process of liberation from involuntary to voluntary control that permits the child to physically explore its environment. It also allows the practice of increasingly fine reaching and grasping activities and lays the groundwork for such self-help skills as beginning feeding (Gorga, 1976).

THE SPECIFICS OF MOTOR DEVELOPMENT

Motor control begins with the head and eyes and gradually extends downward and outward to the rest of the body (Johnston, 1976). By age 3 months, the head can be held erect, and the eyes can follow an arc of 180 degrees. At 6 months, control has extended to the upper trunk and arms, and the child is beginning to sit, reach, and creep. At 9 months, the lower trunk has come under control, and the child can now crawl and pull to standing. Finally, the end of the first year finds control extended to the legs, and walking begins. This head-to-foot developmental pattern (so-called cephalocaudal progression) is paralleled by another developmental sequence which relates to the outward or lateral dimension of the body. This sequence reveals earliest control of the parts of the body closest to the midline (proximal) and later control of those parts farthest away (distal). This is the proximodistal progression principle. Thus, lateral control begins with the shoulder and elbow and gradually extends to the fingers. Within the hand, however, control begins with the little and ring fingers (called the *ulnar* grasp pattern), proceeds to the mid palm and middle finger (producing the *palmar* grasp), and finally includes the thumb and index finger—the *radial* or *pincer* grasp.

Ambulatorywise, at 1 year the child is taking his first awkward and hesitant steps, but by $2\frac{1}{2}$ he will walk in adult fashion and run with assurance. There rapidly develop abilities to walk stairs—first placing both feet down at the same time and then progressing to alternate-foot placement—then to jump, hop, and balance on one foot. By 4, there is beginning ability to throw and catch a ball and to broad-jump. By kindergarten age, the child has added such skills as skipping with alternate feet and beginning roller skating and bicycling (Johnston, 1976; Vulpé, 1977).

In the use of hands, the 1-year-old can pick up and release objects easily and, during the next year, acquires the kind of hand-eye coordination that enables the building of towers of up to 10 blocks. In the first year, one also sees progress in the grasping of objects—from a crude, raking movement to a fine, pincer movement. In the years that follow, refinement in grasp will be reflected in the holding of writing implements—from a total hand grasp and only arm control to a gradual involvement of the fingers and ending with the prominence of the thumb and index and/or forefinger (Johnston, 1976).

ABNORMAL MOTOR DEVELOPMENT

Motor activity has been described in terms of three major dimensions— elements, functions, and skills (see Table 24). The *elements* are the basic building blocks for all motor activity: tone, control, and strength. They permit the execution of basic functions which are then combined into various motor skills. It is abnormality in these three elements that underlies the motor problems seen in retardation.

Tone

Tone refers to the degree of tension or contraction of a muscle. It is important in the maintenance of any given position; it is change in tone that permits movement. Our two types of body muscle, flexors and extensors, perform their functions by increasing in tone (contracting), though any given movement reflects their reciprocal relationship—the contraction of one muscle and the simultaneous relaxation of its antagonist. Thus the bending or flexing of the elbow requires an increase of tone in the elbow flexor muscle and a corresponding relaxation or reduction of tone in the muscle used for elbow extension.

Control

Although movement depends on muscle activity, the quality and direction of that activity are governed by the brain. The initiation of any voluntary movement begins with the brain and results from the transmission of that intention via the nervous system to the muscles. The area of the brain that controls voluntary movement is a part of its uppermost layer, the cortex. Lower brain centers (the cerebel-

TABLE 24   Basic Aspects of Motor Activity

Elements	Functions	Skills
Tone	Postural stability	Sitting
Control	Movement	Walking
Strength	Coordination	Running
	Balance	Reaching
		Manipulating

Source: Johnston (1976).

lum, basal ganglia, and vestibular apparatus) are involuntary or unconscious contributors to motor activity. When the upper brain initiates a movement, the signal passing through the lower centers causes them to refine the movement—to give it the proper degree of smoothness, precision, and fluidity. The lower brain centers are also responsible for the unconscious aspect of postural control. When we suddenly lose our balance, the automatic movements we make to regain it originate there. At birth, muscle and movement control lie primarily in the lower brain centers, and this is why that behavior is largely involuntary or reflexive in nature. It is as the upper brain matures that motor control shifts to the cortex and thus becomes more controlled and voluntary.

Strength

Strength refers to the amount of force a muscle exerts to maintain a given posture (e.g., force against gravity, which enables one to remain standing) or to produce movement. Contrary to popular belief, muscle size is only a relatively minor determinant of muscle strength. *Coordination* of muscle activities is the more important, and it is impairment in coordination due to brain injury that can cause muscle weakness.

DISORDERS OF RATE AND/OR PATTERN

Motor disorders are manifest in either the rate of motor development or in deviant motor patterns.

Rate

Children may show the normal sequence of motor development but progress at a very slow rate. In some, the motor delay is often simply another manifestation of an overall developmental lag. In others, early lag is eventually made up, and motor development is normal.

Deviant Movement Patterns

Abnormalities in movement patterns are caused by deficits in any of the three motor elements. For example, the rigidity or spasticity of the child with cerebral palsy is due to an abnormally heightened muscle tone.

DISORDERS OF TONE, MOVEMENT, BALANCE, AND STRENGTH

Tone

Both increase (hypertonicity) and decrease (hypotonicity) of muscle tone are seen. As just noted, the rigidity in the spastic form of cerebral palsy is an example of hypertonicity. Two types of rigidity are found—"clasp knife" and "lead pipe." In the former, like a jackknife, there is an initial resistance to opening; this is then followed by a sudden cessation of resistance and a springing open. In "lead pipe" rigidity, however, the limb resists movement throughout its total range. Too little muscle tone results from muscles that are so flaccid that they are unable to maintain tension or resistance to stretch. The effect is a floppy "rag doll" quality. Coordination is also poor; there is little movement, and there is a lack of postural stability.

Movement

One of the effects of injury to the motor cortex is to diminish its control of movements generated by the lower brain centers. In the case of the basal ganglia, for example, the loss of cortical control of its activity results in the release of involuntary movements. These take two forms—*choreiform* (rapid, jerky movements) and *tremors* (fine quivering of arms, fingers, and legs).

Balance

Problems of balance are associated with damage to the cerebellum or to its pathways. Balance disorder is one of the main symptoms of cerebral palsy; it is found in children with choreiform movements and occurs as the main symptom of the ataxic form.

Strength

For the most part, muscle strength itself is not a major contributor to the motor problems seen in retardation. Injury to the brain leads to a lack of muscle control rather than to specific muscle weakness. Where there is spinal cord injury, however, specific muscle weaknesses are found (Harryman, 1976).

ROLE OF PRIMITIVE (TONIC) AND AUTOMATIC (RIGHTING) REFLEXES IN MOTOR DISORDERS

We earlier noted that normal motor development depends on the gradual waning of the influence of neonatal "primitive" reflexes and the simultaneous acquisition of "automatic" or protective ones. The primitive reflexes tend to cause the infant to lie in a position of flexion when on its stomach (prone position) and in one of extension when on its back (supine). The automatic ones provide for the kind of adjustments for balance and equilibrium that are necessary to the maintenance of erect postures. The influence of these reflexes on motor development is related to whether or not there is specific brain injury. In the child with delayed motor development but no apparent brain injury (grossly normal physically), the lag in motor development is attributed to a slowness in the appearance of the automatic (postural) reflexes, the primitives ones losing their influence at the proper time, by about age 6 months (Molnar, 1974; Paine, 1964). Contrariwise, delays in motor development that involve brain injury, as in cerebral palsy, result in *both* the persistence of the primitive reflexes and delay in the attainment of the automatic ones (Bobath, 1971; Paine, 1964).

The interfering effect of prolonged persistence of the primitive reflexes is seen, for example, in difficulty in holding the head erect in the prone position. By age 1 month, the normal infant, on its stomach, is able to lift its head. But if one of the primitive reflexes is too powerful, its tendency is to force the infant into a flexion position and to counter attempts to raise the head. (For a description of how primitive and automatic reflexes affect motor development see Johnston, 1976).

TREATMENT: PHYSICAL THERAPY

Treatment procedures focus on the brain-injured child. For the non-brain-injured ones, a motor delay will be dealt with by a program of general motor stimulation. It is the brain-injured child in whom one finds special motor problems.

Status of Postural Reflexes

When the child not only is dominated by primitive reflexes but has not yet developed *any* postural ones, treatment involves *inhibition* techniques. These are intended to reduce heightened muscle tone and thus to ease management. On the other hand, if at least some automatic postural reflexes are present, treatment is designed to strengthen them while also inhibiting the primitive ones. The sequence of treatment is such that it should begin with activities that inhibit the tonic (primitive) reflexes and should gradually follow with the facilitation of the postural ones.

Inhibiting Primitive Reflexes

The two reflexes that are most often modified by inhibition are the *asymmetric tonic neck* and the *tonic labyrinthine* reflexes (see Fig. 31). In the asymmetric tonic reflex, turning of the child's head to either side results in the extension of the arm on that side and flexion of the other arm. This produces the commonly seen "fencing" position. This reflex can interfere with self-feeding training, because if the child turns its head to look at the hand that is holding its food, the hand moves away (extends) rather than moving toward the mouth (flexes). This reflex is less strong when either the head is flexed or the child is in prone. It also has no effect when the head is in the midline and only slightly if in a side-lying position. The tonic labyrinthine reflex causes the child to assume an extensor posture on its back (head arched back) and a flexion posture on its stomach. In either position the reflex interferes with attempts to raise the head. In the normally developing infant, this reflex usually loses its influence between 1 and 3 months, thus permitting the lifting of the head from prone at 1 month and from supine at 2–3 months (Johnston, 1976). Its effect in the supine position can be lessened by flexing the head (thereby relaxing or inhibiting the extensors). It is also eased by placing the child in a side-lying position or, if being held or otherwise supported, in a position of flexion.

Facilitating Automatic Reflexes

Where automatic responses are present to some degree, they can be facilitated through proper handling techniques (Harryman, 1976). The procedures employed reflect application of the behavior principle of "successive approximation." The several types of automatic reflexes are shown in Figure 32. *Head-righting reactions* (keeping head erect without support) can be strengthened

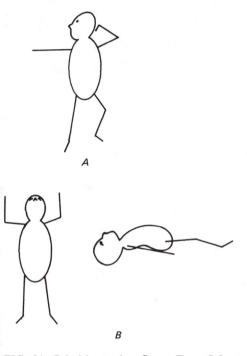

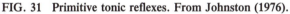

FIG. 31 Primitive tonic reflexes. From Johnston (1976).

by freeing the head from external support while simultaneously providing support at the shoulder girdle. When head-righting reactions are well developed, *equilibrium reactions* of the trunk in the sitting position are fostered by providing support at the next lower level, below the shoulder girdle. As the level of external support moves down the trunk, the child is required to use more and more equilibrium responses to maintain an erect position. Similarly, equilibrium reactions are facilitated when in sitting, crawling, or standing by either gently and slowly tilting the child or by slowly moving the support on which the child rests (e.g., a tilt board). In contrast, sudden changes in the child's position will encourage *protective reflex* extension of the arms. As the automatic responses mature, the amount of inhibition of primitive reflexes necessary to permit these positions is gradually reduced.

Using These Procedures in the Home

Techniques of inhibition and facilitation should be a part of the home management program. This will involve instruction of the parents in carrying, lifting, holding, bathing, dressing, feeding, and positioning (see Finnie, 1975).

Assistive Devices

Physical therapy may not eliminate all motor problems, and aids are then employed to help the child function as independently as possible. If the child is unable to achieve independent sitting, a special chair can provide external support

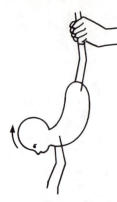

Head righting reflex. There is an attempt to maintain the head
in such a position that the face is vertical and the mouth is
horizontal to the ground.

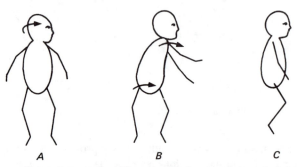

Derotative reaction. When the head and neck are rotated (A) there
is a segmental sequence of movements from the shoulder, trunk, and
legs (B) to "derotate" the body and maintain normal alignment (C).

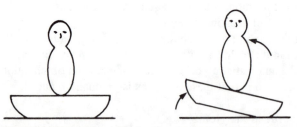

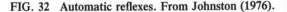

Equilibrium responses in sitting. In response to tilt, the body
will adjust to maintain its upright position.

FIG. 32   Automatic reflexes. From Johnston (1976).

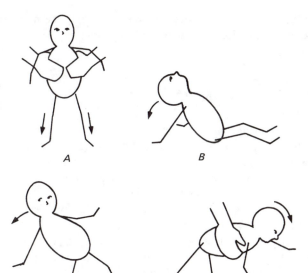

Protective reflexes. These are a series of responses to changes in
body position. *A*, downward; *B*, posterior; *C*, lateral; *D*, forward.

FIG. 32   Automatic reflexes. From Johnston (1976). *(Continued)*

while freeing the hands for manipulative activities. The child who is unable to
learn to walk freely can use several types of assistive devices—short leg braces for
a more stable base of support, canes for balance, and wheelchairs.

TREATMENT: OCCUPATIONAL THERAPY

The focus of occupational therapy is to help the child acquire basic self-care
skills by circumventing the motor problems. In infancy, attention is particularly
directed to feeding skills. Use is made of special assistive devices and the modification of standard objects (e.g., utensils and cups) to enable the child to learn self-
feeding. These were illustrated in Figure 28 in the earlier section on the self-help
curriculum. That section also included a description of special procedures for
improving, swallowing, tongue control, and chewing.

In addition to the use of adapted utensils, comparable modifications can be
made in clothing. Examples of adapted clothing are elastic waistbands, enlarged
neck openings, and loose-fitting garments (Gorga, 1976).

Social-Emotional Development

We now concern ourselves with the retarded child as a "social" being. This
refers to the nature of the child's relationship to others, the management of feelings, and the acquisition of appropriate social behaviors. Preschool programs are

especially important to the socialization of retarded children, especially the more severely impaired, because the child's handicap may seriously limit exposure to nonfamily adults and children.

SOCIAL DEVELOPMENT IN INFANCY AND EARLY CHILDHOOD

The social nature of the human animal is evident even in early infancy. Expressions of pleasure in the form of kicking, smiling, and waving of arms are seen when others are present (Hurlock, 1964). By six months, the infant can distinguish between familiar and strange faces and shows different emotional reactions to each. There is smiling to the familiar and fear to the strange.

During the first year, the infant's predominant relationships are with caretakers. It is they, after all, who meet all of the child's biological needs and who provide various experiences of pleasure. It is out of this relationship that dependency on others for need fulfillment develops. This relationship also serves as the basis for all future needs of winning the approval of others.

During the second year, there begins to be the establishment of a sense of self as separate from caretakers. With it and the simultaneous development of the capacity for independent locomotion, one sees initial forays of independence, though these combine with episodes of clinging. It is also not until the second year that awareness of and interest in other children appears. This can take the form of "exploration" in which they pull each other's hair or clothes or of imitation of each other's actions and vocalizations. Less friendly "toddler" interactions involve blind attempts to take another's toy, the victim responding with anger, fighting, and crying. Snatching objects, pushing, and kicking are common forms of aggression at this age (Breckenridge & Vincent, 1960; Hurlock, 1964; Yarrow, 1960). As the second year ends, interactions become more social. There is less fighting over toys, and children play in proximity to each other (parallel play). Even some mutual play becomes possible (Landreth, 1958; Stone & Church, 1957).

In the years following infancy, adult attachments weaken as involvements with other children increase. Psychological separation is most dramatically seen in the independence and self-assertiveness of the 3-year-old. The storm around self-determination (autonomy) then subsides, and the 4- and five-year-old again relates to adults in a friendly, cooperative manner (Hurlock, 1964). Although interest in other children is growing, the 2-year-old's play is still largely solitary in nature or, at most, parallel. Although they may seek each other's company, there is relatively little interaction except as they watch and imitate each other or try to take another's toy (Hurlock, 1964). It is not until about 3 that children begin to be sufficiently "social" to be able to play *with* one another. They show playmate preferences and, during play, talk to each other. They prefer to play in small groups, usually with just one child, and their interactions consist of watching each other, talking, and making suggestions (see Table 25) (Hurlock, 1964; Hynes, 1960; Mussen, Conger, & Kagan, 1963).

TABLE 25   Mental Age and Some Aspects of Social-Emotional Development

Mental age (years)	Social skills
0–1	Shows attachments and differential responses to adults. Shows desire to be with adults and imitates them. Is capable of being restrained at the verbal level.
1–2	Shows increasing interest in other children but most play is solitary or parallel (in the company of but not with other children). Is influenced by older children as they are imitated in play and behavior. Some beginning resistiveness to adults.
2–3	Increasing ability for cooperative play though most play is still parallel. Beginning playmate preferences. Can participate in simple team games. Capable of showing sympathy. Period of heightened resistiveness to adults—assertive, independent, negativistic.
3–4	Participates in cooperative play. Understands sharing and the taking of turns. Resistiveness to adults diminishes. Conscious of the opinions of others. Tries to gain attention by "showing off." Some mobility outside the home. Can now do errands. Can take some responsibility for keeping things orderly.
4–5	Fears of infancy diminish as new ones arise. Less fear of strange objects, situations, and persons but replaced somewhat by imaginary fears.
5–6	Understands needs for rules. Can play complicated floor games. Respects property. Chooses own friends.

EMOTIONAL DEVELOPMENT

The process of socialization cannot be considered apart from emotional development, because it is in social situations that emotions are commonly generated. Ultimately, it is the impulse to *action* created by *emotions* that the child must learn to control in order to achieve social adaptation. The emotional behavior of young children is quite different from that of adolescents and adults. Their emotional states tend to be intense and short-lived and to show rapid fluctuations. The worker with retarded children may, initially, be struck by the child's apparent emotional immaturity. In fact, the retarded child's level of social and emotional maturity reflects its general level of mental development, and it is the *cognitive* lag relative to chronological age that gives the behavior its immature quality.

Fear and anger are two of the potentially troublesome emotions seen in normal and retarded preschoolers. Young children are especially made uneasy by the unfamiliar (lack of structure), and the retarded child, in particular, benefits from a gradual introduction of new activities. Here, however, the resistance may stem from a lack of confidence in the ability to carry them out (fear of failure and the need for success). The instructional guidelines offered early in the chapter are a means of minimizing such fears.

Of all of our emotions, none is more threatening to effective socialization than anger. Anger is a normal response to frustration, and frustration is an inevitable consequence of existence. The role of the teacher and parent is to try to anticipate and prevent unnecessary frustrations and to teach directly, and by example (modeling), how anger can be discharged in relatively nondestructive ways. The foundation upon which intervention rests, however, is the recognition of the child's *right* to his *feelings*—though not, of course, to all of the actions they impel. If anger is understood as a normal by-product of frustration, attempts to deny its reality and to dissuade the child from his feelings will be avoided.

SOCIAL-EMOTIONAL DEVELOPMENT IN RETARDED PRESCHOOLERS

Of all phases of the preschool program, social and emotional dimensions are probably the most difficult to conceptualize in curriculum terms. We think of socialization as a natural consequence of certain kinds of experience with a lesser emphasis on the kind of direct instruction that typifies the teaching of self-help or academic skills. In fact, the opportunity to foster social and emotional growth pervades every aspect of the preschool program. What is especially important with retarded children, however, is to take an active stance toward encouraging the kind of social and emotional behaviors that will enable the child to function in as wide a range of settings as possible. This means continuous encouragement of the kind of child-adult and child-child interactions that themselves will foster additional development (Sneed, 1978).

Social Behaviors

The range of social behaviors in retarded preschoolers will vary from states of solitariness and predominantly self-stimulatory behavior to beginning "cooperative" play. The latter refers to interactions that require some mutuality, such as playing ball with each other or pushing each other on a swing. Since the level of social interaction is related to mental development, its nature is affected by the degree of handicap. In a study on the effects of integrating normal and handicapped children in the same preschool (Fredericks et al., 1978), a great difference was seen between the spontaneous social behaviors of the two groups of children. The spontaneous activity of the retarded children was primarily solitary in nature. A somewhat more advanced behavior was also occasionally seen—watching other children. For the most part, however, time was spent in self-stimulation (e.g., rocking) or in just doing nothing. There was little involvement with other children, normal or delayed. In contrast, the normal children engaged primarily in play that was at least in close proximity to other children (parallel play) or in which there were such interactions as exchanging play materials (associative play). It is presumed that at least part of this difference in social behavior is related to the differences between the two groups of children in mental age. The normal youngsters were operating at about the 5-year mental age level, whereas the retarded children were probably at the less than 1 year to the 3-year level. When delayed and nondelayed children appear to be at similar mental age levels, as in another study of an integrated preschool (Ispa & Matz, 1978), no differences in social play were observed.

Social Interaction Between Normal and Retarded Preschoolers

Of particular interest in the latter study was that when groups of children were of comparable mental age they did not segregate themselves according to whether or not they were handicapped. In absolute terms, this group of retarded children was much less delayed than those in the Fredricks et al. (1978) study. Their chronological age was 5, they were not more than mildly retarded, and they were operating at the 2- to 3-year mental age level. Thus they were capable of some cooperative play. Interestingly, normal children are said to first show awareness of others' physical handicaps at about age 4, and, during the next few years, their attitudes waver between acceptance and rejection. This would seem to be a propitious time to provide the kind of integrated social experience that could encourage future positive attitudes.

The Severely Handicapped Preschooler

Within the retarded preschool population, special attention must be given to fostering the social development of its most impaired segment. These are children whose retardation often includes significant sensory and/or motor disabilities. The social behavior of the more severely impaired preschoolers is not wholly explicable in developmental or mental age terms. The same is true for similarly affected youths and adults. The perpetual solitariness and stereotypies seen in severely and profoundly retarded individuals have no genuine counterpart in normal development, though some rocking and head banging is found in normal infants. This is most likely to occur at about 8 months of age and usually disappears by age 3 years (DeLissovoy, 1962; Kravitz & Boehm, 1971; Kravitz et al., 1960). What can account for the prominence of these patterns of social isolation? It might be suggested that the absence of language would block communication, but children who lack speech because of deafness are not necessarily social isolates. They may have to communicate with each other through natural gesture, as do some Down syndrome children, but they communicate! We can speculate that this social isolation results from a degree of cognitive and/or sensory impairment whose severity limits the child's capacity to be aroused or stimulated by sources of excitation outside its own body. The normally developing infant, like its severely retarded counterpart, is responsive to experiences of touch, taste, smell, and movement but is also stimulated by visual and auditory experiences. This requires two elements—intactness of the senses of hearing and/or vision and sufficient mental development to make sense of what is seen or heard. For the solitary and self-stimulating child, sensory experiences that do not involve direct physical contact (e.g., sight and sounds) may have no more meaning and stimulation potential than the sounds of a language that is not understood. We shall return to the problem of self-stimulation in Chapter 10.

Promoting Social-Emotional Development

The encouragement of social-emotional growth in retarded preschoolers involves several types of activities—direct cognitive and motor stimulation, the teaching of toy play and group play, and the discouraging of undesirable behavior (Garwood, 1982; Johnson & Werner, 1975).

1. Direct stimulation: Since the cognitive and motor impairments of some retarded preschoolers may be of such severity as to much restrict the child's capacity to respond to general sources of stimulation in its environment, it falls to the

teacher (and parent) to reach out to the child and provide stimulation that is both meaningful and pleasurable. Our goal is to *awaken* interest in sources of pleasurable stimulation provided by others. These will include tactual kinesthetic experiences—stroking and rocking the child, holding and talking to him, and more active forms of physical stimulation, such as bouncing. While these activities will include experiences not unlike those produced by the child through his own forms of self-stimulation, the agent is another human being. The intent is to create interest in *others* as sources of pleasurable stimulation. At another level, parents and teachers can influence the degree of imaginative play in handicapped preschoolers (Strain, 1975; Yawkey, 1982), and the use of normal peers can increase social behaviors (McHale & Olley, 1982).

2. Teaching toy play: The teaching of toy play, too, is intended to foster interest in sources of pleasure outside the self. Utilizing such teaching methods as direct manual guidance, modeling, and reinforcement, we provide the child with objects that can produce developmentally relevant experiences. Of particular interest should be toys that produce an effect. This was touched on in Chapter 5 in defining the ingredients of a healthy child-rearing experience. It has been suggested that activities in which the child directly influences events are important to development; they relate specifically to needs for success and autonomy. Suggestions as to appropriate toys include those that produce sound and movement (e.g., a jumping jack) (Wehman, 1977).

3. Teaching group play: Group play emerges as other children and their activities begin to be a source of interest. This requires exposure to other children and to activities that are developmentally close to the child's level. The earliest signs of some readiness for group play will be occasions where solitary play is mixed with periods of watching the activity of other children. This watching of other children can be a basis for imitating them and, through this, achieving greater physical proximity to them (Wenar, 1971). Teacher-initiated activities that can foster group play include recognizing and pointing to other children when they are named, and play that involves sharing and taking turns. Peterson and Maralick (1977) found that handicapped preschoolers interacted more with peers during block play and manipulative floor play then during art and table activities. Another means of encouraging child interactions is the occasional pairing of children who are at different developmental levels. The more advanced child is asked to temporarily assume a "teacher" role.

4. Imitation: The potential for the less developed child to learn from the more developed one stems from propensities for imitation of behavior of children who are perceived as performing an activity at a higher level of competence than one's own (Strichart & Gottlieb, 1975). Observations of a child who may serve as a model can teach a variety of behaviors including reducing overt fear response (Bandura, Grusec, & Menlove, 1967), language (Guess, Sailor, Rutherford, & Baer, 1968), and learning to apply rules (Zimmerman & Rosenthal, 1974). In addition to competence, other factors encouraging imitation are the activity's novelty, a positive attitude toward the model, and an observer child who is in an active rather than passive mode (Bricker, 1978).

5. Integrated preschools: It is out of this potential for children learning from children that there has been the encouragement of integrating handicapped and normal children in the same preschool setting. In addition to the potential developmental benefits to the delayed child, it offers the possibility of helping normally developing children and their parents to achieve more accepting attitudes toward children who are "different." In the case of the handicapped child, the greatest benefits are likely to be observed in the older and less impaired preschooler (Field, Roseman, De Stafano, & Koewler, 1982; Fredericks et al., 1978; Ipsa & Matz, 1978), those with mental ages of at least 2 years. Such integration may also be more easily achieved in motor play (Fredericks et al., 1978). There is a developmental sequence in the direction of play in normal children: first to the adult, then to a toy, and finally to peers. This same sequence is seen in handicapped children (Field, 1980) thus indicating the children who will be most likely to respond to peer play opportunities. It is clear, however, that positive social interactions between children who are at different developmental levels will not occur spontaneously (Snyder, Apolloni, & Cooke, 1977). They are most likely to occur where the models, whether normal or retarded, are only slightly more advanced developmentally (Apolloni & Cooke, 1978) and when the teacher creates the conditions for interaction (Bricker, 1978). One concern about integrated preschools is that the normally developing child might imitate some of the less desirable behaviors of the handicapped ones. For example, there is natural anxiety that children should not mimic self-stimulatory patterns. Apolloni and Cooke (1978) reassure us that "regressive imitation" only occurs when it is reinforced.

6. Discouraging undesirable behavior: The development of social skills requires not only the provision of appropriate learning experiences but also the discouragement of inappropriate behaviors. A therapeutic preschool environment is one that provides consistency, offers appropriate alternatives to problem behavior, and does not ignore undesirable behavior (except the attention-getting variety described in the early part of the chapter). For the preschool retarded child, Johnson and Werner (1975) suggest such admonishing adult behaviors as pairing a clear "No" with an interruption of the activity, startling the child, providing verbal reprimands, and brief physical restraint.

PARENTS AND SIBS

In Chapter 1 we discussed the impact of the retarded child on the family. Retardation was seen as creating a major stress on the family and one with both short- and long-term consequences. In the past, to the extent that social agencies were sensitive to the needs of such families, services tended to be of a "counseling" nature. This was and is intended to encourage parents to express painful feelings (Heifetz, 1977) or to try to work through the natural kinds of defenses that crisis can engender (e.g., denial or presumption of future cure). It is only after the parents have received some emotional relief through acknowledgment of their own pain that they can begin to think about the needs of their child. While this aspect of the impact of retardation cannot be ignored, a feeling-oriented counseling approach *alone* often fails to provide parents with the kind of concrete assistance or "tools" that would enable them to progress from the status of an "injured party" to one in which they could feel some control over future events. With the advent of behavior modification and its widespread adoption in the training of retarded children, there has been a shift toward giving the parent a more active role in the management of the child. By introducing parents to behavioral principles and offering activities that can stimulate development, parents (and sibs) can become an important adjunct to formal training efforts.

Formats of Parental Involvement

The preferred methods of helping the parent(s) to assume teaching functions involve either direct assistance in the home, as in the home-based infant programs described earlier in the chapter, or parental attendance at the preschool and participation there in the child's learning experience. Parental involvement with the preschool should include both teaching sessions with the child and periodic group meetings with other parents (Baker, 1977; Bristol, 1977; Jeffree, McCookey, & Hewson, 1977). Instructional experiences should begin with teacher demonstration and follow with gradual involvement of the parent as teacher. Ideally, parental attendance should be at least weekly, with parent group sessions occurring every second week. Such programs have varied in length from a minimum of eight to a maximum of 20 individual sessions. Training materials have been specifically developed for parents, such as the READ Project Series (Baker et al., 1973, 1976). The READ manuals are intended to be used without direct teacher assistance, but it is evident that parents feel more comfortable when they have ready access to a regular teacher (Baker, 1977). Of particular interest in the READ program was the finding that once formal parent participation in preschool training ceased their continued use of the skills acquired was sporadic (Baker, 1977). Though the READ Project had encouraged parents to continue planned and formal teaching at the end of their training experience, few persisted. They were, however, much more likely to engage in "incidental" teaching—that is, using their skills around some teaching goal that came up in their child's normal day-to-day experiences. In this sense, it would seem that they were functioning in just the same way as parents of normal children.

Sources of Conflict between Center and Parents

The failure of the READ Project parents to continue the systematic training of their children is likely to be perceived by center staff as a lack of cooperativeness on the part of the parents. Even more common would be the failure of parents to support ongoing training efforts by allowing children to persist in immature behaviors that are not manifest in the preschool. Some of the most common sources of friction between day care staff and the parents have been described by Larrabee (1969). While these pertain to general day care settings, the concerns are not different from those of specialized preschool.

A SENSE OF MATERNAL LOSS OR GUILT

Mother experiences placement of the child outside the home as a loss or as a situation about which she should feel guilty. There may be a sense of inadequacy as a parent, a feeling of rivalry with the day care staff. One mother in a well-functioning home became so jealous of her child's teacher in day care, a feeling that was obviously communicated to the child, that the child stopped talking about what went on in the center and wished to stop going. In this instance the center, through its social worker, helped the mother to understand and accept their respective roles in relation to the child.

CONFLICTS ARISING FROM DIFFERENCES BETWEEN THE LIVING STANDARDS IN THE HOME AND IN THE CENTER

An overburdened low-income mother may resent the child's wanting things he's seen at the center but which she is hard put to provide. Or the living standards in the center may cause the child to press the mother for a different level of care—cleaner clothes, good hot meals, and so forth. It is important that the center help the family to understand the origin of the child's wishes without, at the same time, further undermining an already probably diminished level of maternal self-esteem. The center may also be able to bring to bear the services of other community agencies in obtaining what child, school, and parents, too, really want.

CONFLICTS OVER DIFFERENCES BETWEEN BEHAVIOR PREFERENCES OF THE HOME AND CENTER

The activities encouraged in the center may conflict with what mother prefers or to what she has become accustomed. An inhibited child with little speech and poor mobility blossomed under center stimulation and, in the home, was much more active, talkative, and occasionally mischievous. The "new" child was not necessarily what the mother was comfortable with, and she needed to be worked with in order to keep her from taking the child out of the program. Other common areas of potential friction are differences in expectations with regard to self-help, impulse control, and discipline. In the matter of self-help, for example, the preschool strives for greater independence in the child and is prepared to take the time necessary to teach the needed skills. The mother, however, may have become so frustrated at the child's slowness in acquiring such skills that efforts to teach them have been abandoned and she is resigned to doing these things for him. But the center expects that the home will encourage the skills being taught in the preschool, and this will mean that the mother will have to reexpose herself to the nuisance and strain of watching the child struggle to do for himself what she can do for him so much more easily. But the preschool staff can do more than simply encourage; it can materially aid the family by offering direct teaching assistance. The basic principles of behavior modification—task analysis, successive approximation, and reinforcement—can be applied in the home as well as in the school.

Numerous materials are available that are appropriate to parents as well as teachers. Using parent groups, Galloway and Galloway (1970) assisted families in identifying behavioral goals in the home and implementing programs in carrying them out. Larsen and Bricker (1968) have developed a manual specifically for parents and teachers of moderately and severely retarded young children, and references to other appropriate materials are presented in a footnote to the section on behavior modification offered earlier in the chapter.

Another potential source of conflict is discipline. Do parents set behavioral limits for the child, and, if so, to what extent are they consistent in implementing them? The experience of the parents of Down syndrome children is again instructive. During the early childhood years, Down syndrome children presented such problem behaviors as incessant demands for attention, stubbornness, and temper tantrums. The parents recognized that the training of these children required much patience and that it was important to establish and *adhere* to routines rather than "giving in" *because* the child was handicapped:

> Within his limitations we are treating Jack like a normal little boy and discipline him. When he misbehaves we make him sit in his chair for a while [presumably an undesirable consequence]; we explain why he is having to sit in his chair.

> I had to handle each of my children differently—talk to some, demand of others. I must admit I had to have more patience with Frank than with the others. Toilet training was quite an ordeal. To me he doesn't behave too abnormally. He's just like all boys—runs, plays. I don't like to be harsh or holler at him. Children copy a lot [imitation] and I don't want him to get into bad habits. Of course, sometimes I'm more impatient than other times—or than I should be. I always try to reason with him—to impress on him what he should or should not do (Kramm, 1963).

Both sets of parents did set limits for their retarded child and insisted on offering verbal explanations when punishment was necessary. While it is certainly desirable to make such explanations if the child is capable of understanding what is expected of him, what one *does* in child training is more important than what one *says*.

In contrast to these parents, others were less consistent in handling the child and also treated him quite differently from how they treated his normal sibs. Parenthetically, these parents reported a greater frequency of behavior problems.

> Rose is sometimes so good and sometimes so bad. She runs around in the stores touching everything and calling attention to herself [and to mother!]. Her father wants to protect her. *He never says no to her. He's strict with the boys and he lets Rosie get away with everything.* Sometimes the younger boy teases her. Once he called her a "Nosy Rosy." My husband got very angry and said "Don't let me ever hear

you say that again!'' I told him that if he took that stand the boys would get to hate Rose (Kramm, 1963).

The mother offers a picture of a very overprotective father who, in his zeal to shelter his retarded daughter, assures the continuation of the kind of misbehavior that angers the younger brother and demands the father's intervention. It is no wonder that Rose is teased; she is seen as a "privileged character" who is subject to a different set of rules from her sibs. Although she is not expected to behave in a manner identical to that of her nonretarded sibs when they were the same age, she should be expected to maintain at least that degree of control which corresponds to her general developmental level. If, for example, she is functioning at the level of a 2- or 3-year-old, it is appropriate to expect her to exercise whatever behavioral constraints are achieved at that age.

The situation that the mother describes also reveals how the family fails to meet Rosie's need for structure. She is exposed to two very different sets of rules within the same general setting. Her mother and brothers have behavioral expectations for her that are contradictory to those of the father. What works with Daddy does not work with other family members. Rosie probably does not recognize that she is, in effect, playing a game with two sets of rules and she must often be frustrated because she is sometimes punished for the same things that at other times are ignored. This is the essence of *inconsistency* in child training. Although no situation or person can have perfect consistency—in the case of a person it might not even be a desirable trait—to borrow from a simple arithmetic analogy, how can a child learn that $2 + 2 = 4$ if he is also told that $2 + 2 = 3$! Just as center staff can aid the family in carrying out self-help objectives in the home, so can it lend assistance in helping parents to adopt general child-rearing procedures that will foster the child's social and emotional growth.

Involvement with Other Parents, Siblings, and Other Family Members

PARENTS

The placement of the child in a preschool program opens the family to the possibility of meeting and sharing with others who have similar concerns. The psychological wound associated with being the parent or sib of a child with unwelcome characteristics gradually heals with time and with the support of interested and knowledgeable people. But while parents are appreciative when friends and professionals want to help, it is only *other* parents of handicapped children who are seen as really capable of understanding their feelings and problems. Parent groups can serve as vehicles for the communication and sharing of feelings and for discovering how others have dealt with similar problems. It can diminish the sense of isolation that some families experience. In reviewing their work with parent groups, Cummings and Stock (1962) noted the tremendous need of mothers to ventilate their feelings. Emotions that were previously bottled up now spill out.

Fear and sorrow were expressed but also anger, and guilt over the anger. The child had realistically placed severe demands on their physical and emotional resources, but their image of the "good" mother compelled them to swallow their frustration and to be enduringly loving and accepting. Other concerns were sadness at the child's limitations, feelings of having been deserted or unaided by others, and a sense of personal inadequacy (lowered self-esteem). Those who benefited most from group counseling were mothers who could acknowledge angry feelings toward the child but also, ultimately, direct their attention away from themselves and to the child's needs.

SIBLINGS

Siblings as well as parents are affected by the presence of a retarded child in the family. They, too, may have negative as well as positive feelings toward a brother or sister whose deviance is, by association, perceived as a threat to *their* need for peer acceptance and self-esteem. As a result of experiences with groups of normal adolescent sibs of retarded children, Kaplan (1969) observes that their primary goal is to avoid identification with their retarded brother or sister. Undoubtedly the adolescent's intense preoccupation with self and tremendous need for peer approval can have the effect of heightening negative feelings toward the retarded sib and, often, its accompanying feelings of guilt as well. Nonetheless, most siblings of retarded children manage to cope successfully with these conflicts (Graliker, Fisher, & Koch, 1962; Kramm, 1963), and, in her study of Down's families, Kramm observes that the majority were helpful and sympathetic. In almost half of the Down syndrome families, sibs were said to love their retarded brother or sister and to take pride in their accomplishments. When the retarded child learned a new word, for example, it was a topic of family interest. This is not to minimize sib problems—you have just read of the effect of a parent who is guilty of favoritism. Other problems faced by normal children were fear of embarrassment (loss of self-esteem) by the behavior of their retarded sib (Baum, 1962), accidental destructiveness, excessive demands for attention, pressure to assume parental roles, and concern with their role vis-à-vis their retarded sibling when the parents could no longer care for the child. Sibs of marriageable age wondered, too, about the likelihood of their having a retarded child.

With reference to attitudes toward the responsibilities of normal sibs toward the retarded child the following excerpts from Kramm (1963) are of interest:

> Keith thrives on love. Our family does everything together. When we drove to an institution to look it over, the children all said that they wanted Keith home with them. Sam, my son-in-law, said that Keith would always have a home with him and Mary. Of course, we could never consider having our children assume the care of Keith. But wasn't it nice of Sam to offer. [The creation of a variety of living and working situations *in the community* should give sibs a wider range of options than either assuming full care or seeking institutionalization.]

When the children were younger my husband and I never left Hugh to be cared for by them. On trips we always took him along. [Parents can go to extremes here and respite or short-term care facilities are becoming available as a means of freeing families for activities that would, ordinarily, be more difficult with the retarded child along.] One woman I know said that Hugh should be put in a home because it would affect Eileen's chances to be married. Eileen used to get so upset when Hugh made noises. It embarrassed her when she had friends over. But she got over it. The boys didn't seem to pay attention.

Most families did not expect the normal children to assume a substitute parent role, but the predominant relationship between normal sibs and the retarded child was parental in nature. Even younger brothers and sisters could be protector and teachers as well as playmate.

I have very responsible children. Both are better with the baby than either my husband or myself. I feel I don't give full time to the other two. I try but often feel drained. They accept this [perhaps]. Everything about their little brother is all right with them. He can climb all over them, mess up their schoolwork, do anything. They don't mind [perhaps].

A mother describes her teenage daughter Mandy's relationship with her younger retarded brother.

Mandy is very serious, very deep. She possesses rare gifts. She lives for her little brother. They bring out the best in each other [see below]. She says she's learning from her little brother. Since she shows such interest in him, I think she should go into special education. [A not infrequent consequence of close association with a retarded child.]

When the mother speaks of Mandy and her retarded brother bringing out the best in each other, she is conveying a sentiment similar to that of parents who come to view the child as a positive force in the family. Unquestionably the retarded child can stir deep tenderness, enhance patience, and teach us that a person of value is not limited to individuals who are mirror images of ourselves.

At first I was afraid of the effect John might have on my younger children. Dick [a younger brother] is very sensitive to other children's afflictions and problems; he's only five but already he's protective of John and bawls out other children if they touch him. Then again, he'll say to his playmates, "Come on, let's get away from Johnnie." I can't blame him. Sometimes Johnnie sweeps down something the children have made.

The boys are all very good to him. Al and Stan have always played with him more. They showed him how to play basketball, how to box and wrestle. Sometimes when Larry gets balky they have to force him. Walter is stricter with him than the others are; also he teases him more. Myrtle, the youngest, sits with him a lot—and shows him how to write.

Let us listen to the words of a college student who describes her personal growth experience as a result of working for one semester as a tutor-volunteer to a mentally retarded and cerebral palsied child.[10]

Working with Toni this semester has been quite an experience for me. In the past, I had never worked with, or been around to any degree, anyone who was retarded. I must admit that my first feeling toward her was shock. I was really surprised that I, an inexperienced college junior, was being presented with a severely retarded child to tutor. I feel that as the sessions with Toni continued . . . *I gained a great deal of confidence in myself.* I completely lost my feeling of shock and uneasiness and developed an assured, satisfied, confident feeling in just being around Toni and in working with her. *I came to realize that she was a person, just as I,* but that her physical and mental nature, being as limited as it was, made her stand out in needs. I came to realize some of those needs as my work with Toni advanced. She was a young girl who was in great need of love, attention, and patience. But, above all else, she needed a means of developing self-esteem [awareness of Toni as a "person"]. . . .

It was a strange experience to work with Toni. Advancements, if any, came so slowly and gradually that they almost go unrecognized until one surveys the entire tutoring segment of the semester. *This taught me one thing that I feel is very important—patience* [self-growth]. . . .

This is probably the most unique relationship that I have ever had—and one of the most *rewarding.* By rewarding I do not mean gratifying in terms of academic success [the tutorial experience is a part of a college course]; but rather, I mean the pleasure of knowing that I have reached this girl as a person [increased self-esteem] (emphasis added).

To summarize this aspect of services to the family, although attention to the needs of parents is a well-established role of preschool programs, there has been little concern with the siblings. The center should seek to learn through the parents how the retarded child and his sibs get along, determine parental expectations with regard to sib relationships, and then meet the siblings themselves and inquire of their concerns. The center may ultimately establish sibling groups comparable to those for parents.

[10]Final summary of tutorial experience of Ms. Ann Kelly, Chapel Hill, NC.

OTHER FAMILY MEMBERS

Though the focus has been on parents and sibs, other family members can also play important roles. Gabel and Kotsch (1981) describe how a preschool center can reach out to grandparents and other significant family members to help them understand the nature of the child's difficulties. They can be crucial in helping *their* children, the new parents, to deal with the psychological blow to self-esteem and, later, the child-care demands that are often increased in such children (e.g., Beckman-Bell, 1981; Winton & Turnbull, 1981). In a related paper, Foster et al. (1981) point out the need to be sensitive to the impact of the child on all members of the family, because their impact on each other ultimately affects how the child is treated.

School-Age and Adult Programs: Educational and Recreational

OVERVIEW

This chapter describes two major programming areas for school-age youths and adults—education and recreation. The educational domain is focused on: (a) special education and mainstreaming, (b) direct attempts to improve cognitive functioning, and (c) educational methods for the most severely impaired of the retarded population. This second major topic is "recreation"—an oft-neglected area in the development of retarded youths and adults. Attention is directed to (a) the need for recreational skills, (b) recreational interests of retarded youth, (c) special interests, and (d) special programs.

SPECIAL EDUCATION: EFFICACY AND MAINSTREAMING

Of all services to retarded persons and their families, perhaps none has shown as dramatic a change as those to the school-age population. As recently as the mid-1970s only about half of all retarded youths had access to public education. By the end of the decade, virtually all were receiving some form of education. The key to this doubling of educational opportunities and their nearly universal availability in only 5 years was the enactment in 1975 of the federal legislation "Education for All Handicapped Children Act" (P.L. Public Law 94-142).[1] It affirmed the right of all handicapped children to a free and appropriate education and within the "least restrictive environment." The latter established the rationale for "mainstreaming"—the provision of education to handicapped students within

[1]To receive federal education funds under this law, the state is required to serve all such children.

regular classes and in physical settings that are integrated as much as possible with those of nonhandicapped ones. Among retarded children mainstreaming has primarily affected those with mild impairment. Formerly placed in self-contained "special" (educable) classes and restricted thereby in their contacts with nonhandicapped youths, these students now typically spend at least part of their school day in regular classes. For more seriously impaired youths, self-contained special classes continue to be the rule though, preferably, in the same school rather than in a separate one.

Concern has been expressed regarding the effect of regular class placement on the pursuit of the traditional educational objectives for mildly retarded children (Childs, 1978; Gottlieb, 1981). Since "regular" class objectives are usually "academic," there is fear that the mainstreamed student may lose out in a curriculum that necessarily has a greater emphasis on acquiring skills related to activities of daily living and preparation for employment. But the goals of mainstreaming, essentially social in nature, and access to an educational experience that takes into account the students' special academic needs are not incompatible. The mildly retarded youth will, of necessity, be eventually required to spend significant portions of the school day in special settings (e.g., the "resource" room), and it is here that the traditional curriculum can be delivered.

Efficacy

The impetus for mainstreaming lay, in part, in the finding that traditional self-contained "educable" classes produce no academic advantages and uncertain social ones.

EDUCATIONAL FINDINGS

Children in special classes were frequently found to achieve *less* gradewise in basic academic skills than their counterparts in regular classes (Cassidy & Stanton, 1959; Carwell, 1967; Elenboger, 1957; Hoeltke, 1966; Thurstone, 1959; Welch, 1966), or no difference at all was seen (Blatt, 1958; Goldstein et al., 1965; Jordan, 1965; Mullen & Itkin, 1961; Schell, 1959; Smith & Kennedy, 1967; Warren, 1962; Welch, 1966). Even granting the methodological perplexities surrounding so-called "efficacy" research—issues pertaining to comparabilities of students and instructional components in both settings (Sparks & Blackman, 1965)—special educators have been forced to recognize the absence of academic benefits (Johnson, 1962; Sparks & Blackman, 1965). Whether school achievement as measured by grade level of reading and arithmetic should be the only educational criterion is another matter. After all, the emphasis of special education has been social and vocational rather than academic (Goldstein, Moss, & Jordan, 1962). If we can agree that the general purpose of education is preparation for effective adulthood, then this criterion has yet to be addressed. At the vocational level, for example, it is personality characteristics rather than academic skills that are most relevant to job success in retarded persons (Cohen, 1960; Deno, 1966; Kolstoe & Shafter, 1961).

BEHAVIORAL FINDINGS

The traditional rationale for special class was that it provided a setting in which the educationally handicapped child could achieve success (Cegelka & Tyler, 1970). We can recognize that prolonged exposure to failure would be devastating to self-esteem and lead to avoidance rather than engagement. The author's students working as volunteers with youths who are daily frustrated in school by failure rather than success encounter attitudes of indifference and resignation. But the question arises as to whether special-class placement itself, opportunities notwithstanding, could cause diminished self-worth. The concern here is with the social consequences of educational separation (segregation) when the separation is based on an acknowledged deficit (Jones, 1972). This issue takes on additional significance in light of the typical overrepresentation of disadvantaged minority groups in educable classes. In California, ethnic overrepresentation was *the* basis for judicial decisions pertaining to educable class placement (MacMillan & Meyers, 1980).

In contrast to educational effects, special-class placement does seem to have some impact on behavior. Children in special classes tend to be rated as better adjusted than those in regular ones (Glett, 1958; Cassidy & Stanton, 1959; Elenbogen, 1957; Hoeltke, 1966; Johnson, 1962; Thurstone, 1959). This determination has been made either through teacher evaluation of student behavior or through personality tests. There is some question, however, as to whether the special-class child is really better behaved or whether that setting may simply be more tolerant of behaviors that would be less acceptable in regular classes (Quay, 1963; Specker & Bartel, 1968).

SELF-ESTEEM

The possibly adverse effect of special-class placement on self-esteem has been an important element in the thrust for mainstreaming. In Chapter 2, in the section on personality, we discussed how psychological needs for "intimacy" are affected by separate or integrated class placement. It was concluded that the effects of "labeling" or of special-class placement are not unidimensional. The label and the setting can be protective as well as prejudicial; chronological age seems to be the differentiating factor. Elementary-age children do not seem to be negatively affected by such groupings, but at the junior and senior high levels, special-class placement is perceived as an embarrassment. At the latter ages, integration rather than separation is to be sought.

Mainstreaming

ACADEMIC EFFECTS

Studies on the effect of mainstreaming have typically involved elementary or junior high level children who spend a part of their school day in a "resource room." It is here that their academic deficiencies can be addressed. Major reviews of the mainstreaming literature (Corman & Gottlieb, 1978; Gottlieb, 1981; Keogh & Levitt, 1976) indicate either no difference between integrated and special-class children (e.g., Budoff & Gottlieb, 1976) or a higher level of achievement for the integrated student (Carroll, 1967; Meyers, MacMillan, & Yoshida, 1975; Rodee, 1979; Walker, 1972). Where higher achievement levels were found, they were confined to reading; no differences were found in arithmetic.

SOCIAL AND BEHAVIORAL EFFECTS

It will be recalled that the premainstreaming "efficacy" research generally indicated a better social adjustment in the special-class setting. This is itself peculiar, since the special class was likely to be used for children with behavioral as well as intellectual impairments. Indeed, as just noted, the question is raised as to whether the behavior is *really* better or the teacher is simply more accepting of it. In any case, there is some indication that a change from segregated to integrated classes can directly affect student behavior such that it comes to more closely resemble that of nonhandicapped peers (Gampel, Gottlieb, & Harrison, 1974; Gottlieb, Gampel, & Budoff, 1975). There do appear to be behavioral benefits from mainstreaming, though these do not necessarily translate into full social acceptance. Integrated or not, retarded children have a lower social status than their nonhandicapped peers (Goodman, Gottlieb, & Harrison, 1972; Gottlieb & Davis, 1973). Indeed, under some circumstances, the visibility produced by integration may adversely affect the child (Gottlieb & Budoff, 1973; Gottlieb, Cohen, & Goldstein, 1974). But this lesser social status does not have to translate into diminished self-worth. The retarded youngster like his normal counterpart has access to a range of peer group relationships within or without his own class. The integrated youth appears well able to establish peer group relationships, and, especially at the high school level, expresses preference for the integrated setting (Warner, Thrapp, & Walsh, 1973). In their review of the research on integrated class placement and self-esteem, Sammel and Snell (1979) conclude that placement alone has little effect. The *teacher* rather than the peer group is seen as crucial. The teacher can create the classroom conditions that foster either acceptance or rejection. Even a sensitivity to cooperative rather than competitive classroom activities can assist in this process (Johnson & Johnson, 1980).

ATTITUDES OF EDUCATORS

Inevitably, the potential of mainstreaming depends on its acceptance by teachers and administrators, and this in turn depends on *how* it is implemented (MacMillan, Jones, & Meyers, 1976; Zigler & Muenchow, 1979). Mainstreaming is not merely the physical transfer of mildly retarded students to regular classes; it also requires "support" from the system (Kaufman et al., 1975). As has been expressed in Chapter 1, the academic learning difficulties of mildly retarded pupils are real, they are not the product of a label, and they must be addressed in whatever the class setting. This point has also been made by MacMillan and Meyers (1980) in connection with the delabeling and regular class placement of former "educable mentally retarded" (EMR) children in California. Given the pressures on teachers in recent years, it is not surprising that their attitudes toward mainstreaming are at least mixed. Nevertheless, they are united in feeling that their training has not prepared them for their new responsibilities (Gickling & Theobald, 1975; Guerin & Szatlocky, 1974; Shotel, Iano, & McGettigan, 1972). In a period of economic constraint and general teacher dissatisfaction, the schools will be particularly challenged to provide the resources that will enable mildly retarded youths to feel welcome in the educational community. In this respect, inservice guidelines offered by Paul et al. (1977) should be helpful.

CURRICULUM CONCERNS

It has been noted that mainstreaming might adversely affect curriculum goals. The mildly retarded child will need special assistance throughout the school years, and the standard educational objectives can be accomplished through a blend of regular class, "adapted" or modified regular class, and resource room experiences. The essence of the blend is to increase the degree of *individualization* and *intensification* (Meyen & Lear, 1980) necessary to maximize educational potential. The *goals* of that education relate to *competencies* in the *personal, social,* and *vocational* spheres and a reduced concern for traditional "academic" ones. If the educational experience of the retarded student is not ultimately "useful," what is its purpose?

While a focus on "integration" rather than on "education" can threaten the traditional social-occupational emphasis of educable programs, this is not inevitable. Rather, mainstreaming at its best, while placing the child in a setting that typically points up his inadequacies, offers the possibility of a greater sense of identification with nonhandicapped peers while still preserving access to the instructional experiences necessary to maximizing personal competency.

MAINSTREAMING AND SEVERER LEVELS OF RETARDATION

The disequilibrium created by the requirements of mainstreaming is less evident in children who are more than mildly retarded. They have traditionally been served in self-contained special classes, either in regular schools or in special ones. These pupils continue to be educated in special classes (e.g., trainable), though mainstreaming has increased the likelihood that these classes will be in regular rather than special schools. For moderately retarded students, the focus of education is largely nonacademic, though there is the goal of teaching elementary but functional "academics"—word recognition and basic time and number concepts. Much effort is devoted to self-care skills, functional language, socialization, recreation, and prevocational preparation. At levels of severe and profound retardation, functional academic skills are not anticipated, and emphasis will be on basic self-care: feeding, dressing, grooming, and toileting; acquiring some functional communication ability, verbal or nonverbal; and motor development (Myers, Sinco, & Stalma, 1973). There has also been recent interest in the teaching of some vocational skills to this population, and this is discussed in the next chapter. Appropriate educational programs for profoundly retarded individuals, especially at adolescent and adult levels, have been a source of controversy, and this is treated later in this chapter.

EDUCATION OF THE INTELLECT

A perennial goal of special education has been the provision of an educational experience adapted to the student's learning limitation. More recently, however, there have been attempts to alter these limitations. These efforts are intended to literally change the way in which the retarded person thinks—to seek to directly modify the cognitive deficits that are the essence of mental retardation.

Instrumental Enrichment

This is an educational method that is directed toward cognitive processes deemed to underlie logical thinking. Developed in Israel (Feuerstein, 1970), it was intended to address cognitive characteristics of immigrants from some non-Western cultures. These included a nonanalytical approach to problem solving; indifference to precision; impulsiveness; deficit in temporal, spatial, and verbal concepts; and difficulty in considering multiple sources of information at any one time (Narroc & Bachur, 1975). The last mentioned refers to dealing with complex problems in piecemeal fashion rather than in terms of multiple considerations. In Feuerstein's view, these characteristics were the consequence of inadequate exposure to "mediated learning experience" during the developmental years. The concept of mediated learning was discussed in Chapter 5 in connection with psychological factors in mental development. In "instrumental enrichment," the classroom teacher attempts to encourage a more analytic and logical problem-solving approach by functioning as the "mediator." She introduces concepts, provides verbal labels, stimulates discussion, and written exercises. The full program consists of 300 classroom hours offered over a 2-year period—3–4 hours per week.

The research evidence of the program's effectiveness is unclear. Some gains in spatial abilities and in arithmetic were reported for an Israeli population of adolescents and young adults (Feuerstein et al., 1979). These were individuals with IQs in either the borderline or mildly retarded range; we do not know its specific impact on the retarded population. A U.S. study found no significant IQ gains for several populations—educable mentally retarded, learning disabled, and behavior disordered (Haywood & Arbitman-Smith, 1979). Over a 1-year-period the educable group had increased its IQ of 69 to 76, but no specific gains were found on tests of analytic reasoning. As in the Israeli study, there was a significant gain in spatial abilities (10%) but none in arithmetic.

In evaluating the early evidence of the promise of this method, the investigators concluded that producing cognitive change in mildly retarded adolescents is possible but difficult. They add that the pace of instruction may need to be slowed.

Strategy Training

Interest in "strategy training" grew out of research on memory. The memory deficit of retarded individuals relative to normal ones was attributed to a failure to spontaneously employ the kinds of strategies that help us to remember (Anders, 1971; Ellis, 1963, 1968). Two such strategies are (1) simple repetition or *rehearsal* of what we are trying to recall and (2) *organizing* the material to be remembered according to a principle that reduces its complexity. For example, the four digits 1 9 2 6 can be reduced to two—19 26. Attempting to remember a series of discrete items can be eased if they lend themselves to a smaller number of categorical groupings. For example, the nine items apple, wagon, table, strawberry, car, chair, banana, bicycle, and desk are readily grouped into three categories—fruit, furniture, and vehicles. If we only remember the categories, we can then use their associations to recall all of the items covered by them.

Interest in strategy training also follows from of a view of man as an information-processing organism. It is thought that learning and recall are best understood in terms of the flow of information through perceptual and memory systems (Atkinson & Shiffrin, 1968, 1971; Bray, 1979). The "flow chart" for information involves a four-step sequence—sensory impression, encoding (usually verbal) of the sensory stimulus, storage of the encoded stimulus in short-term and then long-term memory, and then retrieval of the stored information on command. Let us illustrate the process. Suppose we go to a window, sit down, and close our eyes. Now we open our eyes, look out the window for an instant, and then close them again. Suppose in that instant we had seen a tree, the sensory impression. When we close our eyes, the visual image, its literal representation in our mind's eye, disappears in seconds (Neisser, 1967). But even as we saw the tree we were encoding the visual experience, usually with a verbal label, the words "a tree." The encoded experience "a tree" enters our short-term memory, and its subsequent fate depends on what we now do. If our attention turns to something else, the tree event is quickly forgotten; presumably most of our innumerable daily sensory experiences suffer this fate. On the other hand, if for some reason we decide that we want to remember what we have seen, or at least its verbal representation, we can perform mental actions such as using memory strategies that will have the effect of transferring the encoded event into our long-term memory. Once there, it is potentially available for future retrieval or recall.

Research suggests that there are no major differences between normal and retarded persons, at least those with mild retardation, in the first two stages. These are events that occur in a fraction of a second and are presumed to be beyond conscious control or training (Stanovich, 1978). It is the third phase of this process, the mental actions taken to aid retention, that is regarded as deficient in retarded persons—hence the focus on strategy training.

As has been stated, the memory difficulties of retarded individuals have been attributed to the lack of *spontaneous* employment of mnemonic strategies (Belmont & Butterfield, 1969). It has also been found that with specific training in the use of such strategies the differences between retarded and nonretarded populations were significantly diminished (Belmont & Butterfield, 1971; Brown, Campione, Bray, & Wilcox, 1973).

Following the demonstration of benefits of training, strategy research has taken several directions—more intensive training in specific strategies (e.g., Butterfield, Wambold, & Belmont, 1973), a view of retardation as a deficit in "planning"[2] (Brown, 1974), and attempts to generalize training effects. The need for generalization results from the finding that strategy use tends to be time- and situation-specific (Campione & Drawn, 1977). Although a specific strategy can be taught, the learner is at best likely to apply it *without prompting* only in situations very comparable to that in which it was learned. The learner has not understood the implications of what was learned or how to recognize new situations in which the skill could be employed. It is not knowledge per se that is seen as crucial to intelligent behavior but rather one's understanding of what one knows especially as this relates to solving any particular problem (Campione & Brown; Moore & Newell, 1974). Attempts to teach this kind of skill, "evaluation" in Guilford's "structure of intellect model" (Guilford, 1967), involves encouraging the examination of task requirements, relating these requirements to one's capacities (e.g. memory), selecting an appropriate strategy, and then monitoring or evaluating one's performance. (This illustrates the "planning" function in problem solving and the "metacomponents" in Sternberg's view of mental retardation presented in Chapter 1.)

While such "evaluation" can involve the most complex kinds of intellectual functions, some strategies are capable of use by cognitively impaired individuals. Thus a simple "stop-check-and-study" procedure was taught to educable children who were required to learn a list of items that could not be memorized at a single exposure (Brown & Barclay, 1976). The children were to study the items until they were sure that they could recall all of them, and they were taught strategies for accomplishing it. One of these was self-testing, the children learning to test themselves in order to determine whether continued study was necessary. Interestingly, the training not only led to much improved retention but, more significantly, was later generalized to a different task—the gist recall of prose passages (Brown, Campione, & Barclay, 1978).

Can retarded individuals learn to evaluate task demands, implement strategies, and monitor their own progress? Certainly the capacity to generalize or transfer a strategy requires recognition of the similarity between the trained and untrained task. This involves the same process as solving "similarities" problems on intelligence tests—for example, "In what way are a dog and a lion alike?" It requires abstracting from nonidentical conditions their underlying similarity.[3] This question also relates to the nature of mental retardation and to the apparently permanent differences in intellectual functioning between retarded and nonretarded persons at the end of the mental age growth period. It appears that the use of strategies is a developmental phenomenon. The normal 6- or 7-year-old is no more likely to use strategies than his retarded mental age counterpart. It is not until about age 9 that the normal youngster begins to *understand* and employ strategies. Neimark (1976) found age-related changes in memory strategies between ages 9

[2]Both "planning" and "generalizing" were referred to in Chapter 1 in connection with an information-processing view of mental retardation.

[3]The task also involves the essence of Spearman's view on the nature of intelligence as presented in Chapter 1. This was the "educing" or perceiving of relationships—deductive reasoning.

and 17. There was a decrease in talking aloud, note taking, and rote rehearsal and an increase in manipulation of material, self-testing, and categorization. All of this implies that the lack of *spontaneous "strategizing" in retarded youths and very limited evidence of generalization reflects their limited mental age development.* At best, only mildly retarded children achieve mental age scores of 9 and 10 years. Nevertheless, training does produce enhanced memory, and *some* generalization has been found. In the view of Borkowski and Cavanaugh (1979), attempts to train for generalization will be a major focus of future research in mental retardation. Their recipe for generalization calls for identifying multiple strategies, training in each including when and how they are to be applied, and encouraging self-generated task analysis.

BASIC SKILLS TRAINING FOR THOSE WITH PROFOUND RETARDATION

As programs for retarded persons have expanded, there has been an ever increasing awareness of their learning potential. The deinstitutionalization thrust has made it clear that hitherto institutionalized individuals could function in community settings. With growing recognition of the adaptive potential of this population and of the relationship of that potential to *access to services*, attention has necessarily shifted to that portion of the population that appears to be least amenable to education and training—those with profound retardation. Increasingly, it is this segment of the retarded population, often multiply handicapped, along with those with severe retardation who continue to reside in institutions (Scheerenberger, 1982). This is not to say that such persons cannot be served in the community. In the early 1970s, 73 percent of the population of California's day center population—ages 3–21—were severely or profoundly retarded (Levine et al., 1979). Nor were such programs serving only the least impaired of this population. More than one-third (37%) were nonambulatory (unable to walk even with assistance). Thus community programs were serving those with severe motor as well as cognitive impairment.

Effective Training Procedures

There are two elements essential to maximizing the adaptive potential of profoundly retarded individuals: (1) the physical nature of their living and learning environment, and (2) the use of systematic instructional procedures that also incorporate meaningful incentives (appropriate reinforcers).

MODIFYING THE PHYSICAL ENVIRONMENT AND TASK SIMPLIFICATION

The physical environment itself has two aspects—the material and objects that must be mastered (e.g., clothing in dressing and utensils in eating), and the physical setting in which training occurs. The reader cannot recall the difficulties of his own early childhood in acquiring basic self-care skills—feeding, dressing, and toileting—but they can be formidable challenges to those with extreme cognitive impairment, especially when this is also often combined with sensory and/or motor deficits (Payne, 1971).

SIMPLIFYING THE TASK

Roos (1965) described several simple procedures used to ease learning in a then-institutionalized population of severely and profoundly retarded persons. Color cues helped to discriminate between bathrooms, clothing was altered to produce larger head and arm holes, and spoons were modified to reduce spilling. We have earlier referred to "adapted" clothing and utensils in the chapter on preschool programs.

IMPROVING THE PHYSICAL ENVIRONMENT

With regard to the usual living and day room unit housing severely and profoundly retarded persons, there is speculation that its design may contribute to the chaotic and zoolike quality so often encountered, at least, in the past. Gorton and Hollis (1965) provide a vivid picture of the "before" and "after" of such a unit, and their suggestions about modifications are applicable to both day and residential settings (see Fig. 33).

The unit housed 18 profoundly retarded girls aged 6–12. Because of its original similarity to the usual institutional setting, the design is shown prior to and after alteration. The original unit (see Fig. 33) was divided into a sleeping and day area with separation achieved by a lattice divider. Cottage staff were located in a hallway *outside* the unit and could monitor the girls' activities only by leaving their desk. The furnishings of the dayroom consisted of a built-in bench and a television set. The bath had regular tubs and standard toilet fixtures.

The description of the residents before unit alteration is one that is familiar to visitors to "back wards" of institutions for the retarded. It more than justifies public outcry and judicial intervention.

> None of the girls could dress themselves, . . . a few could feed themselves and were toilet trained. The girls manifested such behavior as: minimal response to stimuli, lying on the floor . . . , stereotypies, preoccupation with minutiae, smearing of feces, masturbation, overt aggression, and self-destructive biting, scratching, hair-pulling, and head banging. [The only omission in the description is of the smell.]
>
> It was noted that aides tended to attach great importance to housekeeping tasks and to paper work [preference for nonresident-oriented activities!]. Contact between the aides and the girls which would serve to stimulate learning and social interaction was minimal. For the most part, the aides attended to girls who were in imminent danger from self-destructive acts, . . . overtly aggressive, . . . objects of aggressive acts, . . . had soiled themselves, or . . . who tore or otherwise were destroying their clothing [note that attention was primarily given for undesirable behavior]. Bathing the girls appeared to

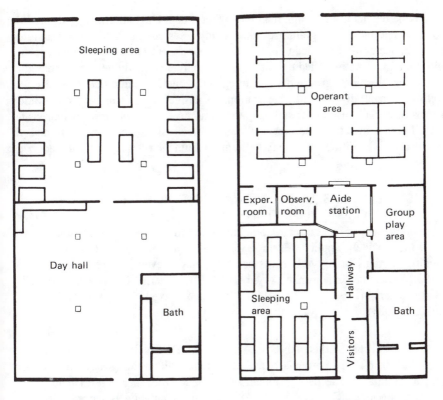

Before modification   After modification

FIG. 33 Cottage unit for severely retarded persons before and after redesign. After Gorton and Hollis (1965).

be a problem . . . [apparently due to the time and effort involved]. In many cases girls had to be lifted in and out of the tub. [This] task which required the aid to stoop and bend was further complicated by the girls who feared the water.

Attempts to toilet train . . . had met with little success. Many cried and struggled when placed on the toilet. The standard size [toilet], open front seat, which did not provide adequate support for some, was an invitation to others to play in the water. The height of the fixture was such that the feet of many . . . could not rest on the floor . . . *the aides resorted to diapering the girls rather than attempting to toilet train them* [and so inadvertently assured that they never would be trained!] (emphasis added).

In considering the horrendous conditions in the unit, it was thought that the limited interest of the aides in attempts at training and interaction might be due to inappropriate physical facilities and to the absence of any formal training program.

It became the goal to redesign the unit so that it could be better managed, provide for training, and the program itself objectively assessed. The result was a unit that was architecturally modified to provide seven areas, each of which fulfills a particular function. The modified unit has a large subdivided "activities" area and other areas for sleeping, group play, bathing and toileting (modified bathtubs and toilets), a centrally located aide station, experimental training and observation rooms (especially useful for staff or parent training), and a place for parent visitation. For the first time the unit also had control of its own temperature and air circulation. Conditions essential to a more humanized environment had been created.

SYSTEMATIC SELF–HELP TRAINING THROUGH BEHAVIOR MODIFICATION

In no area of mental retardation have the principles of behavior modification been more widely applied. From reviews of related research it is evident that significant gains in *self-help* skills can be achieved even in profoundly retarded adults (Berkson & Landesman-Dwyer, 1977; J. Gardner, 1969; W. Gardner, 1973; Nawas & Braun, 1970a, 1970b, 1970c; Watson & Uzzell, 1981; Whitman, Stibak, & Reid, 1983).

SELF-HELP SKILLS AND PLACE OF RESIDENCE

Self-help skills, particularly ambulation and toilet training, have been important in facilitating the deinstitutionalization of retarded persons (Windle, 1962; Eyman, Tarjan, & Cassady, 1970). Of the two, ambulation is the more critical, although, as just noted, more than one-third of the California day center population were nonambulatory. Gains in toileting ability appear to be more easily achieved than those in ambulation, and the likelihood of major gain in mobility for those who are not walking by age 5 is poor (Eyman, Silverstein, & McLain, 1975). In the material that follows, programs are described that report effecting significant gains in each of these self-help domains as well as in the related ones of dressing and eating. In the description of the programs we will see ample use of such behavioral techniques as task analysis, successive approximation, chaining, and reinforcement.

Motor Skills

Utilizing sensorimotor activities originally designed to promote body image, laterality, and directionality (Kephart, 1960), training over a 3-year period of a group of 16 children, predominantly under age 6, resulted in full ambulation in 12 of them. Of these, 5 had been nonambulatory at the program's inception (Eyman et al., 1975). All of those who were only partially ambulatory (walking only when assisted) or who were unsteady in their walking were ultimately able to walk independently and without difficulty. Though the program of training is not described, it is presumed that the activities were comparable to those earlier employed with a group of severely retarded 5-year-olds (Edgar, Ball, McIntyre, &

Shotwell, 1969). These included the use of mattress walking for those unable to maintain balance, and walking and balance boards.

Toilet Training

A large study of an institutionalized series revealed that, with only routine scheduling of toileting, from one-half to nearly two-thirds of those with IQs of less than 30 achieved independent toilet usage (Eyman, Tarjan, & Cassady, 1970; Lohman; Eyman, & Lask, 1967). Delay in the age at which training was achieved was characteristic; it was not until age 12 that the rate reached 50 percent. In contrast, of those with IQs greater than 30, 71 percent were fully trained by age 12, and virtually all were fully trained thereafter.

Within the profoundly retarded group itself, 63 percent were fully trained (using toilet independently), 6 percent were "partially trained" (used toilet when taken), but 31 percent remained untrained (Lohman, Eyman, & Lask, 1967). The totally untrained segment appears to have been the most profoundly retarded, IQs of 10 and under, and with disturbed behavior and medical problems. Presumably, a number were nonambulatory as well.

SPECIAL TRAINING AIDS

In Chapter 7 a toilet-training method was presented appropriate to the preschool-age retarded child. It consisted of placing them on the commode at appropriate intervals and rewarding its use. For profoundly retarded individuals at whatever age, however, there are additional aids that can be employed—automated signal devices and use of penalties as well as rewards.

Automated Signal Devices

Two kinds of signaling devices are found—either worn by the trainee or placed in the commode. They are moisture-sensitive and produce an auditory signal when either urination of defecation has occurred. Worn by the trainee (See Fig. 34), so-called "wet-alarm pants" alert both staff and wearer to the onset of voiding and cause its interruption and subsequent movement of the trainee to the toilet. Its special advantage is to free caretakers of more or less continuous monitoring of the trainee; attention is called to the person only when it is necessary. The signaling device in the commode works similarly and permits prompt reinforcement. This makes continuous monitoring while on the toilet unnecessary and eliminates the need for "visual inspection."

Reinforcement and Punishment

The original toilet-training model limited its incentives to rewards (Ellis, 1963b). While positive reinforcement may indeed increase toilet use (Hudziak et al., 1965; Spencer et al., 1968), it does not necessarily do away with incontinence; it is only that the toilet is used more frequently! But the purpose of training is to limit excretory behavior to the toilet, and the addition of aversive consequences is likely to hasten its achievement. Penalties have included not changing wet clothes immediately (Smith, 1979; Waye & Melnyr, 1973), verbal reprimand (Azrin &

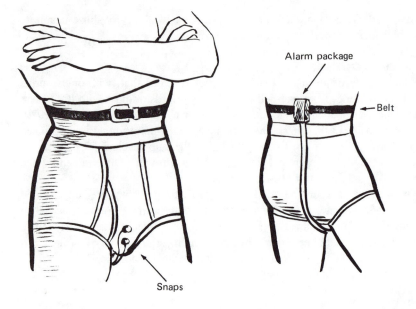

Front view   Rear view

FIG. 34   Alarm pants apparatus. The pants are seen from front and back. Moisture-sensitive snaps are shown in front; the back shows wires leading to the "alarm package." Regular clothing is worn over the training pants and a tone sounds when either urine or feces moisten the area between the snaps. From Azrin and Foxx (1971).

Foxx, 1971; Smith et al., 1975), denial of a preferred activity (Luiselli, 1977), and time out (Ando, 1977; Azrin & Foxx, 1971; Bettinson et al., 1976; Doleys & Arnold, 1975; Smith et al., 1975; Trott, 1977).

RAPID DAYTIME BLADDER TRAINING

Children

Utilizing an auditory signaling device, Van Wagenen et al. (1969) bladder-trained eight formerly incontinent children aged 5–9. Most had no speech but could follow directions. At the onset of voiding, an alarm signal was emitted at which the trainer called "Stop!" and then led the child to the toilet. The combination of a startle produced by the alarm and gesturing by the trainer is reported to have interrupted urination. Once on the toilet, resumption of voiding was encouraged by a gentle stroking of the back. Under this regimen, all children were using the toilet on their own within 3 weeks.

Training included the teaching of related dressing skills and was conducted with three children at a time for 4 hours a day. The trainees were *always* within easy reach of the bathroom. To hasten the learning of the association between voiding and the commode, the frequency of urination was increased by continually offering the children as much water as they would take. During the early phase of training the alarm device was worn continuously, and this meant that the tone also sounded when the child was actually using the toilet. Here, of course, the trainer reacted to the sound with expressions of approval!

A subsequent modification of this procedure involved teaching the association between bath alarm and commode approach and undressing *prior* to actual toilet use. This allowed for intensive practice of the activity unrelated to the frequency of voiding itself (Mahoney et al., 1971).

Adults

A somewhat more complex program, developed by Azrin and Foxx (1971), is reported to have effected rapid and dramatic gains in toilet usage by long-time incontinent adults. Like that of Van Wagenen et al., (1969), the procedure included an auditory signal device, encouragement of high fluid intake, and the teaching of related dressing skills. Its major difference was in the handling of accidents. In the Van Wagenen program there were no consequences for accidents; in Azrin and Foxx, an overcorrection procedure was employed.

Caution is needed in encouraging high fluid intake. So-called "overhydration" can produce serious medical problems (Thompson & Manson, 1983). A guide that relates fluid intake to age and weight is offered by Weisberg (1982).

Under Azrin and Foxx, training was even more intensive; it was conducted on an 8-hour basis and, again, close to a bathroom. When an accident occurred, the trainee's pants alarm was disconnected and an overcorrection procedure called "full cleanliness training" followed. The trainee had to undress, shower, and then dress. He was required to clean any soiled area and then to hand-wash his soiled pants, wring them out and hang them up to dry. Finally, there was a subsequent 1-hour time-out period, denial of access to one's usual chair, and mealtime was delayed! Within one week, accidents had fallen from an average of nearly two per day to only about one every fourth day. Moreover, continence was maintained after training had ended. Noteworthy was the observation that a 90 percent reduction in daytime accidents did not affect nighttime control. The effects of training were specific to the conditions under which they occurred, a phenomenon that is again encountered in the management of behavior problems, the subject of the last chapter.

Subsequent employment of the Azrin and Foxx procedure and its later version (Foxx & Azrin, 1973a) by others serves to confirm its effectiveness (Bettison et al., 1976; Murphy & Zahn, 1975; Sadler & Merkert, 1977; Smith et al., 1975; Smith, 1979). An 80–90 percent reduction in accidents accompanies training, though some regression usually occurs at its cessation. Periodic restoration of training contingencies should quickly restore the earlier rate.

NIGHTTIME TRAINING

Several programs have been used—traditional "home" type nighttime training, the use of bed-wetting alarms, and an Azrin et al. (1973a) adaptation of their daytime method.

Traditional

This involves the reduction of fluid intake in the evening (e.g., none within $1\frac{1}{2}$ hours of bedtime), toileting prior to bedtime, awakening about $1\frac{1}{2}$ hours after bedtime, and then periodic checking. Once a time pattern of accidents has been determined, the trainee is awakened prior to the time of bed-wetting and sent to the toilet for at least 5 minutes. Sleep intervals should be gradually lengthened so as to increase bladder retention, and dryness should be reinforced (Fredericks et al., 1975; Linford et al., 1972).

Bed-wetting Signal

Bed-wetting alarm devices have long been used to treat enuresis, and some success has been reported with moderately and severely retarded individuals, though relapse is common (Sloop & Kennedy, 1973).

Nighttime Training Adaptation

Adapting their daytime program to nighttime, Azrin et al. (1973a) reported a 95 percent decrease, or virtually total nighttime continence, within 5 weeks in a group of 13 profoundly retarded individuals. There was no relapse during a 3-month follow-up. As in daytime training, they used a urine alarm signal and overcorrection.

Contrary to the traditional approach of reducing nighttime fluid intake, they *encouraged* fluid consumption before bedtime, presumably to increase the frequency of voiding pressure and the consequent number of potential learning experiences involving the alarm signal and bladder control. The urine alarm was placed in the bed, and a "potty alert" was put in the commode. The trainee was awakened hourly and placed on the toilet for up to 5 minutes. If no urination occurred, the trainee was offered more fluid and returned to bed. Accidents were followed by disconnection of the urine alarm, a verbal reprimand, requirement to change the linen, and then repeated practice of lying down for 3 minutes and being returned to the toilet. This sequence of toilet visitations would continue for 30 minutes, so it was not until about 45 minutes after an accident that the trainee was allowed to return to sleep for at least an hour. Though initially employed with an institutionalized population, a modification of it has been used in the home (Bollard & Woodroffe, 1977). (Was it initially employed by the Spanish Inquisition!)

Dressing and Grooming Skills

Literature review indicates that systematic instructional methods have been used to teach a wide range of dressing and grooming skills to persons with severe and profound retardation (Berkson & Landesman-Dwyer, 1977; Snell, 1978; Watson & Uzzell, 1981). The technique of *backward chaining* was illustrated in the prior chapter. It is reported to be an easily learned and effective method (Watson & Uzzell, 1981), one for which parent training materials have been developed (Baker et al., 1976; Devore, 1977; Watson & Bassinger, 1974). *Forward chaining*, the teaching of dressing-related movements in their natural sequence, is said to work well with trainees who can follow verbal directions (Watson, 1978) but to be less useful with those who are profoundly retarded. Whether employed in conjunction with either backward or forward chaining, the technique of "graduated guidance" is particularly appropriate to the teaching of skills that require physical prompting. It involves the physical guidance of the trainee through the act being taught and its gradual replacement with verbal and gestural cues as the skill is acquired. It is illustrated in the dressing and dining programs developed by Azrin and his colleagues. These have the Azrin stamp of rapid learning through massed trials.

RAPID DRESSING TRAINING

A group of seven profoundly retarded adults were taught independent dressing within 20 hours. Instruction was conducted in 2- to 3-hour training periods and began with the teaching of undressing before dressing. Training was done "forward" fashion and was based on manual guidance and, through it, the prevention of error. The procedure was as follows:

Position

Trainee seated to prevent unsteadiness. *Hands*: Both of the trainee's hands were used to prevent interfering movements with the usually nonutilized hand (e.g., stereotypy). *Clothing taught*: Underpants, shoes, socks, pants, and shirt; all were slip-on type and without laces, buttons, zippers, belts, or snaps in order to ease mastery. *Clothing size*: Training began with clothing two sizes too large. *Sequence*: First taught to undress in sequence—removal of shoes, socks, pants, underpants, and shirt (shirt was the most difficult). Trainers (2 were used) then dressed the trainee for the next undressing trial. *Session length*: 2–3 hours. *Prompts*: In sequence—verbal, gestural, and manual (graduated guidance).

> Gentle manual guidance was used . . . in the early stages of training. The trainer's hands were molded around the student's hands but not touching the . . . clothing. *A student who resisted guidance was never forced and guidance began again when the student was relaxed.* The trainer's touch was lightened as the student began to respond more on his own . . . near the end of training, the trainer did not maintain touch contact all the time, rather he lightly and momentarily touched the student's hands only when he was not responding . . . or when he had difficulty.

Learning Difficulties

For a garment hard to put on, such as a shirt, intensive training on just that garment alternated with training in the full sequence. Appropriate reinforcers were determined through interviews with caretakers. Short-duration reinforcers (e.g., snacks) were given after each garment was put on or removed; reinforcers that involved longer time periods were given at the end of each undressing-dressing sequence. Noninterruptive reinforcers such as praise and back stroking (tactile stimulation) were given continuously.

An attempt to use this procedure with children indicated the need for some modification. Food "finickiness" limited the use of snack treats, and children were more prone to temper tantrums.

WASHING AND DRYING HANDS AND FACE

Treffry et al. (1970) taught 11 profoundly retarded girls, ages 10–20, to wash and dry their hands and faces. The girls all tested below IQ 30 but could follow simple directions and had no major motor impairments of the hands and arms. The task was broken down into 11 steps (see Table 26), and prior to training none of the girls could perform all steps without assistance. Gains were most rapid during the first 3 weeks, and by the ninth week, seven of the 11 girls were able to wash and dry themselves completely when instructed to do so, though some needed occasional reminding. Training was conducted after each meal, with up to 15 minutes spent on teaching each step. Learning was encouraged by the use of praise and candy, and failure to follow directions resulted in a sharp "No!" and a 15-second period during which the girl was totally ignored. Aggressive forms of resistance such as throwing soap or bothering other girls led to a sharp slap on the fingers. (We report this, although our reservations about physical punishment have been continuously noted.) In teaching each new step, the trainer first told the girl what to do while simultaneously guiding her through it. Over several trials the physical guidance was gradually eliminated until the step was performed with only verbal prompts (fading). The criterion for mastery of any single step was 10 correct responses, presumably consecutive ones. As each step was achieved it was added to the chain of previously mastered ones with reward then limited to completion of the total chain to that point.

ATTENTION SPAN

Teaching any task clearly depends on getting and holding the attention of the learner, and problems of attention span are particularly acute in this population.

TABLE 26   Training Steps in Washing and Drying Face and Hands

Training steps (backward chaining)	Observations
1. Drying face	Steps 1–9 had to be broken down into smaller
2. Drying hands	components. Step 9, for example, consisted of
3. Rinsing soap from face	turning on the hot water tap, turning off the hot
4. Rinsing soap from hands	water tap, turning on the cold water tap, and
5. Washing face with cloth and soap	turning off the cold water tap (forward chaining
6. Wetting face with cloth	is appropriate in this step).
7. Washing hands with cloth and soap	
8. Wetting hands with cloth	
9. Placing water in the sink	
10. Placing the plug in the sink	
11. Pointing to cold water tap on command	

Source: Treffry et al. (1970).

They must be worked with before actually beginning skill instruction. Attention-span training consisted of teaching the girls to pay attention to an item of clothing (dressing skills were to be taught) by rewarding their attention with candy. At first it was the candy itself to which attention was addressed. The candy was held in front of the trainee at eye level until it was attended to for 3 seconds; she was then praised and given it. Over a number off trials, the attention period required for reinforcement was gradually increased to 15 seconds. The next step was to intro-duce the clothing item and hold it next to the candy. The girl was required to attend to both clothing and candy for 10 seconds and then to name it (pointing to it would serve the same purpose in nonspeaking individuals). When this was accomplished, the clothing and candy were gradually shifted from eye level to a table top. At the conclusion of this procedure the girl had learned to attend for a least a brief period and could also follow the trainer as directions were given with regard to various parts (e.g., pointing to a tag on the inside of a sweater).

Training in dressing skills usually involved work with only one piece of clothing at a time, and success was defined in terms of three consecutive correct responses. The sessions were conducted on a one-to-one basis and ran from 15 to 30 minutes each. The trainers were regular aides who had previously had a 30-hour in-service course on behavior modification. As in the teaching of "washing and drying hands and face," the individual steps are shown because of their actual use in the training of severely and profoundly retarded individuals.

PUTTING ON A SWEATER

The instructions for this task were given in forward chaining order and are left in that fashion, although they have been somewhat modified.

1. *Identifying inside and outside of sweater.* The sweater is placed on a table *inside out*, making the seams visible. The seams are felt as well as pointed out (tactile cue) and identified as "bad side." When the trainee has learned to make this discrimination, the actual task of learning to put on a sweater is begun. This was the most difficult step in the chain. Presumably the task begins in this fashion because of easy reversibility in sweater removal.

2. *Turning the sweater right side out.* The sweater is again presented inside out, and the trainee is expected to recognize this, either verbally or by gesture. Having identified the side correctly, the trainee is then taught to turn the sweater to the "good side" by (1) picking it up at the bottom, (2) placing hands in the sleeves, and (3) pulling both hands and sleeves out back through the bottom.

3. *Proper positioning of tag.* The tag at the base of the head hole is used to discriminate the front and back of the sweater (like "inside" and "outside," this is another discrimination that we take for granted). Since the tag is always at the base of the head hole, the trainee must merely learn that tag bottom is "good" and tag top is "bad."

4. *Pulling sweater overhead.*

5. *Placing arms in sleeves.*

6. *Pulling down sweater.*

LACING AND TYING SHOES

Lacing and tying were first taught with a shoe that is not on the trainee's foot but rather on a table with its front facing away from the trainee as it would be on the foot. Teaching with a shoe on the foot was only undertaken after lacing and tying were mastered with the shoe on the table. The directions are presented in backward chaining order, and a different method is shown for completing the more difficult part of making a bow knot. The trainee begins with the shoe completely laced except for the last eyelet. Tying a bow know is based on learning the simple crossover knot. The bow knot is a variant of the latter. Because of the reverse order of teaching, the worker should first make simple one-loop knots and observe the sequence of movements. The sequence accords with the instructions, beginning at step 5 and proceeding to step 1.

Simple Knot

1. Ends of laces are pulled to make simple crossover knot.
2. Trainee's left hand is guided to grab the laces where they form a loop, and then the right hand puts the top lace (left lace) around and through the loop from under.
3. The left end of the lace is placed across the right.
4. The right end of the lace is placed on the table and points straight out and away from the trainee.

Bow Knot

1. Pull loops apart, reducing hole and tightening knot.
2. Bend right loop through the hole under the crossover and push through.
3. Cross over loops in exactly the same way as making the simple knot—left loop across right loop.
4. Form small loops with the ends of each lace.
5. Make simple knot.

The dressing skills described thus far are familiar to all of us; of particular interest are two training regimens that relate to more specialized skills—putting on a brassiere and tending to personal hygiene.

PUTTING ON A BRASSIERE (FORWARD ORDER)

1. The girl is first helped to put the bra around her waist so that the shoulder straps hang down behind her (inside out, upside down, and backwards). This makes it easy for her to hook the fastener, which is now at her midsection. During this step the girl is guided to find the name tag sewn inside the backstrap and to place the bra so that the tag is on her right ribs and facing outward. She is then helped to reach around behind her back with the left hand and to grasp the free end of the bra.
2. The trainee is taught to hook the fastener.

3. The girl is guided to turn the bra to the correct position so that the fastener is at her back, though the bra is still upside down and inside out.
4. The girl is taught to place her hand through the shoulder straps and to pull them over her shoulders. This turns the bra right side up and out.

FEMININE HYGIENE

Current methods for managing menstruation involve adhesive strips, sanitary belt and pad, and Tampax. Of the three, adhesive strips appear to be the easiest to use.

Teaching involves a simple two-choice discrimination of the sticky side to panties, wrapping of a used napkin, and its disposal. Training in its use need not await menstrual periods, and coloring can be used to simulate bleeding. Of particular importance is the need to teach individuals that menstruation occurs in all women and that menstrual blood is meant to be lost, unlike bleeding following an injury (Bender & Valetutti, 1976). Educational materials may be obtained from product manufacturers.

OTHER GROOMING SKILLS

Training programs have been developed for the entire range of grooming skills. Examples include tooth brushing and dental hygiene (Abramson & Wunderlich, 1972; Horner et al., 1975), complexion care (Keilitz et al., 1975), use of deodorant (Lewis et al., 1975), and even nose blowing (Ingethron et al., 1975). Comprehensive training materials are found in such sources as in Wehman (1979), Bender and Valletutti (1976), Snell (1978), Mori and Masters (1980), and in a manual of programs developed by an institution (Wheeler et al., 1977).

Eating and Cooking Skills

Grossly inappropriate eating habits are often seen in retardation—using fingers instead of utensils, oversized bites, eating too fast, taking another's food, and throwing food and utensils. The persistence of such clearly unacceptable dining behavior has been attributed to ineffective instruction and inadequate motivation (O'Brien, Bugle, & Azrin, 1972). It is clear that such behavior is alterable, and training has typically incorporated the use of manual guidance ("graduated guidance") and the penalizing of inappropriate behavior with temporary interruption of eating. Interruption has taken various forms: physical restraint of the diner's hands (Henrickson & Doughty, 1967), removal of a food tray for at least 10 seconds (Groves & Carrocio, 1971), movement of the diner's hands back from the table for at least 15 seconds (Martin, McDonald, & Omichinski, 1971), and termination of the meal and removal from the dining room (Edwards & Lilly, 1966).

PECULIAR EATING HABITS

One also sees, particularly in children, extraordinarily narrow food preferences; the child has become accustomed to particular foods and rejects all others. The author has observed such preferences in blind retarded children who at 8 and 9· years of age were still accepting only baby food. When they were placed in a setting where other foods were offered, they rebelled and refused to eat. Fingado et al. (1970) describe a retarded child who would eat only certain kinds of strained baby foods and drink only one brand of chocolate milk. This youngster was admitted to an institution on a 30-day basis for the treatment of this eating pattern. He was offered only normal foods, and, after an initial period of rejection, he accepted them. At the end of the 30-day period he was eating all foods without hesitation. It is clear that the parents of this child had allowed the problem to persist and inadvertently made the problem worse by being unwilling to accept the upset necessary to change it. Of course, they could not know for how long the child would "fuss" and go hungry.

RAPID MEALTIME TRAINING

In reviewing earlier work, Azrin and Armstrong (1971) saw the need for a procedure that would achieve rapid results and reach hitherto recalcitrant trainees. They developed a program that, within 2 weeks, is purported to have enabled a group of profoundly retarded adults to eat in a socially appropriate manner. The chief features of the training were "minimeals," graduated manual guidance, and overcorrection. Its elements are as follows. *Minimeals*: Regular meals are divided into smaller portions and are served throughout the day. The effect is to increase the training period beyond that ordinarily limited to mealtime. *Graduated guidance*: As described in the section on "Rapid Dressing Training". *One food—one utensil*: During any one meal use only one utensil. *Hand in lap*: The hand not being used is kept in the lap; this prevents food-grabbing. A feeding trial does not begin until the hand is placed in the lap voluntarily or no resistance is shown to trainer's gentle restraint of the hand. *No incorrect responses*: Attempts to use fingers instead of the utensil are physically prevented. *No distractions*: Training is conducted in the dining room but *not* during regular mealtimes. *Reinforcers*: Verbal praise and rubbing of shoulders and back (tactual). *Correction of errors*: Once reasonable proficiency has been demonstrated with the spoon (and, presumably the fork), spilling errors are required to be cleaned by the trainee ("restitutional overcorrection"). Similarly, the trainee is required to clean up any mess created by throwing of food or utensils. *Positive practice*: Following correction for errors (e.g., spoon spilling because of overloading), the student is given several trials of loading very small amounts of food. *Multiple trainers*: Two trainers were used on the first day and until the trainee could be managed by one. One trainee guides the utensil hand while the other restrains the lap hand and controls the head posture. *Simple to complex*: Training begins with relatively simple skills—drinking from a glass and using a spoon—and gradually progresses to fork and knife. Though each minimeal focuses on a single utensil, over the course of a day there is exposure to all utensils.

> Eating skills were taught in the following sequence . . . (1) napkin, (2) glass, (3) spoon, and (4) fork were taught by guiding the student to hold the utensil in the correct manner and then perform the appropriate

action . . . wiping, drinking, scooping, or piercing; (5) holding . . . knife correctly for transferring butter from . . . butter dish to . . . bread; then spreading . . . butter; and (6) cutting meat with knife and fork . . . dividing the complex behaviors into smaller units. *Buttering* The student was taught to pick up the knife, load it. . . , then direct . . . butter to a *pre-cut bite-sized piece of bread*. At first, any attempt to touch the butter to the bread was followed by a bite ("successive approximation" and "reinforcement"), then progressively more spreading was required. Finally, the whole bread slice was introduced. *Cutting* First the student was taught to pierce and immediately eat *pre-cut, bite-sized pieces of meat* with fork tines facing down. Then the student pierced and ate these bites as they were cut by the trainer. The student was then taught to pick up the knife . . . each approximation to a sawing motion was completed by the trainer who immediately gave the cut piece to the student. Gradually more pressure for sawing was required . . . until he could separate the meat himself. The student ate "continental" style (fork remaining in left hand for right handers).

The criterion for successful completion of training was three consecutive correct performances of the skill being trained and not more than three errors in a standard test meal. This consisted of a commercial TV Dinner and was served at noon, when it was felt that the trainee could meet the test meal criterion. The transfer of these skills and their maintenance in the regular dining room required some continued supervision and overcorrection for inappropriate behavior.

COOKING SKILLS

Training in meal preparation has generally been limited to those with not more than moderate retardation (Kaman, 1974; Steed, 1974), though picture recipe cards have been developed for those with severe retardation (Robinson-Wilson, 1976). A pictorial approach to meal preparation is described by Spellman et al. (1978) that includes suggestions for teaching through pictures meal planning, shopping, food preparation, and cooking. It also includes picture instruction in general housekeeping skills. One group of workers actually sought to develop "independent cooking skills" in a profoundly retarded woman (Schleien et al., 1981). The student was a 28-year-old woman attending a day program and living at home. Three skills were taught—boiling an egg, broiling an English muffin and cheese, and preparing a TV Dinner. The targeted activities each represented a different use of a kitchen stove and thus had the potential for teaching skills that could be applied to other similarly prepared food. "Boiling" requires use of the top stove burner; broiling the English muffin and cheese, the oven broiler; and the TV Dinner, the baking oven. The program is described in some detail because it illustrates the kind of instructional aids that can be employed to teach skills to individuals that were hitherto thought to be beyond their reach. Perhaps most remarkable was that the trainee had epilepsy and actually had some seizures during the course of training! One of the trainers was always in close proximity to her so that danger of seizure-related kitchen accidents was minimized.

Skill Sequence
Chosen on the basis of the presumed order of difficulty, from least to most, were boiling of egg, broiling of muffin, and baking of TV Dinner. Each skill was task analyzed and taught in natural sequence, and five trials were given for each targeted step.

Teaching Method
Instructions, in sequence, began with a *verbal* cue. This was followed by trainer *modeling* if the response was inadequate, and, if this was unsuccessful, manual guidance. Training was conducted 4–5 days a week for 15 minutes in the late-morning prelunch time. The training period was tied to a mealtime but, presumably, could have been extended to nonmealtimes à la Azrin and Armstrong (1973).

Teaching Materials
The materials employed, the special adaptation of equipment, and the use of color codes to circumvent reading problems are of particular interest. They are indicated in Table 27.

Results
All three skills were learned and were able to be transferred to comparable equipment in another day center and the home. She was also able to generalize boiling and baking in connection with a cooking packet and pizza. Interestingly, generalization of broiling hot dogs was at least initially a problem, because they were typically boiled in her home.

RECREATIONAL AND LEISURE TIME ACTIVITIES
The need for recreational skills and outlets in retarded youths and adults is no less than in nonhandicapped individuals. Indeed, the inability to make constructive use of leisure time is often a source of behavioral difficulty in adolescence and adulthood (Blum, 1967; Denny, 1965). We tend to equate recreation with leisure time and fun, but it is also an important medium for skill development—*learning* through fun—and for enhancing feelings of self-worth (Carlson & Ginglend, 1961, 1968; Fait, 1967; Freeman & Mundy, 1971; Pomeroy, 1964; Wehman, 1977). And while participation in the Special Olympics does not assure developmental growth (Bell et al., 1977), it certainly does offer children and youths opportunities for mastery and increased self worth. At a more adult level, Fitzimmon's (1970) description of a bowling program offers a beautiful example of how an activity that is inherently pleasurable can also contribute to personal growth. It will be presented shortly.

TABLE 27   Materials and Special Adaptations for Three Cooking Skills

Skill	Materials/equipment	Modification
Boil egg	Egg	Hard-boiled egg to prevent breakage
	Saucepan full of boiling water	Place egg into empty saucepan; then fill with water
	Water	
	Stove: top stove burner	Color-coded dial and burner, cover extraneous dials with placemats to facilitate matching to sample.
	Kitchen timer	Red tape strip to mark appropriate calibrations
	Spoon	Slotted spoon to prevent scalding, easier to recover egg
	Bowl	Extra-large plastic salad bowl to prevent breakage, simplify accuracy
Broil English muffin and cheese	English muffin	
	Cheese slice	Presliced American cheese
	Aluminum foil	Pie pan to simplify manipulation of muffin
	Stove: broiler	Color-coded dial and broiler door; cover extraneous dials with placemats
	Kitchen timer	Red tape strip
	Pot holder	Gloved pot holder to ensure more complete safety
Bake TV Dinner	TV Dinner	Empty TV Dinner tray covered with aluminum foil (economically feasible)
	Stove: oven	Color-coded dial and over door; cover extraneous dials with placemats
	Kitchen timer	Red tape strip
	Pot holder	Gloved pot holder

Source: Reprinted from Schleien et al. (1981).

Recreational Interests of Retarded Persons

The recreational interests of retarded persons will reflect the activities to which they have been exposed and their general level of cognitive, motor, and social maturity. Activities employed will usually reflect developmental levels that are intermediate between mental age and chronological age. This is particularly characteristic of mildly retarded individuals. A 16-year-old youth with a mental age of 10 years, IQ 60, could have recreational interests that more closely approximate those of a teenager than those of a preadolescent 10-year-old. As the degree of retardation increases, recreational interests appear to parallel mental age more closely.

ENCOURAGING CHRONOLOGICAL AGE–APPROPRIATE ACTIVITIES

Especially at the severer levels of impairment one observes interests that are more typical of younger persons. But recognizing the immaturity imposed by the cognitive deficit does not mean that only activities engaged in by nonhandicapped younger persons of that developmental level are appropriate. The aim of "normalization" is to provide experiences that enhance the image of the devalued individual, and the challenge here is to find recreational activities that are both within his ken and not demeaning. Adults rolling balls across the floor at each other is incongruous, but a similar activity can be conducted in age-appropriate fashion through bowling. Wehman et al. (1980) show how through the modification of standard recreational equipment even severely physically handicapped individuals can participate in age-appropriate activities (e.g., bowling, picture taking, fishing, etc.).

INSTRUCTIONAL GUIDELINES

Recreators will note that many retarded individuals do not *spontaneously* use recreational materials. The materials need to be introduced, and their use has to be demonstrated. The lack of spontaneous play has been partly attributed to a greater difficulty in learning through observation and imitation (Carlson & Ginglend, 1961). Apart from the need for recreators to take an active role in getting the retarded person to participate, the recreator will need to (a) to recognize a shorter attention span and a need to vary what is being presented, (b) to break up an activity into its simplest elements, (c) to demonstrate precisely what is expected, (d) to practice each component with greater than usual frequency, (e) to encourage and praise or otherwise reward at each step, and (f) only *gradually* to introduce more complex elements or chains of activities.

DEMONSTRATION

In teaching recreational skills stress is placed on demonstration and physical guidance, because retarded individuals, like the rest of us, learn best by doing—only more so! Since much recreation is motor in nature, it is natural that demonstration and doing take precedence over verbal instruction. The special difficulty of retarded persons in understanding at only the verbal level makes teaching through doing particularly essential.

RECREATIONAL ADAPTATIONS

Adaptations or modifications of standard recreational activities are most likely to be necessary for individuals with more than mild retardation. Four types of adaptations are described: equipment, rules, skill sequences, and architectural (Wehman, Schleien, & Kiernan, 1980).

Equipment

Returning to our bowling example, equipment can be modified to enable persons to bowl who have major physical limitations. Figure 35 shows three

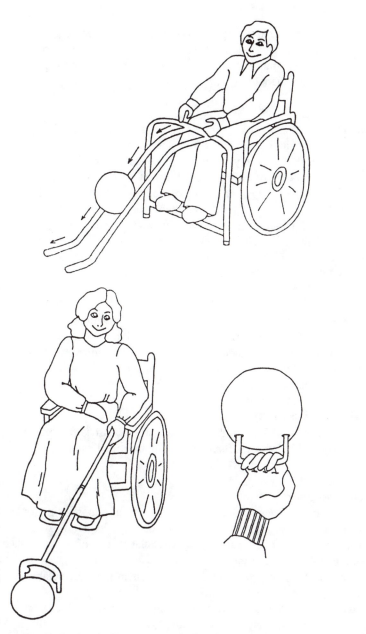

FIG. 35   "Adaptive" equipment for bowling. From Wehman et al. (1980).

equipment adaptations: a bowling "ramp," a ball "pusher," and a "gripper." In the last named, a handle snaps back flush into the ball, allowing it to roll to the pins.

Rules
Where physical and/or cognitive impairments affect the capacity to adhere to the standard rules for any activity, modification is in order. The essence of rule changing is to create the opportunity for the handicapped person to participate at whatever level possible and then to try to move toward approximation to the standard.

Skill Sequences
The order with which individual steps in a skill sequence are taught may benefit from alteration. For the severely handicapped person interested in learning some cooking skills, the process of boiling an egg might be reversed. Instead of requiring the student to place an egg into a pot of boiling water, the egg might more safely be placed in a pot of cold water and then later boiled. An interesting modification is suggested for picture taking. Usually we raise our camera to eye level, sight, and then depress the shutter release. Individuals with problems of motor coordination could be trained to position their finger over the release mechanism prior to raising the camera (Wehman et al., 1980).

Architectural
Architectural barriers to the use of community accommodations are gradually diminishing. Wheelchair ramps permitting access to public buildings are now common, and other modifications include enlarged doorknobs and extended handles on drinking fountains. Suggestions are also offered for making fishing from piers accessible to wheelchair-bound individuals.

Recreational Content
There is now presented the kind of recreational activities used with retarded youths and adults—physical activities, arts and crafts, music, and camping.

PHYSICAL ACTIVITIES
Motor Skills and Sports
Studies of the motor abilities of retarded youth, especially those with some organic involvement, indicate significant impairment (Cratty, 1967; Rarick, Dobbins, & Broadhead, 1976). This appears to be particularly true of movements involving precision and speed and is more prominent in females than males. Both sexes are also more likely to be overweight, a condition in part attributable to lesser participation in physical activities (Rarick et al., 1976).

Physical educators recommend activities that will develop muscular strength and power (e.g., tumbling, gymnastics, and running), coordination (e.g., throwing, catching, and kicking), balance (e.g., balance beam and hopping), flexibility, (to improve range of motion on spine and hip) and provide enough exercise to reduce tendencies to obesity. These are gross motor activities; fine motor skills can be addressed through programs of arts and crafts (Rarick et al., 1976). Within the limitations imposed by motor difficulties, retarded individuals enjoy the usual range of popular sports—softball, skating, swimming, bowling, and so on. Swimming in particular is a good recreational outlet (Brown, 1959).

Physical Activities and the Severely Impaired

Even persons with severe and profound retardation can participate in and profit from physical education. In this population abnormalities of posture and gait are characteristic. The most common posture ones are flat feet, feet pointed and elevated outward, a forward thrust of head and neck, protruding and sagging abdomen, and lordosis (sway back) (Stoker, 1977). Lordosis is a forward curvature of the lower spine (lumbar region) and is especially prominent in teenage and adult females (Bunker, 1978). To a lesser degree one observes kyphosis, a curvature of the upper spine (thoracic region), which causes round shoulders and a forward-leaning head. Both of the curvatures can result from muscular imbalance and are modifiable through appropriate exercises (Bunker, 1978). Sherill (1980) notes how these abnormalities call attention to retarded persons in normal community settings and encourages the practice of activities that call for the full extension of trunk, head, neck, and limbs—activities that involve reaching, lifting of the chest, and upward stretching.

Wehman and his colleagues have several recreational programs specifically for this group (Wehman, 1979; Wehman, Renzaglia, Schutz, & Karan, 1976). Recognizing poor muscle tone of severely and profoundly retarded adults in a sheltered workshop, undoubtedly affecting endurance (Bunker, 1978), it was decided to teach basic physical fitness exercises such as push-ups and sit-ups. It is very likely that the muscle problems in these individuals are at least partly due to the sedentary nature of their daily lives. Wehman (1979) has also suggested play activities for those with sensory as well as physical handicaps.

Adapted Physical Education

Stein (1962) describes an "adapted" physical education program for educable high school students. Mental age was the most useful guide to activities. They included (a) gymnastics—apparatus and tumbling, side horse, trampoline, balance beam, parallel bars, horizontal ladder; (b) individual and dual games—archery, shuffleboard, tetherball, modified handball and bowling, croquet, and horseshoes; (c) games and relays—cageball, kickball, and so on; and (d) team sports—fundamentals, relays, and lead-up games in basketball, volleyball, touch football, softball, and so forth. Much emphasis was placed on physical fitness and weight training.

The Cerebral Palsied Individual

David (1969) outlined an individualized program for cerebral palsied youth. It is directed toward (a) increasing the interaction of the impaired limbs with the unimpaired ones (e.g., in hemiplegia), (b) improving ambulation, (c) sharpening hand-eye coordination, and (d) strengthening laterality and directionality (see Pomeroy, 1964).

Bowling

Bowling has been an extremely popular recreational outlet for retarded persons. Fitzimmons (1970) describes a program in which more than 1300 individuals participated in tournament play. Bowling was valued not only for its recreational aspect but also for activities surrounding it. Participation enhanced social maturity, mobility and independence. The impact of the program is best conveyed in Fitzimmons' own words:

> Any child living in a community has a chance to participate. We were not interested in only developing skills of bowling. It was everything that goes with it: proper dress, proper actions, expanding their world, motivating them. . . .
>
> We were always told, they will learn to bowl in one bowling lane, and they will become highly confused [referring to cross-lane bowling]. We do cross-lane bowling. We are now teaching them to use foul lines which they said would really foul the whole thing up, but it doesn't. They do just as well [the old story of exceeding the expectations that we set for them].
>
> They progress [in tournaments] from county to district. . . . They go on to state. But as they do this, they are learning to travel, learning to go by bus . . . [increasing mobility]. They are learning to *plan* other things. If we are in the San Francisco area, they see the zoo; if we are in Los Angeles, they take in Disneyland and Marineland. They are expanding their world. They have learned proper behavior in public. They have learned how to go to the bowling alley and order shoes for their size, watch for dangers at the ball returns, how to take turns at proper times.
>
> To begin with, we used college and high school students to help create enthusiasm for what they were doing. When we started you had to lead some of them up to the alley. They dropped the ball, turned around and went back and sat down. They did not know that the ball was even aimed at anything [these would be severely retarded persons]. Now, you do not find very many bowling lane managers that will allow you to let them walk up on the alley bed. If you can you are fortunate because then you can let them follow the ball and they can acquire the association faster [ball and pin]. But most will not allow this.
>
> Through the enthusiasm of the college and high school students working with them [an example of the use of volunteers], one girl who at first made no connection at all, finally found out that her ball occasionally knocked down a pin. It did something when it got to the other end of the lane. This girl is now bowling over 100. This is just fantas-

tic. I cannot do that—mine always go down the gutter. This was a girl who sat at home. Her mother was in a depressed state because she followed her around, or she whined all the time. The doctor contacted us because they were afraid the mother was going to commit suicide and kill the girl, too. Through bowling the girl became interested in other things. . . . She is now involved in a workshop [sheltered workshop] sorting IBM cards. She has learned to iron.

When they go bowling, these people also learn to order snacks [reduced dependence]. This is introducing the mentally retarded to the community. When we first started bowling, some of the operators were a little reluctant about letting us bring groups in. When they saw how well behaved they are, they are now almost fighting to have us come.

What we first became aware of is the fact that they could go as a group, but when they tried to go out individually, they were not accepted. We felt that as the program grew, it had to be something that they could do alone [increasing independence], with their family, with a small group, or with a large group. It was something that those in institutions could participate in when they came into the community and family-care homes. They were already familiar with a lane in the community and it was something they could do [building "bridges" from the old to the new—from the "structured" to the "unstructured"].

The parents became aware of their acceptance. Often parents would never go out and observe their children in public [shame and lowered self-esteem]. When they saw them accepted on a tournament basis . . . they became proud of their children [association with their children was no longer experienced as diminishing worth in the eyes of others]. The EMR's [educable retarded persons] in turn could take their trophies back to school and have them on display to show what their bowling team did.

The TMR's [trainable retarded persons] have gained a great deal from bowling . . . it is something that they can participate in.

It is thrilling to watch a bus load come up to motels and now be able to handle their key [independence]. They can . . . match their key number to their room [using number skills], change into their swimming clothes and go swim [swimming *is* an excellent recreational outlet for retarded persons], go back and get ready for the tournament. *The bowling tournament is just a vehicle for creating these experiences* [the essence of the habilitative or "therapeutic" aspect of recreation; emphasis added].

Competition . . . is no problem [at least here] because they soon learn that first they are competing against themselves and then they learn to compete against one another [a principle that could be applied in other recreational settings]. Someone once said that *everyone* must have a trophy ["infantilizing" rather than "normalizing"]. So we let a state tournament chairman try this out one year. One boy, however, said to us, I do not know what you are giving me that for, I did not win!

The Fitzimmons description epitomizes the educational benefits of a good recreational experience. These young people, apparently of all degrees of retardation, gained in self-confidence, mobility, maturity, and increased acceptance by others including their own parents. Truly such a program met needs for self-esteem and self-expression.

ARTS AND CRAFTS

Arts and crafts are an important recreational outlet for retarded persons (Carlson & Ginglend, 1961, 1968). Although they tend to be less creative, perhaps because of greater tie to what *is* rather than to what *might be*, much satisfaction is available through this medium. Arts and crafts can be enjoyed at all levels of complexity, from coloring a balloon to simple woodworking. They can be pursued in the home as well as in the classroom and are a source of pleasure at any age. In view of the special problem of retarded adults in the effective use of leisure time, it is the belief here that an intensive effort should be made during the school years to interest retarded students in activities that can be pursued as hobbies.

From a psychological standpoint, arts and crafts furnish a means of achieving self-esteem and self-expression. At the self-esteem level, one's creations can bring recognition and the approval of others, a sense of personal accomplishment, and an opportunity to give as well as to receive. Too often, retarded persons are only at the "receiving" end. To the child or youth who is struggling to master basic reading, writing, and number skills, the product of his own creation is incontrovertible evidence of his own worth and competence.

But arts and crafts are not only a source of self-affirmation; like other forms of recreation, they can also be a valuable medium for skill training. In the manipulation of tools and materials, one is learning about their properties and functions. Materials have texture, color, weight, odor, and even taste, and they can be used in a variety of ways. In their very handling, visual-motor coordination is strengthened. Drawing, cutting, pasting, folding, and stitching all require some degree of dexterity, and these hand-eye skills will be the basis of future vocational activities for virtually all retarded persons. Whether in regular competitive employment, sheltered workshops, or activity centers, most of the work done by retarded individuals is manual in nature, and anything that contributes to dexterity can only enhance vocational potential.

Arts and crafts, like the physical activities described in the previous subsection, can also serve as a tension or energy outlet. The child with seemingly inexhaustible energy or the youth with pent-up feelings can find constructive release in such activities as manipulation of paint brush or hammer or in punching clay. The following is a list of arts and crafts activities enjoyed by retarded persons:

1. Coloring, drawing, printing, painting: coloring, crayon, wet chalk drawing, string painting, finger painting, comb painting, brush painting.

2. Making things (paper play, wire making, mobiles): pasting, cutting, tearing, and folding (e.g., medallions, papier-mâché, cutting pictures, bracelets, lanterns, hats).
3. Weaving and sewing: mats, sewing cards, baskets, towels, knitting, weaving on simple looms, rug braiding, and embroidery.
4. Clay craft and other media: Retarded persons need much preliminary experience with Plasticene or other commercial clays that can be used again and again. Once familiar with them, one can shift to self-hardening clay that is permanent (Carlson & Ginglend, 1961). Other media are copper foil, ceramics, candlecraft, and leathercraft.
5. Woodworking: hammering, sanding, and simple woodworking.

MUSIC

Music can provide a variety of satisfactions for retarded persons. In a group setting one can see the pleasurable contagion of a shared musical experience: elevation of spirits and a sense of well-being. Choral work, in particular, offers the opportunity to be a part of a larger group in which individual units, separately and together, combine to produce a sound that is pleasing to any ear.

For the retarded child, songs and rhythms are also an effective instructional medium. Learning the names of fingers through a song like "Where is Thumbkin?" is a source of pleasure to the child. Group singing also enables the verbally reticent child to be less self-conscious in self-expression.

The musical interests of retarded individuals reflect their general level of maturity, although the tie to mental age is much less strong. Moderately retarded as well as mildy retarded teenagers enjoy the same music as normal adolescents.

Songs

In the selection of singing material to be used for instructional purposes with children, Carlson and Ginglend (1961) recommend songs that vary in mood (some lively and some slow), songs that are within an octave range, and songs whose words are "meaningful." These would be songs that relate to the child, to the people and objects about him, and to his feelings.

Rhythms

Rhythms are an extremely popular activity especially with preadolescent retarded youth. Rhythm activities include marching, playing rhythm instruments, and rhythm sticks.

Musical games and dances

Musical games and dances are joyous contributors to the musical experience of retarded persons of all ages. There is pleasure in its social aspect—a sense of camaraderie in the cooperative behavior necessary to carry out the activity well. This particular type of musical experience also provides a wealth of skill training. These activities require concentration and teach leadership. Physical and motor skills are practiced while also serving as good energy outlets. Some examples of appropriate games and dances for preteenagers follow.

1. Music—"stop" games: Participants march, dance, or play a rhythm instrument, stop when the music does, and then follow a direction, such as "Freeze," "Squat," "Do as I do," musical chairs.
2. Singing games: The group acts out a simple story in time to a catchy tune—for example, "Ring around the Rosie," "Did You Ever See a Lassie?," "Farmer in the Dell," "London Bridge."
3. Folk dances: Carlson and Ginglend indicate that most folk dances have to be simplified. Square dancing and the Mexican Hat Dance are much enjoyed.

CAMPING

Perhaps the greatest involvement of organized recreation in mental retardation has been in day and residential camping. A good camping program offers unparalleled opportunities for combining fun and learning; residential ones, in particular, can much advance independence and self-care. Whether day (Ginglend & Gould, 1962) or residential, camping programs will include the same range of activities found in camps for nonhandicapped children: arts and crafts, nature lore, music and drama, sports and games, and waterfront.

A Statewide Program of Regional Residential Camps

A statewide summer camp program was organized that serves retarded youngsters from both institutions and the community (Rourke, 1971). Regional camps were established and served both institutional and community children. The program is both recreational and habilitative in its focus. The recreational component includes hikes, cookouts, swimming, boating, dancing, song festivals, hayrides, and ballgames; its training aspect is concerned with increasing skills in activities of daily living and in interpersonal relationships.

Camping for Preadolescent Orthopedically Handicapped Children

Of particular interest is a camp that serves preadolescent children with physical disabilities, primarily orthopedic in nature (Programs for Handicapped, 1971). The camping experience is integrated so that half of the youngsters are physically impaired and half are normal. The goals of an integrated camping experience are identical to those proposed earlier in connection with the integration of preschool-age retarded children in day care centers for normal youngsters. We can only learn about and begin to identify with people who are "different" by spending time with them.

Because of physical handicaps, the emphasis of the camping program is on outdoor living rather than on athletics. It is also necessary to modify integrated group activities so as to minimize the effect of major differences in physical abilities. To create group cohesion on a hike, for instance, the counselor deliberately slows the pace by pointing out aspects of nature as the group proceeds. This gives the slower-moving campers a chance to keep up and lessens the likelihood of excessive fatigue. At cookouts, jobs are assigned to all, but those that might be hazardous for physically handicapped youngsters are quietly given to able-bodied youth. In the water, however, where one's body is lighter, the physically disabled camper is less disadvantaged and not uncommonly outdoes his nondisabled buddy.

The camp's physical facility is adapted to the special needs of disabled youngsters. The camp terrain is fairly level, and ramps permit wheelchair access to all activity areas. Ramp grades not only must allow for easy wheelchair movement, but they must also be mild enough for ambulatory children who use crutch and brace. Toilets have arm supports, and doors are wide enough for wheelchairs.

The camp has a large specially equipped pool; a craft shop (ceramics, photography, weaving, woodworking); an outdoor and indoor recreation area; a barn, nature house, and garden; and an overnight lodge. Games consist of croquet, paddle ball, volleyball, basketball (short court and with lower hoop), softball (short bases), horseshoes, badminton, and tetherball.

The campers are underprivileged city youth, boys and girls, ages 8–11, whose parents cannot provide them with a summer vacation. The physically handicapped child is required to have basic self-care skills—presumably feeding, dressing, and toileting—and must have some facility with whatever appliance is used.

Year-Round Camping

A special program of year-round camping has been developed for the residents of Brainerd State Hospital, an institution for retarded persons in Minnesota. Its emphasis is on learning through concrete experiences, with the primary medium being small-unit camping and nature itself (Endres, 1968). The institution has its own camp site, and its staff perform the typical counselor functions. Together with the usual summertime activities, there is a full program of winter sports.

Nonambulatory Campers

The Brainerd camp site is also used by nonambulatory institutional residents who require wheelchairs. The program for these physically as well as mentally handicapped campers centers in four areas: (a) water sports: swimming, floating on inner tubes, playing catch with beach balls, and water basketball; (b) pontoon boat riding; (c) fishing; and (d) listening to and identifying birds (Jentsch, 1971). Of the various physical activities provided for persons in wheelchairs, swimming is most preferred. The nonambulatory physically disabled individual can often achieve greater "body" pleasure in the water, because the body is lighter and more easily manageable.

THE ROLE OF LOCAL RECREATION DEPARTMENTS

With emphasis on the development of services to retarded persons at the community level, recreation or parks and recreation departments are adding to their basic programs a component for ill and handicapped individuals. There follows a brief description of one such program in a community of about 125,000 people.

During the school year, weekly evening activities are held in six of its nine community centers. An area of each center is set aside for persons with special recreational needs, and the activities presented are selected on the basis of both chronological and mental age. Depending on the facility, instruction is offered in bowling, swimming, physical fitness, arts and crafts, archery, music, sports, and games. In addition to these evening programs, a special physical fitness class is provided on an after-school basis to primary and intermediate-age educable children. All of these programs are staffed by local college students who are majoring in related fields. The parks and recreation department also co-sponsors a Boy Scout troop for retarded youth between the ages of 11 and 18.

Together with its programs to school-age retarded youths, recreational services are offered to the residents of a halfway house, to older persons in nursing and boarding homes, to homebound blind individuals, to crippled children in conjunction with the local Easter Seal Society, and to youths enrolled at the local cerebral palsy school.

During the summer, a day camp program is offered on a 10-acre park tract located about 10 miles from the community. The camp operates for 10 weeks, and its facilities include activity cottages, a ballfield, and an equipped playground. Use is also made of other park facilities such as lakes, paddle boats, riding and nature trails, and shelters. The camp serves more than 150 mildly and moderately retarded youths, age 6 and older. Special camp programs are also provided to cerebral palsied youths, blind youths, and adults in nursing and boarding home care.

This year-round community recreation program is under the direction of a special supervisor in the parks and recreation department. He is assisted by the regular community center staff, by 25 part-time summer and winter workers, and by more than 100 youth and adult volunteers.

RECREATIONAL PROGRAMS FOR ADULTS

The recreational needs of retarded adults, like their normal counterparts, will generally have a lesser "physical" emphasis. The activities described thus far are in some cases "adult-appropriate," and to these are added those that should be the focus of retarded persons in their place of residence. Caretakers in adult family care and group homes will particularly want to try to provide these recreational outlets along with some mentioned earlier.

Indoor Activities

Table games: Wehman (1979) has called attention to card and table games as recreational outlets. Of particular interest is the use of such games with even severely retarded individuals. Wehman details table games developed by Rakin et al. (1975) that involve spinning dials and matching puzzle pieces, moving pieces on game boards, and interpreting numbers. Simple card games are also appropriate with this population. Each of these activities can be tied to an educational goal and also be a source of fun. Bingo is widely played in classrooms as a pleasurable way of teaching number recognition. Bingo could be adapted to teaching *any* kind of visual material. *Creative homemaking activities*: baking and cooking, canning and preserving, sewing, knitting, crocheting, embroidery, macrame. *Hobbies*: candlemaking; clay and copper craft; decopage and collage; woodwork and furniture refinishing; linoleum block printing; flower craft and flower arranging; model building; mosaics—tiles, seeds, and macaroni; bead making; printing and drawing papier mâché, "pen palling"; terrarium gardening; puppet making; musical instrument; singing and dancing; pet care—bird, fish, turtle, dogs, cats, and hamsters; newspapers and magazines; TV.

Outdoor Activities

Walking, shopping movies, sports—bowling, roller and ice skating, fishing, running, biking, hiking, picnicking, horseshoes, swimming, shuffleboard, badminton, volleyball, basketball, frisbee, soccer, kiting—attending sports events and county fairs, visiting, dating, dining out, church, "Y," traveling, tours.

Adolescent and Adult Concerns: Vocational, Sexual, and Residential

OVERVIEW

In this chapter three topics are addressed that are of particular relevance to the retarded adolescent and adult: vocational, sexual, and residential. In the vocational domain, the work potential of retarded individuals at all levels of cognitive impairment will be examined. In recent years there has been increased interest in achieving some vocational productivity among those with even severe and profound retardation, and we will consider the evidence for their work potential as well as that of those with lesser degrees of impairment. Concerns about sexual manifestations in retarded youth have been "historical" as well as contemporary. Early in this century the mildly retarded were regarded as a "reproductive menace." More recently, with the thrust toward normalization and community living, manifestations of sexuality evoke concern on the part of the family caretakers and the general community. We will try here to address fundamental issues arising from the reality of retarded persons as sexual beings. The last topic presented deals with the rapidly developing array of community-based residential options to the family home or to the state institution. The creation of such an array is crucial to enabling retarded persons to spend their lives in settings that can most fully realize their adaptive potential. We will also consider the current status of our public institutions and the population they increasingly serve.

VOCATIONAL STATUS

Preparing for the World of Work

The link between formal education and later employment is often tenuous, but it is particularly important to youths whose formal education will generally end with high school. Vocational education for non-college-bound students has long been recognized as a valid if "lesser" educational goal, though the youths traditionally served have not been those with major mental or physical handicaps. Attention to the vocational preparation of retarded students in the 1960s grew as federal and state agencies sought to encourage their participation in the work force. In recent decades we have learned that *retarded persons are employable and can be found working in both the public and private sectors and in regular competitive work settings as well as in "sheltered" ones*. The conditions that determine their role as "workers" relate not to *capacity* but to *opportunity*. The latter is dependent on both the economic health of the general society and its concern for the well-being of its handicapped members. Before describing the vocational potential of retarded youths and the process through which that potential can be realized, it is important for us to consider the significance of this aspect of our adult lives.

A principal means of achieving self-esteem in adulthood is through "work." Though its significance has varied with social and economic conditions, the "work ethic" still has a powerful hold on our society. To a considerable degree we *are* what we *do*. Beyond its power to provide us the economic means of meeting daily living expenses, work offers opportunities for participation in culturally valued activities which can bring approval (intimacy) from "significant others"—family, friends, employers, and co-workers—and can give us a sense of our own competence (success). Work provides us with a sense of purpose, usefulness, and worth; its importance to our psychological health is no more clearly evident than in the emotional distress that follows prolonged unemployment or, as in the case of older people, enforced retirement.

Of course, attitudes toward work in our society are not uniform. Certainly, among those for whom poverty has been a multigenerational experience, work in its usual sense has a different meaning. For now, however, consider the experience of several retarded young people who were given the opportunity to work in a retail pet shop. This was a special project conceived by a young couple who had worked with retarded youths in a sheltered workshop but felt that many of their charges could, with proper supervision, function in the regular work world (Graham & Poling, 1963):

> In a store—under proper supervision—kids are in the daily stream of life. And the constant challenge of new problems, new customers, different jobs . . . stretches their minds . . . instead of stagnating at lowest common denominator tasks [simple repetitive assembly operations], our kids are constantly stimulated—and they grow, amazingly.

Johnny Robertson was 22 years old, unemployed, and considered unemployable except in a sheltered workshop. He attended a private school until age 16 and then returned home where for 6 years he lived a life of "intolerable emptiness." Other young people shunned or baited him; he grew morose and hostile, lost what confidence he had gained in school, and finally spent his time locked in his room with a television set. Though sheltered workshop placement was recommended, the family rejected what they viewed as "recreational" rather than "real" work—a problem in some sheltered workshops—and sought regular (competitive) but somewhat sheltered employment for him. For a time he worked at cleaning stalls at a riding academy—he loved horses—but the job ended when the academy closed. Johnny's parents then learned of the pet shop opportunity and, together with parents of other retarded young men, helped to get it started. His mother made the following remarks:

> I still find it hard to believe. Twenty-two years of heartbreak and despair, and suddenly, you gamble fifty dollars on two people who you suspect are impractical dreamers. And what do you get? A small miracle. Our Johnny who had no life, now has a full and happy one—a job and a place to go everyday. A place where he is actually needed [self-worth], a place where he has puppies and people to love and be loved by [intimacy]. The change is unbelievable. Now he goes to the movies alone, eats by himself in restaurants, buys his own clothes, does everything he was afraid to do before. And he laughs! So do Clarke and I, now. Believe me, it's a welcome sound in a house that heard none for years. . . .

The development of retarded youths like Johnny into competent employees was not achieved overnight. It took weeks to teach the fact that pets had to be fed every day. Initially, youngsters were given only simple jobs; this built their confidence and provided an opportunity to explore their specific interests and work potential. Once determined, "stretching" of that potential began. Danny, age 27, mental age 10 years (IQ 60), was interested in handling money and was given the job of taking the daily receipts to the bank. Then the shop owners began to pretend that they too busy to prepare the deposit slip for him. Very slowly, Danny learned to count money, to enter the sum in the ledger, and to fill out the deposit slip. The job took him an hour, but his confidence and self-esteem soared.

One of the youths was very frightened of the animals, and his continued employment was in doubt. On this particular morning he brought to work a cake he had baked for his co-workers. His employers, recognizing that he enjoyed cooking, put him to work preparing food for the animals. It involved mixing food in specified proportions for different breeds of puppies. With obvious pride, he soon began serving his "dishes" to animals that had earlier frightened him.

The shop had been initially supported through small contributions from the parents of the young men employed there. There was no assurance that the shop would be successful, and early pay schedules appear to have been impromptu. But with the progress of the youths, the board of directors voted each a modest monthly salary. Said one father, "That five dollars meant more to my girl than a thousand dollars would have to me." Though receiving a regular salary clearly nourished self-esteem, even more important in this respect was earning a key to the store. At the end of the first year, keys were given to the four young people who had shown the greatest initiative and responsibility. Thereafter they were expected to open the store on time each morning. Winning one of these keys and the tremendous status it signified became the greatest ambition of the employees. The manager commented that when these keys were first passed out he never dreamed that they would become that store's equivalent of Phi Beta Kappa!

The vocational success story of these retarded young adults did not end with the pet shop. Some of them went on to work in jobs of comparable complexity in a large department store. Others would have to remain in the more relatively sheltered setting of the shop. But at whatever level of employment (and this includes the sheltered workshop), work had been the vehicle for dramatically changing self-images. It gave these handicapped young men and women a chance to be a part of life's mainstream; to feel a sense of value and worth as human beings.

Apart from its inspirational aspect, such a story reveals the kinds of problems encountered by retarded youths once beyond the protected status of "pupil" and our need to prepare them educationally as best we can. The money or arithmetic problems of Danny are no surprise and, at least for mildly retarded students, become an important focus of our educational effort. Let us now look at the vocational potential of retarded persons. We will consider the kinds of jobs they perform, the skills that underlie them, their common work difficulties, and the responsibility of the school in preparing them for the role of "worker."

Vocational Potential of Mildly Retarded Youths and Adults

Any consideration of the employability or job potential of retarded youth begins with recognition that vocational potential is closely related to the degree of retardation. It is chiefly among mildly retarded individuals that we find persons functioning in regular (competitive) employment. At greater degrees of retardation, one is likely to find individuals working in sheltered workshops or in adult day activity centers. The latter may not, in fact, be a work setting at all but primarily provide educational and recreational activities. Though mildly retarded persons are *capable* of competitive employment, their attainment of this depends much on the commitment to this goal of the agencies concerned with placing handicapped people in employment (e.g., vocational rehabilitation). Thus many such individuals can be found in sheltered workshops where, in a sense, they can be viewed as "underemployed." In any case, in the following we will distinguish between two broad levels of work potential—(1) competitive employment and the mildly retarded and (2) sheltered and work activity levels of employment and those with at least moderate retardation.

EMPLOYABILITY

Numerous studies reveal that about 80 percent of mildly retarded youths find employment in regular jobs (Deno, 1966; Goldstein, 1964). A recent study of largely mildly retarded former sheltered workshop employees ($\overline{X}$ IQ 59, range 42–70) who had placed in regular jobs found a third (34%) still employed after a period of 4 to 5 years (Brickey, Campbell, & Browning, 1985). Particularly influential in their continued employment were supportive attitudes of their parents.

The "service" sector has become the predominant employment area, with smaller numbers found in industry, simple office work, and labor (Brolin, Durand, Kromer, & Muller, 1975; Clark, Kivitz, & Rosen, 1968). The jobs performed are usually "unskilled" in nature. This is to be expected from workers with very limited reading and numbering skills and who have difficulties in making complex judgments. The reader may be surprised that even in our technologically sophisticated economy persons with mental retardation are still employable. True, the proportion of jobs that are "unskilled" has declined from 60 percent in 1900 to about 25 percent today. But, for the foreseeable future, at least 20 percent of jobs will still be at the unskilled level (Nixon, 1970).

The reason for continued availability of employment here lies in the rapid increase of jobs in the service sector. This has been our fastest-growing employment area and includes such settings as hospitals, hotels and motels, restaurants and cafeterias, and nursing homes. Here retarded and nonretarded unskilled workers are employed as aides, orderlies, kitchen workers, food servers, dishwashers, housecleaners, and janitorial aides. In the industrial domain retarded workers are found in warehouses, in laundries, and in simple assembly operations. Even the white-collar sector provides some opportunities, with retarded workers functioning as messengers and office machine operators. Wherever jobs are found or can be redesigned so that they are *well defined, highly routinized,* and *fairly constantly paced*, retarded persons are employable (Peterson & Jones, 1964).

Well-defined jobs are clear as regards expectations. The tools, equipment, and procedures are well specified. There is a minimum of decision making, and no special skills are required beyond those necessary to the procedures. But even well-defined jobs are not free of some subjectivity. If, for example, the task is "cleaning," when is a room "clean"? People clearly have different standards, and the worker must learn what the employer means by "clean." We also need to guard against the tendency to assume that words have the same meaning for all of us. To "clean the room" for one person might mean making beds, sweeping, and light dusting. For another it could also mean vacuuming, mopping, cleaning hard-to-reach areas, washing windows, and more. Failure to meet employer expectations may result from lack of specificity as to just what was expected. Sleith (1966), in advising prospective employers of retarded workers, stressed this need:

1. Talk to the retarded employee on a person-to-person level, as you would to anyone else. Only try to be more specific, more precise and more crystal clear—as if you were speaking to someone in the upper levels of grade school. [But] don't "talk down" to him as though he were a small child. He's not.

2. Speak in concrete terms, not abstractions. If, for example, you want him to put the pail away, show him exactly where "away" is.

3. Demonstrate what you want him to do. Just don't tell him.

4. Show him where things are—time clock, lockers, restrooms,

cafeteria or lunch area, drinking fountain, supply room—as you would for any new employee. But take your time, don't rush, and be sure he understands.

5. Take extra care to explain about working hours, proper clothes on the job, his work station, whom he reports to, what his pay will be (inform him of the various deductions from his total paycheck), and where the bus stops. It's doubly important for him to know these . . . points.

The second characteristic of jobs appropriate to retarded workers is that they are highly routinized, repetitive in nature. The task is performed in essentially the same way each time, and once the basic job skills have been acquired, only minimum supervision is necessary. While repetitive work is probably more acceptable to retarded than to nonretarded individuals, it would be a mistake to assume that the former cannot experience boredom. Retarded workers, like the rest of us, enjoy variety in their daily activities, and their job satisfaction will be increased if given the opportunity to expand horizontally, if not vertically. That is, the retarded employee, and nonretarded employee as well, should have an opportunity to learn a number of tasks within his range of competence so that variety in the form of periodic rotation from one task to another is possible.

The third attribute of jobs retarded people can perform is that they are fairly constantly paced. There are at least two dimensions to pace. First, there is the problem of adjusting one's work tempo to that of co-workers. The employee who cannot modulate his work rate so that it fits into the tempo of those with whom he is involved will need to be placed in settings where he is free to set his own pace. The second aspect of pace relates to worker capacity to adapt to variation in work rate. The retarded worker may have more difficulty in coping with periodic increases in work tempo, because the effect of an increased rate is to make the task more difficult. The story of a young man who worked in a hamburger shop is recalled. During slow periods he had no difficulty in meeting the orders of the countermen, but during rush hour he became confused and frustrated.

The following is a list of jobs that can be performed by mildly retarded persons.

Services (domestic)
  Child Care
  Cleaning and room preparation: house, motel, hotel, hospital, rest home

Services (food)
  Bus boy or girl
  Dishwasher: hand and machine
  Helper (in cafeteria, restaurant and hospital): cook, baker, general kitchen, steam table

Industry (general)
  Small-parts assembly
  Soldering

Construction
  Laborer: highway, dam, and bridge work; building construction

Sales
  Helper: retail, pet shop
  Stock clerk
  Packer, wrapper

Services (building—
Helper: janitor, custodian, general maintenance, porter, watchman
Elevator operator

Services (personal)
Hospital, nursing, and rest home aide and orderly, nurse's aide, companion
Helper: barber and beauty shop
Washroom attendant

Industry (textiles)
Helper: yard goods clothing manufacturing
Sewing machine operator

Industry (lumber and lumber products)
Helper: furniture factory, upholstery, toy factory, framing shop, box factory

Industry (paper and paper products)
Helper: pulp mill, newsprint factory, stationery manufacturing

Industry (printing)
Helper: newspaper, greeting card, printing, book binding

Industry (leather and leather goods)
Helper: leather manufacturing, leather accessories manufacturing, shoes and boot manufacturing

Industry (stone, glass, and clay products)
Helper: glass production, brick yard, drain-tile-pipe, pottery, cement block, quarry

Industry (food products)
Helper: poultry, slaughter house, frozen foods, cannery, bake shop, candy factory, dairy products

Public Service
Helper: road maintenance, garbage and trash collection, park and grounds maintenance, painting, maintenance

Trades and services
Helper: auto body repair, bricklayer, carpenter, concrete finisher, dry wall, electrician, mechanic, painter, pipe fitter, plumber, roofer, sheet metal, solderer, steam fitter, stonemason, tile setter, upholsterer, wiper (machine), welder
Helper: cleaning establishments, laundries, rug cleaning, diaper service, service station, car wash, parking garage
Machine operator: punch press, drill press, trimmer, buffer, grinder, sprayer, gluing, leather cutting, foot-power printing press, tenoner, straightener, wire bending, gear cutting

Office Work
Clerk: general, filing, mail handler, mail/messenger
Office machine operator: copier, mimeograph, multilith

Farmwork
Hand: general farming, ranch, poultry, lumbering, forestry
Helper: nursery, gardener, greenhouse

Fishery
Hand: shell fishing, hatchery
Helper: fishing boats

Miscellaneous
Delivery man
Helper: all vehicles
Warehouse

EDUCATIONAL IMPLICATIONS

For mildly retarded students an appropriate secondary education should offer a combination of *related* educational and vocational experiences. So-called "work-study" programs were designed to provide actual work experience to senior high school students (Kolstoe, 1975; Orzack, Cassell, & Halliday, 1969; Shawn, 1964; Syden, 1963). The goals of the work experience for retarded students may vary from that of nonretarded ones in that there will be a greater emphasis on "work habit" training than on craft skill development. The jobs held by retarded youths are unskilled. These jobs do not require specialized abilities, and those that are needed can usually be taught quickly. What cannot be taught so quickly are the *social skills* and *work habits* that are essential to virtually all employment (e.g., Cohen, 1960; Deno, 1966; Kolstoe, 1975; Rosen, 1971). In a study of the causes of termination of employment in a group of mildly retarded adults, the most common reason was social or interpersonal inappropriateness (Greenspan & Shoultz, 1981). Examples were excessive talking, ignoring directions, and inappropriate interrupting, aggressiveness, lateness, and irregular attendance. Employability requires regular job attendance, punctuality, getting along with co-workers and supervisors, accepting direction and correction, maintaining an adequate work rate, and showing concern for work quality. "Dependability" encompasses these behaviors and, if not present at initial employment, can only be expected to develop over time. The school years, including the elementary and junior high periods, provide the *time* during which it can be fostered. This is not to imply that the process cannot be speeded up in the older adolescent or young adult through the appropriate use of reinforcers.

Work-study programs ordinarily consist of a half-day of academics and a half-day of work experience. Academics focuses on consumer- and work-related skills (e.g., units of measure, tools, filling out job applications, job vocabularies). Vocational activities can initially involve assisting in various school functions (e.g., messenger and library) and should begin in the junior high school years, if not earlier. It is then when work-related behaviors begin to develop. Later there should be participation in vocational classes, and at least rudimentary tool skills can be acquired. Though these students will lack the reading and arithmetic skills necessary to most crafts, they may be able to achieve enough tool facility to function as "helpers." The final phase of work-study programs involves actual placement in work settings. These may be developed independently by the school or jointly in cooperation with the local vocational rehabilitation agency.

Vocational Potential of Moderately, Severely, and Profoundly Retarded Youths and Adults

The work capacity of mildly retarded individuals is well established; more recently we have recognized work potential at more severe levels of retardation (Bellamy, 1976; Brickey, Campbell, & Browning, 1985; Crosson, 1969; Gold, 1973; Revell, Wehman, & Arnold, 1984; Wehman, 1981; Wehman et al., 1982). In the earlier-cited study of successfully employed former sheltered workshop employees (Brickey et al., 1985), 7 of the 18 who were still on the job after some 5 years were moderately retarded. Particularly notable has been the demonstration of job potential in some who are even profoundly retarded (e.g., Bellamy, Peterson, & Close, 1976).

VOCATIONAL SKILLS

Mithaug and his colleagues have conducted a number of studies designed to identify competencies necessary to employment at the level of the sheltered workshop. Initial investigations consisted of surveys of workshop supervisors in order to determine their views of the minimal competencies necessary to entry level sheltered workshop employment (Johnson & Mithaug, 1978; Mithaug & Hagmeier, 1978; Mithaug & Haring, 1977). Nine competencies were identified and subsequently incorporated in a scale, the Prevocational Assessment and Curriculum Guide (Mithaug, Mar, & Stewart, 1978). They were attendance/endurance, independence, production, learning, behavior, communication skills, social skills, grooming/eating skills, and toileting skills.

Having determined what supervisors said were minimal competencies, Mithaug et al. then looked at those of 89 employees of a sheltered workshop and compared them with those of 41 clients of that same facility's work activities center (Mithaug, Mar, Steward, & McCalmon, 1980).[1] They found that sheltered employees did indeed largely function at or above the minimum reported by supervisors. These employees mostly exceeded the minimum in production and social skills and actually fell below it in communication and grooming/eating skills. Interestingly, the work activity group differed relatively little; they were functioning at better than 90 percent of the sheltered workshop minimum. In only three areas was there a significant difference: they were somewhat less productive, were less independent, and had poorer attendance and endurance. Even here, however, they were still within from 75 to 85 percent of the sheltered workshop minimum. The largest single difference between the two groups was in production, a dimension of primary concern to most employers and one that will be discussed later.

VOCATIONAL POTENTIAL
OF A SCHOOL POPULATION

A second facet of this study entailed the rating of these competencies in a population of 179 moderately to profoundly retarded individuals enrolled in educational programs in schools, institutions, and community centers. The average age was 18, most were under 22, and the group included a substantial number of profoundly retarded persons. Of the 179, 70 were profoundly retarded, 79 severely retarded, and 30 moderately retarded. The large number of profoundly retarded subjects is of special interest, because there is a tendency in the literature

---

[1]"Sheltered employment" and "work activity" employment are distinguished by levels of productivity and earnings. "Sheltered" employees earn at least one-half of the commensurate wage for that same job in regular employment. "Work activity" employees produce and earn at less than one-half of that standard.

to use the term "severely retarded" to encompass both the severely and pro-foundly retarded, as if there were no real differences between them. In fact, the differences between them in adaptive potential are not insignificant and were illus-trated in Chapter 1.

First let us look at the total group, and then we will consider them in terms of degree of retardation. Figure 36 shows the profile of prevocational competen-cies in the nonworking (largely student) group as compared with those of the earlier-described sheltered workshop and work activity groups. The difference between the nonworkshop population and the other two groups is striking. Relative to the two employed groups, the nonworkshop (largely student) one is least devel-oped in learning, independence, and grooming/eating. In relation to entry level

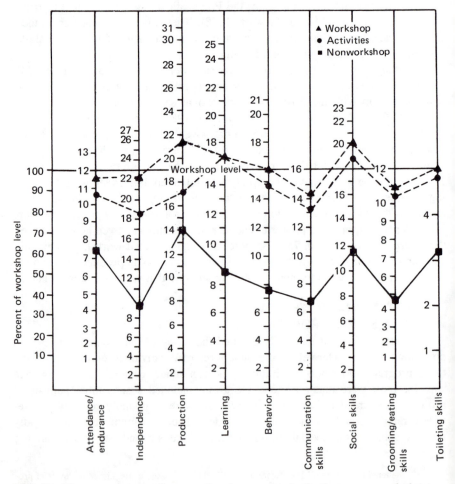

FIG. 36 Mean percentage of prevocational competencies in three groups relative to minimum necessary to entry level employment in a sheltered workshop. From Mi-thaug, Mar, Stewart, & McCalmon (1980).

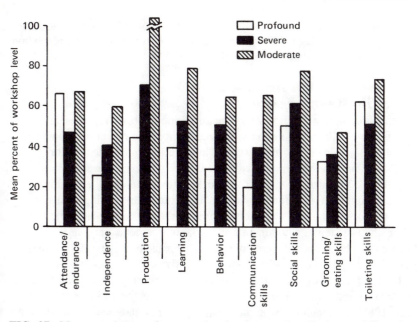

FIG. 37   Mean percentage of prevocational competencies relative to sheltered workshop minimum in a nonworkshop and largely student population grouped by degree of retardation. From Mithaug et al. (1980).

sheltered workshop requirements they were least prepared in the communication and grooming/eating areas (37%) and independence (38%).[2] They lagged least in production.

Figure 37 shows the prevocational competency profiles by degree of retardation. In all but two of the categories, attendance/endurance and toileting, there is a consistent relationship between level of retardation and vocational readiness. Note that the moderately retarded group is already exceeding the sheltered workshop minimum at production. But even with the effect of intellectual impairment the profoundly retarded subgroup is still functioning at an average of 50 percent of that minimum. The severely retarded are at 60 percent and the moderately retarded at 76 percent. This study enables us to conceptualize the vocational potential of even the most seriously impaired individuals as representing a point on a *continuum of employability* and implies that, with appropriate procedures, some measure of meaningful productivity is achievable.

TRAINING IMPLICATIONS

As with mildly retarded youths, this research reveals the importance of training in skill areas not specific to work itself. In preparing youth for employment at some level, teachers will want to address the areas of *communication* (some ability

---

[2]The category "independence" is said to refer to "inappropriate behavior, adaptation to new work settings, (and) motivation to work."

to communicate and to follow directions), *grooming/eating* (personal hygiene, appropriate dress and eating behavior), *independence* (work motivation, adaptation to new work settings), and *behavior* (disruptiveness).

Competitive Employment with Sheltered Features

Although competitive employment has traditionally been regarded as accessible only to those with not more than mild retardation, the recent development of "work stations" and "supportive work" in regular employment settings has opened this possibility for those with moderate and even severe retardation (Wehman, 1981; Wehman et al., 1982). Work stations represent a combining of sheltered and competitive features by using the actual work setting as a training area. Selected jobs within the work setting are chosen as training sites and can be regarded as the last step in a continuum of work environments varying from adult activity programs to competitive employment. Under the tutelage of a "counselor/supervisor," and at no cost to the employer, workers are trained and then employed. Employment is associated with continued monitoring by the trainer for at least 30 days. Food and janitorial services seem to be the most popular areas (Wehman, 1981), although the manufacturing sector has also been used. In some manufacturing settings, a whole department may be manned by handicapped workers. In the regular work area they perform jobs that are commonly contracted for in sheltered workshops.

Whereas "work stations" may involve relatively permanent supervision of a group of employees, "supportive work" is intended to achieve a fully independent employee status (Revell, Wehman, & Arnold, 1984). Both moderately and mildly retarded persons have benefited from this approach, which involves careful job placement, on-the-job training, and extensive follow-up. Food and custodial services are potential job sites, and long-term studies of such placements have shown that moderately as well as mildly retarded persons can perform at this level (Wehman et al., 1982).

Apart from the satisfaction of being of genuine assistance to others, employers gain tax advantages by hiring handicapped persons. For the handicapped person himself there is the possibility of either permanent full-time employment or a lesser level of employment, one that does not threaten assured federal benefits under the Supplemental Security Insurance (SSI) system.

WORK PRODUCTIVITY IN SEVERE AND PROFOUND RETARDATION

One of the more dramatic vocational developments has been the teaching of the capacity to work to individuals who were regarded as incapable of such activity. Under the tutelage of imaginative and dedicated researchers, severely and profoundly retarded adolescents and adults have been taught a variety of manual assembly tasks of which the bicycle brake (Gold, 1972) and the cable harness and cam switch activator (Bellamy, Peterson, & Close, 1975; Hunter & Bellamy, 1976; Ivin, 1976) are the best known. Admittedly, the time required to master such assemblies may far exceed that needed to learn the assembly operations common to sheltered workshops or work activity programs. For example, it required a total of 44.5 hours for a severely retarded woman to learn a 47-step saw chain assembly (O'Neill & Bellamy, 1978). *The time required to learn the task may well be the predominant difference between the retarded and nonretarded worker.* With enough time and/or the right reinforcer(s), the retarded worker may eventually reach normal production standards. An example of this is shortly illustrated (Bellamy, Inman, & Yeates, 1978).

Given the demonstration of unforeseen capacities, their likelihood of being realized is another matter. Wehman (1979) has identified four major impediments to productivity—unawareness of relevant perceptual cues (e.g., size, color, form, location), sensory and motor impairments, slow motor behavior, and disruptive behaviors. He offers the following suggestions regarding their remediation.

Perceptual Problems

These can be addressed by procedures that give greater prominence or visibility to the relevant dimension. Such prominence is attained through such methods as explicit verbal instruction, using colors to clarify an assembly sequence (color coding), or further task simplification.

Sensory and Motor Impairments

In this population are found many multihandicapped persons. Motor disorders are particularly common, but one also encounters severe deficits of vision and hearing. The visually impaired individual is likely to be particularly disadvantaged in manual activities, and instructors will need to substitute the cues of touch, location, and sound for sight. For individuals with significant movement limitations, special jigs (Hollis, 1967) can be developed.

Slow Motor Behavior

Slow motor behavior directly affects productivity, and methods of speeding up worker movements include verbal prompts (Bellamy, Peterson, & Close, 1975) and peer modeling (Wehman, 1979). Slow work rates lend themselves to the use of reinforcing contingencies. After all, "piecework" is a standard means of determining individual worker earnings. Work rate can be expected to accelerate by reducing the time period between achieving target rates and reinforcement and by increasing the frequency and amount of reinforcement (e.g., Schroeder, 1972; Wehman, Renzaglia, Schutz, & Karan, 1976).

An interesting example of the use of reinforcers to increase productivity is found in a study of three profoundly retarded female sheltered workshop employees (Bellamy, Inman, & Yeates, 1978). They ranged in age of from 19 to 26 years and had mental ages of from 2 to 3 years. Their work consisted of assembling a cable harness, a task that required the attaching of 11 wires. To facilitate assembly, each wire was color-coded, and cues were provided to assist the assembler in recognizing where each wire began and ended. Prior to attempts to speed up cable assembly, these workers were completing units at a rate far slower than the industrial standard of 17 minutes. Figure 38 shows that for S_1 and S_2, baseline rates averaged about 40 and 130 minutes, respectively. And S_3 was initially taking from 70 to 90 minutes per unit. For S_1 and S_3, the new reinforcement contingency was to double wages to two pennies for each cable assembled in less than the worker's average baseline time. A timer was sounded for each worker, and it was that worker's job to beat the bell! The period of the graph marked "timer" indicates when this contingency was initiated. For S_2, the first new contingency was to permit her to spend her penny as soon as it was earned (increasing "proximity" of reinforcement). Later she was given the opportunity to increase her unit earnings as well.

For S_1 the doubling of pay (increasing the amount of reinforcement) is associated with a steady decline in the time needed for an assembly. By 6 weeks she was producing at the industrial standard! S_3 also appears to have benefited, as her work rate reached the industrial standard within about 3 weeks. She had already shown a steady decline in unit assembly time but, until the doubling of her pay, her rate had remained a consistent 10 minutes slower than standard. Only S_2 failed to reach the standard, though her rate increased under both contingencies: The lapse at the end of the S_2 recording is not explained, but she then returned to what had become her average rate of about 60 minutes. This was still better than twice as fast as prior to the program.

What is striking is that even profoundly retarded persons were capable of achieving an industrial standard. It is so easy for us to underestimate the potential of such severely impaired persons. *We keep equating their disability with their potential.* We forget that what *we* are is at least as much a product of our opportunities as it is the product of the capacities or limitations we bring to these opportunities.

Disruptive Behavior

Low productivity may also result from competing disruptive behaviors. Ideally, a powerful positive reinforcer can automatically reduce disruptiveness, because the goal toward which the worker aspires is simply incompatible with disruptiveness. For example, if out-of-seat or other off-task behavior has reduced productiveness, then fixing a time period by which the task must be completed and the reinforcer earned will, almost necessarily, increase on-task behavior. While the use of positive reinforcers is the ideal approach, alone, it may not have enough power to affect the client's disruptiveness. One will want to combine positive reinforcement with negative consequences, contingencies the client perceives as unwelcome. Examples include "response cost" (e.g., the loss of previously earned reinforcers—pennies, tokens, points, privileges), time out (e.g., physical isolation or temporary loss of the opportunity for reinforcement), physical restraint, and overcorrection (Thompson & Grabowski, 1977; Wehman, 1979). Special care is needed in using negative contingencies (punishment), and more will be said about this in the next chapter, when we address some especially disturbing behavior problems seen in this population.

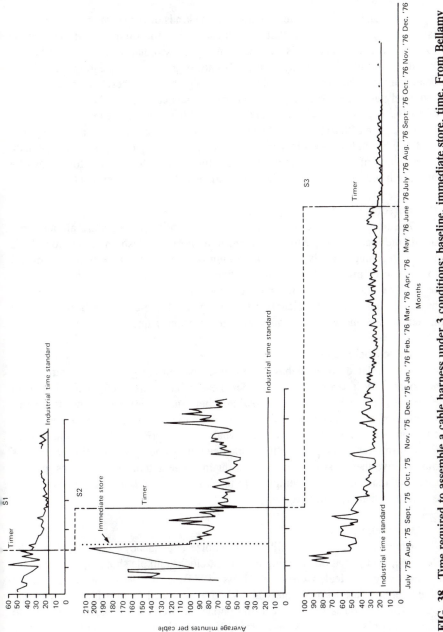
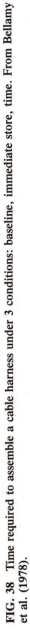

FIG. 38 Time required to assemble a cable harness under 3 conditions: baseline, immediate store, time. From Bellamy et al. (1978).

FOSTERING WORK–RELATED
SOCIAL BEHAVIORS

Wehman has also directed attention to the kinds of nonvocational deficiencies that affect employability and that were illustrated in the studies of Mithaug et al. (1978, 1980). A "social skills" curriculum is proposed that focuses on four behaviors important to work settings: personal care (e.g., grooming/eating etc.), basic social interactions, community skills, and judgment. Of these, he believes that moderately and some severely retarded individuals can master the first three; the fourth is "cognitively oriented" and perhaps beyond current training capacities. Of course, even "basic social interactions" involve judgment. The retarded youth or adult who shakes hands inappropriately (e.g., too frequently) is showing a lack of awareness of the principle that governs this social behavior; the forms may be taught, but unless they are applied appropriately the person seems odd.

Personal Care

Assuming that basic feeding, dressing, and toileting skills are already possessed, the focus is on performing them in as normal a fashion as possible. This includes teaching socially acceptable dining behavior, such as eating with mouth closed, use of proper utensils, and picking up correct amounts of food. "Minimeals" are suggested as a teaching method; this was described in the previous chapter. Grooming skills, cleanliness, and personal hygiene have been taught to this population and were also discussed in the prior chapter.

Basic Social Skills

Work-related social behaviors include appropriate greeting, postures, and eye contact. Wehman does not consider these behavior as "complex," though in describing "conversation" and knowing when and where not to interject comments, reference is made to sensitivity to subtleties. But these subtleties depend on cognition—our capacity to recognize what is appropriate. Clearly, some *behaviorial* forms can be taught, but their practice without adequate social *awareness* is going to give them a stilted and deviant quality. The author would suggest putting at least as much effort in attempting to teach *understanding* of these behaviors as he would in their practice.

Community Skills

Under this rubric are skills that minimize dependency—learning to use the telephone, transportation, vending machines, clocks, simple shopping, and managing money (e.g., Heal, Colson, & Gross, 1984). Leff (1974) was able to teach some telephone use to moderately and severely retarded ("trainable") school-age youth. The method is shown for a dial phone but would be equally applicable to pushbutton ones. Visual cues were provided through a modification of the standard numbers (see Fig. 39). Students with a mental age of 5 years were able to use a device which simply enlarged the numbers and showed no letters. For students with mental ages in the 3.5- to 5-year range, a second cue was added: each number had a different color. A separate device was employed to assist the student in

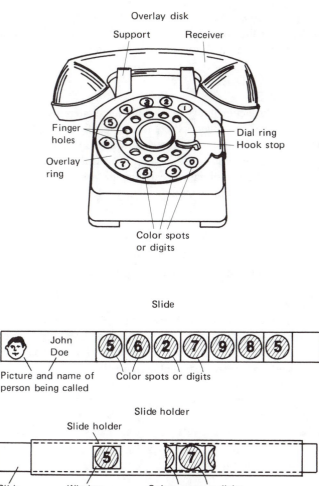

FIG. 39   "Adapted" telephone and adapted "directory." From Leff (1974), Copyright © Instructo/McGraw-Hill. Distributor: Crestwood Company, P.O. Box 04606, Milwaukee, WI 53204. U.S. Patent No. 3878623.

learning the sequence of numbers to be dialed. The generalization of this skill to the pay telephones would involve some money concepts but not more than coin discrimination and elementary counting. These competencies should be attainable with mental ages of 5 years or more. Indeed, they may be attainable at lesser mental ages as well.

Similarly, trainable adolescents have acquired some independent community mobility by learning how to ride a bus (Certo & Schwartz, 1975). Prerequisite skills, identified through task analysis, were making change (again, simple number and coin recognition), acquiring sight words relevant to bus designation, learning the appropriate stop, and telling time. Task analytic approaches have been successful in teaching time telling (Pierce, 1972) and also simple money management (Certo & Swetlik, 1976) to trainable youths. It is the chaining of individual skills that enables all of us, retarded and normal, to carry out seemingly complex tasks.

"VOCATIONALIZING" ADULT DAY CARE PROGRAMS

Retarded youths and adults lacking entry level skills for sheltered workshops are found in day care programs. These may operate independently or be part of a sheltered workshop. Day care programs tend to focus more heavily on educational and recreational activities than on vocational ones; yet it is clear that, with current training technology, many of these individuals can acquire some work skills. Wehman (1979) has described some of the conditions that can foster a more work-oriented atmosphere.

Physical Space

Need is seen for at least one large room that can serve as a general work area and for smaller rooms or cubicles that can be used for special training purposes.

A "Work" Atmosphere

A setting that is conducive to developing work skills will be at least 6 hours in length (9–3), provide normal work rhythms in the forms of breaks and lunch period, use a time clock, and provide incentives. Within this 6-hour period, time can also be allotted to educational and recreational activities.

Appropriate Tasks

These will generally be of the "sit-down" variety and involve packaging, collating, and assembly. Other "domestic-related" tasks should also be taught (e.g., bed making and dishwashing). Clients should be exposed at one time to several tasks and ones that range in difficulty.

WORK TEAMS

Of particular interest is the suggestion that clients be grouped into work teams. These would be organized on the basis of homogeneity of work abilities. As clients demonstrate adequate functioning on the tasks assigned to their particular team, they can be moved from their team to one at the next higher level.

Job Enrichment

Although cognitive impairment restricts the range of jobs that can be performed, long-term involvement in simple assembly tasks may produce some of the same kind of boredom found in automobile assembly line employees. In Sweden, the answer to monotony was to assign production goals to *teams* rather than to *individuals*. Here, workers could alternate with others on their team and work could be daily performed on a number of activities rather than on only one. An analogous attempt at "job enrichment" in mental retardation involved simply adding to the number of elements handled in a ball-point pen assembly task (Morris, Martin, & Nowak, 1981). Two groups of workers were studied, one in the moderate to mild range ($\overline{X}$ IQ 52) and the other in the severe to profound range ($\overline{X}$ IQ 29). The brighter group responded with an increased level of productivity, but the more impaired one did not. Their productivity actually declined.

Apart from this differential effect, one must also consider whether the task modification actually constituted "enrichment" in the eyes of the worker. It may make little difference to people who do not regularly use pens or, for that matter, those who do, whether they assemble part of the pen or all of it! Enrichment is likely to be of special benefit on tasks that are themselves sources of satisfaction. Admittedly, these may be difficult to develop in activities that are largely "assembly". in nature—hence the use of multiple tasks rather than only one and the exposure of workers to more prestigious ones (e.g., operating power tools).

SEXUALITY

Of the curriculum areas, none is so fraught with difficulty for educators and the family as that of sexuality; yet it is a matter of intense interest to mildly and moderately retarded youths if not to those with more severe deficit. In characterizing the concerns of retarded young adults, Edmonson et al. (1977) observed that "the quality of their lives is surely more dependent upon the ability to satisfy the universal human need for social approval, acceptability, companionship, and love ('intimacy'). It can be no wonder that they attach so much importance to marriage and parenthood."

Traditional Views of Sexuality in Retarded Persons

Early in this century sexual expression in retarded individuals was a source of dread (Kanner, 1964). Apart from moral concerns about promiscuity, there was a genuine fear that retarded adults would have larger-than-average families and that this would have the effect of depressing the average level of intelligence in the general population. These fears led during the 1920s to the widespread enactment of state laws pertaining to marriage among retarded individuals and to sterilization (Kindred, Cohen, Penrod, & Shaffer, 1976). Although population fears were to prove groundless (in Chap. 1 we noted that although their families tend to be larger, a much smaller proportion of retarded adults marry and become parents), active sterilization was the rule until the 1950s. Indeed, prior to 1950, sterilization of institutionalized persons was often a prerequisite of community return. After 1950, however, laws regarding sterilization became much more restrictive. Formerly compulsory sterilization gave way to voluntary procedures and the requirement of judicial approval when the individual was not deemed capable of giving legal consent.

Normalization and Deinstitutionalization

The tightening of sterilization laws was a small but significant step away from the earlier view of retarded persons as a social threat, but the 1960s were to witness extraordinary changes in public perception. Once seen as a "menace," the retarded individual began to be seen as a victim, discriminated against in such domains as education, employment, housing, marriage, and parenthood. This was to lead to the assertion of "rights" and to federal laws protecting those rights (see Chap. 6).

Of the various abuses, the one getting the greatest attention is related to institutional life. National exposés described horrendous physical and psychological conditions in many large institutions (e.g., Blatt & Kaplan, 1960). The consequence was to create the impetus for "deinstitutionalization" and the affording to retarded persons of residential life *within* rather than *apart from* the general community. But it is precisely in the more open setting of the community that the sexuality of the retarded individual attains a greater level of visibility. Exposed to peers in educational, recreational, residential, and vocational settings, sexual impulses are aroused that could be more readily ignored or contained by the physical restrictions of institutional life.

Sexual Concerns
in Mental Retardation

The combination of sexual feelings and intellectual impairment causes difficulties for the retarded person and his family and, as we have just seen, concerns in the general society.

"PERSON" PROBLEMS

For the individual there is society's resistance to the acknowledgment of the reality of sexual feelings and a policy of restricting social and educational experiences. One effect is to block communication about feelings and to compound the usual confusion, distortion, and plain misinformation about sexuality (Edmonson & Wish, 1975; Gordon, 1973a). Moreover, when institutionalization was *the* residential option, its sexually segregated nature fostered behaviors that were much less acceptable in the community (Money, 1973; Rosen, 1972).

"FAMILY" PROBLEMS

No less involved than the person himself are his parents. Parents of mildly and moderately retarded adolescents either deny their child's sexuality (Nigro, 1975) or acknowledge their need for sex instruction (Goodman, Budner, & Lesh, 1971; Hall, Morris, & Barker, 1973). Like parents of nonhandicapped youth, these parents are uncomfortable about the discussion of sex with their children. The ambivalence that sex creates is illustrated in the remarks of the mother of a 16-year-old girl with Down syndrome:

> I don't know how to approach the subject of sex. Why should we explain it if there's no reason she'll ever need the information [denial]. I don't know. Do kids really have the idea or do we put ideas in their head? Why should we explain it if there's no reason she'll ever need the information? On the other hand [ambivalence], I wouldn't want her to think it would be all right for her to go to bed with someone because

she sees John and me in bed. . . . I'll tell Cindy about sex when she asks [implying that her daughter will take the initiative]. I'm probably living in a fool's paradise" [probably!] (Nigro, 1975).

"SOCIETY'S" PROBLEMS

The ambivalence of the parents is, of course, shared by the rest of society, including the professionals. After all, we are all the product of a culture in which there is a strong taboo about sex. Some brief observations on the origins of the taboo are of interest.

Psychoanalytic Theory

Freud, of course, gave sex a prominent role in his theory of neurosis. He noted that "in the course of cultural development no other function has been so energetically and extensively repudiated. . . ." Freud regarded the origin of our sexual behavior as being the Oedipal experience, childhood sexual feelings for the opposite-sex parent, and the conflict and fears growing out of it (Fromm, 1953). For Fromm (1953), the cultural anxiety related to sex stems not from incestuous impulses but rather from parental prohibition of normal sexual activity of the child. The child's *physical* functions—first of defecation and later of sexual desires and actions—are given *moral* weightings. The child is made to feel guilty about natural feelings and, since the sexual urge is present in all of us from childhood on, it becomes a permanent potential source of guilt.

Religious Tradition

One sex educator (Johnson, 1973) sees the root of the association between sex and morality as lying in ancient Judeo-Christian beliefs. He notes that the influential St. Augustine wrote that the gateway to hell lay between a woman's thighs and that it was St. Augustine who permanently fixed the sex-sin guilt association in the Christian mind. Henry VIII brought ecclesiastical law under the jurisdiction of civil law and so provided the basis for the later transmission of Judeo-Christian morality and law to our shores by the Puritans. In Johnson's view, in the sexual sphere there has been no real separation of church and state in our country. The ancient religious-moral tradition persists in the precepts that govern our present behavior. Admittedly, the decade of the 1960s shook those precepts!

"See No Evil, Hear No Evil"

Given our tradition it is hardly surprising that all of us involved with retarded persons have commonly "overlooked" their sexuality (Nigro, 1975). It has been suggested that, like our ambivalent mother, the less they know the better off they are (Gordon, 1973b). (Certainly, that could be paraphrased as the less *we* know, the better off *we* are!) Nevertheless, efforts to encourage a full life within the community rather than in physically segregated settings make clear the need for assisting them in *understanding* their sexual feelings and in learning how they can be expressed in fulfilling and socially acceptable ways.

Sexual Behavior
in Retarded Individuals

Given our cultural ambivalence, we cannot expect to assist retarded persons and their families if we reject the reality of their sexuality. Are retarded people really sexual? Apart from personal observation and anecdotal reports, research on this is meager—a not surprising condition since the topic itself is inherently less open to study. What is available primarily relates to those with mild retardation, though some descriptive data are also offered on more severely impaired individuals.

MILDLY RETARDED

Community and Institutional

Gebhard (1973) surveyed 84 white male adolescents and young adults, the great majority of whom were mildly retarded. They all had institutional histories—about two-thirds in correctional settings and the remainder in mental retardation ones. Though the sexually segregated quality of their lives while institutionalized can be assumed to have affected the nature of their sexual experiences, it cannot be held responsible for sexual behavior itself. No difference was found between this population and a nonretarded comparison group; both attained puberty at age 13, and over 90 percent of each acknowledged some masturbation. Within the retarded population was reported the full range of sexual behaviors—petting, premarital coitus, and homosexuality. As one might have anticipated, the frequency of homosexuality was greater in the group with the institutional history, and, interestingly, its persistence in postinstitutional adult life was related to the length of prior institutionalization or incarceration. About one-quarter of the adults were exclusively homosexual, but Gebhard concludes that in spite of their institutional histories, retarded persons seem remarkably heterosexual in their orientation.

Of the adult portion of the group, about half had married, but two-thirds of these marriages were broken either by separation or divorce. We can speculate that *any* population that largely consists of members with correctional histories is likely to have less stable marriages than the general population. Within the marriages the frequency of coitus was comparable to that of the controls.

Edgerton (1963) enriches our picture of sexuality in such a population by describing the sexual attitudes of male and female residents of an institution. They were physically normal and generally mildly retarded, and their average age was 21. They perceived themselves as the elite group within the residential hierarchy and would, today, be found in much smaller numbers, if at all, in institutional populations. Among males there was much evidence of heterosexual interest. Girls were judged in terms of their attractiveness, and there was a desire for exclusiveness in dating relationships. Necking was an early expectation, but a "traditional" morality was professed. Boys would not date girls who were sexually active and expressed repugnance at oral sex and at male and female homosexuality.

We are told that "romance" for the girls was as important as "fighting" for the boys. "Elite" girls achieved status through romantic appeal, were committed to exclusiveness in their male relationships, and were very jealous of their boyfriends. They also expressed traditional sexual values but were more tolerant of homosexuality.

What emerges is a portrayal of male-female attitudes that appear to mirror those of their nonretarded contemporaries. Their intellectual limitations do not seem to have affected their sexual selves. Indeed, this may have increased their compliance with institutional rules regarding sexual behavior, their being less ready intellectually to challenge the rules conveyed to them by institutional staff—persons in authority.

Sexual Behavior in a Large Community Residential Facility

A much "quieter" picture of sexual life is reflected in impressions gained of male and female residents of a 48-bed facility located in the community (Carruth, 1973). Characterized as "high borderline retarded," these young adults (mean age 24, range 18–40) seemed to share something of a "family" relationship. They dined together and worked in the same sheltered workshop. Their social relationships were almost exclusively with each other, perhaps because they were not within easy access to a population center.

The seemingly more restrained quality of their sexual lives may relate to the fact that their social activities were well monitored. Though they were allowed to visit each other's rooms, they were required to inform counselors of these visits and to keep the doors open. Over the course of a year, only one sexual episode, a homosexual one, was observed. It can be presumed that the "open-door policy" would have discouraged sexual behavior in even the most ardent of them (and us)! It was reported that only a small proportion of the residents were dating and only with other residents. Their major social interactions involved watching television together in a day room; at the sexual level, intimacies consisted of some touching and pinching.

Marriage

Among them there had been one marriage. A newspaper story reports on the prospective wedding of another retarded couple. They had met in the group home where they lived and had fallen in love. Because of house rules that forbade the closing of doors, they took walks in order to be alone. On the streets, they often drew hostile stares. She had lost an arm in an accident, and he had cerebral palsy. He observed, "People don't like or trust the mentally disabled. Given enough time, maybe people will understand we're trying to live a normal life. We have sexual feelings like everybody else. Of course we do," angry that people would think otherwise.

MODERATELY TO PROFOUNDLY RETARDED

We are probably not too surprised at the apparent normality of the sexuality of mildly retarded individuals. Even the reported absence of sexual behavior in the 48-bed community facility does not mean a lowered level of drive. Under conditions of constant scrutiny, it can be assumed that only bathrooms provide some measure of privacy and that masturbation becomes the primary sexual outlet. But what of those with more severe impairment?

The population studied by Gebhard (1973) included 15 males with IQs in the 41–50 range. The major finding was a somewhat reduced level of sexual activity, but even here the frequency of masturbation is reported at 80 percent. Interviews revealed that sexual arousal could be produced by thinking about females and seeing pictures of unclothed women. Their response to potentially erotic stimuli were seen as "surprisingly . . . very like the responses of the retarded group as a whole."

The Gebhard study also indicated a normal range of sexual behaviors in a moderately retarded subgroup, an observation also made by Edgerton (1975). In persons with IQs in the 36–51 range, there was manifest "every conceivable form of sexual behavior. . . ." And even in individuals with profound retardation sexual behavior was seen, seemingly chiefly masturbatory in nature.

Sexual Knowledge

If the reality of sexual feelings in retarded persons is acknowledged, then the manner of their expression becomes relevant. The goal for them, as for the rest of us, is for culturally appropriate and thus adaptive expression of these most intimate feelings. And this begins with their understanding of these feelings and socially acceptable modes of expression. This brings us to the question of what knowledge retarded people have about sex and some information is available for those with mild and moderate impairment. They are likely to be familiar with common sexual terms, recognize such activities as masturbation and intercourse, and to understand the relationship between intercourse and pregnancy. They are also aware of such social customs as dating and marriage and recognize the tie between marriage and parenthood (a tie that may be loosening in our culture). They are less likely to be aware of methods of birth control and of venereal hazards (Edmonson, Wish, & Fiechtl, 1977; Hall & Morris, 1976; Hall, Morris, & Bricker, 1973). Interestingly, moderately retarded *adults* do not seem to differ in any major way from their mildly retarded counterparts, though the latter are, as might be expected, somewhat more knowledgable (Edmonson et al., 1977). Major differences in sexual knowledge began to be evident in the below-40 IQ range.

Although at the adult level, moderately and mildly retarded individuals are described as roughly comparable in sexual knowledge, this appears to be less true at school age. In one study (Fischer & Krajicek, 1974), trainable youth, ages 10–17, were reported to have little understanding of intercourse, pregnancy, and childbirth. Only about half recognized a picture of a male masturbating or had some awareness of the relationship between intercourse and childbirth.

Sexual Attitudes and Behavior

ATTITUDES

Based on responses to pictorial representations of sex, mildly and moderately retarded young adults express attitudes that reflect relatively traditional mores (Edmonson et al., 1977). Indeed, they appear to be much more conservative than many of their nonretarded contemporaries. There is strong disapproval of homosexuality and of relationships between married and unmarried persons. In the sexual domain itself there is disapproval of masturbation (though it appears to be widely practiced by them) and apparent acceptance of folklorish admonitions regarding its consequences. Similarly, they are negative toward intercourse among unmarried individuals, though there does seem to be some acceptance of it among persons who have a relationship. In this respect, they seem to mirror the increased acceptance in contemporary youth of sexual intimacy as a component of a serious relationship. Toward marriage for themselves, they were strongly positive, an observation often made about retarded adults (e.g., Edgerton, 1967).

In his study of formerly institutionalized and predominantly mildly retarded adults, Edgerton (1967) noted the importance placed on marriage. Sex, marriage, and parenthood were of central concern. For individuals whose former institutional status was something to be hidden, the assumption of the roles of spouse and parent was visible evidence of their "normalcy." For sterilized females, the preclusion of the possibility of parenthood was especially frustrating (Edgerton & Sabagh, 1963). Those who were more accepting of sterilization doubted their ability to properly care for children. We will return shortly to the vexing issue of the retarded person as "parent."

BEHAVIOR

Within the context of serving retarded individuals in the community, the attitudes of caregivers toward sexuality become extremely important. Even though the retarded individual is likely to express conservative ideas regarding sexual behavior, the behavior itself exists. Yet whether in small community residential facilities or in large institutions, open manifestations of sexuality are generally unwelcome (Deisher, 1973), though, in some sexually segregated settings, homosexuality may be ignored or, where heterosexual control is possible, contraceptive pills provided (Narot, 1973). Though our culture is now much more accepting of sex before or outside of marriage (Reiss, 1973), we are not yet comfortable enough with our own sexuality to sanction the same behavior in persons who are not sufficiently free to handle their own needs for privacy. In the author's view, it is the distinction between public and private expressions of sexuality that creates the greatest conflict, not the sexual behavior itself. As long as care givers severely limit opportunities for normal sexual expression, socially acceptable behavior is precluded. If, ethically and morally, we cannot deny retarded individuals the human gratification we demand for ourselves (Narot, 1973), then care givers must begin to create the conditions that can allow for normal expression.[3]

---

[3]For provocative discussions of religious and sociological aspects of sexuality, the reader is referred to chapters by Narot, Hoffmeyer, and Davis in *Human Sexuality and the Mentally Retarded* (De la Cruz and LaVeck, 1973).

Marriage

NATURE

Research studies on the marriages of retarded individuals, typically mildly retarded, though few in number and commonly limited to small numbers of families, provide some impressions of their general character. The predominant one is that they are not particularly different from those of nonretarded persons in terms of general stability and feelings of satisfaction (Andron & Sturm, 1973; Edgerton, 1967). Given the greater obstacles that are likely to confront such families—lower income, job security, and job status; minimal social education, and, in the case of institutionalized persons, the absence of a model of what spouse roles entail—they appear to have done better than might have been predicted (Andron & Sturm, 1973; Edgerton, 1973; Floor, Baxter, Rosen, & Zisfein, 1975; Mattinson, 1973; Peck & Stephens, 1965). Doing better than everyone expects seems to be the rule in retardation! In commenting on the appropriateness of marriage but not parenthood for retarded adults, Bass (1964) saw the relationship as meeting needs for sexual expression, affection, and mutual support. The companionship aspect was particularly valued and was contrasted with their social isolation before marriage.

Given the reality of some prospect of marriage, researchers see the need for providing sex education, contraceptive information, and premarital counseling (Floor, et al., 1975). Another area of concern is financial (Andron & Sturm, 1973). Money management problems were referred to in Chapter 1, and prospective partners may need assistance in budgeting and in understanding and using credit and banks. In one study the average amount of debt was 10 times greater than the savings!

Another important adjunct to successful marriage for some retarded couples was access to other "helping" adults—parents, other relatives, neighbors, or social workers (Andron & Sturm, 1975). This is another reminder of the "benefactor" (advocate) role referred to in the first chapter. There is need for a human service mechanism under which individuals with *some* dependency needs can receive *selective* assistance—only as much as is necessary. Partial or limited guardianship, described in an earlier chapter, is one example in another sphere of an attempt to tailor supervision such that the ward retains as much autonomy as possible.

In the Andron and Sturm series, 11 of the 12 couples were childless. Seven of the 11 women had been sterilized, either during an earlier institutionalization or later at their families' insistence. Of the seven sterilized women, five were unhappy about their inability to bear children. Their feelings ranged from disappointment to bitterness. In some cases they had not been told the true nature of the operation (e.g., "appendectomy"). Presumably, current laws regarding "consent" make such deceptions less likely. Among these childless couples there was interest in adoption; their nurturing desires seem to have been quite strong.

RETARDED PERSONS AS PARENTS

Whatever the optimism regarding the potential of retarded adults to fulfill spouse roles, at least for those with mild retardation, there seems to be little enthusiasm for their assuming parental ones (Bass, 1964; Goodman, Budner, & Lesh, 1971; Edgerton, 1973; Peck & Stephens, 1965). Though our knowledge of the quality of life experienced by children of retarded parents is very limited, what is known should make us cautious about attempts at social planning for this population as a "group."

Floor et al. (1975) studied a large series of formerly institutionalized young adults among whom there were 54 marriages and 32 children. Borderline in intelligence ($\overline{X}$ IQ 76), their findings are certainly relevant to a mildly retarded population. Of the 32 children, one had been removed from the family by the courts because of "neglect." The researchers commented, "While the care of some children would be questionable by middle-class standards, there are others who appear to be receiving proper medical attention and affection from both parents." Even one investigator who appears to feel strongly about the undesirability of retarded individuals as parents (Scally, 1973) indicates that at least one-third of such children were being reared satisfactorily. That two-thirds were seen as in undesirable child-rearing settings should give us pause, however.

A study of a group of 15 mildly retarded adolescents and their parents is also instructive (Goodman, Budner, & Lesh, 1971). Eleven of the 15 wanted both marriage *and* parenthood. The parents were supportive of their children's desire for marriage but were mixed in response to the wish for children. Those who visualized their children as suitable parents felt that their affectional and nurturing feelings would compensate for the intellectual limitations, a view considered unrealistic by the researchers. Those parents who questioned their child's capacity to function as a parent had several reservations. They wondered about the impact of intellectual impairment on planning and decision making. They also wondered whether the children of such a marriage would be normal. And if they were normal, how would they feel about having retarded parents? What would be the emotional impact on them? Clearly, here the parents are projecting the impact of their own experience.

A questioning of the capacity of retarded adults to function effectively as parents is not limited to the nonretarded observer. As just stated, some retarded individuals also express doubts about their abilities to meet the responsibilities of parenthood. Ironically, those with sufficient self-awareness to look at themselves in relation to the demands of parenting probably have the best potential for actually fulfilling that role!

A married male in another study (Sabagh & Edgerton, 1962), said, "I can understand why they did [referring to sterilization] as they have to have parents who will take care of their kids and sometimes these people . . . couldn't do that." He added, however, "They should not sterilize everybody because some of us would take care of our kids and now we don't have no chance to have any." Among the couples studied by Andron and Sturm (1973), several acknowledged limitations as potential parents. One women felt that she was too nervous, another that she was simply incapable of caring for children, and a third quite candidly observed that although she wanted children she knew that her mother would end up caring for them!

EFFECTIVE PARENTING

It is apparent that the retarded adult is generally regarded as lacking in the qualities that make for effective parenting, though the nature of the presumed deficit is not always made explicit. It is the view here that it is in the role of "teacher," a role detailed in Chapter 5, that the retarded person is necessarily going to be limited. But we do not require that nonretarded individuals meet some test of potential parent effectiveness in order to bear children. Do we unfairly discriminate against retarded persons when we discourage their becoming parents?

If "effective parenting" involves both an affective and teaching dimension (see Chap. 5), then it is incumbent upon society to create the means through which such outcomes can be realized. At a minimum this involves consideration of the responsibilities of parenthood taught within the framework of family-life education programs. It means awareness of alternative life-styles within marriage and recognition that parenting involves demands as well as satisfactions. At the most basic level, the retarded adolescent should understand the relationship between sex and pregnancy and the means of preventing unwanted pregnancy through contraception. Earlier-reported research reveals that it is precisely in the contraceptive or family planning area that the retarded adolescent is least knowledgeable. Since the school years are the last time that society can be certain to have prolonged involvement with any of its citizens, it is crucial that these issues are addressed then.

A PHILOSOPHY OF INTERVENTION

All of the aforementioned measures are *educational* and *voluntary*. They constitute the most conservative (least restrictive) courses of action a society can take toward a matter of general concern. While the intent is to encourage *rational* choices, by their voluntary nature we accept the reality that people whom we would question as would-be "effective" parents are *free* to make their own choices. Though freedom carries with it the recognition of making choices with which we might disagree, the a priori prevention of such choices starts us down a dangerous road. Others would determine who shall survive. Once established, such a principle has no absolute limits; all ends can be rationalized. This does not mean that we are not free to use the legal system to attempt to impose our solution by preventing pregnancies in individuals who seem unable to make "rational" choices. But the courts provide a basis for dealing with this problem on an *individual* rather than a *class* basis, and it is this procedure that assures the greatest likelihood of individual equity and fairness.

Sex Education

It is ironic that the individuals about whom we have the most ambivalence regarding sex education are in the greatest need of it. Whether in community or institutional settings, they have less opportunity to acquire a realistic understanding of their sexual selves than do their nonretarded peers. Without proper sex education, there is the risk of sexual exploitation or of sexual rejection (Edmonson, 1980).

THE TEACHER

Because the need for sex education has only recently been acknowledged, teachers are often unprepared. They are uncertain about what to teach, unfamiliar with teaching materials, and, most important, frequently uncomfortable with the topic itself (Johnson, 1973). Regarding "comfort," Johnson discusses the need for the teacher to come to terms with the "language" of sex. He is referring to our sexual slang and sees teachers as often failing to communicate because they persist in using terms that are foreign to their students.[4]

Apart from the anatomical terminology of sex, it is the behavioral aspect that is of particular concern. A well-known educator (Gordon, 1973c) suggests that the following sexual guidelines need to be communicated:

1. Masturbation is a normal sexual expression no matter how frequently it is done and at what age. It becomes a compulsive, punitive, self-destructive form of behavior largely as a result of suppression, punishment, and resulting feelings of guilt.

2. All direct sexual behavior involving the genitals should take place only in privacy. However, since institutions for the retarded (or group homes) are not designed or operated to ensure privacy, the definition of what constitutes privacy . . . must be very liberal. Bathrooms, one's own bed, bushes [!], and basements are private domains.

3. Anytime a girl and a boy who are physically mature have sexual relations, they risk pregnancy.

4. Unless both members of a heterosexual couple clearly want to have a baby and understand the responsibilities involved in childrearing, they should use an effective method of birth control.

5. Until a person is about 18 years old, society holds that he or she should not have intercourse. After that age, the person can decide for himself.

6. Adults should not be permitted to use children sexually.

7. The only way to discourage homosexual expression is to risk heterosexual expression.

Although Gordon seems to be sanctioning parenthood, his encouragement of a greater acceptability of abortion and of voluntary sterilization indicates his reservations about retarded persons in this role.

---

[4]A useful package for teacher trainers is *Guidelines for Training in Sexuality and the Mentally Handicapped* (Kempton & Forman, 1976). See also Edmonson (1980) for a description of a variety of training materials.

EFFECTS OF SEX EDUCATION

A study of the impact of a sex education program on retarded youths indicates a greater readiness to discuss sexual feelings and some increase in masturbation (Kempton, 1978). A similar finding with regard to masturbation was reported in a sex education study with a nonretarded group (Kirby, Alter, & Scales, 1979).

Of particular interest was a program for trainable adolescents, ages 12–18, IQs 35–54, conducted over a 2- to 3-year period (Hamre-Nietupski & Williams, 1977). No behavioral data are reported, as the emphasis was on teaching-related cognitive content. Virtually all of them were capable of understanding such content as bodily distinctions, family relationships, and acceptable social behaviors. Concepts of personal hygiene were well understood, though those pertaining to reproduction seemed more difficult.

Because parents are often anxious and unclear about an adult role for their retarded child and certainly ambivalent about sex education, efforts to win their support are essential. One means of accomplishing this can be "parental groups," in which parents can be encouraged to explore their oft-unspoken fears and begin to face the reality of their child's sexuality.

RESIDENTIAL SERVICES

Increase in Community Facilities

In Chapter 6, there was a description of the variety of out-of-home residential options. The focus was on the rapidly expanding base of community alternatives to the traditional state institution. During the 1970s these programs grew at an extraordinary rate (Janicki, Mayeda, & Epple, 1983). From about 600 group homes in the early 1970s (O'Connor, 1976), the number had grown to 5700 by 1982. These were facilities serving not more than 15 residents; if those group homes serving more than 15 are included, the total in 1982 was about 6300. These community programs housed 58,000 individuals, 74 percent of whom (43,000) were in the smaller ones. The great majority of the residents, 85 percent, were 18 years of age and older (Bruininks, Hauber, & Kudla, 1980; Janicki et al., 1983).

In spite of their tremendous growth, the group homes have not been without problems, chief of which in the late 1970s pertained to staffing and funding (Bruininks, Kudla, Wieck, & Hauber, 1980). Recruitment and retention of qualified staff are characteristic concerns. Wages are low, advancement opportunities limited, and turnover is high. Funding of group homes has also always been marginal. They have not had equal access to federal and state funds, the state-operated institutions particularly benefiting from federal support. Another concern has been for the services provided to residents. The kind of continuum described in Chapter 6 is often lacking. There may be inadequate programming for residents; a detailed description of life in group homes studied by Landesman-Dwyer et al. (1980) makes clear how little time is actually used for training purposes. The program may also lack other supportive community services such as respite care, transportation, other residential alternatives, advocacy, follow-along, and nutrition.

By the late 1970s, in addition to the group homes, there were also 5000–7000 family care beds (Bruininks, Hill, & Thersheim, 1980) and perhaps half again as many apartment beds (Janicki et al., 1983).

During this same decade, under the thrust of "deinstitutionalization," there was a 54 percent reduction in the national institutional population (Scheerenberger, 1982). Whether this trend continues depends on our capacity to serve the most impaired segments of the retarded population in community programs. They make up the great majority of the current institutional population but are also receiving services in community programs.

The "Community" Rationale

Proponents of normalization and deinstitutionalization were initially reflecting outrage at gross abuses in living conditions in some institutions (Blatt & Kaplan, 1966; Blatt, 1970). Smaller and more homelike community programs were seen as likely to be more responsive to individual resident needs, to avoid "herd" treatment, and to foster growth. But research bearing on the presumed advantages of community living had yet to be done. This is no longer the case. There is a rapidly growing body of research that reveals that more normalizing environments produce increased competency at all levels of retardation. There are two streams of research that pertain: one compares the "quality of care" in large and small residential facilities, and the other considers comparative behavioral competencies in settings that differ in size and location.

QUALITY OF CARE

This domain has primarily involved the study of the degree to which residential programs individualize client care. On management practice or care scales that vary from resident-oriented to institution-oriented, larger facilities *tend* to be less resident-oriented than smaller ones (King, Raynes, & Tizard, 1971; MacEachron, 1983; McCormick, Balla, & Zigler, 1975; Pratt, Luszcz, & Brown, 1980). But there is no simple relationship between size and quality of care (Balla, 1976; Baroff, 1980; Landesman-Dwyer, Sackett, & Kleinman, 1980). While smaller settings are likelier to be more individualized in their care, care practices vary widely across settings of all sizes. On related dimensions, overprotective practices that can stifle greater independence are not uncommon in smaller family settings (Campbell, 1971; Bjaanes & Butler, 1974), and some group homes may be as isolating of the resident from the broader community as the physically more removed institution (Edgerton, 1975). Nonetheless, one consequence of this research has been to encourage the development of more individualized or familylike groupings, even within larger residential settings (MacEachron, 1983; Raynes, 1977, Zigler & Balla, 1977).

What is perhaps improbable in any large setting, irrespective of groupings, is the nurturing of the sense of freedom, autonomy, and lack of regimentation, which *can* be the subjective experience of formerly institutionalized persons now living in small group homes (e.g., Scheerenberger & Feldenthal, 1977). Clearly, not all offer such freedom (e.g., Campbell, 1971; Bjaanes & Butler, 1974), but it is only when numbers are small that individualization is *possible*!

ADAPTIVE BEHAVIOR

The second strand of research relates to behavioral competency under a variety of residential conditions. The findings have been unusually consistent. Higher levels of adaptive behavior are associated with (a) movement from large institutions to the community (Conroy, Efthimiou, & Lemanowicz, 1982; Kleinberg & Galligan, 1983; Thompson & Carey, 1980), (b) continued residence in the community (Aanes & Moen, 1976), and (c) movement from larger to smaller units within the same institution (Hemming, Lavender, & Pill, 1981; MacEachron, 1983; Witt, 1981). Within a picture of enhanced behavioral competence, several skill areas seem to be particularly responsive to deinstitutionalization or to residential change within larger settings. They are language, domestic (household) skills, and socialization (Kleinberg & Galligan, 1983). In considering these adaptive gains, especially domestic skills in community settings, Kleinberg and Galligan note that there is obviously greater *opportunity* to engage in such activities in community residences than in institutions (see Figs. 40 and 41). Community settings also seem to foster social skills. Increased resident-to-resident verbal interactions appear to be encouraged (Pratt, Luszcz, & Brown, 1980), strengthening the language area, and one observes more cooperative social behavior. Pratt et al. (1980) also found that the degree of "controlling" speech of caretakers tended to be lower in community settings and, in an earlier study, that "controlling speech" and "stimulating care" were inversely related (Pratt, Bumstead, & Raynes, 1976).

OPPORTUNITY

In reviewing the factors that seem to underlie the behavioral advantages of community residence, that of *opportunity* appears to be particularly relevant. Residents of small group homes can learn a variety of cooking skills, for instance, because the residence is feeding six people, not 60 or 600! Cooking is done in a regular "family" kitchen, using the kind of cooking equipment found in the home and in amounts that are appropriate to a family. There is time to teach, to learn, to practice, to make mistakes. The caretakers are not operating under the kind of pressures that require cooks in institutions to prepare meals for hundreds or even thousands of persons. Moreover, shopping is done at neighborhood food stores. Residents can accompany caretakers and participate in the selection and purchase of food. Residential facilities serving large numbers of people do not buy their groceries at the local supermarket; they are trucked in!

Similarly, by virtue of its location in the community rather than physically remote from it, there is easier access to its educational, vocational, and recreational resources. Eyman et al. (1979) studied changes in adaptive skills of residents within community facilities over a 3-year period. In general, older and less retarded individuals tended to improve in adaptive behavior irrespective of where they resided. But within these community programs those that particularly fostered

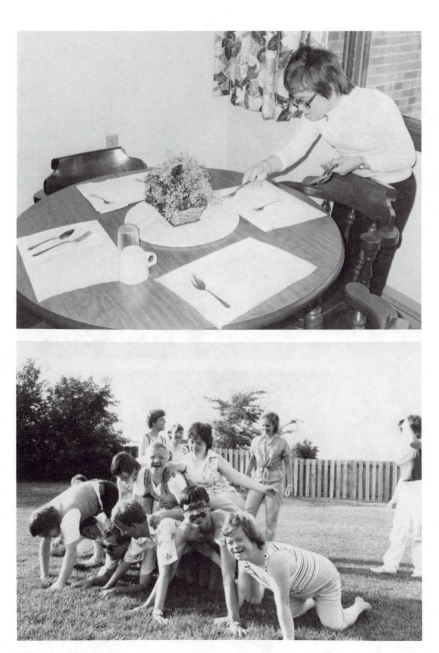

FIG. 40 Residents of a group home for youths with Down syndrome. Photos are courtesy of REM, Inc.

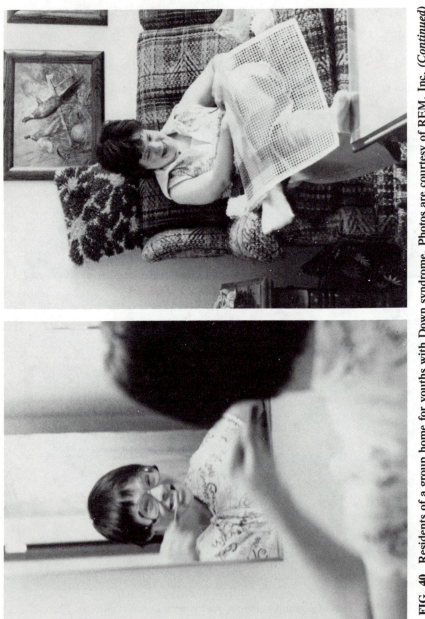

FIG. 40 Residents of a group home for youths with Down syndrome. Photos are courtesy of REM, Inc. *(Continued)*

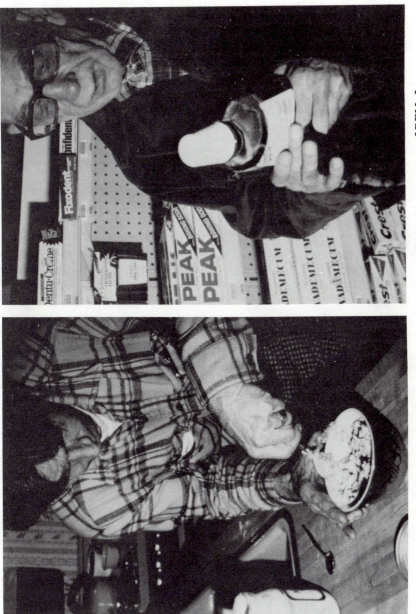

FIG. 41 Acquiring community living skills in an adult group home. Photos are courtesy of REM, Inc.

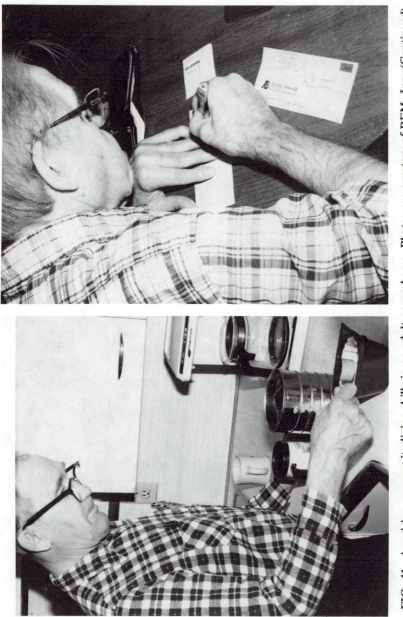

FIG. 41 Acquiring community living skills in an adult group home. Photos are courtesy of REM, Inc. *(Continued)*

greater independence ("personal self-sufficiency") were (a) easy to get to and near community services, (b) fitted well within their neighborhood (group homes in residential rather than in nonresidential neighborhoods), and (c) were physically attractive and comfortable places in which to live.[5] Hull and Thompson (1980) also found that the location of a group home with regard to its convenience of access (e.g., via public transportation) was an important predictor of resident adaptive behavior. Other enhancing care-giver activities were the promotion of interactions with nonhandicapped persons and activities that encouraged self-sufficiency and independence. To the extent that the retarded person is *exposed* to opportunities for encountering and coping with a wider range of environments, there is the possibility of change and personal growth. This is the essence of the observation of Roger, the mildly retarded young adult described in Chapter 1, who is quoted as saying, "People are retarded by what they don't know." Only through *exposure* can new learning occur and the "don't know" diminish.

Comparison of Group Homes and Family-Care Homes

NATURE AND IMPACT OF COMMUNITY LIVING

It appears that about 10 percent of the community residential population were living in family-care homes. Here, the individual actually resides with a family in their own home. Several studies have compared the residential experience in family-care and group homes. Baker et al. (1974) found family-care homes to be more protective and less training-oriented than group homes. Group homes offered greater autonomy, demanded more in the way of household responsibilities, and involved greater community outreach. But Scheerenberger and Felsenthal (1977) regarded the family-care home as less regimented and as a more individualized environment. Nevertheless, resident satisfaction was nearly universal in both settings. These were formerly institutionalized adults who had been living in the community for at least 1 year. Only about 11 percent indicated a wish to return to the institution. Another group studied had been place in nursing homes and intermediate-care facilities, possibly larger than the average group home. They were a considerably older population, average age 44 compared to an average of 13 for the family-care residents and 27 for the group home residents, and were somewhat less positive about their current placement. Nevertheless 74 percent expressed satisfaction with it, 29 percent indicating a desire to return to the institution. In the upcoming section on the institutions we will discover that there has been a sharp reduction in the population of deinstitutionalized individuals placed in nursing homes.

The most comprehensive of the studies examined the behavioral effects of at least 2 years of postinstitutional community residence in family-care and group

---

[5]These are representations of factors derived from an unpublished factor analytic study of PASS 3 by Demaine, Wilson, Silverstein, and Mayeda.

home settings (Willer & Intagliata, 1982). Growth in self-care and community skills occurred in both settings and at all levels of retardation. Although the group homes were particularly strong in increasing community skills (meal preparation, traveling, money management, shopping), family-care homes tended to reduce behavior problems. Family-care residents differed from those in the group homes in being more passive and less impulsive. But they were comparable in level of involvement with the wider community and in out-of-home contacts with friends and family. Group home staff were seen as benefiting from training in managing behavior problems, whereas family-care homes were cautioned against "sheltering," the concern of Baker et al. (1974), and urged to provide their residents with greater skills in community living.

Institutions

In spite of a dramatic reduction in the institutional population in the 1970s and an overall decline of 35 percent from its peak of 195,000 in 1967 (Lakin et al., 1982), in the early 1980s there were still more than twice as many individuals in state-operated "public residential facilities" (PRFs) than in community homes. A view of that population is now presented as it appeared in 1981 (Scheerenberger, 1982).

NUMBER AND SIZE

In 1981 there were 282 PRFs serving a population of about 126,000. This represented a reduction of some 64,000 from the 1970 census of 190,000. Paradoxically, this population decline has not been mirrored by a reduction in the *number* of state PRFs. Their number appears to have continually grown; it is their average *size* that has decreased (Epple, Jacobson, & Janicki, 1985). In 1981 the median PRF housed 393 individuals, a 22 percent reduction in size over the PRF of the mid-1960s (median 506). Prior to 1960, the average PRF housed more than one thousand persons (1160). There has been a 66 percent reduction in the size of PRFs since the 1960s, but in 1981 there were still 32 with capacities in excess of 1000 and three with capacities exceeding 2000. PRFs in 1981 ranged in size from a "group-home-like" 12 to a giant of 2446.

SEX DISTRIBUTION

Of the PRF population, 57 percent were male and 43 percent female. The proportion of males has increased by 3 percent since 1976. This may reflect the tendency of institutions to serve individuals whose behavior is less manageable in community facilities.

LEVEL OF RETARDATION

The 1981 population distribution by level of retardation was 7.1 percent mild, 13.0 percent moderate, 24.4 percent severe, and 55.5 percent profound. There has been a reduction in the proportion of all levels of retardation served except for the profound. In the 1960s about 27 percent of the institutional population was profoundly retarded; that number has more than doubled in recent years.

AGE

The average age was 32 years, and there was little difference in average age by degree of retardation—mild 37, moderate and severe 34, and profound 30. The somewhat lower average age of the profound segment is presumed to reflect their lower life expectancy (e.g., Baroff, 1974; Cleland, Powell, & Tarkington, 1971).

ADAPTIVE BEHAVIOR

Consonant with the population change, the proportion of current PRF residents who could independently feed and toilet themselves was reduced. In 1981, 65 percent could feed themselves and 61 percent were toilet-trained, reductions of about 25 percent since the mid 1970s. There was also a major decline in language skills, a domain of particular deficit in the profoundly retarded. Only 51 percent of the institutional population could communicate verbally as compared with 84 percent in the mid-1970s. There was also a drop of from 93 percent to 76 percent in those who could understand speech. There was no change in ambulation. The proportion who could walk without assistance remained at 74 percent.

MULTIPLE HANDICAPS

Again, in keeping with the population change, the proportion of multihandicapped persons increased. They were 38 percent of the institutional population in 1981 as against 34 percent in the mid-1970s. It would appear that the most pronounced increase was in the number of residents classified as emotionally disturbed—a whopping 150 percent. As community programs have grown and institutions have been depopulated, retarded persons with severe behavior problems have become increasingly visible. They have often fallen between the cracks of service agencies—rejected by mental health because of the retardation and frustrating to mental retardation workers because of their "mental health" problems (e.g., Rowitz, 1980; Reiss, Levitan, & McNally, 1982). It is out of this growing concern for the humane management of severe behavior problems in the retarded population that an entire chapter, the final one, has been devoted.

ADMISSIONS, READMISSIONS, AND DISCHARGES

Admissions

Admission rates also reflect the population decline. In 1981 there were 5733 new admissions, a 33 percent drop relative to the mid-1970s. Interestingly, admission rates were down for *all* levels of retardation and for persons below age 22. The average ages at admission by level of retardation were mild 20 years, moderate 25 years, severe 27 years, and profound 21 years. Since admission rates were down even for the profoundly retarded, their growth in the population must reflect less likelihood of subsequent discharge. Most new admissions came from the family home (40%) or from another mental retardation residential setting (37%). In a subsequent study (Lakin et al., 1983), behavior that injured others or was unusual or disruptive was the chief cause of admission (in 1982). The significance of behavior problems for both admission and readmission has also been noted in a national survey of public and community residential facilities (Hill & Bruininks, 1984).

Readmissions

Readmission rates have also declined. There were 2312 in 1981, a 28 percent decrease from a mid-1970s rate of 3227. The average age at readmission was only slightly higher than that of first admissions—mild 21, moderate 29, severe 28, and profound 27. Again, behavior disorders were the chief cause (Lakin et al., 1983).

Discharge

Even with an institutional population that is increasing in degree of retardation, movement of residents out of the facility continued at a pace unchanged from the mid-1970s, though a decline was projected for 1982. In 1981 nearly 12 percent of the PRF population was moved—to group homes (24%), to other PRFs (23%), to own home (19%), and to community intermediate care facilities (14%). Interestingly, some 16% were actually ready for placement, reflecting a lag in the creation of alternative residences. On a more optimistic note, there was a very significant decline in the use of nursing homes as a placement alternative. In 1976, 16 percent were so placed in contrast to only 4 percent in 1981.

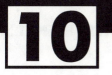

Management of Behavior Problems Prominent in Severe and Profound Retardation

OVERVIEW

The management of behavior problems of severely and profoundly retarded persons involves the same behavioral strategies applied to less handicapped individuals, but the degree of retardation does affect the kinds of reinforcers that will be appropriate. This is addressed in the section on positive reinforcement. In Chapter 6, the basic principles underlying the "behavioral" approach were described; they reflect, in essence, the only kinds of contingencies that can be applied to behavior—reward, punish, or ignore. Singly or in combination, these are the methods used to influence behavior, and in this chapter they are redefined and described in some detail. The chapter includes (a) a review of the application of these contingencies to behavior problems in the severely and profoundly retarded population, (b) presentation of a behaviorally oriented problem-solving strategy that can be applied to any behavior disorder, and (c) a discussion of treatment procedures, behavioral and otherwise, for problems prominent in this population—aggression, stereotypy (self-stimulation), self-injurious behavior, rumination, and pica. Apart from the material presented here, comprehensive reviews of this literature are found in Johnson and Baumeister (1981), Matson and McCartney (1981), Schroeder, Mulick, and Schroeder (1979), Thompson and Grabowski (1972, 1977),[1] and Whitman, Stibak, and Reid, (1983).

---

[1] A good how-to-do-it text.

BEHAVIORAL CONTINGENCIES (CONSEQUENCES)

Positive Reinforcement

This is a rewarding consequence. It may be provided for the absence of undesired behavior or the presence of that which is desired. It is the most culturally preferred contingency (e.g., Harris & Ersner-Hershfield, 1978), because it avoids those that are intended to be unpleasant. (In Chap. 6, our concerns about punishment were indicated.)

Four types of positive reinforcement have been identified. They are distinguished from each other by their degree of compatibility with the behavior one seeks to modify. They are differential reinforcement of (1) compatible behavior (DRC), (2) incompatible behavior (DRI), (3) *any* other behavior (DRO), and (4) lower rates of the undesired behavior (DRL).

Although each has shown some effectiveness, DRI appears to be the most useful (Johnson & Baumeister, 1981). One of its limitations, also true of DRO, is that it does not require the presence of any *specific* behavior for reinforcement to occur, only the *absence* of the targeted negative behavior (NB).[2] In dispensing positive reinforcement there may be the inadvertent reinforcement of *other* NBs that are occurring at that time! The potential of positive reinforcers *alone* depends on such elements as their general availability, variety, and strength. As regards availability, while a given reinforcer may be available in a special treatment setting, it may be absent in nontreatment ones—hence the importance of combining social reinforcement (approval, praise, a smile) with whatever other reinforcers are used. Social reinforcers can be easily dispensed anywhere! With respect to variety, the range of reinforcers will include objects, preferred activities, pleasant edibles, the aforementioned approval, stars, tokens, and money. The power of each of these will be influenced in part by the client's intellectual level and prior history. With respect to intellect, one is apt to find a significant narrowing of the range of reinforcers in persons with profound retardation. There may be limited interest in others, hence reduced responsiveness to social reinforcement, and in objects and activities that are enjoyed at higher levels of mental development. As we shall see, here there is likely to be dependence on "primary" (physiological) reinforcers (e.g., edibles) or on such experiences as pleasant tactile and kinesthetic stimulation.

Withdrawal of Positive Reinforcement

EXTINCTION

This method assumes that if the consequences presumed to be maintaining NB are eliminated, the behavior will disappear. It is accomplished by either deliberately ignoring NB (when it is assumed that "attention" to the behavior has been

---

[2]For convenience, we shall hereafter refer to negative behavior under treatment as NB and desired or appropriate behavior as AB.

reinforcing it) or by creating settings where the presumed reinforcers cannot be experienced (e.g., reducing off-task behavior by arranging an environment in which there is less likelihood of distraction). A distinction is drawn between extinction and time-out. In the former, the occurrence of the targeted NB elicits no response; in the latter it does.

Extinction has been widely employed with "nuisance" behaviors such as excessive attention getting (Ayllon & Michael, 1959), tantrums (Allen, Turner, & Everett, 1970), and spitting (!), (Forehand, 1973). It has also been used in dealing with more disruptive behaviors—property destruction (Martin & Foxx, 1973), aggression (Allen et al., 1970; Martin & Foxx, 1973), and self-injurious behavior (SIB) (Jones, Simmons, & Frankel, 1974; Lovaas & Simmons, 1969). Extinction obviously has serious limitations in the management of genuine physical attacks against others or in physically injurious behavior directed against the self. With reference to SIB, extinction will be effective if the purpose of the hitting is clearly to gain adult attention and the intensity of the hitting is not severe enough to cause physical damage (e.g., Duker [1975] on control of SIB in a Lesch-Nyhan child). The child who hits himself and then looks at the adult for his response is a good candidate for this method. Another limitation is that the results of extinction are usually gradual rather than dramatic, especially with high-frequency NBs, and large amounts of NB may have to occur before it lessens. The author once waited out 5000 self-hits before the behavior finally ceased. It was possible to do this because the individual was wearing a protective guard, which prevented actual injury.

TIME-OUT

This commonly used procedure consists of removal of the possibility of positive reinforcement when NB occurs. A number of time-out variants have been described (Schroeder, Mulick, & Schroeder, 1979). They involve (1) ignoring the "offender" (O) for a specific period of time, thus depriving him of attention; (2) physically removing oneself from O's presence, again depriving him of attention; (3) temporarily preventing participation in ongoing activities (e.g., brief meal deprivation) but not physically removing him from the setting (so-called "nonexclusionary time-out" (Foxx & Shapiro, 1978); (4) physically restraining O but not removing him from setting; (5) secluding —temporary removal to a separate and presumably nonreinforcing setting ("seclusion"); and (6) temporarily covering O's eyes and face ("facial screening"; Lutzker, 1978; Zeigob, Jenkins, Becker, & Bristow, 1973; Zeigob, Alford, & House, 1978).

Time-out has been a very widely used method; the ubiquitous "time-out room" is evidence of its popularity. In its various forms it has been employed with aggression (Poling & Ryan, 1977), SIB (Lucero, Frieman, Spoering, & Fehrenbacher, 1976; Tate & Baroff, 1966), and stereotypy or self-stimulation (Sachs, 1973). The author witnessed the effectiveness of the second of the six variants in connection with SIB in a blind autistic child. Taken for a walk in unfamiliar surroundings, the child needed someone to hold his hand in order to find his way about. When he struck himself we would remove our hands, leaving him standing in a strange setting without means of guidance (Tate & Baroff, 1966). Presumably, the unpleasant consequences of sudden loss of needed physical contact was strong enough "medicine" to cause him to inhibit self-hitting.

Other behaviors treated with this method have been food stealing and that dreaded duo, regurgitation and rumination. Food stealing was decreased by terminating eating and removing the person to a seclusion room for the remainder of the meal (Barton, Guess, Garcia, & Baer, 1970). Regurgitation and rumination was similarly reduced by meal termination and physical withdrawal of the trainer (Smeets, 1970).

There are a number of considerations relevant to time-out. Foremost is the availability of a program sufficiently reinforcing to make its loss unpleasant! We are all aware of the socially unresponsive individual who may *prefer* to be in a seclusion room rather than in contact with a program. For such an individual misbehavior may actually be strengthened if it is followed by seclusion. Another consideration relates to the actual process of physical removal. We focus on this particular form because of its common usage. To avoid equating implementation of time-out of any kind with "attention," there should be only a minimum of explanation. In physical removal the worker will want to avoid force, if possible, since this only models aggressive behavior for O.

Physical exclusion as in seclusion has the advantage of the prevention of accidental reinforcement during time-out, but it also has the disadvantage of removing O from whatever training opportunities are then extant. This is the particular benefit of nonexclusionary time-out. O is temporarily denied access to reinforcement but remains in the learning situation.

Duration of time-out and its termination are also important issues. Very lengthy seclusion periods not only remove O from training but also may result in a gradual adaptation to seclusion. The ethics of long time-out periods have been questioned (e.g., Baumeister & Rollings, 1976; Harris & Ersner-Hershfield, 1978), and some workers suggest the use of short periods (e.g., 5–10 minutes) (Bigelow, 1977; Johnson & Baumeister, 1981). Of course such short time periods would be ill adapted to seclusion, since the use of the method itself can be quite time-consuming. In one institution, the minimum period is about 15 minutes, though the procedure is regarded as especially intrusive and is said to be used only rarely. While a minimum time period for seclusion may be set, it is common to require O to be free of objectionable behavior for at least a brief period of time prior to release (e.g., 3–5 minutes).

Apart from the limitations created by physical removal from ongoing programs, seclusion does not actually prevent the occurrence of NB. This is particularly important for SIB, and O cannot be left in such a setting if serious SIB occurs.

In general, time-out is viewed as most appropriate for tantrums, aggressive behavior, and *mild* behavior problems (Harris & Ersner-Hershfield, 1978).

Overcorrection

Of the methods described, overcorrection has had wide appeal as a procedure for coping with all sorts of NBs (Johnson & Baumeister, 1981; Marholin et al., 1980). It is treated here in some depth because, in combination with positive reinforcement, it appears to be the single most effective and socially acceptable means of dealing with NB.

RATIONALE
The procedure is purported to combine both education and punitive components. It calls for the punishment of NB through activities that are themselves generally more adaptive and socially functional (Foxx & Azrin, 1972, 1973).

FORMS OF OVERCORRECTION
Two types of overcorrection are employed—"restitutional" and "positive practice." *Restitutional overcorrection* is used when the NB has had a damaging effect on the physical environment. It requires O not only to restore the environment to its prior state but also to improve it relative to what prevailed prior to NB. *Positive practice* overcorrection represents an additional educative component or may be used in its own right with nondestructive aberrant behavior.

To illustrate, if O overturns kitchen furniture he might be required to not only to restore it to its proper position but also to clean it and the area around it (restitution). He even might be required to practice setting a table (positive practice). For physically nondamaging NBs (e.g., self-stimulatory or stereotyped hand movements), O might be required to perform hand activities incompatible with them (positive practice) (see Fig. 42).

Names given to specific overcorrection procedures include "household orderliness training" (Foxx & Azrin, 1972), "functional movement training" (Foxx & Azrin, 1973), "autism reversal" (Azrin, Kaplan, & Foxx, 1973), "hand awareness training" (Azrin et al., 1975), and "required relaxation" (Webster & Azrin, 1973).

GRADUATED GUIDANCE
A characteristic feature of overcorrection is the use of "graduated guidance" (Foxx & Azrin, 1972). This refers to the physical prompting that may be necessary to ensure that O performs the requirements of the procedure. Only the minimal amount of force necessary to compliance is to be used and, where possible, should be gradually eliminated ("faded") and replaced by only verbal directions. Since the intensity of O's resistance can vary, there may be situations where much force is needed and the procedure could take a serious physical toll of both worker and O. Its appropriateness under those conditions is questionable.

USES
Positive practice has been commonly applied to stereotypies (Deno, Guttman, & Fullmer, 1977; Epstein et al., 1974; Harris & Wolchik, 1979; Roberts et al., 1979; Rollings, Baumeister, & Baumeister, 1977; Zehr & Theobald, 1978) and to self-injurious behavior (De Catanzaro & Baldwin, 1978; Harris & Romaczyk, 1976; Matson, Stephens, & Smith, 1978; Zehr & Theobald, 1978). "Required relaxation," a form of positive practice, is used to reduce a general state of agita-

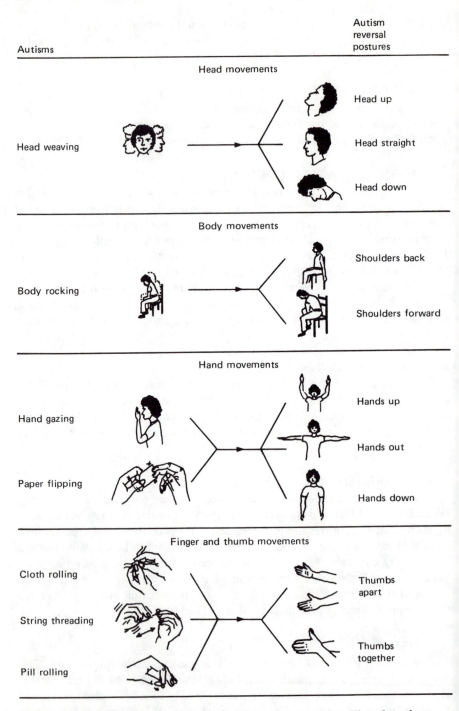

FIG. 42 Examples of positive practice for common stereotypies. These have been dubbed "autism reversal postures." From Azrin, Kaplan, & Foxx (1973).

tion (Webster & Azrin, 1973). The procedure requires O to lie in bed, restrained if necessary, until the agitation passes.

Restitution has been employed to reduce clothes stripping (Foxx, 1976), property destruction and aggression (Foxx & Azrin, 1972), food grabbing (Azrin & Wesolowski, 1974), pica—eating of inedibles (Matson et al., 1978), and regurgitation (Duker & Seysm 1977).

SELECTING APPROPRIATE PROCEDURES

The purpose of these procedures is both to teach and to punish. Teaching involves requiring adaptive (correct) responses in the place of the maladaptive ones. The repetition of this "correct" behavior constitutes positive practice and, in relation to self-stimulatory behavior, commonly consists of practicing nonaberrant arm movements. These movements simulate a forced exercise (e.g., hands up, outward, and down) (Fig. 42). Though these exercises do not seem "adaptive" as such, their pursuit does seem to "teach"!

Positive practice exercise generally uses the "offending" limbs. Deviant hand movements are replaced with nondeviant hand ones, but these forced exercises also seem capable of reducing non-limb-related deviances (e.g., foot movements, mouthing, "growling," and table hitting) although perhaps not to the same degree (Epstein et al., 1974; Roberts et al., 1979).

Restitutional procedures consist of activities that are the natural consequence of a particular NB coupled with the additional element of "improvement." Household cleaning tasks have been used to decrease household object destruction (Foxx & Azrin, 1972), clothes stripping was eliminated by requiring O to re-dress but with additional garments (Foxx, 1976), and pica was treated by contingent tooth brushing. For pica, a mouthwash and lemon juice solution were initially employed, the lemon for its aversive properties. But this proved ineffective, and the experimenter switched to a 10 percent hot sauce and water solution (Matson et al., 1978).

Although restitution and positive practice have usually been employed singly, the furniture overturning and table setting example illustrates how they might be combined. Required relaxation, too, has been coupled with both "apologizing" and "household tasks" to reduce screaming and furniture overturning. Paper shredding was dealt with by straightening of the living area (restitution) and 5 minutes of appropriate "book looking" (Shapiro, 1979).

RELEVANT ISSUES

Feasibility

The complex nature of the procedure, especially restitution, raises questions as to its practicality. For both restitution and positive practice, there is the possibility of *client resistance* and subsequent need for something stronger than "prompting" (Axelrod et al., 1978; Baumeister, 1978; Foxx, 1978; Picker et al., 1979; Richmond & Martin, 1977). We have already noted that the procedure may not be appropriate with Os who will not accept it without much struggle. Another key determinant of its feasibility is *staff attitude* toward procedures that are much more physically taxing than those usually employed. Overcorrection can be also very demanding of staff time (Baumeister, 1978; Heron, 1978; Richmond & Martin, 1977). Its innovators suggest that it should be of *extended duration*—at least 30 minutes (Foxx & Azrin, 1972). Happily, effects have also been produced with much shorter time periods (Marholin et al., 1980). This will be more true of positive practice than of restitution. The very nature of the latter cannot but be time-consuming.

Staff attitudes do seem mixed (Johnson & Baumeister, 1981). It can be physically exhausting (Corbett, 1975) and create unwanted images. Staff, in one setting, said that they would prefer to be seen by visitors using required relaxation than any other of the procedures (Webster & Azrin, 1973). Staff attitudes may clearly not be neutral, and, for serious NBs, because of its long time use, staff may be partial to seclusion time-out.

Topographical Similarity

This important issue was commented on in the section on selecting appropriate procedures. Several research studies make clear that suppressive effects are not limited to overcorrection procedures that use the same body part involved in the NB (Epstein et al., 1974; Dole & Epstein, 1975; Roberts et al., 1929; Ollendick, Matson, & Martin, 1978). The study of Ollendick et al. (1978) is of interest in that the effects of topographically similar and dissimilar procedures were compared although not on the same individuals. For topographically similar overcorrection, the NBs were repetitive hand wringing and nose touching. The overcorrection procedure was an incompatible hand-arm exercise. Each NB resulted in a full 5 minutes of successive 10-second periods of hands at sides, overhead, and straight out. The specific procedure begins with the worker giving a verbal description of the misbehavior—for example, "You're touching your nose." This calls O's attention to the behavior for which he is about to be "overcorrected." Then in sequence, the instructions "hands at sides," "above your head," "straight out front." If O did not comply within 5 seconds, physical prompting followed. (The author went through this exercise himself; it is not really very tiring, as arms at sides gives one a rest every 20 seconds. Arms extended sideways seems more fatiguing than arms extended either upward or forward.) For the topographically dissimilar procedure, the same hand-arm exercise was applied to excessive loud laughing and self-stimulatory head weaving. Thus hand-arm movements were employed to treat unrelated NBs. The results are instructive. The so-called "hand overcorrection" reduced both types of NBs—80 percent reduction for the topographically similar behaviors and 60 percent for the topographically dissimilar ones. The superiority of the topographically similar overcorrection was strikingly seen when the procedure was discontinued. Here a return to baseline (pretreatment condition) resulted in no increase in NB. Contrariwise, when the overcorrection was topographically dissimilar, its termination was followed by a recovery of NB to its full pretreatment strength.

Apart from the implications for treatment strategy, the suppressive effect of the topographically dissimilar procedure indicates that it is the punishing quality of the procedure rather than its purported educative one that is salient (O'Brien, 1981; Ollendick, Matson, & Martin, 1978). The "educative" part is that O learns a lesson!

Time between NB and Overcorrection

Overcorrection is typically conducted immediately following NB. This, of course, helps to fix the connection between NB and its consequence, but there may be situations where this is impractical. In one study comparing the effect of immediate versus delayed overcorrection, the latter proved equally effective (Azrin & Powers, 1975). Having to perform some schoolwork after class as a penalty for earlier misbehavior is a well-known example. To the degree that it is the punitive aspect of overcorrection that produces its effects, the timing is not crucial except for those with severe cognitive impairment. They need the proximity of the two events in order to better grasp their connection.

Negative Side Effects

A perennial concern about procedures that embody punishment is that there may be unwanted side effects. One concern is the attitude of O toward the procedure. It clearly is most useful with reasonably compliant souls. In others it can evoke all kinds of emotional distress, from whining and crying to full-blown physical resistance (Doleys & Arnold, 1975; Matson, Stephens, & Horne, 1978; Doleys, McWhorter, Williams, & Gentry, 1977).

Another concern is that the suppression of the targeted NB may be followed by increases in untreated NBs or in the appearance of new ones. The findings here are mixed. Treatment of one of four self-stimulatory hand movements was not found to affect the rate of the untreated three (Luiselli, Pemberton, & Helfen, 1978). Similarly, treatment of fecal eating (coprophagy) in an individual who also ate trash did not affect trash consumption (Foxx & Martin, 1975). On the other hand, in another study suppression of hand movements was followed by the onset of head bobbing (Harris & Wolchick, 1979). This too was later eliminated. Incidentally, this study also included the suppression of NBs with topographically unrelated overcorrection.

Positive Side Effects

Paradoxically, some of the positive side effects reported by workers using overcorrection or other aversive procedures are heightened interest, responsiveness, and alertness (e.g., Matson & Stephens, 1978; Freeman, Moss, Somerset, & Ritvo, 1977). The author saw this effect in an autistic and retarded child following the use of noninjurious electric shock for SIB (Tate & Baroff, 1966). We should not be surprised at a heightened "awareness" of their environment!

Another hoped-for effect, one that relates to the educative intent of overcorrection, is that O acquires some new socially adaptive behaviors. One may wonder whether O will spontaneously engage in activities that were originally coerced, but there is some indication that this can occur. Some spontaneous appropriate toy play was seen in children whose pretreatment toy play was self-stimulatory in nature (Wells, Forehand, Hickey, & Green, 1977). And where a psychiatric patient was required to pick up trash and deposit it in containers when she threw trash at individuals, she was observed to begin to deposit trash in containers spontaneously (Matson & Stephens, 1977). The author's military experience is a case in point. He certainly did not have habits of reasonable room cleanliness prior to military service but was *required* to keep his personal belongings and quarters neat under penalty of "sergeant retribution." He learned, and though today not a paragon of cleanliness, he is more comfortable in reasonably clean and neat surroundings.

OVERALL EFFECTIVENESS

There seems to be general agreement that overcorrection is an effective method of reducing negative behavior. It appears to be more powerful than any of the forms of positive reinforcement used alone (Johnson & Baumeister, 1981), but in combination with positive reinforcement it can be a potent tool. Relatively few studies provide an opportunity to directly compare alternative procedures for coping with NB; one such is that of Harris and Wolchik (1979). Four boys with autistic features and much self-stimulatory behavior were treated with three of the contingencies described—time-out, DRO, and overcorrection. Overcorrection was consistently the most powerful suppressor, and its effects were immediate and dramatic. Time-out was also effective in two of the children though less so than overcorrection. DRO was the least useful, and in one child it was actually associated with an increase in the NB! A similar observation was made by Foxx and Azrin (1973). The findings of this study are shown in Figure 43.

Aversive Stimulation (Punishment)

Of all of the contingencies used to influence behavior, none have been as controversial as those involving "punishment"—the deliberate employment of noxious consequences as a means of decreasing NB. The use of punishment has been discouraged on both ethical and practical grounds (Bigelow, 1977; Maurer, 1974). Its power is seductive and its underlying rationale could lead to ever increasing levels of pain delivery. This is the brutalizing process referred to in the earlier discussion of punishment in connection with the preschool child. Concerns are reiterated here because these procedures have been particularly applied to some of the debilitating behaviors seen in severely and profoundly retarded individuals.

The controversy becomes clear when we consider the kinds of aversive stimuli that have been used—hitting (head and hand slaps), cold showers, squirting lemon juice in the mouth, electric shock, and prolonged physical restraint. Though the use of physical restraint was referred to in the section on time-out, it probably ought to be included here as well. It is likely that contingent restraint is more often intended as punishment per se (e.g., Hamilton et al., 1967) than as purely denial of access to positive reinforcement. In one sense the classification of these procedures is fluid and would depend on the intent of the user. Curiously, while lengthy physical restraint would seem to be a fairly aversive contingency, for some SIB

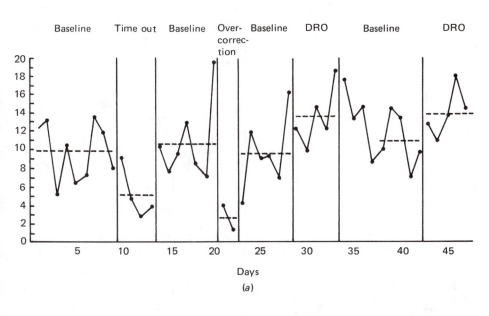

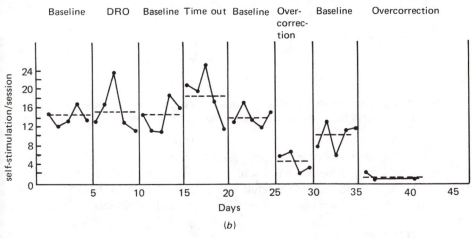

FIG. 43 Comparative effectiveness of time-out, DRO, and overcorrection in reducing self-stimulatory behavior. Adapted from Harris and Wolchik (1979).

individuals it can actually serve as a positive reinforcer (Favell et al., 1978, Favell, McGimsey, Jones, & Cannon, 1981; Foxx & Dufrense, 1984). The author has observed initiation of SIB on the removal of restraints (Tate & Baroff, 1966) and has seen individuals whose restraints are temporarily removed behave as if they wanted them to be restored (Baroff & Tate, 1968). This phenomenon has also been studied by Rojahn et al. (1978).

Before recoiling in horror at such practices, it should be recognized that these contingencies have generally been reserved for behaviors that have not re-

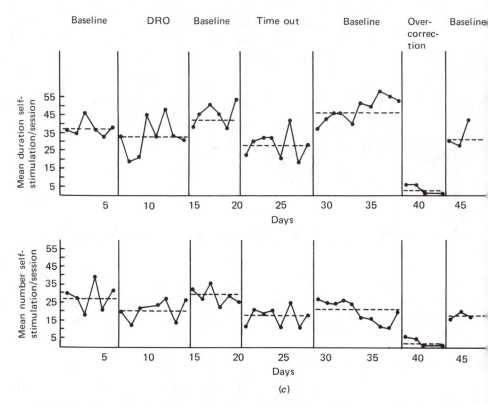

FIG. 43 Comparative effectiveness of time-out, DRO, and overcorrection in reducing self-stimulatory behavior. Adapted from Harris and Wolchik (1979). *(Continued)*

sponded to other forms of intervention and may constitute a physical threat to the person himself. Striking one's forehead, a common form of self-injurious behavior, may cause detachment of the retina and blindness! Chronic voluntary vomiting can create a life-threatening degree of dehydration and weight loss.

USES

Aversive stimuli have proved to be effective reducers of such severe NBs as SIB, ruminative vomiting, and pica. It is their very effectiveness that creates the dilemma of their use.

SPECIAL CONCERNS

The controversy posed by these procedures is revealed in an excerpt of a report on an institutional survey related to their use:

A majority of respondents commented on aversive conditioning usage. Some said that AC is a cruel treatment and should never be used. Others supported AC used as an alternative to mechanical restraints or excessive medication. Many psychologists expressed frustration in their attempts to use AC with some residents and noted their administration's lack of understanding of AC procedures and/or administrative disapproval of this treatment. The potential negative reaction of the lay public was also mentioned as a reason for not using this form of treatment. One psychologist indicated that chemical restraints (psychotropic drugs) are preferred . . . because they 'look' the cleanest, i.e., their effects are less readily observable. Another respondent reported that AC procedures would not be used in this facility even to prevent a resident from literally beating himself to death. (Wallace et al., 1976)

On a nationwide basis almost half of the responding institutions (45%) accepted aversive stimulation as a legitimate treatment for some residents. Guidelines for its employment are now widely available (e.g., Nolley et al., 1980; Richmond & Martin, 1977; Repp & Dietz, 1978; Thompson & Grabonski, 1977). They would limit its use to a treatment of last resort and would require its employment only under strict administrative supervision. Guidelines call for "consent" from parents or guardians and from a facility "human rights" committee, a trained staff; and criteria for termination (e.g., Repp & Diets, 1978; also see Matson & McCartney, 1981). Interestingly, the use of such guidelines in at least one institution resulted in a sharp reduction in the use of mechanical restraints for dealing with aggression (Nolley et al., 1980). Overcorrection and response cost in combination with positive reinforcement for appropriate behavior largely replaced restraint. Of further interest, prior to the guidelines, relatively little use was made of positive reinforcement in conjunction with punishment.

LIMITATIONS
Apart from ethical considerations, the usefulness of these procedures is limited by the specificity of their effects and possible negative side effects.

SPECIFICITY
Characteristic of aversive stimuli is that their suppressive effect is specific to the particular setting in which they are used (Baumeister & Forehand, 1973; Baumeister & Rollings, 1976). Control in the training setting does not spontaneously generalize to nontraining ones—hence the need for generalization. One common method is to couple the use of an aversive contingency with the standard form of disapproval—a loud "No!" The author has had direct experience with this kind of conditioned suppressor (Tate & Baroff, 1966). A shock stick used to curb SIB produced a buzzing sound when shock was delivered. Soon it was only necessary to produce the buzz to interrupt SBI. The buzz had become a conditioned suppressor and the equivalent of a loud and forceful "No" (see also McFarlain et al., 1975; Merdaum, 1973).

SIDE EFFECTS
Unwanted side effects are a common concern in the use of punishment. There are fears of causing disruptive emotional states (Johnson & Baumeister, 1981) and of endowing dispenser and setting with the same aversive quality associ-

ated with the punishment itself (Gardner, 1971; Heron, 1978; Richmond & Martin, 1971). Curiously, *positive* side effects have been reported, and the author was witness to one such instance. The child we worked with, a youngster with strong autistic features, seemed more alert and happier following the use of shock and the very rapid suppression of SIB (Tate & Baroff, 1966). Others have reported decreased avoidance behavior and crying (e.g., Bucher & Lovaas, 1968).

Baumeister (1978) does not think that fears about aversive stimuli have been borne out in the related research literature, (see also Axelrod & Apsche, 1983 and Johnston, 1972), and that concern for misapplication rather than side effects is more relevant. The author would again observe that the "side effects" may be more potent for the *trainer* than for the recipient. The deliberate use of painful contingencies cannot but gradually desensitize one to the pain of others. It is this potentially "brutalizing" effect of the use of such procedures that has concerned the author (Baroff, 1976).

A BEHAVIORAL INTERVENTION STRATEGY

Our goal here is to provide a *systematic* way of thinking about behavior, strengthening AB, and reducing NB. The model is based on a problem-solving[3] approach which provides a *method* of analyzing behavior rather than predetermined treatments. The rationale of this approach lies in the multiplicity of factors that might lead to the same behavioral outcome. Thus disruptive behavior in a given individual might be the outcome of serious health problems, stress in the home, demands in the program setting, needs for attention, or disruptiveness of other clients. Each of these different causes could lead to the same outcome, and unless one is prepared to try to relate outcome to cause, treatment may be of no avail. It would be fruitless, for example, to develop a treatment program that eased demands on a client if, in fact the disruptiveness is ultimately due to client need for greater attention. Reducing demands will not ease the problem; only greater attention will!

Elements of the Problem-Solving Method

The method involves four basic steps—data, analysis, treatment, and evaluation. The author enjoys creating mnemonics as a means of tying together and remembering elements of a system, and "DATE" provides a mnemonic that both organizes the four components and facilitates their recall.

"D"—DATA

Quantitative procedures are stressed. Behaviors of concern are described in sufficient detail to permit their measurement. If it happens, you can count it! The

---

[3]The author is especially indebted to former colleague Rudy Buckman for deepening his understanding of the value of this approach.

occurrence of "target" behaviors (TB) is then recorded over time in terms of such measures as frequency, direction, or intensity. The effectiveness of a given treatment is then determined by a *measurable decline* in the occurrence of target behaviors relative to its pretreatment (baseline) level. Numerous figures in the succeeding sections on specific behavior problems illustrate the recording of behavior.

"A"—ANALYSIS

Having defined our target behavior and determined how to measure it, we now attempt to identify the conditions that evoke it and the consequences that immediately follow. There are three components of analysis, sometimes referred to as the ABCs of behavior: "antecedent" (A), "target behavior" (B) and "consequences" (C). It is this particular sequence, A→B→C, that enables us to begin to understand what triggers TB and maintains it. A common sequence associated with attention-getting behavior is one in which the appearance of a potentially reinforcing staff person is the trigger (antecedent) for the onset of some form of behavior (e.g., inappropriate request for assistance) intended to get that staff person's attention. If the behavior is indeed responded to, the response constitutes the "attention" that reinforces and maintains it. Curiously, even negative responses can be reinforcing if attention is the desired consequence.

The essence of "analysis" is *observation*, itself a remarkable addition to our treatment armamentarium. Paying close attention to a particular behavior reveals aspects of it formerly unnoticed. For example, if you observe over time individuals who are described as chronically misbehaving, you discover they are not *always* misbehaving. Your analysis can then begin to tease out the factors that lead either to NB or AB. Indeed, it is observation that first calls attention to the fact that sometimes the client is behaving appropriately. It is just that attention has been hitherto given only for disruptive behavior. In other words, our perspective and attitude toward the client can be changed just as a result of observation—even before we have actually attempted to treat the behavior. That altered perspective represents a more realistic view of the client and is bound to be therapeutic.

"T"—TREATMENT

Having defined the target behavior(s) and analyzed the conditions under which it occurs, we are now prepared to develop a treatment strategy. Its focus is to encourage AB and to discourage NB. Our analysis will have indicated the kinds of consequences that appear to have maintained the behavior and thus makes clear what we should *not* be doing if we are to produce change. Treatment will consist of providing reinforcement for desired behaviors and contingencies varying from extinction to punishment for undesired ones.

Johnson and Baumeister (1981) provide us with a strategy for selecting appropriate contingencies for NB.

1. *Contingencies for behavior that is dangerous neither to self nor to others.*
   a. *Begin with positive reinforcement*, preferably DRI. Naturally occurring reinforcers are ideal. If the initial effort is not producing desired change, modify

the type, size, and frequency of reinforcement and, where possible, the degree of deprivation.
  b. If still no change, add *time-out* to positive reinforcement.
  c. If the combination of some form of time-out and positive reinforcement is unproductive, replace time-out with overcorrection. Johnson and Baumeister would also consider aversive stimulation for intractable but not dangerous behavior; the author would prefer to limit the degree of aversiveness to that inherent in overcorrection.

2. *Contingencies for physically dangerous behavior.*
  a. Where the behavior constitutes a physical threat to self, others, or the environment, it is ethically justifiable to move rapidly to overcorrection or aversive stimulation.
  b. *Physical restraint.* Referred to earlier, the prominence of physical restraint as a consequence of assaultive behavior deserves some attention. Procedures are being taught that are intended either to temporarily physically control an individual or to restrain the person for varying periods.
  c. *Emergency physical restraint.* Under such designations as response-contingent physical restraint, safety mechanics, and protective intervention technique (PIT), direct-care staff are learning physical procedures for temporarily subduing an individual without risk of injury to client or self. Concerns about its use relate to inadequately trained staff and possible injury and to its possible use as a "punisher" rather than as a means of achieving temporary physical control.
  d. *Planned physical restraint.* Lengthy physical restraint was widely used in the past with individuals who were dangerous to themselves or others and, as illustrated in the following, for other behaviors as well. In a chapter on "behavioral" counseling of parents of retarded children, a parent reports:

> Our sixteen-year-old son is in the state hospital. When we visited last weekend, we discovered he had been tied in restraints twenty-three hours during the last week because of "self-stimulation." We complained to the nursing staff but they said it was a "time-out" procedure to stop his self-stimulation. Is this really a legitimate practice and what can we do to see that his rights are protected? (Thompson & Young, 1977)

   This was clearly not "time-out" but rather a means of obviously preventing self-stimulation and, probably, punishing it as well. Federal courts have ruled that physical restraints can be employed only under special conditions, typically those that pose a serious physical threat and then under a variety of procedural safeguards. It was pointed out earlier that the implementation of such safeguards in one institution has resulted in a marked reduction in the use of restraint and its replacement by overcorrection and increased use of positive reinforcement (Nolley et al., 1980).

3. *Contingencies in general.* Thus far in this section, the focus has been on relating dangerousness of behavior to appropriate contingencies. But it needs to be

remembered that the essence of our capacity to intervene depends on our access to meaningful contingencies per se. If behavior is governed by its consequences, then they must be our focus. A common way of organizing all possible consequences is shown in Figure 44.

"E"—EVALUATION

The fourth element in our problem-solving method speaks to the effectiveness of the treatment procedure. As noted earlier, this will be evident in measurable changes in the occurrence of target behaviors. Reinforced behaviors should increase, and behaviors either ignored or punished should decrease. In the material that follows on treatment of specific behavior problems, there are numerous examples of such effects.

If our planned contingencies prove ineffective, several "trouble-shooting" questions should be considered: (1) Are our contingencies too weak? (2) Have they been applied appropriately? (3) Are our behavioral goals appropriate? and (4) Has the program been carried out consistently? The last of these considerations is probably the most important. Unless staff are prepared to follow the prescribed reinforcement and punishment procedures, our efforts are doomed. If we are satisfied that none of the above can account for our failure to effect significant change, a return to the analysis phase is appropriate. Presumably we have not yet teased out the factors maintaining the target behavior. It is in the nature of the method that we cannot be certain that our initial effort will be successful. "Intervention" is really a kind of experiment in which the correctness of our assumptions will only be known by the changes that do or do not occur. It is, ultimately, the client's behavior that is the means by which our analysis is measured.

Coping with Specific Behavior Problems

In this section we address the major behavior problems seen in severely and profoundly retarded individuals.[4] In this population will be seen all of the milder

---

[4]Excellent reviews of the management of these problems from a behavioral perspective are found in Whitman, Stibak, and Reid, 1983, Matson and McCartney (1981), Thompson and Grabowski (1977), and Baumeister and Rollings (1976).

	Present	Remove
To increase behavior	Positive stimuli DRO, DRI, DRL (positive reinforcement)	Negative stimuli (negative reinforcement)
To decrease behavior	Negative stimuli (punishment)	Positive stimuli via response cost time out extinction

FIG. 44 Contingency table showing all possible consequences intended to increase appropriate and decrease inappropriate behavior.

forms of behavior difficulties found in less handicapped individuals together with a group of disorders that are particularly prominent in those with the severest degrees of cognitive impairment.

AGGRESSION

Consisting of verbal and physical assaults and property destruction, aggression most often occurs in all of us, normal and retarded, following (1) exposure to intense, noxious, and painful events or to situations previously paired with them ("conditioned" aggression) or (2) denial of experiences previously found rewarding (Hutchinson, 1972). Attention is particularly called to "conditioned" aggression, because the reason for an aggressive response may be obscure. Each of our life histories has included the pairing of painful and frustrating experiences with particular people, objects, or situations, and reexposure to them even under conditions intended to be benign can evoke aggression.

Common Antecedents

Specific events that can result in aggression include demands for compliance, crowding, noise, "territorial" intrusions, physical illness, change, and victimization. Aggression may also occur because of unawareness or denial of other means of expressing opposition or because it produces attention. Much aggression (and negative behavior in general) seems motivated by the attention it produces—the proverbial "squeaky wheel" (Talkington, Hall, & Altman, 1971).

Individual Space, Territory, and Aggression

Within a population that may be limited in general mobility, the physical setting itself can contribute to aggression. "Territorial" behavior has been described in this population. Individuals establish specific spatial areas as their own and become aggressive when others enter that space ("turf" wars) (Boe, 1977; Paluck & Esser, 1971a; Rago, 1978). Boe (1977) suggests that one means of reducing aggression without actually increasing space is to plan activities such that groups are split, thus reducing the total number of persons in any one area at any one time. Spacewise, recent standards call for at least 80 square feet of activity space for each member of a residential setting (Accreditation Council, 1978).

Forms of Aggression

The manner in which aggression is expressed is shaped by life experience. In a very real sense aggression is "modeled" (e.g., Bandura, 1973). "Social skills" training reflects efforts to teach more socially adaptive behavior to retarded individuals. This is especially important in populations that lack effective verbal communication skill, a particular characteristic of the severely and profoundly retarded subgroups (Levine, Elzey, & Fiske-Rollin, 1979). In a study of a predominantly severely and profoundly retarded school-age day center population, only 20 percent used some words, the remainder communicating either with speechlike utterances (20%) or only through cries or nonspecific sounds (60%). Though not limited to aggression, attempts to teach prosocial behavior to retarded persons have used prompting, modeling, direct instruction, and feedback (Gibson, Lawrence, & Nelson, 1976; Paloutzian et al., 1971).

Management of Aggression

In keeping with the earlier-described rationale, behavioral contingencies are presented in terms of the least intrusive to the most intrusive.

1. Positive reinforcement alone: Few studies seem to have been successful in coping with aggressive behavior solely through positive reinforcement. One such study is of particular interest because it employed a *DRI group contingency* (Gola, Holmes, & Holmes, 1982). The method was used with four profoundly retarded women, all of whom were severely disruptive. In order for any *one* person in the group to be rewarded (candy), *all* had to initially be seated and, later, both seated and working. Group-oriented contingencies have been used with mildly retarded children in classrooms (Sulzbacher & Houser, 1968) and with moderately and severely retarded adults in a sheltered workshop (Frankosky & Sulzer-Azaruff, 1978). The group contingency was very effective. Not surprisingly, the level of disruptive behavior was lower when the individuals had to work as well as merely sit. Others have noted that simply keeping people quiet and docile without an alternative activity is not a very productive goal (Winett & Winkler, 1972). Indeed, absolutely unjustifiable!

2. Positive reinforcement—Presentation and withdrawal: The most common management practice with aggression has been time-out from positive reinforcement (Bates & Wehman, 1977; Mulick & Schroeder, 1980). Procedures are first identified that specifically combine positive reinforcement and time-out.

DRO and contingent time-out has been used to reduce severely disruptive and aggressive behaviors (Bostow & Bailey, 1969; Repp & Deitz, 1974; Vukelich & Hake, 1971). In individual work with a severely assaultive adult female (a choker!), it was found that even a minimum of 1 hour of contingent restraint alone only partly suppressed her behavior. The assaultiveness disappeared when reinforcing social attention was provided when she was not aggressive.

A combination of *DRI, response cost, and brief physical restraint* was employed with four severely retarded preadolescents (Perline & Levinsky, 1968). DRI consisted of tokens given intermittently for desired behaviors. On the occurrence of a maladaptive one, a token was taken away (response cost). For two of the children, physical restraint was added to response cost. The effect was to produce a major decline in aggression. Interestingly, the addition of physical restraint did not significantly add to the suppressive effect of response cost.

Time-out alone procedures for aggression have most commonly involved seclusion or isolation in a small, relatively unstimulating, enclosed environment; the ubiquitous time-out room (e.g., Burchard, 1967; Calhoun & Matherne, 1975; Pendergrass, 1972; Peniston, 1975). In other cases, time-out has meant restraint in a chair (Hamilton, Stephons, & Allen, 1967; Vukelich & Hake, 1971), sitting in a corner (Doleys et al., 1977), temporary food removal while remaining at the table (Kemp, 1973), wearing a symbol denoting time-out but without physical removal, and exclusionary time-out (Foxx & Shapiro, 1978; Spitalnik & Drabman, 1976).

The method of "required relaxation" (Webster & Azrin, 1973) can also be viewed as a kind of time-out. Negative behavior is interrupted, and the individual is confined to a time-out area—here, his bed! The offender is required to remain in bed, with restraint if necessary, until the agitated state has disappeared. The disappearance of assaultiveness in the Vukelich and Hake study resulted from some positive attention during time-in!

3. Overcorrection: In the case of a 50-year-old profoundly retarded woman who overturned and threw furniture, the individual was required not only to restore and straighten the table(s) overturned but also to straighten all other tables in the room (Foxx & Azrin, 1972). If necessary, physical "prompting" was used to accomplish the task (any other kind of housekeeping chore would also be appropriate).

Biting

Another profoundly retarded woman *bit* other persons. Unresponsive to a 15-minute time-out procedure, she was treated by first cleansing her mouth with an oral antiseptic and then *requiring her to assist the staff in the medical treatment of the attacked person!*

The requirement that the aggressor make specific amends to the victim is also finding its way into our general criminal justice system. Apart from ministering to the needs of one's victim as in the case of the "biter," overcorrection, as in the following example, also may require formal apology.

Inappropriate Sexual Behavior and Aggression

Polvinale and Lutzker (1980) worked with a 13-year-old Down syndrome male (IQ 36) who had a history of severe aggression and sexually inappropriate behavior. The latter consisted of genital self-stimulation and of enticing or coercing classmates into sexual interactions at school. This occurred in an outdoor area during either a teacher-directed exercise period or an unstructured recess. Following baseline observation, there was a brief period of DRO consisting of intermittent praise (attention) when the youth was not misbehaving and what is referred to as "social restitution" when he was. Immediately on the misbehavior, the youngster was required to apologize to each of six different peers, beginning first with his victim. Not only was apology required, but it had to be given within 5 seconds of the verbal prompt or the child had to apologize to still another youngster. At no time were more than eight apologies necessary. The effect is shown in Figures 45 and 46. It can be seen that both genital self-stimulation and aggressiveness were essentially eliminated. DRO alone seems to have been somewhat more useful with the aggressive behaviors, but overcorrection appears to have quickly reduced both negative behaviors. The author does not know if the social act of apology necessarily carried with it a real sense of guilt, but, whatever it meant to the aggressor it seemed to have had some aversive quality.

Clothes Tearing

An interesting variant on negative contingencies is "satiation." Here, the individual is *required* to engage in the *maladaptive* behavior but with a frequency

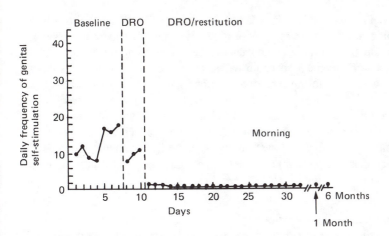

FIG. 45 Frequency of genital self-stimulation during morning observation sessions. Adapted from Polvinale and Lutzker (1980).

presumed ultimately to render that behavior aversive. Any activity that is reinforcing is only reinforcing for a certain time period. After that, it is no longer "fun." This is the self-limiting nature of any pleasurable activity, referred to in connection with the personality model presented in Chapter 2. Satiation has been used to reduce "hoarding" behavior by flooding the hoarder with that which is hoarded. Thus retarded males who hoarded magazines and papers in their clothing had their ward flooded with magazines (Ayllon & Mitchel, 1959). Similarly, a psychotic female hospital patient who continually stole and hoarded towels was "cured" by having towels placed in her room to a point where she began independently to remove them! (Ayllon, 1963). Enough is enough!

Satiation combined with positive practice overcorrection was used with six

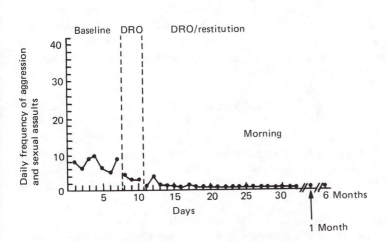

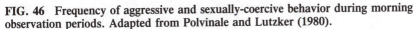

FIG. 46 Frequency of aggressive and sexually-coercive behavior during morning observation periods. Adapted from Polvinale and Lutzker (1980).

"clothes rippers" (Carroll, Sloop, Mutter, & Prince, 1978). Prior to this, onset of clothes ripping resulted in 15 minutes of time-out and a subsequent re-dressing by the staff. Treatment had three components: satiation, overcorrection, and a fixed-interval DRO reinforcement schedule. After each occurrence of clothes tearing, the offender was taken to the time-out room and there instructed to keep ripping the garment into its smallest pieces. This went on for 15 minutes and was followed by a positive-practice dressing and undressing session. This too went on for 15 minutes. In combination with these two negative consequences, the individual had access to candies on a fixed interval[5] that was gradually lengthened from 10 minutes of non-clothes tearing to 60 minutes. The effect of the treatment program was very rapid and long-lasting.

Direct Physical Intervention

An important area of behavior management is concerned with the treatment of the physically aggressive individual (Harvey & Schefers, 1977). Under such labels as "safety mechanics," response-contingent physical restraint, and "preventive" or "protective intervention techniques" (PIT) (e.g., Upchurch et al., 1980[6]), physical control procedures are described that are intended to interrupt dangerously aggressive behavior and to accomplish this without injury to the self or to the aggressor. Emphasis is placed on their use purely for *defensive* purposes, permitting safe physical control, rather than as means of intimidation or physical punishment. These procedures would then be followed by whatever contingencies are ordinarily employed for aggression.

Drugs

Psychotropic drugs have been widely used with disruptive behaviors. Lipman (1971) had earlier noted abuses in their application. Drugs were used to remedy staff shortages, for staff convenience, or as punishment. A decade later Rivinus (1980) concluded that psychotropic drugs were still greatly overused, at least in institutional settings. Simultaneous use of multiple drugs (polypharmacy), overdosage, and inappropriate usage were the most common problems. Causes for overusage and misusage have been laid to probable frustrations of workers and families and to the lack of comprehensive programs at both the institutional and community levels (Kirman, 1975).

A recent study of an institutional population in Ohio reveals a continued high level of inappropriate psychopharmacologic treatment (Bates, Smeltzer, & Arnoczky, 1986). At least half of the medication regimens were inappropriate. The proportions were highest for antidepressants (c. 75%), anxiolytics were second (c. 70%), lithium compounds were third (c. 57%), and antipsychotics were least likely to be inappropriately prescribed (c. 32%). Over a third of those seen as

---

[5]Rewarded for going a predetermined time without targeted NB.

[6]Upchurch et al (1980) provide a manual that has clear illustrations of each of the procedures: blocks, therapeutic holds, releases from holds, and carries.

inappropriately medicated had no psychiatric diagnosis at all, drugs being given for such behaviors as "masturbates too much" or "talks back to staff."

Undoubtedly contributing to the problem is that most of the medication regimens had been prescribed by nonpsychiatrists.

Drugs appear to be most appropriate "where the retarded individual experiences symptoms associated with an acute schizophrenic or affective disorder, in some hyperactive retarded children with major attention and concentration problems, and in persons with seizures" (Rivinus, 1980). While disruptiveness may be reduced, drugs can also impair learning ability (Freeman, 1970). In an interesting study on the effects of drugs on intelligence test performance, it was found that *termination* of medication had particularly striking effects when correct responses were reinforced.[7] Even without reinforcement, some increase in IQ was observed (Breuning & Davidson, 1981).

Within the framework of a carefully reviewed drug regimen and in association with programmatic efforts, aggressive and assaultive behavior has been responsive to treatment with the phenotiazines—Thorazine, Mellaril, Stelazine, and Prolixin. The piperidines are more potent and less likely to cause sedation and hypotension, but they increase the risk of extrapyramidal reactions (Rivinus, 1980).

Behavior Contracting

In a mildly retarded adolescent male, stealing was treated through a contractual agreement (Broadfoot, 1975). He agreed to refrain from stealing for 30 consecutive days in return for a luncheon at McDonalds. (We can add the Big Mac to our armamentarium of reinforcers.) Perhaps, as important, was a daily recording of his rate of stealing on a large calendar in his classroom. Each day without theft brought praise. After 3 stealing episodes he was finally able to complete the consecutive 30-day period and, subsequently, a new contract was negotiated based on 60 days of nontheft. The author views the daily prominent recording of the boy's behavior as a potentially powerful source of positive reinforcement and self-esteem, and, for him, concrete evidence of his own ability to modify his behavior.

STEREOTYPED BEHAVIOR

Behaviors

Among severely and profoundly retarded persons in particular, one sees much stereotyped behavior (Baumeister, 1978). These are repetitive and often rhythmical movements such as rocking, swaying, head and body banging, eye poking, and hand waving and finger movements. Those stereotyped behaviors that involve the striking, hitting, or biting or one's own body are referred to as self-injurious behaviors (SIB) and are treated separately because of the special management problem they pose.

Stereotyped behavior of the noninjurious form is commonplace, occurring in

---

[7]Without medication there was greater sensitivity to reinforcement.

about two-thirds of institutionalized severely and profoundly retarded individuals (Berkson & Mason, 1963; Kaufman & Levitt, 1965). The self-injurious form is much less frequent, but it still occurs in about 10 percent of such populations (Maisto et al. 1978; Schroeder et al., 1978; Smeets, 1971).

Although these behaviors are common in retardation, they are also seen in nonretarded blind individuals ("blindisms") and in children classified as autistic. Stereotyped behavior is also found in some normal infants, principally head banging, rocking, and head rolling, but it usually disappears by age 3 years (Delissovoy, 1962; Kravitz et al., 1960). Its transient appearance in children who are free of mental or sensory handicaps has caused some to regard it as a normal developmental phenomenon (Baumeister, 1978; Berkson, 1967). Perhaps briefly conspicuous around the time of teething or at the transition from sitting and standing (Hollis, 1978), it persists in all of us in the form of such common "movements" as leg swinging and thumb and hair twirling (Baumeister, 1978). It is only that these movements represent a very small proportion of the normal behavioral repertory; they dominate that of the other populations.

Causation

The oddity of stereotyped behavior has evoked much speculation as to its cause. The most common explanations relate it to elevated tension states and/or to self-stimulation in the service of "activity" or "stimulation" needs (Baumeister, 1978; Baumeister & Forehand, 1973; Berkson, 1967). Studies show that the behavior increases under a variety of conditions that seem to reflect either heightened tension or reduced external stimulation. It commonly follows frustration (Baumeister and Forehand, 1973), nonreward of a previously rewarded behavior (Mulhern & Baumeister, 1969), placement in an unfamiliar setting (Berkson & Mason, 1963), removal from restraint (Forehand & Baumeister, 1970b), and exposure to an environment that is restrictive in stimulation (Berkson & Mason, 1963; Davenport & Berkson, 1963; Kauffman & Levitt, 1965; Warren & Burns, 1970). In connection with its increase following the removal of restraint, as earlier noted, there is clear indication that for some individuals prolonged restraint is not aversive (Tate & Baroff, 1966; Favell, McGimsey, & Jones, 1978; Favell, McGimsey, Jones, & Cannon, 1981). Favell et al. (1978, 1981) have actually used restraint as a positive reinforcer, and in the fascinating documentary film "Harry" (Foxx, 1980; Foxx & Dufrense, 1984), Harry's self-injurious behavior is brought under control by employing as a reinforcer access to long-used arm restraints.

Stereotypy has been seen to diminish in some persons when they are provided attention (Moseley et al., 1979), toys, and other objects of interest (Moseley et al., 1970, Rincover et al., 1979) and nonstereotypy is reinforced (Baumeister & Forehand, 1971; Favell, 1973). Stereotypy has also been reduced through positive practice overcorrection (e.g., Azrin et al., 1973; Foxx & Azrin, 1973) and by blocking sensory stimulation associated with the stereotypy (Rincover, 1976; Rincover et al., 1979).

On the Nature of Stereotypy

Although also referred to as "self-stimulatory behavior," the first hard evidence that this does occur as a means of providing the person with desired sensory experience has been found in the work of Rincover (1976) and Rincover et al. (1979). Their research involved identifying sensory experiences presumed to be associated with various forms of stereotypy and then observing the effects of blocking such stimulation. Blocking of such experiences (e.g., visual, auditory, and kinesthetic) produced rapid reductions in the behavior. Even more convincing was the finding that substituting toys for activities that provided the same kinds of sensory stimulation seemed to rapidly escalate their attractiveness.

Given this background, we can conceive of non-stress-related stereotypy as simply reflecting the universal need for maintaining some level of stimulation or activity in individuals whose sensory or cognitive impairments render them generally unresponsive to the usual forms of stimulation. Most of us receive the major portion of our stimulation through our eyes and ears. Sights and sounds are meaningful to us unless we are blind or deaf. But the severely/profoundly retarded person may be unresponsive because the cognitive impairment may have rendered these same sights and sounds meaningless. An equivalent experience might be hearing the sounds of a foreign language that one neither understands nor can make inferences about. It is simply "noise." To maintain some presumed minimal level of sensory stimulation, (input or arousal), the person who is cognitively and/or sensorily impaired will, if necessary, create his own stimulation experience. Thus rocking and hand flapping appear to be a form of self-induced kinesthetic stimulation, finger movements in front of the eyes a form of visual stimulation, and body banging a form of tactual and also, perhaps, kinesthetic stimulation. The degree to which we can be confident of these presumptions relates to the apparent relationship between the blocking of these sensory experiences and a reduction in their occurrence.

Modifying Self-Stimulatory Behavior

Major reviews on the treatment of self-stimulation would suggest that it can be reduced or eliminated by (1) blocking of the relevant sensory experience and (2) providing contingencies that punish its occurrence and reward its absence.

We have just referred to the work of Rincover and his colleagues as providing the strongest basis for assuming that at least some stereotypic behavior can be attributed to the sensory reinforcement it provides. While Hollins (1978) has shown that through reinforcement body rocking could be engendered in a child who never did it spontaneously, it is likely that most stereotypic behavior is engaged in simply because it is pleasurable or tension reducing. Under the circumstances, O'Brien (1978) suggests that the justification for interfering with such behavior must be found in the fact that it either is physically injurious, causes restriction of access to more normalizing kinds of experiences, is severely disturbing to others, or decreases opportunities for reinforcement. Interestingly, O'Brien indicates that if the behavior does not produce serious problems, treatment is unnecessary, and it should be regarded as a "leisure time activity" and a source of reinforcement. As we shall see, the Rincover procedure lends itself to enabling the individual to continue to enjoy the sensory experience though in a more socially appropriate manner.

Rincover et al. (1979) worked with four retarded and autistic children who had high rates of stereotypy. The children, two boys and two girls, ranged in age from 8 to 10, and were functioning in the retarded range. Their mental ages were all below 3 years. They lacked appropriate play skills and were deficient in language. Only one child had any functional speech; two were primarily echolalic, and one was mute. The clinical picture is characteristic of early childhood autism (see Chap. 2). Casual observation of each child for 2 days and consultation with teachers permitted a judgment as to the probable sensory consequences that were reinforcing the stereotyped behavior.

Two children primarily engaged in hand and finger movements. One, Larry, incessantly flapped his hands, apparently producing much *proprioceptive*[8] stimulation. He usually held his arms out to his sides with his fingers, wrists, and arms in constant motion. The other, Janet, would flap her fingers. She would hold her hands up before her eyes and rotate her fingers and wrists back and forth. For Janet it was thought that *visual* stimulation as well as proprioception was involved in her stereotypy. A third child, Reggie, persistently twirled objects (e.g., a plate on a hard surface). When twirling an object he leaned toward it as if listening to the sound the spinning object produced. For Reggie, it was thought that *auditory* stimulation was the reinforcing sensation. The fourth child, Karen, incessantly picked feathers, lint, or a small string from her own or *others'* clothing! She then threw it in the air and waved her arms vigorously as if to keep it aloft. When it fell to the ground she immediately picked another and repeated the sequence. It was presumed that *visual* stimulation was the relevant sensory experience.

The intent of the sensory extinction procedures was to prevent the child from obtaining the particular sensory experience presumed tied to the stereotypy. This was accomplished by literally "masking" the stimulation. For proprioception that involved taping a small vibratory mechanism to the back of the hand. It generated a low-intensity and high-frequency pulsation but did not physically restrict self-stimulation.[9] For the auditory stimulation associated with listening to the spinning plate, the table surface was carpeted. For visual stimulation two methods were employed. In the case of the child with finger and hand movements, a blindfold consisting of a handkerchief was placed over her eyes and tied behind her head. For this child, then, there was both vibration and blindfolding. In the case of the other child who was using visual stimulation, illumination was reduced. Overhead lights were turned off, and though the room was lit sufficiently for most activities,

---

[8]"Proprioception" refers to sensory experience arising from our kinesthetic and vestibular senses. Kinesthetic sense organs provide information about the position of our limbs and body in space. The vestibular sensation refers to our awareness of balance and movement (Morgan & King, 1971).
[9]We are not told how the vibrator masked proprioceptive experience.

several observers found it almost impossible to follow the descent of a floating feather or piece of string. While the specific procedures utilized reflect the creativeness of the researchers, we need not be dazzled by their ingenuity. It is enough for us to understand the principle that has been employed. Once we think we have identified the relevant sensation, each of us will develop our own means for masking it.

Substituting Socially Appropriate Play Experiences

From the author's standpoint, the most significant aspect of this research dealt not with extinction of stereotypy as such but rather with providing a *rationale* for choosing more appropriate activity to substitute for it. In a second phase of the study, socially appropriate play was encouraged by offering toys that provided the same kind of sensation as the stereotypies: a music box to provide a variety of auditory stimuli, interlacing building blocks and beads and string to provide proprioceptive stimulation, and a bubble-blowing kit to approximate the visual stimuli produced by floating feathers and string.

Masking of sensory experience resulted in a dramatic reduction in stereotypy in three of the four children. Only Janet persisted in it. Nor was she able to substitute more adaptive play activities. In the case of the other three children, toys came to be substituted for stereotypy. The gains persisted over several months with no other reinforcers for play or restraints on stereotypy. Toy sensory modality preference was clear for the three children who benefited. Reggie, the spinning-plate listener, played with a music box and Autoharp but not with blocks and beads. Larry, one of the two hand and finger flappers, played with blocks and beads but not with the music box. Karen blew bubbles and showed no interest in blocks and beads. The results of the treatment for three of the four children are shown in Figure 47.

The demonstration of sensory modality preferences in these children is consistent with efforts to teach nonspeaking autistic children to communicate through signs. Here a visual modality is substituted for the auditory and/or speech one. These modality preferences can also be assumed to account for stereotypies in retarded individuals and offer a clue as to how one can approach a child from an educational and training standpoint. The capitalizing on sensory preferences is particularly salient to work with severely and profoundly retarded individuals. Their learning difficulties are so great as to give extraordinary significance to any modality to which they seem capable of responding.

Combining Positive and Negative Consequences

Other than by sensory extinction it appears that stereotyped behavior can be substantially reduced or essentially eliminated by combining inducements for more appropriate behaviors with mild punishment. The "punishment" aspect was described earlier in connection with the use of various forms of positive-practice overcorrection. In the context of stereotypies, this involves required exercises as illustrated in Figure 46. It is assumed that these involuntary exercises are experi-

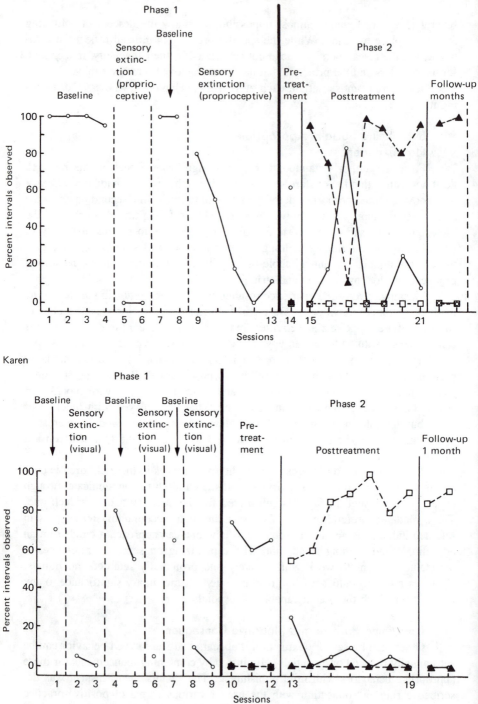

FIG. 47 Reducing self-stimulation by sensory masking and by substituting equivalent sensory experience in appropriate toy play. From Rincover, Cook, Peoples, and Packard (1979).

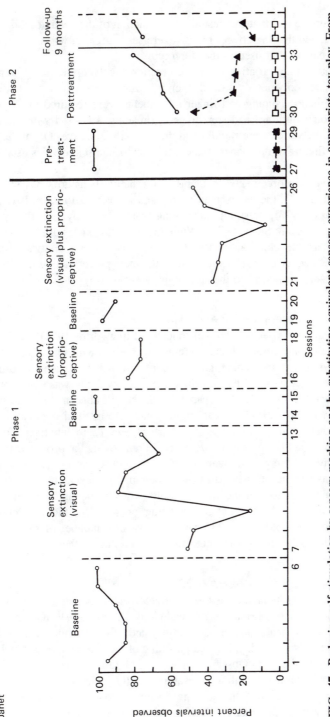

FIG. 47 Reducing self-stimulation by sensory masking and by substituting equivalent sensory experience in appropriate toy play. From Rincover, Cook, Peoples, and Packard (1979). (*Continued*)

enced as aversive and that this results in a reduction of the behavior that evokes it. It was also noted that the effect of these exercises is greatest when they involve the same body part as that used in the stereotypy.

An interesting variation on overcorrection involved the use of some of one individual's stereotypies as forced exercises for others (Roberts et al., 1979). Stereotyped hand clapping and finger movements were required to be performed contingent on mouthing, and stereotyped grimacing was used with the table hitting. Both procedures were rapidly and dramatically effective. Of interest was the subsequent finding of no change in the frequency of the stereotypies used as forced practice.

Positive reinforcement for adaptive alternative behaviors has included toy play (Favell, 1973), the use of educational and recreational materials (Azrin, Kaplan, & Foxx, 1973), or simply abstaining from stereotypy for given periods of time (Repp, Dietz, & Spier, 1974). While these contingencies used alone may lose their effect as the child habituates to previously novel activities (Baumeister, 1978), the Rincover et al. study indicates that their power can be much enhanced through sensory similarity to the stereotypy it seeks to replace.

Treating Stereotyped Toe Walking

Toe walking is seen in normal toddlers (Illingworth, 1971) and in children with retardation and autism. It is also found in children with spastic cerebral palsy, muscular dystrophy, and congenital shortening of the Achilles tendon (Illingworth, 1971). In the 9-year-old child described here, toe walking was of serious family concern (Barret & Linn, 1981). Apart from the child's abnormal appearance it was interfering with normal motor learning and had dire medical implications. It was suggested that surgery would be necessary at age 12 to lengthen the Achilles tendon if physical therapy was unsuccessful in remedying the problem. In conjunction with physical therapy an overcorrection procedure was implemented in which the child was required to perform simple toe-tapping movements with the heel of his foot planted firmly on the floor. Results were again rapid. From a baseline frequency of about 50 percent toe standing or walking, the rate immediately dropped about fivefold. Table 28 provides a list of a number of stereotypies and overcorrection procedures that were effective in reducing them.

SELF–INJURIOUS BEHAVIOR

This aberrant behavior has been characterized as perhaps the most dramatic and extreme form of chronic psychopathology (Carr, 1977). Its most common manifestations are head banging, self-biting, and self-scratching (Schroeder et al, 1978), but one also sees slapping and punching of the face and head, pinching, and even kicking of the self. Observed in autistic children as well as in those with severe and profound retardation, it was originally interpreted in psychoanalytic terms and regarded as self-directed aggression or masochism (e.g., Cain, 1961). The currently used designation "self-injurious behavior" is intended to denote

TABLE 28   Stereotypies Effectively Reduced with Overcorrection

Stereotypy	Related research	Overcorrection procedure	Topographical similarity
Body rocking	Azrin et al., 1973	Maintaining shoulders in fixed positions	Similar
Head and finger movements	Foxx & Azrin, 1973; Harris & Wolchik, 1979	Holding hands and/or fingers in fixed positions	Similar
	Roberts et al., 1979	Exaggerated hand claps with arms stretched overhead	Similar
		Required grimicing— another of this child's stereotypies	Dissimilar
	Ollendick et al., 1978	Holding hands in fixed positions	Similar
Head movements	Foxx & Azrin, 1973	Holding head in fixed positions	Similar
Mouthing	Roberts et al., 1979	Holding hands in fixed positions	Dissimilar
	Roberts et al., 1979	Hand clapping— another of the child's stereotypies	Dissimilar
	Foxx & Azrin, 1973	Finger movements— another of the child's stereotypies	Dissimilar
Toe walking	Barrett & Linn, 1981	Brushing mouth with toothbrush and rinsing with antiseptic	Similar
		Tapping of toes on one foot on prescribed set of cloth footprints while heel is held in floor	Similar
Vocalizations	Roberts et al., 1979	Finger movements— another of the child's stereotypies	Dissimilar
	Higgs et al., 1980; Ollendick et al., 1928	Fixed head positions Holding hands in fixed positions	Dissimilar Dissimilar

only behavior that *results* in injury to the self without implying any willful intent to produce that effect (Tate & Baroff, 1966). Indeed, some children have been observed as apparently trying to protect themselves from their own hitting by engaging in various forms of self-restraint (Baroff & Tate, 1968). Although SIB has usually referred to behaviors that are damaging to tissue, Schroeder et al. (1981) have also included under this category self-induced vomiting and eating of inedibles (pica), behaviors that can also be health hazards.

Case History

Some sense of the extraordinary nature of this behavior is found in the description of Susie, (Tate, 1972) an 18-year-old girl who was the first SIB individual the author encountered. Admitted to an institution for the retarded at age 11, she was battered and bruised. The injuries were attributed to head banging, and within hours after admission, she was placed in restraint. During the next $7\frac{1}{2}$ years she was to remain restrained, in bed, though also receiving drug therapy, physical therapy, and concerned care. All treatment efforts were without avail. She was under 24-hour restraint with the exception of being briefly removed from the bed each day for a bath. Even this was hazardous, as she often had to be held by several attendants to prevent her from banging her head against the bathtub. Physically, Susie was normal in size, had good hearing, but was blind. (SIB is frequently seen in children with blindness, and the blindness is sometimes attributed to the constant hitting of the face and head). She could say a few single words and hum portions of several tunes. She had an extensive variety of SIB, its form limited only by her degree of physical freedom. Our initial work with her involved freeing of one leg; she was typically restrained in bed in spread-eagle fashion on her back.

When her leg was released from restraints, Susie kicked herself and any hard object in reach. She kicked the side of the bed, her other leg and foot, and her crotch. During a 7-hour 33-minute observation period when her right leg was padded to minimize injury and her left leg was free, she kicked 5866 times. Although kicking was a highly predictable behavior, the rate and topography varied. On some days almost all kicks were heel to knee at a steady rate. At other times Susie kicked in bursts with pauses of several minutes. Some kicks were bone-jarring and produced bleeding even when the kicked leg was padded with 4 inch thick polyurethane foam. Occasionally, the kicks were playfully light and accompanied by laughter. In a few instances when she was restrained loosely and one leg was free, she would simultaneously move her head forward and her knee up and back so that the two collided with great force. Several hematomas on the face and head resulted from such action.

When an arm was released from restraints, Susie hit her face and head repeatedly with her fist. One morning her right eye was closed by the swelling of the tissue surrounding it, and blood was oozing from cuts around the eye. She had apparently worked her right hand out of the restraining cuffs during the night. Even when fully restrained in bed with leather cuffs about her ankles and wrists, Susie was able to inflict damage. She bit the inside of her cheeks, cut her fingers with her fingernails, and banged her head against her shoulders. The shoulder damage was controlled by having her wear a 2 inch thick polyurethane foam collar. The cutting and gouging of her fingers, which produced large open sores around her fingernails, could be managed by taping her fingers and taping cotton gloves on her hands. Fortunately she did not often bite the inside of her cheeks, for we never devised a method of controlling this activity. The biting had once been a serious problem and, when Susie was 14, *all her teeth except her molars were removed* as a last resort to stop self biting (emphasis added). Before her teeth were extracted she had severely lacerated her shoulders and cut through her lower lip.

Clearly, Susie had a highly developed repertoire of self-injury. If her behavioral repertoire included any normal behaviors besides the verbal ones, they were effectively masked by self-injury. When free to respond, Susie either injured herself or remained nearly motionless. (Tate, 1972).

Prevalence

As noted earlier, SIB is found in about 10 percent of institutionalized retarded populations. It is also observed in children classified as autistic (Carr, 1970) or schizophrenic (Green, 1967; Shodell & Reiter, 1968). The most detailed study on its prevalence and its associated problems was conducted by Schroeder et al. (1978). They found, with others, that SIB occurred more frequently in the more severely impaired of an institutionalized population: 2 percent of the mildly retarded, 9 percent of the moderately retarded, and 14 percent of the severely and profoundly retarded.

Sex Ratio

SIB occurred with almost equal frequency between the sexes—52 percent in males and 48 percent in females. This finding differs from that of Maisto et al. (1978), who reported higher rates in females, especially younger ones.

Severity

SIB has such a frightening connotation that there is a tendency to think of all of it as "serious" or "severe." In fact, the population could be differentiated by degree of severity, and the great majority, 77 percent, were characterized as "mild." Presumably, this distinction was made on the basis of the frequency and intensity of SIB. In another study, SIB was reported as more severe in males (Maisto et al., 1978).

Seizures and Severity

Seizures were particularly prominent in those with severe SIB—41 percent as against 20 percent of those with mild SIB. The latter was comparable to the frequency of seizures in the non-SIB population—22 percent.

Sensory Handicaps

Visual impairment was especially prominent, irrespective of severity. Whereas only 7 percent of the non-SIB population had visual impairment, 23 percent of SIB individuals were so affected. Unlike vision, there was little evidence of any relationship between hearing loss and SIB. Of the SIB group, 8 percent had hearing impairment as against 5 percent of the non-SIB population.

Speech

The absence of language has been commonly noted. Indeed, some SIB has been thought to be a form of indirect communication in individuals who lack functional speech (Schroeder et al., 1978). In this study about 68 percent of SIB residents lacked speech. Since its frequency is greatest in those retarded individuals who are particularly deficient in speech, it is not clear that the proportion without speech was excessive relative to non-SIB residents with comparable cognitive deficit.

Treatment Modalities and Effects

Of particular interest was the effect of various treatment programs. The Schroeder et al. population had consisted of 208 residents identified over a 3-year period. Of these, almost half (101) were followed for a full 3 years. Of the 101, nearly one-third (31) had been in a behavior modification program, with or without drugs; the remainder had either received psychotropic or seizure medication or no treatment at all. Nearly all of the behavior modification group were judged as improved—29 of 31 (94%). There was no difference between those who received only behavior modification and those who had behavior modification and drugs (seizure or psychotropic).

Of the 42 residents who received only medication, the most common regimen was a combination of seizure and psychotropic drugs. A typical combination was Phenobarbital, Thorazine, Artone, and Tofranil.[10] The psychotropics either singly or in combination were judged to have had a positive effect in about one-third (32%), whereas of those who received either seizure medication alone or no medication of any kind, only 18 percent had improved. Clearly, the behavior modification program had produced the greatest benefits whether applied alone or in conjunction with drugs.

Causation

Among the aberrant behaviors seen in retardation, it is likely that none has evoked as much speculation as SIB regarding cause (Bachman, 1972; Baumeister & Rollings, 1976; Carr, 1977; Durand & Carr; Edelson, 1984; Favell et al., 1982; Frankel & Simmons, 1976). SIB appears to violate the most fundamental principle of human motivation—the need to avoid pain—and seems to be in conflict with the widely accepted principle of self-preservation. With regard to pain, it has been suggested that the pain experience itself is altered in SIB (Edelson, 1984; Mahler et al., 1959); apparent insensitivity to ordinarily painful stimuli has been reported in some autistic children (Wing, 1972). However the SIB person experiences the behavior, the author's research (Tate & Baroff, 1966) made clear that when ordinarily painful stimuli are applied by *other* than the person himself, they are reacted

---

[10]There is recent preliminary evidence that Prolixin may be of special benefit (*Personal Communication*, 1986).

to as if they are painful. Thus electric shock produces avoidance, and even a pinch evokes a normal "ouch." And, as already noted, the tendency for some SIB individuals to seek self-restraint suggests that they, also, find their own behavior aversive. Consistent evidence of altered pain sensitivity is yet to be established.

Theories of causation fall into three categories—organic, psychodynamic, and behavioral.

1. *Organic.* Some SIB may have a medical basis. In the Lesch-Nyhan syndrome, described in Chapter 3, a characteristic behavior is the biting of mouth and fingers. To a lesser degree, SIB also occurs in another mental retardation disorder—the Cornelia de Lange syndrome. Thus far no relationship has been found between the chemical abnormality in Lesch-Nyhan, an elevated uric acid level, and SIB. Perhaps more to the point is the finding that even in these disorders SIB can be reduced through behavior modification. Duker (1975) was able to essentially eliminate self-biting by instructing staff to ignore it and its accompanying whining. In a review of possible precipitants of SIB, Carr (1977) concludes that although organic factors may contribute to its initial development, it is maintained by adult attention. Such was indeed the case in the Duker study. A similar finding is reported for a child with a contact dermatitis (Carr & McDowell, 1980).

2. *Psychodynamic.* Psychodynamic theories have variously attributed SIB to attempts to establish body reality and ego boundaries, to distinguish the self from the external world, and as aggression directed against the self (Cain, 1961). Apart from how the validity of these ideas could be determined, psychotherapeutic treatment approaches have not been effective (Schroeder et al., 1981). Certainly, they are unlikely to be useful with SIB individuals who are also severely retarded.

3. *Behavioral.* Perhaps the most widely accepted view of SIB is that whatever its origin, its persistence is related to the *consequences* it evokes, and, ultimately, these must be rewarding. Thus SIB has been shown to be responsive to (1) *positive reinforcement,* as in the attention provided by caretakers in the Duker study; (2) *negative reinforcement*—its occurrence resulting in the terminating or avoiding of some nonpreferred activity; and (3) changes in *stimulation*—SIB has also been seen as a form of stereotypy or self-stimulation practiced in stimulus-deprived environments (e.g., Baumeister & Forehand, 1973; Berkson, 1967; Collins, 1965). The self-stimulation hypothesis finds some support in studies where the provision of other kinds of sensory stimulation has reduced SIB (Collins, 1965; Favell, McGimsey & Schell, 1982; Myerson et al., 1967; Rincover & Devany, 1982). This work echoes that of Rincover et al. (1979) regarding decreasing stereotypy through sensory blocking and the substitution of sensorily equivalent but more socially appropriate activity.

Since each of the three behavioral hypotheses has some research support, it is likely that SIB is not caused by any *one* factor. It is best conceived of as a multidetermined operant response that is maintained by the consequences it produces and may be particularly strengthened by the absence of speech or other forms of functional communication.

Treatment of Self-Injurious Behavior

A major precipitant of SIB seems to be unwanted demands. Carr et al. (1976) showed systematic change in SIB in a mildly retarded child as a function of demand versus nondemand conditions: SIB increased under demand conditions and decreased under nondemand ones. Indeed, SIB abruptly ceased when merely the signal for impending termination of the demand situation was given. Thus SIB has been used as a weapon for avoiding situations that appear to be aversive to the individual (e.g., Carr, 1977; Myers & Diebert, 1971; Weeks & Gaylord-Ross, 1981; Wolf et al., 1967). This can include simply avoidance of social contacts (Corte et al., 1971; Peterson & Peterson, 1968).

An unexpected antecedent is actual *release* from physical restraint. Researchers have observed that some SIB individuals become extremely disturbed and initiate SIB upon the removal of restraints (e.g., Lovaas & Simmons, 1969; Tate & Baroff, 1966). Moreover, as already noted, one also sees apparent efforts at self-restraint. When Susie's hands were freed of restraint, she would immediately strike her face and then raise her back and place her arm under it as if to hold it. Sam, a preadolescent with autism and retardation, wore arm restraints at home. When they would accidentally loosen, he would put his hands together and approach his mother as if he wanted her to tie them again (Baroff & Tate, 1968). Another youngster was seen to slap his face and then put his hands beneath his undershirt as if to contain them. It was earlier suggested that the SIB individual may actually experience the behavior as aversive but one over which he has little control. In this sense, SIB is like a very powerful habit, and many of us share this fraility (e.g., breaking the cigarette habit).

Recognition of preference for restraint led Favell et al. (1978) to actually use access to restraint as a reward. Rapid reduction of SIB was achieved by providing arm splint restraints as a reward for increasing periods of non-SIB. Moreover, when access to restraint was made contingent on toy play, toy play increased. The dramatic attachment to one's physical restraints is graphically portrayed in the SIB documentary film "Harry" (Foxx, 1980). Of course, the capacity for using restraint as a reinforcer depends on the severity of SIB in the nonrestrained condition.

Favell et al. (1978) speculated that restraint was reinforcing because it was associated with a reduction in aversive stimuli. This could refer to the preceding antecedent "demands." Other investigators (Rojahn et al., 1979) found that the wearing of protective devices tended to decrease social interactions with caretakers. For SIB individuals who shun social contact, restraint may be a powerful reinforcer.

Positive reinforcement alone has not been very effective in suppressing SIB (Schroeder et al., 1981), and it has been suggested that it may be ethically justifiable to move quickly to more *intrusive* procedures—specifically, overcorrection or aversive stimulation (Johnson & Baumeister, 1978). Since the severity of SIB does vary, where it does not pose a threat of significant tissue damage, initial use of less intrusive methods is recommended. Durand and Carr (1985) offer guidelines for nonintrusive approaches in school settings. Stress is placed on teaching nonverbal children who appear to use SIB as an avoidance mechanism to substitute speech for SIB. One could also use gestures or sign language.

Prevention

Apart from physical restraint per se, one approach that takes advantage of apparent efforts at self-control involves the use of adaptive clothing. In the earlier chapter on preschool programs there was illustration of utensils that were modified or adapted for use by children with motor handicaps. In SIB, Rojahn et al. (1978) altered a jacket so that its side pockets were enlarged. The result was to increase *appropriate* self-restraint—keeping hands in pockets as against the former method of wrapping arms and hands in clothing.

Positive Reinforcement

Of the four forms of positive reinforcement described earlier, DRI is generally the most useful. It is the only one that specifically reinforces a behavior that is physically incompatible with the target behavior, and this is particularly relevant to SIB, where even small levels are undesirable. In a study that compared the effectiveness of DRO and DRI in three profoundly retarded head bangers, only DRI was effective (the reinforcers were *edibles*—orange juice and ice cream) (Tarpley & Schroeder, 1979).

In a study that incorporated environmental enrichment, sensory substitution, and positive reinforcement, chronic SIB was much reduced in two nonambulatory and profoundly retarded individuals (Lockwood & Bourland, 1982). Of particular interest was the provision of toys attached by hangers to wheelchairs. This allowed for continued access. The toys were made of rubber and soft plastic, the type that would be chewed by infants, and were intended to substitute for self-biting. Reinforcement consisted of praise and affectionate stroking of face and rubbing of arms. The reinforcer, too, seems to have provided the same sensory experience as the SIB—tactual. Similarly, Favell et al. (1982) were able to substitute toy chewing for hand mouthing.

SIB has also been reduced by reinforcing nonhitting with attention (Carr & McDowell, 1980; Durand, 1984, Lovaas et al., 1965), food (Peterson & Peterson, 1968), sweets (Corte et al., 1971), and access to a change of scene (Rose, 1979) or the restraint itself (Favell et al., 1981). Attention was such a powerful reinforcer that Lovaas et al. (1965) were actually able to *increase* the rate of SIB in a child by making sympathetic comments (providing attention) each time she hit herself. The hitting was not hard enough to do damage; the intent was only to show the lawful nature of the behavior.

Though positive reinforcement alone will be the treatment of choice only where SIB is not severe, it should be a part of any program that also includes negative consequences. It has been frequently noted that the ideal intervention for serious behavior problems will include incentives for adaptive behavior as well as disincentives for negative ones.

Withdrawal of Positive Reinforcement: Extinction and Time-Out

Since extinction involves ignoring the target behavior, it is only feasible in SIB when the behavior is not truly tissue damaging. Extinction is probably the ideal method of dealing with SIB when its use seems to be clearly intended to affect others. Thus some SIB persons hit themselves and then watch what their caretakers do. Duker (1975) used extinction with a child whose SIB was associated with the Lesch-Nyhan syndrome:

> R. often looked at the therapist after biting himself. Once after a session, when he was carried to the ward without washing gloves (gloves to block hand biting), he did not bite himself. However, as soon as he was laid down . . . he started to tremble, asked for his washing gloves (desire for the restraints), bit himself and started to cry. When he bit during the treatment sessions, *the behavior was mostly occasioned by the entrance of a nurse, or by the presence of a strange nurse on the ward. Once he bit when he saw an attendant of his former ward passing by.* (Duker, 1975; emphasis added)

These observations together with the staff's typical response to the SIB lent themselves to the following "functional analysis" (according to the behavioral problem-solving approach):

Antecedents	Behavior	Consequences
Presence of Staff	Self-biting and accompanying whining and crying	Staff responds sympathetically to child and seeks to reduce presumed discomfort

Given the obvious attention-getting nature of R's SIB and its nonsevere nature, treatment consisted of instructing staff to ignore the behavior and its accompanying whining and crying. Staff were told to limit attention, the relevant reinforcer, to only desired behavior (DRO). The effect of this program is shown in Figures 48 and 49. After an initial slight increase in SIB, the rate dropped steadily. The reduction in associated crying was even more dramatic. It dropped rapidly after the first treatment period and disappeared by the seventh. It was clearly being maintained by the attention it had evoked. When that consequence disappeared, so did the behavior. The author is not surprised at the response to extinction. Where the individual clearly shows interest in your reaction to any behavior, its attention-getting intent is obvious. Ignoring it, if feasible, is bound to be effective.

Instructive as the Duker study is, it does not typify the behavior of most SIB "practitioners." The behavior is not usually so blatantly attention getting, and ignoring it is unlikely to result in its rapid decrease. In several studies where SIB was allowed to occur but in which the individual was not in danger, literally thousands of blows have been observed before any reduction was evident (Lovaas & Simmons, 1969; Jones et al., 1974; Tate, 1972) or there was no effect at all (Lovaas et al., 1965). And, of course, extinction cannot be used where SIB is physically damaging.

Time-out during meal times has been effective in reducing SIB. Interruption of access to food for even brief periods—15 minutes (Lucero et al., 1976) and 45 minutes (Corte et al., 1971)—has reduced SIB. A more stringent contingency

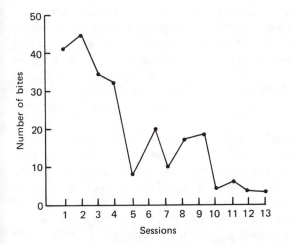

FIG. 48   Number of bites per $2\frac{1}{2}$-hour training sessions. From Duker (1975).

involved a 2-hour delay if there were at least three hits during a meal (Myers & Deibert, 1971). It might be expected that the power of meal interruption will diminish over the course of the meal and that if SIB does tend to increase during its latter part, the delay period should be lengthened. Access to a desired dessert might also be restricted. Another time-out procedure, here used in a classroom, involved the contingent use of materials that served as a blindfold—so-called facial screening (Lutzker, 1978; Zeigob et al., 1976).

Punishment

Forced exercises (see Fig. 41) have been reported effective in SIB as well as with stereotypy. In addition to the usual standing position, Azrin et al. (1975)

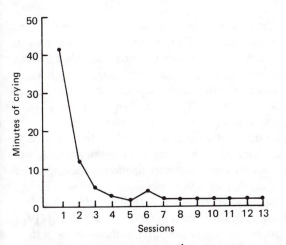

FIG. 49   Minutes of crying per $2\frac{1}{2}$-hour training sessions. From Duker (1975).

implemented them in the sitting position for those who were unable to stand or who became too fatigued or upset at standing. Conducted for 20-minute periods, after 1 day without SIB the exercise period was reduced to 5 minutes, then to 2 minutes, and finally to a simple warning if there had been no SIB on the previous day. A variant of the arm exercise consisted of "arm pumping" in two wheelchair-bound children (DeCatanzaro & Baldwin, 1978). The limb involved in SIB was the one pumped; again illustrating the apparent desirability of "punishing" the limb that offends!

Still another variant, though one that did not involve the offending organ, was brief forced running (Boreson, 1980). The SIB was self-biting, and its antecedents were both instructional demands and attention seeking. SIB had been reinforced by the termination of trainer requests. After exhausting less intrusive alternatives, DRO, DRI, extinction, and even 10-minute periods of contingent restraint, the procedure implemented required the individual to walk up and down stairs at a rapid rate. A training staircase was used in the classroom, and any convenient stairway for SIB occurring outside the classroom. This was a two-person procedure—one "pushing" while the other followed closely and ensured proper foot positioning. The procedure is said to have been very economical time-wise. It required less than a 1-minute interruption of classroom activity (!). Though undoubtedly tiring to the teachers, the effects were immediate. Presumably, the individual found the activity aversive. The person "exhibited some resistance each time the contingency was implemented. He did this by leaning in the opposite direction against which he was being guided" (Boreson, 1980).

Finally, an oral hygiene program was used to reduce hand biting in a 3-year-old with cerebral palsy (Agosta et al., 1980). Following a bite, the child was reprimanded and then taken to the bathroom for 2 minutes of tooth brushing. The toothbrush had been soaked in Listerine! After this, the child was required to engage in an additional 2 minutes of hand washing and toweling. We shall learn more about oral hygiene programs in connection with the treatment of indiscriminate eating (pica).

Though only examples of the effective use of overcorrection are noted here, earlier observations regarding its advantages and limitations are repeated. As with other forms of punishment, its effects are rapid, dramatic, and relatively enduring. But there are also disadvantages. It can evoke undesired modeling, strong negative emotions, counteraggression, escape behavior, and symptom substitution (Harris & Ersner-Hershfeld, 1978; Schroeder et al., 1981). If there is strong physical resistance, its practicability is questioned (Foxx, 1978).

Physical restraint has been the most expedient method of controlling SIB. Recall that Susie had been in restraint for many years prior to our working with her. While preventing SIB, restraint also precludes participation in training activities and creates the possibility of developing attachment to restraints (à la Harry). Prolonged restraint, restraint that is more or less a permanent affair, has been regarded by the courts as violating individual rights. Thompson and Young (1977) would limit its use to SIB that represents a genuine physical threat to the self.

In the earlier section on aversive stimulation, it was reported that this contingency has been effective with SIB, and examples of aversive stimuli were presented. Under current treatment guidelines and with possibilities for intervention available at less intrusive levels (e.g., overcorrection), there has been much reduction in its use (e.g., Nolley et al., 1980).

Drugs

Although an earlier period of SIB was often treated with tranquilizers, Rivinus (1980), in his review of the use of psychotropic drugs with retarded individuals, concluded that these agents were generally ineffective. As indicated earlier, there is preliminary evidence that the psychotropic drug Prolixin may be of benefit. Drugs may be of assistance where a mood disorder is also present, but the effect is primarily on the emotional state (lithium—Cooper & Fowlie, 1973; Rivinis & Harmatz, 1979).

An interesting interaction between a drug and mild punishment is found in a study using the drug haloperidol (Durand, 1982). Neither haloperidol nor mild hand squeezing (the punishment) *used alone* reduced SIB, but the combination seemed to increase the aversiveness of the hand squeeze (see Fig. 50). In light of unwanted side effects—increased drooling and more time spent in bed—a forced arm exercise might very well have accomplished the same purpose.

CHRONIC RUMINATIVE VOMITING

Among some profoundly retarded persons, happily few in number, one encounters the socially repugnant behavior of ruminative vomiting. This consists of self-induced vomiting, chewing of the vomitus (rumination), and swallowing of

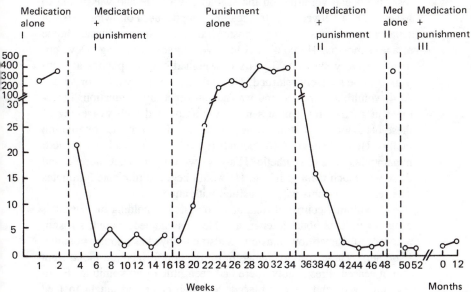

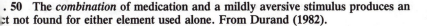

. 50 The *combination* of medication and a mildly aversive stimulus produces an
ct not found for either element used alone. From Durand (1982).

the vomitus. This is a repetitive process which usually occurs in the first hour after a meal and has been observed at all ages (infants—Lange & Melamed, 1969; Sajwaj et al., 1974; preadolescents—Wright & Menolascino, 1966; adolescents— Mulick et al., 1980; adults—Azrin & Wesolowski, 1975; Davis et al., 1980; Jackson et al., 1975).

Of the aberrant behaviors described thus far, this is one that can truly be life-threatening. There is chronic malnutrition and lowered disease resistance (Kanner, 1957; Richmond et al., 1958).

Prior to the advent of behavior modification, treatment was largely psycho-dynamic in orientation. The disorder was viewed as manifestation of a disturbed mother-child relationship, especially around feeding (Richmond & Eddy, 1957; Richmond, Eddy, & Green, 1958; Wright & Menolascino, 1966). Both psychotherapeutic and behavioral approaches have had some success, though the latter is probably much easier to implement and much quicker in its effects. Rivinus (1980) suggests that psychotropic drugs can be helpful and cites a study on the use of lithium to treat cyclical vomiting (Reid & Leonard, 1977).

Psychotherapeutic Approach

Wright and Menolascino (1966) describe the use of "nurturant nursing" in treating four severely retarded boys, ages 6–10. Of the four, two were described in detail, and a recounting of the history and treatment of one of them is presented in order to give a clear picture of the condition:

This is a 6-year-old boy with marked feeding problems and weight loss. He began vomiting on the second day of life and was found to have a fistula between the trachea and esophagus. Following surgical repair and a generally stormy postoperative course, he returned home at age 3 months. He continued to have sporadic vomiting. Development was very slow. At 3 years he weighed only 23 pounds and appeared to be severely retarded. He could neither sit, walk, nor speak. At 4, vomiting increased and was accompanied by rumination. Placement in another residential setting was associated with worsening of these behaviors, and at age 6 he was admitted to a mental retardation facility. He then weighed $16\frac{1}{2}$ pounds (!) and was extremely emaciated, nonambulatory, and apathetic. His jaws were in constant motion, and there was much teeth grinding. He would begin to ruminate 5 minutes after eating, and this was intensified with any stress.

The initial course of treatment consisted of holding him in one's arms for up to 2 hours after meals. He was cuddled, patted, stroked, and rocked. Repetitious music was also employed as another potential "soother." There was no change in rumination for about a month, but then it ceased. Presumably, there had been little or no vomiting. Feeding improved, and he was placed in a high chair and taught to feed himself. He became more active and showed some laughter. He did enjoy being held and would cuddle up closely to the person holding him. At discharge, $4\frac{1}{2}$ months later, he weighed 31 pounds and is described as a totally different child, both physically and mentally. (From Wright & Menolascino, 1966)

Behavioral Approach

Of the several behavioral approaches, *overcorrection* and *satiation* appear to combine feasibility and effectiveness. Satiation has not been previously described. It consists of essentially providing unlimited opportunity to practice the maladaptive behavior or unlimited access to that which is presumed to be reinforcing the behavior. At such high levels of access the activity or its underlying reinforcer loses its rewarding potential; the individual becomes "satiated." Therapeutic effects have also been observed following standard forms of positive reinforcement, extinction, time-out, and aversive stimulation.

1. Positive reinforcement. In a careful study that sought to compare the various types of positive reinforcement and extinction on this behavior (Mulick et al., 1980), all forms of positive reinforcement did reduce though not eliminate it. Extinction had no effect.
2. Extinction. Though extinction (ignoring of the behavior) was not effective in that study, it did apparently terminate it in a child whose vomiting typically resulted in being sent from a classroom where presumably he did not want to be. Here again, we see how a particularly noxious behavior can be used to get the child what he wants. Once the child was no longer permitted to leave the classroom, the behavior ceased (Wolf et al., 1970). Combined with an overcorrection cleaning procedure, an even more rapid disappearance would be predicted. In another study, vomiting was ignored for 30 minutes, after which the individual was cleaned and clothes were changed (Smith & Lyon, 1976). The procedure was effective, though it must have placed a good deal of stress on the staff and peers.
3. Satiation. Food satiation appears to be an effective means of treating the behavior. Food is offered until refused. One criterion of refusal was two refusals within 1 minute. Since ruminators are usually much undernourished, such feeding is not going to cause a weight problem. In one study two profoundly retarded adult ruminators were offered double portions of the standard meal plus cereal, ice cream, and milk shakes. Milk shakes were also provided either 1 hour or $1\frac{1}{2}$ hours after lunch so as to maintain satiation until dinner (Jackson et al., 1975). In another study, the ruminator initially consumed as many as 11 servings; a future limit was set at not more than five. As vomiting decreased so were food portions, and after 6 months the individual was eating a normal portion with an option for seconds. Associated procedures consisted of slowing the rate of eating and taking a 1-hour walk in an area other than that in which postmeal vomiting usually occurred (Pickup & Arsenault, 1976).[11]

---

[11]Another food-related procedure that is purported to be effective is the use of peanut butter. Once swallowed it is said to be resistive to regurgitation.

4. Time-out. Two kinds of time-out procedures have been used. Smeets (1970) interrupted feeding and physically withdrew when S vomited (I can understand that!). Davis et al. (1980) made the playing of desired music in a teaching setting contingent on in-seat behavior and nonvomiting. Either target behavior resulted in a 30-minute interruption of continuous music—instrumental bluegrass. Bluegrass won! Truly, music hath charms.

Punishment

1. Overcorrection: Vomiting was terminated within 1 week in a profoundly retarded female adult by requiring her to clean the area she soiled (Azrin & Wesolowski, 1975).

2. Aversive stimulation: In the 1960s several studies reported the control of vomiting through contingent electric shock (Lang & Melamed, 1969; Luckey, Watson, & Musick, 1968; White & Taylor, 1967). More recently, life-threatening rumination in an otherwise normal 6-month-old infant was controlled by the squirting of lemon juice in her mouth at the onset of a ruminating gesture (Sajwaj, Libet, & Agras, 1974). Mulick et al. (1980) consider that aversive procedures may still be warranted when the behavior becomes life threatening.

Summary

Of all of the formidable behavior problems, chronic ruminative vomiting may be the most resistant to total suppression (Schroeder et al., 1981). Like SIB, it seems to serve multiple purposes. Conditions that maintain it include social reinforcement, task avoidance, and the reinforcing property of the ruminated food itself (!). Indeed, it is the assumption that "continued eating" is the intent of the behavior, at least around mealtime, that is the rationale for serving extra portions of food. The extra portions substitute for the food that has been eaten, vomited, ruminated, and then reconsumed.

SCAVENGING BEHAVIOR: PICA AND COPROPHAGY

Among profoundly retarded individuals one encounters some with extraordinary eating behaviors. The previous section described the reconsumption of vomit; the present one depicts the scavenging and chronic consumption of substances ordinarily not used as food. The term "pica" is generic for the eating of nonedibles. It comes from the Latin for magpie, a bird with a predeliction for consuming a diversity of things (Danford & Huber, 1982). Coprophagy is a special form of pica and refers to the ingestion of feces.

Pica

The most extensive study on pica is that of Danford and Huber (1982). In a population of nearly 1000 institutionalized retarded persons, predominantly adults, 26 percent showed pica. Its frequency was much related to the degree of retardation, occurring in one-third of the profoundly retarded, a rate twice as great as that of those with even severe retardation (16%). In the remainder its frequency was about 10 percent. The picas observed in the population survey were divided into two groups—nonfood and food. The three most common nonfood picas were eating of strings and rags; feces, vomit, and urine; and paper, cigarettes, and soil. Of the food picas, consumption of water, coffee and coffee grounds, and food from trash cans were the most frequent.

Practitioners of pica are not indiscriminate in their tastes! They tend to prefer a single food or nonfood and spend a good deal of time looking for their preference. The selectivity of their pica indicates that the behavior cannot be attributed to a simple failure to discriminate between edibles and nonedibles. They know what they want!

Nonfood pica was the most frequent form; it represented two-thirds of all picas, the remaining third being about equally divided between food and a combination of food and nonfood pica. Food picas predominated in those with less than severe retardation; nonfood picas were virtually absent here. Only in the severe and profound subgroups did nonfood picas predominate, and this was particularly true of those with profound retardation.

In children and younger adults, nonfood pica was much more common than food pica. After age 40 this was much diminished, and food picas increased.

Individuals with pica are at risk for medical problems. These include constipation, pin worms, vomiting after eating the nonedible, and intestinal obstructions. Surgery for such obstructions is commonplace. Obstructions are found in "persons who swallow rocks, razor blades, towels, screens, safety pins, etc." (Schroeder et al., 1981) and may require surgery for their removal. A well-known form of pica and one that can actually *cause* retardation is the eating of flaking leaded paint (lead encephalitis). This was referred to in Chapter 4. Finally, vitamin C and D deficiencies are possible consequences (Kalisz, Ekvall, & Palmer, 1978).

It is not easy to write about the kinds of behavior described in ruminative vomiting and pica. We are confronted with the jarring reality of individuals whose behavior is utterly repulsive in terms of normal standards. But such behavior is encountered in mental illness as well as in retardation. Feces smearing is a common acute psychotic symptom. *These behaviors are manifestations of altered brain functioning. Though their origin often lies outside our understanding, it is essential to recognize that we, too, have the capacity to engage in such aberrant activity. More important, these behaviors can be modified.*

Coprophagy

Of the picas, coprophagy, the consumption of feces, own or others', must be extraordinarily difficult to tolerate. Ruminative vomiting cannot be far behind! Such individuals are commonly kept in isolation, or their arm and head movements are restrained—to prevent rectal digging (Foxx & Martin, 1975).

At least some picas seem to be intrinsically reinforcing. Compulsive consumption of coffee, cigarette butts, and oak leaves (!) may relate to their drug effects (Danford & Huber, 1982). Schroeder (personal communication) thinks that the eating of tobacco from cigarette butts is probably just a substitute for chewing tobacco. It has also been suggested that permanent finger feeding may encourage pica and that early learning of utensil use is important (Albin, 1977). Where finger feeding has persisted, even subsequent learning of utensil use may not be effective in reducing pica.

Apart from encouraging early use of utensils, prevention has taken the form of devices that block pica. Camisoles (straitjackets), mesh restraining bags, and face masks (e.g., fencing masks) have all been employed. Two of the problems associated with their use are the creation of vulnerability to aggression from others because of one's own hand immobility (Foxx & Martin, 1975) and an increased social distance from staff (Rojahn, Schroeder, & Mulick, 1980).

Treatment

Three types of treatment are discussed.

1. *Positive reinforcement.* The aversiveness of some of the picas and the attendant health hazards have lent themselves to treatments that are generally more stringent than purely positive reinforcement.
2. *Time-out.* Time-out in the form of contingent restraint has been employed (Ausman et al., 1974; Bucher et al., 1976). In one study, a helmet with a Plexiglas window and ventilating vent was used as time-out along with DRO (Ausman et al., 1974). Both studies achieved at least short-term reduction of pica.
3. *Punishment.* In their review of this behavior under the general rubric of SIB, Schroeder et al. (1981) conclude that overcorrection has been the most successful method of control (Foxx & Martin, 1975; Matson, Stephens, & Smith, 1978; Rojahn et al., 1979; Rusch et al., 1976; Singh & Winton, 1985). Overcorrection here has typically involved oral hygiene and personal grooming contingencies as well as cleaning up the environment. Foxx and Martin (1975) described in some detail their procedures for treating coprophagic adults. When such behavior was observed, the offender (a truly apt description), was (a) taken to a toilet and required to spit out what was in the mouth (b) required to brush teeth and gums with a toothbrush that had been immersed in a mouth wash and to wipe lips with a washcloth dampened with antiseptic, (c) required to wash hands, fingernails, and anal area (feces are commonly obtained through "rectal digging"), and (d) made to clean and/or disinfect the area where pica had occurred. The oral hygiene and washing procedures were each 10 minutes in length as was the later cleanup time. Staff accomplished this by wearing rubber gloves and a hospital gown or apron. Apart from immediate treatment effects, biweekly stool specimens were eventually free of the intestinal parasites, medical evidence of increased control. Over a 3-month follow-up period, nearly complete suppression was maintained, though occasional episodes still occurred.

Bibliography

Aanes, D., & Moen, M. (1976). Adaptive behavior changes of group home residents. *Mental Retardation, 14,* 36–40.

Abel, T. M. (1953). Resistances and difficulties in the psychotherapy of mental retardates. *Journal of Clinical Psychology, 9,* 107–109.

Abeson, A., Burgdorf, R. C., Jr., Casey, P. J., Kunz, J., & McNiel, W. (1975). Access to opportunity. In N. Hobbs (Ed.), *Issues in the classification of children* (Vol. II). San Francisco: Jossey-Bass.

Abramowicz, H. K., & Richardson, S. A. (1975). Epidemiology of severe mental retardation in children: Community studies. *American Journal of Mental Deficiency, 80,* 18–39.

Abramson, E. E., & Wunderlich, R. A. (1972). Dental hygiene training. *Mental Retardation, 10,* 6–8.

Abramson, P. R., Gravink, M. J., Abramson, L. M., & Sommers, D. (1977). Early diagnosis and intervention of retardation: A survey of parental reactions concerning the quality of services rendered. *Mental Retardation, 15,* 28–31.

Accreditation Council for Services for Mentally Retarded and Other Developmentally Disabled Persons. (1978). *Standards for services for developmentally disabled individuals.* Chicago: Joint Commission on Accreditation of Hospitals.

Achenbach, T. M. (1970). Comparison of Stanford-Binet performance of nonretarded and retarded persons matched for MA and sex. *American Journal of Mental Deficiency, 74,* 488–494.

Adams, M. (1971). *Mental retardation and its social dimensions.* New York: Columbia University Press.

Agosta, J. M., Close, D. W., Hops, H., & Rusch, F. R. (1980). Treatment of self-injurious behavior through overcorrection procedures. *Journal of the Association for the Severely Handicapped, 5,* 5–12.

Alberman, E., Polani, P. E., Roberts, J. A. F., Spicer, C. C., Elliott, M., Armstrong, E., & Dhadial, R. K. (1972). Parental X-irradiation and chromosome constitution in their spontaneously aborted fetuses. *Annals of Human Genetics, 36,* 185–194.

Albin, J. (1977). The treatment of pica (scavenging) behavior in the retarded: A critical analysis and implications for research. *Mental Retardation, 15,* 14–18.

Alexander, D., Ehrhardt, A. A., & Money, J. (1966). Defective figure drawing, geometric and human in Turner's syndrome. *Journal of Nervous and Mental Disorders, 142,* 161–167.

Alexander, D., & Money, J. (1965). Reading ability, object constancy, and Turner's syndrome. *Perceptual and Motor Skills, 20,* 981–984.

Allen, G. (1958). Patterns of discovery in the genetics of mental deficiency. *American Journal of Mental Deficiency, 62,* 840–849.

Allen, G., & Baroff, G. S. (1955). Mongoloid twins and their siblings. *Acta Genetica et Statistica Medica, 5,* 294–326.

Allen, G., Kallmann, F. J., Baroff, G. S., & Sank, D. (1962). Etiology of mental subnormality in twins. In F. J. Kallmann (Ed.), *Expanding goals of genetics in psychiatry.* New York: Grune & Stratton.

Allen, J., DeMyer, M. K., Norton, J. A., Pontius, W., & Yang, E. (1971). Intellectuality in parents of psychotic, subnormal and normal children. *Journal of Autism and Childhood Schizophrenia, 1,* 311.

Allen, K. E., Turner, K. D., & Everett, P. M. (1970). A behavior modification classroom for Head Start children with problem behaviors. *Exceptional Children, 37,* 119–129.

Almeida, G. M., & Barros, N. G. (1964). Megalencefalia, consideracoes a respeito de 7 casos diagnosticados em vida. *Arquivos de Neuro-psiquiatria, 22,* 25–32.

Alper, A. E., & Horne, B. M. (1959). IQ changes of institutionalized mental defectives over two decades. *American Journal of Mental Deficiency, 64,* 472–475.

Alpern, G. (1967). Measurement of "untestable" autistic children. *Journal of Abnormal Psychology, 72,* 478–486.

Alter, M. (1962). Anencephalus, hydrocephalus, and spina bifida. *Archives of Neurology, 7,* 411.

American Medical Association. (1964). *Mental retardation: A handbook for the primary physician.* Report of the American Medical Association Conference on Mental Retardation, Chicago.

Amidon, A., & Brim, O. G. (1972). What do children have to gain from parent education? Paper prepared for the Advisory Committee on Child Development, National Research Council, National Academy of Sciences.

Ainsworth, M. D., & Wittig, B. A. (1969). Attachment and exploratory behavior of one-year-olds in a strange situation. In B. M. Foss (Ed.), *Determinants of infant behavior,* Vol. 4. New York: Wiley.

Anastasi, A., & Levee, R. F. (1960). Intellectual defect and musical talent: A case report. *American Journal of Mental Deficiency, 64,* 695–703.

Anastasi, A. (1961). *Psychological testing* (2nd ed.). New York: Macmillan.

Ando, H. (1977). Training autistic children to urinate in the toilet through operant condition techniques. *Journal of Autism and Childhood Schizophrenia, 1,* 151–163.

Anders, T. (1971). Short-term memory for presented supraspan information in nonretarded and mentally retarded individuals. *American Journal of Mental Deficiency, 75,* 571–578.

Anderson, J. D. (1980). Spatial arrangement of stimuli and the construction of communication boards for the physically handicapped. *Mental Retardation, 18,* 41–42.

Andron, L., & Sturm, M. L. (1973). Is "I do" in the repertoire of the retarded? *Mental Retardation, 11,* 31–34.

Apolloni, T., & Cooke, T. P. (1978). Integrated programming at the infant, toddler, and preschool levels. In M. J. Guralnick (Ed.), *Early intervention and the integration of handicapped and nonhandicapped children.* Baltimore: University Park Press.

Apolloni, A. H., & Triest, G. (1983). Respite services in California: Status and recommendations for improvement. *Mental Retardation, 21,* 240–243.

Apthekar, N. H. (1953). *Dynamics of casework and counselling.* Boston: Houghton Mifflin.

Arthur, G. (1947). *A point scale of performance tests. Revised form II.* New York: Psychological Corporation.

Ashurst, D. I., & Meyers, C. E. (1973). Social system and clinical model in school identification of the educable retarded. In R. K. Eymans, C. E. Meyers, & G. Tarjan (Eds.), Sociobehavioral studies in mental retardation [Special issue]. *Monographs of the American Association on Mental Deficiency, 1.*

August, G. J., Stewart, M. A., & Tsai, L. (1981). The incidence of cognitive disabilities in the siblings of autistic children. *British Journal of Psychiatry, 138,* 416–422.

Ausman, J., Ball, T. S., & Alexander, D. (1974). Behavior therapy of pica with a profoundly retarded adolescent. *Mental Retardation, 12,* 16–18.

Ausman, J., & Gaddy, M. (1974). Reinforcement training for echolalia. *Mental Retardation, 12,* 20–21.

Axelrod, S., & Apsche, J. (1983). *The Effects of Punishment on Human Behavior.* New York: Academic Press.

Axelrod, S., Brantner, J. P., & Meddock, T. D. (1978). Overcorrection: A review and critical analysis. *Journal of Special Education, 12,* 367-391.

Ayllon, T. (1963). Intensive treatment of psychotic behavior by stimulus satiation and food reinforcement. *Behavior Research and Therapy, 1,* 53-61.

Ayllon, T., & Michael, J. (1959). The psychiatric nurse as a behavioral engineer. *Journal of the Experimental Analysis of Behavior, 2,* 323-334.

Azrin, N. H., & Armstrong, P. M. (1973). The "mini-meal"—A method for teaching eating skills to the profoundly retarded. *Mental Retardation, 11,* 9-13.

Azrin, N. H., & Foxx, R. (1971). A rapid method of toilet training the institutionalized retarded. *Journal of Applied Behavior Analysis, 4,* 89-99.

Azrin, N. H., Gottlieb, L., Hughart, L., Wesolowski, M. D., & Rahn, T. (1975). Eliminating self-injurious behavior by educative procedures. *Behavior Research and Therapy, 13,* 101-111.

Azrin, N. H., Kaplan, S. J., & Foxx, R. M. (1973b). Autism reversal: Eliminating stereotyped self-stimulation of retarded individuals. *American Journal of Mental Deficiency, 78,* 241-248.

Azrin, N. H., Sneed, T. J., & Foxx, R. M. (1973a). Dry bed: A rapid method of eliminating bedwetting (enuresis) of the retarded. *Behavior Research and Therapy, 11,* 427-434.

Azrin, N. H., Schaeffer, R. M., & Wesolowski, M. D. (1976). A rapid method of teaching profoundly retarded persons to dress by a reinforcement-guidance method. *Mental Retardation, 14,* 29-33.

Azrin, N. H., & Wesolowski, M. D. (1974). Theft reversal: An overcorrection procedure for eliminating stealing by a retarded person. *Journal of Applied Behavior Analysis, 7,* 577-581.

Azrin, N. H., & Wesolowski, M. D. (1975). Eliminating habitual vomiting in a retarded adult by positive practice and self-correction. *Journal of Behavior Therapy and Experimental Psychiatry, 6,* 145-148.

Bachman, J. A. (1972). Self-injurious behavior: A behavioral analysis. *Journal of Abnormal Psychology, 80,* 211-224.

Bailey, J. S. (1981). Wanted: A rational search for the limiting conditions of habilitation. *Analysis and Intervention in Developmental Disabilities, 1,* 45-52.

Baird, P. A. (1983). Mental retardation in B.C. The scope of the problem. *British Columbia Medical Journal, 25,* 134-136.

Baird, P. A., & Miller, J. R. (1968). Some epidemiological aspects of Down's syndrome in British Columbia. *British Journal of Preventive and Social Medicine, 22,* 81-85.

Baird, P. A., & Sadovnick, A. D. (1985). Mental retardation in over half-a-million conservative livebirths: An epidemiological study. *American Journal of Mental Deficiency, 89,* 323-330.

Baker, B. L. (1977). Support systems for the parent as therapist. In P. Mittler (Ed.), *Research to practice in mental retardation: Vol. I. Care and intervention.* Baltimore: University Park Press.

Baker, B. L., Brightman, A. J., Heifetz, L. J., & Murphy, D. M. (1973). *The READ Project Series.* Cambridge, MS: Behavioral Education Projects.

Baker, B. L., Brightman, A. J., Heifetz, L. J., & Murphy, D. M. (1976). *Steps to independence: A skills training series for children with special needs.* Champaign, IL: Research Press.

Baker, B. L., Seltzer, G. B., & Seltzer, M. M. (1974). *As close as possible: Community residences for retarded adults.* Boston: Little, Brown.

Baker, D. B. (1980). Applications of environmental psychology in programming for severely handicapped persons. *Journal of the Association for the Severely Handicapped, 5,* 234-249.

Baker, D., Telfer, M. A. Richardson, C. E., & Clark, G. R. (1970). Chromosome errors in men with antisocial behavior. *Journal of the American Medical Association, 214,* 869-878.

Balla, D. (1976). Relationship of institution size to quality of care: A review of the literature. *American Journal of Mental Deficiency, 81,* 117-124.

Balla, D., Styfco, S. J., & Zigler, E. (1971). Use of the opposition concept and outerdirectedness in intellectually average, familial retarded, and organically retarded children. *American Journal of Mental Deficiency, 75,* 663-680.

Ballard, R. (1977). The overgrown infant. In A. M. Rudolph (Ed.), *Pediatrics* (16th ed.). New York: Appleton-Century-Crofts.

Baller, W., Charles, D., & Miller, E. (1966). *Midlife attainment of the mentally retarded. A longitudinal study.* Lincoln: University of Nebraska Press.

Balow, B., & Bloomquist, M. (1965). Young adults ten to fifteen years after severe reading disability. *Elementary School Journal, 66,* 44–48.

Balthazar, E. E. (1971). *Balthazar scales of adaptive behavior for the profoundly and severely mentally retarded: A system for program evaluation and development: Sec. 1. The scales of functional independence.* Champaign, IL: Research Press.

Bandura, A. (1973). *Aggression: A social learning analysis.* Englewood Cliffs, NJ: Prentice-Hall.

Bandura, A., Grusec, J., & Menlove, F. (1967). Vicarious extinction of avoidance behavior. *Journal of Personality and Social Psychology, 5,* 16–23.

Banerdt, B., & Bricker, D. (1978). A training program for selected self-feeding skills for the motorically impaired. *AAESPH Review, 3,* 222–230.

Bank-Mikkelsen, N. E. (1969). A metropolitan area in Denmark: Copenhagen. In R. Kugel & W. Wolfensberger (Eds.), *Changing patterns in residential services for the mentally retarded,* Washington: President's Committee on Mental Retardation.

Barclay, A., & Yater, A. C. (1969). Comparative study of the Wechsler Preschool and Primary Scale of Intelligence and the Stanford-Binet Intelligence Scale, Form L–M, among culturally deprived children. *Journal of Consulting and Clinical Psychology, 33,* 257.

Bardon, L. M. E. (1964). Siccacell treatment in mongolism. *Lancet, 2,* 234.

Barefield, J. B. (1976). Aversive control of self-injurious behavior by use of ammonia inhalants. Master's thesis, Northeast Louisiana University, Monroe.

Barker, J., Goldstein, A., & Frankenburg, W. (1972). *Denver Eye Screening Test (DEST).* Denver: University of Colorado Press.

Baroff, G. S. (1958). Current theories on the etiology of mongolism. *Eugenics Quarterly, 5,* 212–215.

Baroff, G. S. (1959). WISC patterning in endogenous mental deficiency. *American Journal of Mental Deficiency, 64,* 482–485.

Baroff, G. S. (1974). *Mental retardation: Nature, cause, and management.* Washington: Hemisphere.

Baroff, G. S. (1976). On the use of aversive techniques in controlling self-injurious behavior. *American Psychologist, 31,* 616.

Baroff, G. S. (1980). On "size" and the quality of residential care: A second look. *Mental Retardation, 18,* 113–117.

Baroff, G. S. (1982). Predicting the prevalence of mental retardation in individual catchment areas. *Mental Retardation, 20,* 133–135.

Baroff, G. S., & Tate, B. G. (1968). The use of aversive stimulation in the treatment of chronic self-injurious behavior. *Journal of the American Academy of Child Psychiatry, 7,* 454–470.

Barrett, R. P., & Linn, D. M. (1981). Treatment of stereotyped toe-walking with overcorrection and physical therapy. *Applied Research in Mental Retardation, 2,* 13–21.

Bartak, L., Rutter, M., & Cox, A. (1975). A comparative study of infantile autism and specific developmental receptive language disorder. I. The children. *British Journal of Psychiatry, 126,* 127–145.

Bartel, N. R., & Guskin, S. L. (1971). A handicap as a social phenomenon. In W. M. Cruickshank (Ed.), *Psychology of exceptional children and youth* (3rd ed.). Englewood Cliffs, NJ: Prentice-Hall.

Barton, E. S., Guess, D., Garcia, E., & Baer, D. M. (1970). Improvement of retardates' mealtime behavior by timeout procedures using multiple baseline techniques. *Journal of Applied Behavior Analysis, 3,* 77–84.

Bass, M. S. (1964). Marriage for the mentally deficient. *Mental Retardation, 2,* 198–202.

Bates, P., & Wehman, P. (1977). Behavior management with the mentally retarded: An empirical analysis of the research. *Mental Retardation, 15,* 9–12.

Bates, W. J., Smeltzer, D. J., & Arnoczky, S. M. (1986). Appropriate and inappropriate use of psychotherapeutic medications for institutionalized mentally retarded persons. *American Journal of Mental Deficiency, 90,* 363–370.

Baum, M. H. (1962). Some dynamic factors affecting family adjustment to the handicapped child. *Exceptional Children, 28,* 387–392.

Baumeister, A. A. (1967). The effects of dietary control on intelligence in phenylketonuria. *American Journal of Mental Deficiency, 71,* 840–847.

Baumeister, A. A. (1978). Origins and control of stereotyped movements. In C. E. Meyers (Ed.), *Quality of life in severely and profoundly mentally retarded people: Research foundation for improvement.* Monograph of the American Association of Mental Deficiency, No. 3. Washington: American Association on Mental Deficiency.

Baumeister, A. A. (1981). The right to habilitation: What does it mean? *Analysis and Intervention in Developmental Disabilities, 1,* 61–74.

Baumeister, A. A., & Forehand, R. (1971). Effects of extinction of an instrumental response on stereotyped body rocking in severe retardates. *Psychological Record, 21,* 235–240.

Baumeister, A. A., & Forehand, R. (1973). Stereotyped acts. In N. R. Ellis (Ed.), *International review of research in mental retardation* (Vol. 6). New York: Academic Press.

Baumeister, A. A., & Rollings, P. (1976). Self-injurious behavior. In N. R. Ellis (Ed.), *International review of research in mental retardation* (Vol. 9). New York: Academic Press.

Baumeister, A. A., & Williams, J. (1976). Relationship of physical stigmata to intellectual functioning in mongolism. *American Journal of Mental Deficiency, 71,* 586–592.

Bax, M. C. O. (1964). Terminology and classification of cerebral palsy. *Developmental Medicine and Child Neurology, 6, 295–297.*

Bayley, N. (1969). *Bayley Scales of Infant Development.* New York: Psychological Corp.

Bayley, N. (1970). Development of mental abilities. In P. M. Mussen (Ed.), *Carmichael's manual of child psychology* (3rd ed., Vol. I). New York: Wiley.

Bazelon, M., Paine, R. S., Cowie, V., Hunt, P., Houck, J. C., & Mahanand, D. (1967). Reversal of hypotonia in infants with Down's syndrome by administration of 5-hydroxytryotophan. *Lancet, 1,* 1130–1131.

Bean, F. X. (1961). The effect of classroom instruction upon the class inclusion behavior of the educable mentally retarded. Unpublished doctoral dissertation, Teachers College, Columbia University, New York.

Beck, H. L. (1969). *Social services to the mentally retarded.* Springfield, IL: Charles C Thomas.

Becker, W. C., & Gersten, R. A. (1982). A follow-up of Follow Through: The later effects of the direct instruction model on children in fifth and sixth grades. *American Education Research Journal, 19,* 75–92.

Beckman-Bell, P. (1981). Child-related stress in families of handicapped children. In R. R. Fewell (Ed.), Families of handicapped children [Special issue]. *Topics in Early Children Special Education, 1*(3), 45–54.

Behrman, R. (1973). *Neonatology: Diseases of the fetus and infant.* St. Louis: Mosby.

Beliles, R. P. (1975). Metals. In L. J. Casarett & J. Dowll (Eds.), *Toxicology, the basic science of poison.* New York: Macmillan.

Bell, N. J. (1976). IQ as a factor in community lifestyle of previously institutionalized retardates. *Mental Retardation, 14,* 29–33.

Bell, N. J., Kozar, B., Martin, A. S., Morris, B. R., & Morris, J. L. (1977). *The impact of Special Olympics.* Lubbock, TX: Texas Tech. University.

Bellamy, G. T. (Ed.). (1976). *Habilitation of severely and profoundly retarded adults.* Eugene, OR: University of Oregon Press.

Bellamy, G. T., Inman, D. P., & Yeates, J. (1978). Workshop supervision: Evaluation of a procedure for production management with the severely retarded. *Mental Retardation, 16,* 317–319.

Bellamy, G. T., Peterson, L., & Close, A. (1975). Habilitation of the severely and profoundly retarded: Illustrations of competence. *Education and Training of the Mentally Retarded, 10,* 174–186.

Beller, E. K. (1972). Impact of early education on disadvantaged children. In S. Ryan (Ed.), *A report on longitudinal evaluations of preschool programs.* Washington: U.S. Office of Child Development.

Bellugi, U. (1972). The development of language in the normal child. In J. E. McLean, D. E. Yoder, & R. L. Schiefelbusch (Eds.), *Language intervention with the retarded: Developing strategies.* Baltimore: University Park Press.

Belmont, J. M. (1971). Medical-behavioral research in retardation. In N. R. Ellis (Ed.), *International review of research in mental retardation* (Vol. 5). New York: Academic Press.

Belmont, J. M., & Butterfield, E. C. (1969). The relation of short-term memory to development and intelligence. In L. P. Lipsitt & H. W. Reese (Eds.), *Advances in child development and behavior* (Vol. 4). New York: Academic Press.

Belmont, J. M., & Butterfield, E. C. (1971). Learning strategies as determinants of memory deficiencies. *Cognitive Psychology, 2,* 411–420.

Benda, C. E. (1954). Psychopathology of childhood. In L. Carmichael (Ed.), *Manual of child psychology* (2nd ed.). New York: Wiley.

Benda, C. E. (1960). *The child with mongolism.* New York: Grune & Stratton.

Bender, M., & Valletutti, P. J. (1976). *Teaching the moderately and severely handicapped* (Vol. 1). Baltimore: University Park Press.

Berger, S. L. (1972). A clinical program for developing multimodal language responses with atypical deaf children. In J. E. McLean, D. E. Yoder, & R. L. Schiefelbusch (Eds.), *Language intervention with the retarded.* Baltimore: University Park Press.

Bergner, L., & Yerby, A. S. (1968). Low income and barriers to use of health services. *New England Journal of Medicine, 278,* 541–546.

Berkson, G. (1967). Abnormal stereotyped motor acts. In J. Zubin & H. F. Hunt (Eds.), *Comparative psychopathology—animal and human* (pp. 76–94). New York: Grune & Stratton.

Berkson, G., & Landesman-Dwyer, S. (1977). Behavioral research on severe and profound mental retardation. *American Journal of Mental Deficiency, 81,* 428–454.

Berkson, G., & Mason, W. A. (1963). Stereotyped movements of mental defectives. III. Situation effects. *American Journal of Mental Deficiency, 68,* 409–412.

Berlyne, D. E. (1970). Children's reasoning and thinking. In P. H. Mussen (Ed.), *Carmichael's manual of child psychology* (Vol. 1). New York: Wiley.

Berman, J. (1970). Sex ratio in hyperphenylalanimemia. *New England Journal of medicine, 283,* 491.

Berman, P. W., Graham, F. K., Eichman, P. L., & Waisman, H. A. (1961). Psychologic and neurologic status of diet-treated phenylketonuric children and their siblings. *Pediatrics, 28,* 924–934.

Berry, H. K., O'Grady, D. J., Perlmutter, L. J., & Bofinger, L. H. (1979). Intellectual development and academic achievement of children treated early for phenylketonuria. *Developmental Medicine and Child Neurology, 21,* 311–320.

Bettison, S., Davidson, D., Taylor, P., & Fox, B. (1976). The long-term effects of a toilet training program for the retarded: A pilot study. *Australian Journal of Mental Retardation, 4,* 18–35.

Bialer, I. (1961). Conceptualization of success and failure in mentally retarded and normal children. *Journal of Personality, 29,* 303–320.

Bialer, I. (1969). Psychotherapy and other adjustment techniques with the mentally retarded. In A. A. Baumeister (Ed.), *Mental retardation: Appraisal, education, and rehabilitation.* Chicago: Aldine.

Bialer, I. (1970). Emotional disturbance and mental retardation. In F. J. Menolascino (Ed.), *Psychiatric approaches to mental retardation.* New York: Basic Books.

Bice, H. V. (1947). Mental deficiency, moron level. In A. Burton & R. E. Harris (Eds.), *Case histories in clinical and abnormal psychology.* New York: Harper.

Bigelow, G. (1977). The behavioral approach to retardation. In T. Thompson & J. Grabowski (Eds.), *Behavior modification of the mentally retarded* (2nd ed.). New York: Oxford University Press.

Bigelow, G., & Griffiths, R. (1977). An intensive teaching unit for severely and profoundly retarded women. In T. Thompson & J. Grabowski (Eds.), *Behavior modification of the mentally retarded* (2nd ed.). New York: Oxford University Press.

Biken, D. (1977). Myths, mistreatment, and pitfalls: Mental retardation and criminal justice. *Mental Retardation, 15,* 51–57.

Bilovsky, D., & Share, J. (1965). The ITPA and Down's syndrome: An exploratory study. *American Journal of Mental Deficiency, 70,* 78–82.

Bilsky, L. (1976). Transfer of categorical clustering set in mildly retarded adolescents. *American Journal of Mental Deficiency, 80,* 588–594.

Bilsky, L., Evans, R. A., & Gilbert, L. (1972). Generalization of associative clustering tendencies in mentally retarded adolescents: Effect of novel stimuli. *American Journal of Mental Deficiency, 77,* 77–84.

Binet, A., & Simon, T. (1911). *Le mesure du développement de l'intelligence chez les jeunes infants.* Paris: A. Coneslant.

Birch, H. G. (1956). Theoretical aspects of psychological behavior in the brain damaged. In M. Goldstein (Ed.), *Psychological services for the cerebral palsied* (pp. 48–61). New York: United Cerebral Palsy Associations of New York State.

Birch, H. G., & Cravioto, J. (1966). Infection, nutrition and environment in mental development. In H. V. Eichenwald (Ed.), *The prevention of mental retardation through the control of infectious disease* (Public Health Service Publication No. 1692) (pp. 227–248). Washington: U.S. Government Printing Office.

Birch, H. G., Pinuro, C., Atcalde, E., Toca, T., & Cravioto, J. (1971). Relation of kwashiorkor in early childhood to intelligence at school age. *Pediatric Research, 5,* 579–585.

Birch, H. G., Richardson, S. A., Baird, D., Horobin, G., & Illsley, R. (1970). *Mental subnormality in the community: A clinical and epidemiological study.* Baltimore: Williams & Wilkins.

Birch, H. G., Thomas, A., Chess, S., & Hertzig, M. E. (1962). Individuality in the development of children. *Developmental Medicine and Child Neurology, 4,* 370–379.

Bjaanes, A. T., & Butler, E. W. (1974). Environmental variation in community care facilities for mentally retarded persons. *American Journal of Mental Deficiency, 78,* 429–439.

Black, D. B., Kato, J. G., & Walker, G. W. (1966). A study of improvement in mentally retarded children accruing from Siccacell therapy. *American Journal of Mental Deficiency, 70,* 499–508.

Blacketer-Simmonds, D. A. (1953). An investigation into the supposed differences existing between Mongols and other mentally defective subjects with regard to certain psychological traits. *Journal of Mental Science, 90,* 702–708.

Blank, C. E. (1960). Apert's syndrome (a type of acrocephalosyndactyly) observations on British series of thirty-nine cases. *Annals of Human Genetics, 24,* 4–32.

Blatt, B. (1958). The physical, personality, and academic status of children who are mentally retarded attending special classes as compared with children who are mentally retarded attending regular classes. *American Journal of Mental Deficiency, 62,* 810–818.

Blatt, B. (1970). *Exodus from pandemonium. Human abuse and a reformation of public policy.* Boston: Allyn and Bacon.

Blatt, B., & Kaplan, F. (1966). *Christmas in purgatory: A photographic essay on mental retardation.* Boston: Allyn and Bacon.

Blinick, G., Wallach, R. C., Jerez, E., & Ackerman, B. D. (1976). Drug addiction in pregnancy and the neonate. *American Journal of Obstetrics and Gynecology, 125,* 135–142.

Bliss, C. K. (1965). *Semantography.* Sydney, Australia: Semantography Publications.

Bloom, B. S. (1964). *Stability and change in human characteristics.* New York: Wiley.

Bloom, L. (1970). *Language development: Form and function in emerging grammars.* Cambridge, MA: M.I.T. Press.

Bloom, L. (1975). Language development. In F. D. Horowitz (Ed.), *Review of child development research* (Vol. 4). Chicago: University of Chicago Press.

Blount, W. (1968). Concept usage research with the mentally retarded. *Psychological Bulletin, 69,* 281–294.

Blumberg, B. S., Sutnick, A. I., & London, W. T. (1970). Australia antigen as a hepatitis virus. *American Journal of Medicine, 48,* 1–8.

Bobath, B. (1971). *Abnormal postural reflex activity caused by brain lesions* (2nd ed.). London: Heinemann.

Boe, R. B. (1977). Economical procedures for the reduction of aggression in a residential setting. *Mental Retardation, 15,* 25–28.

Bollard, R. J., & Woodroffe, P. (1977). The effect of parent-administered dry-bed training on nocturnal enuresis in children. *Behavior Research and Therapy, 15,* 159–165.

Bonvillian, J. D., Nelson, K. E., & Rhyne, J. M. (1981). Sign language and autism. *Journal of Autism and Developmental Disorders, 11,* 125–137.

Borberg, A. (1951). Clinical and genetic investigations into tuberous sclerosis and Recklinghausen's neurofibromatosis. *Acta Psychiatrica et Neurologica, 71,* 239.

Borkowski, J. G., & Cavanaugh, J. C. (1979). Maintenance and generalization of skills and strategies by the retarded. In N. R. Ellis (Ed.), *Handbook of mental deficiency, psychological theory and research* (2nd ed.). Hillsdale, NJ: Lawrence Erlbaum.

Borreson, P. M. (1980). The elimination of a self-injurious avoidance response through a forced running consequence. *Mental Retardation, 18*, 73–77.

Bortner, M., & Birch, H. G. (1970). Cognitive capacity and cognitive competence. *American Journal of Mental Deficiency, 74*, 735–744.

Bostow, P. E., & Bailey, J. (1969). Modification of severe disruptive and aggressive behavior using brief time-out and reinforcement procedures. *Journal of Applied Behavior Analysis, 2*, 31–37.

Boullin, D. J., Coleman, M., & O'Brien, R. A. (1970). Abnormalities in platelet 5-hydroxytryptamine efflux in patients with infantile autism. *Nature, 226*, 371.

Boullin, D. J., Coleman, M., O'Brien, R. A., & Rimland, B. (1971). Laboratory predictions of infantile autism based on 5-hydroxytryptamine efflux from blood platelets and their correlation with the Rimland E-2 score. *Journal of Autism and Childhood Schizophrenia, 1*, 63.

Bowlby, J. (1940). The influence of early environment. *International Journal of Psychoanalysis, 21*, 154–178.

Bowlby, J. (1952). Maternal care and mental health. *WHO Monographs, 2.*

Bowlby, J., Ainsworth, M., Boston, M., & Rosenbluth, D. (1956). The effects of mother-child separation: A follow-up study. *British Journal of Medical Psychology, 29*, 211–247.

Bowman, P. W., & Hoffman, J. L. (1969). *An investigation of factors contributing to successful and non-successful adjustment of discharged retardates.* Pownal, ME: Pineland Hospital and Training Center.

Braddock, D., Hemp, R., & Howes, R. (1986). Direct costs of institutional care in the United States. *Mental Retardation, 24*, 9–12.

Bradley-Johnson, S., & Travers, R. M. (1979). Cardiac change of retarded and nonretarded infants to an auditory signal. *American Journal of Mental Deficiency, 83*, 631–636.

Brady, R. O. (1977). Lipidoses. In A. M. Rudolph (Ed.), *Pediatrics* (16th ed.). New York: Appleton-Century-Crofts.

Brassell, W. R. (1977). Intervention with handicapped infants: Correlates of progress. *Mental Retardation, 15*, 18–22.

Bray, N. W. (1979). Strategy production in the retarded. In N. R. Ellis (Ed.), *Handbook of mental deficiency, psychological theory and research.* Hillsdale, NJ: Lawrence Erlbaum.

Brazelton, T. B. (1973). *Neonatal behavioral assessment scale.* Philadelphia: Lippincott.

Breckenridge, M. E., & Vincent, E. L. (1960). *Child development* (4th ed.). Philadelphia: Saunders.

Brennand, J., Chinault, A. C., Konecki, D. S., Melton, D. W., & Caskey, C. T. (1982). Cloned cDNA sequences of the hypoxanthina/guanine phosphororibosyltransferase gene from a mouse neuroblastoma cell line found to have amplified genomic sequences. *Proceedings of the National Academy of Sciences, 79*, 1950–1954.

Breuning, S. E., & Davidson, N. A. (1981). Effects of psychotropic drugs on intelligence test performance of institutionalized mentally retarded adults. *American Journal of Mental Deficiency, 85*, 575–579.

Bricker, D. *Early intervention: The criteria of success.* Paper presented at Gatlinburg Conference on Mental Retardation, Gatlinburg, TN, 1978.

Bricker, D. (1978). A rationale for the integration of handicapped and nonhandicapped preschool children. In M. J. Guralnick (Ed.), *Early intervention and the integration of handicapped and nonhandicapped children.* Baltimore: University Park Press.

Bricker, W. A. (1972). A systematic approach to language training. In R. L. Schiefelbusch (Ed.), *Language of the mentally retarded.* Baltimore: University Park Press.

Bricker, W. A., & Bricker, D. D. (1970). A program of language training for the severely language handicapped child. *Exceptional Child, 37*, 101–111.

Brickey, M. P., Campbell, K. M., & Browning, L. J. (1985). A five-year follow-up of sheltered workshop employees placed in competitive jobs. *Mental Retardation, 23*, 67–73.

Bristol, M. M. (1977). Continuum of service delivery to preschool handicapped and their families. In P. Mittler (Ed.), *Research to practice in mental retardation: Vol. 1. Care and intervention.* Baltimore: University Park Press.

Broadfoot, B. (1975). Use of a positive reinforcer to eliminate stealing. *Bulletin of Behavior Modification in Mental Retardation, 1,* 9–11.

Brolin, D. E., Durand, R., Kromer, K., & Muller, P. (1975). Postschool adjustment of educable retarded students. *Education and Training of the Mentally Retarded, 10,* 144–149.

Bronfenbrenner, U. (1972). The roots of alienation. In U. Bronfenbrenner (Ed.), *Influences on human development.* Hinsdale, IL: Dryden.

Brown, A. L. (1974). The role of strategic behavior in retardate memory. In N. R. Ellis (Ed.), *International review of research in mental retardation* (Vol. 7). New York: Academic Press.

Brown, A. L. (1978). Knowing when, where, and how to remember: A problem of metacognition. In R. Glaser (Ed.), *Advances in instructional psychology.* Hillsdale, NJ: Lawrence Erlbaum.

Brown, A. L., & Barclay, C. R. (1976). The effects of training specific mnemonics on the metamnemonic efficiency of retarded children. *Child Development, 47,* 71–80.

Brown, A. L., Campione, J. C., & Barclay, C. R. (1978). Training self-checking routines for estimating test readiness: Generalization from list learning to prose recall. Unpublished manuscript, University of Illinois, Urbana.

Brown, A. L., Campione, J. C., Baay, N. W., & Wilcox, B. C. (1973). Keeping track of changing variables: Effects of rehearsal training and rehearsal prevention in normal retarded adolescents. *Journal of Experimental Psychology, 101,* 123–131.

Brown, A. L., Campione, J. C., & Murphy, M. D. (1974). Keeping track of changing variables: Long-term retention of a trained rehearsal strategy by retarded adolescents. *American Journal of Mental Deficiency, 78,* 446–453.

Brown, A. L., & DeLoache, J. S. (1978). Skills, plans, and self-regulation. In R. Siegler (Ed.), *Children's thinking: What develops.* Hillsdale, NJ: Lawrence Erlbaum.

Brown, B. S., & Courtless, T. F. (1967). *The mentally retarded offender.* Washington: The President's Commission on Law Enforcement and Administration of Justice.

Brown, E. S., & Warner, R. (1976). Mental development of phenylketonuric children on or off diet after the age of six. *Psychological Medicine, 6,* 287–296.

Brown, L., Branston, M. B., Hamre-Nietupski, S., Pumpian, I., Certo, N., & Gruenewald, L. (1979). A strategy for developing chronological-age-appropriate and functional curricular content for severely handicapped adolescents and young adults. *Journal of Special Education, 13,* 81–90.

Brown, L., Nietupski, J., & Hamre-Nietupski, S. (1976). The criterion of ultimate functioning and public school services for severely handicapped students. In L. Brown, N. Certo, K. Belmore, & T. Crowner (Eds.), *Papers and programs related to public school services for secondary age severely handicapped students* (Vol. VI, Part 1). Madison, WI: Madison Metropolitan School District.

Brown, L., & Pearce, E. (1970). Increasing the production rate of trainable retarded students in a public school simulated workshop. *Education and Training of the Mentally Retarded, 5,* 15–22.

Brown, R. (1973). *A first language: The early stages.* Cambridge, MA: Harvard University Press.

Brown, R. A., Gunzburg, H., Johnston Hannah, L. G. W., MacColl, K., Oliver, B., & Thomas, A. (1971). The needs of patients in subnormality hospitals if discharged to community care. *British Journal of Mental Subnormality, 17* (Part 1, No. 32), 7–24.

Brown, R. L. (1959). *Swimming for the mentally retarded.* New York: National Association for Retarded Children.

Brown, W. T., Jenkins, E. C., Friedman, E., Brooks, J., Wisniewski, K., Raguthu, S., & French, J. (1982). Autism is associated with the fragile-X syndrome. *Journal of Autism and Developmental Disorders, 12,* 303–308.

Browning, P. L., & Keesey, M. (1974). Outcome studies on counseling with the retarded: A methodological critique. In P. L. Browning (Ed.), *Mental retardation: Rehabilitation and counseling.* Springfield, IL: Thomas.

Bruininks, R. H., Hauber, F. A., & Kudla, M. J. (1980). National survey of community residential facilities: A profile of facilities and residents in 1977. *American Journal of Mental Deficiency, 84,* 470–478.

Bruininks, R. H., Hill, B. K., & Thorsheim, M. J. *A profile of specially licensed foster homes for mentally retarded people in 1977* (Project Report No. 6). Minneapolis: University of Minnesota, Department of Psychoeducational Studies.

Bruininks, R. H., Kudla, M. J., Wieck, C. A., & Hauber, F. A. (1980). Management problems in community residential facilities. *Mental Retardation, 18,* 125–130.

Bruininks, R. H., Rynders, J. E., & Gross, J. C. (1974). Social acceptance of mildly retarded pupils in resource rooms and regular classes. *American Journal of Mental Deficiency, 78,* 377–383.

Bryant, K. N., & Hirschbert, J. C. (1970). Helping parents of a retarded child. *American Journal of Diseases of Children, 102,* 52.

Bucher, B., & Lovaas, O. I. (1968). Use of aversive stimulation in behavior modification. In M. R. Jones (Ed.), *Miami: Symposium on the prediction of behavior, 1967: Aversive stimulation.* Coral Gables, FL: University of Miami Press.

Bucher, B., Reykdal, B., & Albin, J. (1976). Brief physical restraint to control pica. *Journal of Behavior Therapy and Experimental Psychiatry, 1,* 137–140.

Budoff, M., & Corman, L. (1976). Effectiveness of a learning potential procedure in improving problem-solving skills of retarded and nonretarded children. *American Journal of Mental Deficiency, 81,* 260–264.

Budoff, M., & Gottlieb, J. (1976). Special class students mainstreamed: A study of an aptitude (learning potential) × treatment interaction. *American Journal of Mental Deficiency, 81,* 1–11.

Budoff, M., & Siperstein, G. N. (1978). Low-income children's attitudes toward mentally retarded children: Effects of labeling and academic behavior. *American Journal of Mental Deficiency, 82,* 474–479.

Bumbalo, T. S., Morelewicz, H. V., & Berens, D. L. (1964). Treatment of Down's syndrome with the "U" series of drugs. *Journal of the American Medical Association, 178,* 361.

Bunker, L. K. (1978). Motor skills. In M. E. Snell (Ed.), *Systematic instruction of the moderately and severely handicapped.* Columbus, OH: Merrill.

Burchard, J., & Tyler, V. (1965). The modification of delinquent behavior through operant conditioning. *Behavior Research and Therapy, 2,* 245–250.

Burde, B., & Choate, M. S. (1975). Early asymptomatic lead exposure and development at school age. *Journal of Pediatrics, 87,* 638.

Burt, C. (1966). The genetic determination of differences in intelligence. A study of monozygotic twins reared together and apart. *British Journal of Psychology, 57,* 137–153.

Butterfield, E. C., Wambold, C., & Belmont, J. M. (1973). On the theory and practice of improving short-term memory. *American Journal of Mental Deficiency, 77,* 654–669.

Byers, R. K., & Lord, E. E. (1943). Late effects of lead poisoning on mental development. *American Journal of Diseases of Children, 66,* 471.

Byrnes, M. M., & Spitz, H. H. (1977). Performance of retarded adolescents and nonretarded children on the tower of Hanoi problem. *American Journal of Mental Deficiency, 81,* 561–569.

Bzoch, K. R., & League, R. (1970). *Receptive-Expressive Emergent Language Scale for the measurement of language skills in infancy.* Gainesville, FL: Tree of Life Press.

Bzoch, K. R., & League, R. (1971). *Assessing language skills in infancy* (Handbook for the Receptive-Expressive Emergent Language Scale). Gainesville, FL: Tree of Life Press.

Cabalska, B., Duczynska, N., Borzymowska, J., Zorska, K., Koslacz-Folga, A., & Bozkowa, K. (1977). Termination of dietary treatment in phenylketonuria. *European Journal of Pediatrics, 126,* 253–262.

Cain, A. C. (1961). The presuperego "turning inward" of aggression. *Psychoanalytic Quarterly, 30,* 171–208.

Cain, L. F., Levine, S., & Elzey, F. F. (1963). *Manual for the Cain-Levine Social Competency Scale.* Palo Alto, CA: Consulting Psychologists Press.

Caldwell, B. M. (1970). The rationale for early intervention. *Exceptional Children, 36,* 717–726.

Calhoun, K. S., & Matherne, P. (1975). The effects of varying schedules of time-out on aggressive behavior of a retarded girl. *Journal of Behavior Therapy and Experimental Psychiatry, 6,* 139–143.

Cameron, N., & Margaret, A. (1951). *Behavior pathology.* Boston: Houghton Mifflin.

Campbell, A. C. (1971). Aspects of personal independence of mentally subnormal and severely subnormal adults in hospitals and in the local authority hostels. *International Journal of Social Psychiatry, 17,* 305–310.

Campbell, L. W. (1968). *Study of curriculum planning.* Sacramento, CA: State Department of Education.

Campione, J. C., & Brown, A. L. (1978). Toward a theory of intelligence: Contributions from research with retarded children. *Intelligence, 2,* 279–304.

Campione, J. C., & Brown, A. L. (1977). Memory and metamemory development in educable retarded children. In R. V. Kail, Jr., & J. W. Hagen (Eds.), *Perspectives on the development of memory and cognition.* Hillsdale, NJ: Lawrence Erlbaum.

Campos, J. (1976). Heart rate: A sensitive tool for the study of emotional development. In L. Lipsitt (Ed.), *Developmental psychobiology: The significance of infancy.* Hillsdale, NJ: Lawrence Erlbaum.

Cantu, J. M., Scaglia, A., Medina, M., Gonzalez-Diddi, M., Morato, T., Moreno, M., & Perez-Palacios, G. (1976). Inherited congenital normofunctional testicular hyperplasia and mental deficiency. *Human Genetics, 33,* 23–33.

Carlson, B. W., & Ginglend, D. R. (1961). *Play activities for the retarded child.* New York: Abingdon Press.

Carlson, B. W., & Ginglend, D. R. (1968). *Recreation for retarded teenagers and young adults.* Nashville, TN: Abingdon Press.

Carlson, J. S., & Wiedl, K. H. (1978). Use of testing the limits procedures in the assessment of intellectual capabilities in children with learning difficulties. *American Journal of Mental Deficiency, 86,* 559–564.

Carr, D. H. (1970). Chromosome abnormalities and spontaneous abortions. In P. H. Jacobs, W. H. Price, & P. Law Eds.), *Human population cytogenetics.* Edinburgh, Scotland: Edinburgh University Press.

Carr, J. (1976). The severely retarded autistic child. In L. Wing (Ed.), *Early childhood autism.* New York: Pergamon Press.

Carr, E. G. (1977). The motivation of self-injurious behavior: A review of some hypotheses. *Psychological Bulletin, 84,* 800–816.

Carr, E. G., & McDowell, J. J. (1980). Social control of self-injurious behavior of organic etiology. *Behavior Therapy, 11,* 402–409.

Carr, E. G., Newsom, C. D., & Binkoff, J. A. (1976). Stimulus control of self-destructive behavior in a psychotic child. *Journal of Abnormal Child Psychology, 4,* 139–153.

Carr, J. (1970). Mental and motor development in young mongol children. *Journal of Mental Deficiency Research, 14,* 205–220.

Carr, J. (1974). The effect of the severely subnormal on their families. In A. M. Clarke & A. D. B. Clarke (Eds.), *Mental deficiency: The changing outlook* (3rd ed.). New York: Free Press.

Carr, J. (1976). The severely retarded autistic child. In L. Wing (Ed.), *Early childhood autism.* New York: Pergamon Press.

Carrier, J. K. Jr. (1976). Application of a nonspeech language system with the severely language handicapped. In L. Lloyd (Ed.), *Communication assessment and intervention strategies.* Baltimore: University Park Press.

Carrier, J. K., Jr., & Peak, T. (1975). Program manual for Non-SLIP (Nonspeech Language Initiation Program). Lawrence, KS: H. & H. Enterprises.

Carroll, A. W. (1967). The effects of segregated and partially integrated school programs on self-concept and academic achievement of educable mental retardates. *Exceptional Children, 34,* 93–99.

Carroll, S. W., Sloop, E. W., Mutter, S., & Prince, P. L. (1978). The elimination of chronic clothes ripping in retarded people through a combination of procedures. *Mental Retardation, 16,* 246–249.

Carrow, E. (1973). *Test for auditory comprehension of language.* Austin, TX: Urban Research Group.

Carruth, D. G. (1973). Human sexuality in a halfway house. In F. F. de la Cruz & G. D. LaVeck (Eds.), *Human sexuality and the mentally retarded.* New York: Brunner Mazel.

Carswell, H. (1973). Amniocentesis: Balancing the risks and benefits. *Medical Post, 9,* 13.

Carter, C. O. (1958). A life table for Mongols with the causes of death. *Journal of Mental Deficiency Research, 2,* 64.

Casler, L. (1961). Maternal deprivation: A critical review of the literature. *Monograph of the Society for Research in Child Development, 26*(2), [Special issue].

Cassidy, V. M., & Stanton, J. E. (1959). *An investigation of factors involved in the educational placement of mentally retarded children.* Columbus: Ohio State University Press.

Cattell, P. *The measurement of intelligence of infants and young children.* New York: Psychological Corp.

Cattell, R. B. (1971a). *Abilities: Their structure, growth, and action.* Boston: Houghton Mifflin.

Cattell, R. B. (1971b). The structure of intelligence in relation to the nature-nurture controversy. In R. Cancro (Ed.), *Intelligence: Genetic and environmental influences.* New York: Grune & Stratton.

Cegelka, W. J., & Tyler, J. L. (1970). The efficacy of special class placement for the mentally retarded in proper perspective. *Training School Bulletin, 67,* 33–68.

Certo, N., & Schwartz, R. (1975). *Teaching trainable retarded students to ride a community bus.* Madison: Department of Studies in Behavioral Disabilities, University of Wisconsin.

Certo, N., & Swetlik, B. (1976). Making purchases: A functional money use program for severely handicapped students. In L. Brown et al. (Eds.), *Madison's alternative to zero exclusion: Papers and programs related to public school services for secondary school age severely handicapped students.* Madison, WI: Madison Public Schools.

Centerwall, S. A., & Centerwall, W. R. (1960). A study of children with mongolism reared in the home compared to those reared away from the home. *Pediatrics, 25,* 678–685.

Centerwall, W. R., Centerwall, S. A., Armon, V., & Mann, L. B. (1961). Phenylketonuria. II. Results of treatment of infants and young children: Report of 10 cases. *Journal of Pediatrics, 59,* 102–118.

Chamberlin, H. R. (1975). Mental retardation. In T. W. Farmer (Ed.), *Pediatric neurology* (2nd ed.). New York: Harper & Row.

Chao, D. H. C. (1959). Congenital neurocutaneous syndrome in childhood. II. Tuberous sclerosis. *Journal of Pediatrics, 55,* 447–459.

Chao, L., Carter, S., & Gold, A. P. (1977). In A. M. Rudolph (Ed.), *Pediatrics* (16th ed.). New York: Appleton-Century-Crofts.

Chatorian, A. M. (1977). Tumors of the central nervous system. In A. M. Rudolph (ed.), *Pediatrics* (16th ed.). New York: Appleton-Century-Crofts.

Chess, S. (1970). Emotional problems in mentally retarded children. In F. J. Menolascino (Ed.), *Psychiatric approaches to mental retardation.* New York: Basic Books.

Chess, S., & Hassibi, M. (1970). Behavior deviations in mentally retarded children. *Journal of the American Academy of Child Psychiatry, 9,* 282–297.

Chess, S., Korn, S. J., & Fernandez, P. B. (1971). *Psychiatric disorders of children with rubella.* New York: Brunner Mazel.

Childs, R. E. (1979). A drastic change in curriculum for the educable mentally retarded child. *Mental Retardation, 17,* 299–301.

Chow, T. J., & Earl, J. L. (1970). Lead aerosols in the atmosphere: Increasing concentrations. *Science, 169,* 577.

Churchill, J. A., Berendes, H. W., & Nemore, J. (1969). Neuropsychiatric disorders in children of diabetic mothers. *American Journal of Obstetrics and Gynecology, 105,* 257–268.

Clarke, A. D. B., & Clarke, A. M. (1954). Cognitive changes in the feeble-minded. *British Journal of Psychology, 45,* 173–179.

Clark, G. M. (1980). Career preparation for handicapped adolescents: A matter of appropriate education. *Exceptional Education Quarterly, 1,* 11–18.

Clark, G. R., Kivitz, M. S., & Rosen, M. (1968). *A transitional program for institutionalized adult retarded.* Elwyn, PA: Elwyn Institute.

Clarke, A. M., & Clarice, A. D. B. (1974). *Mental deficiency: The changing outlook* (3rd ed.). New York: Free Press.

Clarren, S. K., & Smith, D. W. (1978). The fetal alcohol syndrome. *New England Journal of Medicine, 298,* 1063–1067.

Clausen, J. A. (1967). Mental deficiency: Development of a concept. *American Journal of Mental Deficiency, 71,* 727–745.

Clausen, J. A. (1972). Quo vadis, AAMD. *Journal of Special Education, 6,* 51–60.

Cleary, T. A., Humphreys, L. G., Kendrick, S. A., & Wesman, A. (1975). Educational uses of tests with disadvantaged students. *American Psychologist, 30,* 15–41.

Cleland, C. C., Powell, H. C., & Talkington, L. W. (1971). Death of the profoundly retarded. *Mental Retardation, 9,* 36.

Clements, P. R., Bates, M. V., & Hafer, M. (1976). Variability within Down's syndrome (trisomy-21): Empirically observed sex differences in IQs. *Mental Retardation, 14,* 30–31.

Clements, S. D. (1966). *Minimal brain dysfunction in children: Terminology and identification, phase one of a three-phase project.* Washington: U.S. Department of Health, Education, and Welfare (NINDB Monogram No. 3).

Cobb, H. V. (1972). *The forecast of fullfillment.* New York: Teacher's College Press.

Cofer, C. N., & Appley, M. H. (1967). *Motivation; Theory and research.* New York: Wiley.

Cohen, J. S. (1960). An analysis of vocational failures of mental retardates placed in the community after a period of institutionalization. *American Journal of Mental Deficiency, 65,* 371–375.

Coleman, M. (1975). The use of 5-hydroxytryptophan in patients with Down's syndrome. In R. Koch & F. de la Cruz (Eds.), *Down's syndrome (mongolism): Research, prevention and management.* New York: Brunner Mazel.

Cohen, F. (1976). Advocacy (principal paper). In M. Kindred, J. Cohen, D. Penrod, & T. Shaffer (Eds.), *The mentally retarded citizen and the law.* New York: Free Press.

Cohen, H. J. (1979). Community health planning. In P. R. Magrab & J. O. Elder (Eds.), *Planning for services to handicapped persons: Community, education, health.* Baltimore: Paul H. Brookes.

Cohen, J. (1966). The effects of blindness on children's development. *Children, 13,* 23–27.

Coleman, M. (1978). Down's syndrome. *Pediatric Annals, 7,* 90–103.

Collins, D. T. (1965). Head-banging: Its meaning and management in the severely retarded adult. *Bulletin of the Menninger Clinic, 29,* 205–211.

Collmann, R. D., & Newlyn, D. (1958). Changes in Terman-Merrill IQs of mentally retarded children. *American Journal of Mental Deficiency, 63,* 307–311.

Conger, J. J. (1957, June). The meaning and measurement of intelligence. *Rocky Mountain Medical Journal.*

Conen, P. E., & Erkman, B. (1966). Frequency and occurrence of chromosomal syndromes. II. E-trisomy. *American Journal of Human Genetics, 18,* 387.

Conley, R. W. (1973). *The economics of mental retardation.* Baltimore: Johns Hopkins University Press.

Conley, R. W. (1976). Mental retardation—an economist's approach. *Mental Retardation 14,* 20–24.

Connolly, B., & Russell, F. (1976). Interdisciplinary early intervention program. *Physical Therapy, 56,* 155–158.

Conroy, J.W., & Derr, K. E. (1971). *Survey and analysis of the habilitation and rehabilitation status of the mentally retarded with associated handicapped conditions.* Washington: Department of Health, Education, and Welfare.

Conroy, J., Efthimiou, J., & Lemanowicz, J. (1982). A matched comparison of the developmental growth of institutionalized and deinstitutionalized mentally retarded clients. *American Journal of Mental Deficiency, 86,* 581–587.

Cook, J. J. (1963). Dimensional analysis of child-rearing attitudes of parents of handicapped children. *American Journal of Mental Deficiency, 68,* 354–361.

Cooke, S. A., Cooke, T. A., & Apolloni, T. (1976). Generalization of language training with the mentally retarded. *Journal of Special Education, 10,* 299–304.

Coop, R. H., & Sigel, I. E. (1974). Cognitive style: Implications for learning and instruction. In R. L. Jones & D. L. MacMillan (Eds.), *Special education in transition.* Boston: Allyn and Bacon.

Cooper, A. F., & Fowlie, H. C. (1973). Control of gross self-mutilation with lithium carbonate. *British Journal of Psychiatry, 122,* 370–371.

Cooper, L. Z. (1968). Rubella: A preventable cause of birth defects. *Birth Defects Original Article Series, 4,* 23–25.

Cooper, L. Z. (1977). Rubella. In A. M. Rudolph (Ed.), *Pediatrics* (16th ed.). New York: Appleton-Century-Crofts.

Cooper, L. Z., Ziring, P. R., Ockerse, A. G., Fedun, B. A., Kiely, B., & Krugman, S. (1969). Rubella: Clinical manifestations and management. *American Journal of Diseases of Children*, *118*, 18–29.

Coopersmith, S. (1967). *The antecedents of self-esteem*. San Francisco: W. N. Freeman.

Corbett, J. (1975). Aversion for the treatment of self-injurious behavior. *Journal of Mental Deficiency Research, 19*, 79–95.

Corbett, J. A., Harris, R., & Robinson, R. G. (1975). Epilepsy. In J. Wortis (Ed.), *Mental retardation and developmental disabilities* (Vol. VIII). New York: Brunner Mazel.

Corman, L., & Gottlieb, J. (1978). Mainstreaming mentally retarded children: A review of research. In N. R. Ellis (Ed.), *International review of research in mental retardation* (Vol. 9). New York: Academic Press.

Cornwell, A. C., & Birch, H. G. (1969). Psychological and social development in home-reared children with Down's syndrome (mongolism). *American Journal of Mental Deficiency, 74*, 341–350.

Corsale, K. (1977). Developmental changes in the use of semantic information for recall. Doctoral dissertation, University of North Carolina, Chapel Hill.

Corte, H. E., Wolf, M. W., and Lolke, B. J. (1971). A comparison of procedures for eliminating self-injurious behavior of retarded adolescents. *Journal of Applied Behavior Analysis, 4*, 201–213.

Corter, H. M., & McKinney, J. D. (1966). *Cognitive training with retarded children* (Vol. I) (Cooperative Research Project No. 32-43-0530-5028). Washington: U.S. Department of Health, Education, and Welfare.

Cowen, E., Zax, M., Klein, R., Izo, L., & Trost, M. (1965). The relation of anxiety in school children to school record, achievement, and behavioral measures. *Child Development, 36*, 685.

Cowie, V. A. (1970). *A study of the early developmental of mongols* (Institute for Research into Mental Retardation Monograph No. 1). Oxford: Pergamon Press.

Craft, M. (1959). Mental disorder in the defective: A psychiatric survey among in-patients. *American Journal of Mental Deficiency, 63*, 829–834.

Cratty, B. (1967). *Movement behavior and motor learning*. Philadelphia: Lea & Febiger.

Cravioto, J., & DeLicardie, E. R. (1972). Environmental correlates of severe clinical malnutrition and language development in survivors from kwashiorkor or marasmus. In *Nutrition, the nervous system and behavior*. Washington: Pan American Health Organization.

Creak, M. (1961). Schizophrenic syndrome in childhood. Progress report of a working party (April 1961). *Cerebral Palsy Bulletin, 3*, 501–504.

Creak, M. (1964). Schizophrenic syndrome in childhood. Further progress report of a working party (April 1964). *Developmental Medicine and Neurology, 6*, 530–535.

Creak, M., & Ini, S. (1960). Families of psychotic children. *Journal of Child Psychology and Psychiatry, 1*, 156–175.

Cromwell, R. L. (1963). A social learning approach to mental retardation. In N. R. Ellis (Ed.), *Handbook of mental deficiency*. New York: McGraw-Hill.

Crosson, J. E. (1964). A technique for programming sheltered workshop environment for training severely retarded workers. *American Journal of Mental Deficiency, 73*, 814–818.

Crothers, B., Paine, R. S. (1959). *The natural history of cerebral palsy*. Cambridge, MA: Harvard University Press.

Crowe, F. W. & Schull, W. J. (1952). Phenylketonuria: Studies in pigment formation. *Folia Hereditaria et Pathologica, 1*, 259–268.

Crowe, F. W., Schull, W. J., & Neill, J. V. (1956). *A clinical, pathological and genetic study of multiple neurofibromatosis*. Springfield, IL: Charles C Thomas.

Cruickshank, W. M., Bentzen, F. A., Ratzeburg, F. H., & Tannhause, M. T. (1961). *A teaching method for brain-injured and hyperactive children: A demonstration pilot study*. New York: Syracuse University Press.

Curtis, L. A. (1965). A comparative analysis of the self-concept of the adolescent mentally retarded in relation to certain groups of adolescents. *Dissertation Abstracts, 25*, 2846–2847.

Cytryn, L., & Lourie, R. S. (1967). Mental retardation. In A. M. Freedman & H. I. Kaplan (Eds.), *Comprehensive textbook of psychiatry*. Baltimore: Williams & Wilkins.

Dalton, A. J., Crapper, D. R., & Schlotterer, G. R. (1974). Alzheimer's disease in Down's syndrome: Visual retention deficits. *Cortex, 10,* 366–377.

Dameron, L. E. (1963). Development of intelligence of infants with mongolism. *Child Development, 34,* 733–738.

Danes, B. S. (1977). Mucopolysaccharidoses. In A. M. Rudolph (Ed.), *Pediatrics* (16th ed.) New York: Appleton-Century-Crofts.

Danford, D. E., & Huber, A. M. (1982). Pica among mentally retarded adults. *American Journal of Mental Deficiency, 87,* 141–146.

Daniel, A. N. (1969). An example of individual instruction in developmental education, *Journal of Health, Physical Education, and Recreation, 40,* 56.

Das, J. P., & Pivato, E. (1976). Malnutrition and cognitive functioning. In N. R. Ellis (Ed.), *International review of research in mental retardation* (Vol. 8). New York: Academic Press.

Davenport, C. B. (1911). *Heredity in relation to eugenics.* New York: Henry Holt.

Davenport, R. K., Jr., & Berkson, G. (1963). Stereotyped movements of mental defectives. II. Effects of novel objects. *American Journal of Mental Deficiency, 67,* 879–882.

Davis, K. (1947). Final note on the case of extreme isolation. *American Journal of Sociology, 52,* 432–437.

Davis, W. B., Wieseler, N. A., & Hanzel, T. E. (1980). Contingent music in management of rumination and out-of-seat behavior in a profoundly mentally retarded institutionalized male. *Mental Retardation, 18,* 43–45.

Dawson, G. (1982). Cerebral lateralization in individuals diagnosed as autism in early childhood. *Brain and Language, 15,* 353–368.

Dawson, G. (1983). Lateralized brain function in autism: Evidence from the Halsted-Reitan neuropsychological battery. *Journal of Autism and Developmental Disorders, 13,* 269–286.

De la Cruz, F. F., & LaVeck, G. (1962). Tuberous sclerosis: A review and report of eight cases. *American Journal of Mental Deficiency, 67,* 369–380.

DeCatanzaro, D. A., & Baldwin, G. (1978). Effective treatment of self-injurious behavior through a forced arm exercise. *American Journal of Mental Deficiency, 82,* 433–439.

DeCharms, R. (1968). *Personal causation: The internal affective determinants of behavior.* New York: Academic Press.

Decker, H., Herberg, E., Haythornthwaite, M., Rupke, L., & Smith, D. (1968). Provision of health care for institutionalized retarded children. *American Journal of Mental Deficiency, 73,* 283–293.

Dedrick, P. (1974). Premenstrual training. In L. Brown, W. Williams, & T. Crowner (Eds.), *A collection of papers and programs related to public school services for severely handicapped students.* Madison, WI: Madison Public Schools.

Deisher, R. W. (1973). Sexual behavior of retarded in institutions. In F. F. de la Cruz, & G. D. LaVeck (Eds.), *Human sexuality and the mentally retarded.* New York: Brunner Mazel.

DeLissovoy, V. (1962). Headbanging in childhood. *Child Development, 33,* 43–56.

Demaine, G. C., & Silverstein, A. B. (1978). MA changes in institutionalized Down's syndrome persons: A semi-longitudinal approach. *American Journal of Mental Deficiency, 82,* 429–432.

Dember, W. N. (1974). Motivation and the cognitive revolution. *American Psychologist, 29,* 161–168.

DeMyer, M. K. (1976). Motor, perceptual-motor and intellectual disabilities of autistic children. In L. Wing (Ed.), *Early childhood autism* (2nd ed.). New York: Pergamon Press.

DeMyer, M. K., Barton, S., Alpern, G. D., Kimberlin, C., Allen, J., Yang, E., & Steele, R. (1974). The measured intelligence of autistic children. *Journal of Autism and Childhood Schizophrenia, 4,* 42.

DeMyer, M. K., Norton, J. A., & Barton, S. (1971). Social and adaptive behaviors of autistic children as measured in a structured psychiatric interview. In D. W. Churchill, G. D. Alpern, & M. K. DeMyer (Eds.), *Infantile autism: Proceedings of the Indiana University Colloquium.* Springfield, IL: Charles C Thomas.

DeMyer, M. K., Pontius, W., Norton, J. A., Barton, S., Allen, J., & Steele, R. (1972). Parental practices and innate activity in normal, autistic, and brain-damaged infants. *Journal of Autism and Childhood Schizophrenia, 2,* 49–66.

Dennis, K. (1976). Children of the Creche: Conclusions and implications. In A. M. Clarke & A. D. B. Clarke (Eds.), *Early experience: Myth and evidence*. London: Open Books.

Dennis, W. (1960). Causes of retardation among institutional children. *Journal of Genetic Psychology, 96*, 47–59.

Dennis, W., & Najarian, P. (1957). Infant development under environmental handicap. *Psychological Monographs, 71*, No. 7 [Special issue].

Deno, E. (1966). Vocational preparation of the retarded during school years. In S. G. DiMichael (Ed.), *New vocational pathways for the mentally retarded*. (pp. 20–29). Washington: American Personnel and Guidance Association.

Deno, S. L., Gutman, A. J., & Fullmer, W. (1977). Educational programs for retarded individuals. In T. Thompson & J. Grabowski (Eds.), *Behavior modification of the mentally retarded*. New York: Oxford University Press.

Dentler, R. A., & Mackler, B. (1962). Ability and sociometric status among normal and retarded children: A review of the literature. *Psychological Bulletin, 59*, 273–283.

DesLauriers, A. M., & Carlson, C. F. (1969). *Your child is asleep*. Homewood, IL: Darsey.

Despert, J. L. (1951). Some considerations relating to the genesis of autistic behavior in children. *American Journal of Orthopsychiatry, 21*, 335–350.

Deutsch, C. P. (1964). Auditory discrimination and learning: Social factors. *Merrill-Palmer Quarterly, 10*, 277–296.

Deutsch, M. (1967). The role of social class in language development and cognition. In M. Deutsch (Ed.), *The disadvantaged child: Selected papers of Martin Deutsch and associates* (pp. 357–369). New York: Basic Books.

Deutsch, M., et al. (1971). *Regional research and resource center in early childhood: Final report*. Washington: U.S. Office of Economic Opportunity.

DeVore, S. M. (1977). *Individualized learning program for the profoundly retarded*. Springfield, IL: Thomas.

Dewey, M. A. (1973). Vocational guidance for former autistic children. *Communication, 4*, 67.

Deykin, E. Y., & Macmahon, B. (1975). Seizures among autistic children. *American Journal of Psychiatry, 136*, 1310–1312.

Dicks-Mireaux, M. J. (1972). Mental development of infants with Down's syndrome. *American Journal of Mental Deficiency, 77*, 26–32.

Diggs, E. A. (1963). A study of change in the social status of rejected mentally retarded children in regular classrooms. Unpublished doctoral dissertation, Colorado State College, Fort Collins.

DiMichael, S. G. (1964). Providing full vocational opportunities for retarded adolescents and adults. *Journal of Rehabilitation, 30*, 11–14.

Dingman, H. F., & Tarjan, G. (1960). Mental retardation and the normal distribution curve. *American Journal of Mental Deficiency, 64*, 991–994.

Dobson, J., & Williamson, M. (1970). Provocative observation in the PKU collaborative study. *New England Journal of Medicine, 282*, 1104.

Dobson, J., Williamson, M., & Koch, R. (1970). Sex ratio in hyperphenylalaninemia. *New England Journal of Medicine, 283*, 491.

Dobzhansky, T. (1955). *Evolution, genetics and man*. New York: Wiley.

Dobzhansky, T. (1962). *Mankind evolving*. New Haven, CT: Yale University Press.

Dobzhansky, T. (1973). *Genetic diversity and human equality*. New York: Basic Books.

Dodd, B. (1975). Recognition and reproduction of words by Down's syndrome and non-Down's syndrome retarded children. *American Journal of Mental Deficiency, 80*, 306–311.

Doke, L. A., & Epstein, L. H. (1975). Oral overcorrection: Side effects and extended applications. *Journal of Experimental Child Psychology, 20*, 496–511.

Doleys, D. M., & Arnold, S. (1975). Treatment of childhood encopresis: Full cleanliness training. *Mental Retardation, 13*, 14–16.

Doleys, D. M., & McWhorter, A. Q., Williams, S. C., & Gentry, W. R. (1977). Encopresis: Its treatment in relation to nocturnal enuresis. *Behavior Therapy, 8*, 77–82.

Doll, E. A. (1941). The essentials of an inclusive concept of mental deficiency. *American Journal of Mental Deficiency, 46*, 214–219.

Doll, E. A. (1964). *Vineland Scale of Social Maturity.* Minneapolis: American Guidance Service.

Domino, G., Goldschmid, M., & Kaplan, M. (1964). Personality traits of institutionalized mongoloid girls. *American Journal of Mental Deficiency, 68,* 498–502.

Domino, G., & Newnam, D. (1965). Relationship of physical stigmata to intellectual subnormality in mongoloids. *American Journal of Mental Deficiency, 69,* 541–547.

Donnar, S. (1980). Venous thromboembolism and pregnancy. *Clinics in Obstetrics and Gynecology, 8,* 455–473.

Donnell, G. N., Alfe, O. S., Rublee, J. C., & Koch, R. (1975). Chromosomal abnormalities. In R. Koch & F. de la Cruz (Eds.), *Down's syndrome (mongolism): Research, prevention, and management.* New York: Brunner Mazel.

Down, J. L. H. (1867). Observations on an ethnic classification of idiots. *Journal of Mental Science, 13,* 121–123.

Drayer, C., & Guzman-Neuhaus, G. (1971). Pediatrics. In J. Wortis (Ed.), *Mental Retardation III.* New York: Grune & Stratton.

Dreger, R. M., & Miller, K. S. (1968). Comparative psychological studies of Negroes and whites in the United States: 1959–1963. *Psychological Bulletin, 70* (3, pt. 2) [Special issue].

Drews, E. (1962). The effectiveness of homogeneous and heterogeneous ability grouping in ninth grade English classes with slow, average and superior students. Unpublished manuscript, Michigan State University, East Lansing.

Drillien, C. M. (1967). The incidence of mental and physical handicaps in school age children of very low birth weight. II. *Pediatrics, 39,* 238–247.

Drillien, C. M., & Wilkinson, E. M.,(1969). Mongolism: When should parents be told. In Wolfensberger, W. & Kurtz, R. A. (Eds.), *Management of the family of the mentally retarded.* Chicago: Follett.

Drumwright, M. A., Drexler, H., Van Natta, P., Camp, B., & Frankenburg, W. (1973). The Denver Articulation Screening Exam. *Journal of Speech and Hearing Disorder, 38,* 3–14.

DuBose, R. F. (1977). Predictive value of infant intelligence scales with multiple handicapped children. *American Journal of Mental Deficiency, 81,* 388–390.

DuBose, R. F. (1981). Assessment of severely impaired young children: Problems and recommendations. *Topics in Early Childhood Special Education, 1,* 9–18.

Dugdale, R. L. (1877). *The Jukes.* New York: Putnam.

Duker, P. C. (1975a). Behavior control of self-biting in a Lesch-Nyhan patient. *Journal of Mental Deficiency Research, 19,* 11–19.

Duker, P. C. (1975b). Behavior therapy for self-injurious behavior: Two case studies. *Research Exchange and Practice in Mental Retardation, 1,* 223–232.

Duker, P. C., & Seys, D. M. (1977). Elimination of vomiting in a retarded female using restitutional over-correction. *Behavior Therapy, 8,* 255–257.

Dunn, L. M. (1959). *Peabody Picture Vocabulary Test.* Minneapolis: American Guidance Service.

Dunn, L. M. (1968). Special education for the mildly retarded—is much of it justifiable? *Exceptional Children, 35,* 5–22.

Dunn, H. G., McBurney, A. K., Ingram, S., & Hunter, C. M. (1977). Maternal cigarette smoking during pregnancy and the child's subsequent development: II. Neurological and intellectual maturation to the age of $6\frac{1}{2}$ years. *Canadian Journal of Public Health, 68,* 43–50.

Dunst, C. (1974). Patterns of cognitive skill acquisitions in developmentally delayed infants. Paper presentation at American Association of Mental Deficiency, Toronto.

Dunst, C. J. (1976). The handicapped infant: Is there justification for cognitive intervention. Paper presented at American Association of Mental Deficiency, Chicago.

Durand, V. M. (1982). A behavioral/pharmacological intervention for the treatment of severe self-injurious behavior. *Journal of Autism and Developmental Disorders, 12,* 243–251.

Durand, V. M. (1984). Attention-getting problem behavior: Analysis and intervention. Unpublished doctoral dissertation, State University of New York, Stony Brook.

Durand, V. M., & Carr, E. G. (1985). Self-injurious behavior: Motivating conditions and guidelines for treatment. *School Psychology Review, 14,* 171–176.

Dusek, J. B., & O'Connell, E. J. (1973). Teacher expectancy effects on the achievement test performance of elementary school children. *Journal of Educational Psychology, 65,* 371–377.

Earl, C. J. C. (1934). The primitive catatonic psychoses of idiocy. *British Journal of Medical Psychology, 14*, 3–11.

Edelson, S. M. (1984). Implications of sensory stimulation in self-destructive behavior. *American Journal of Mental Deficiency, 89*, 140–145.

Edgar, C. L., Ball, T. S., McIntyre, R. B., & Shotwell, A. M. (1969). Effects of sensory-motor training on adaptive behavior. *American Journal of Mental Deficiency, 73*, 713–720.

Edgerton, R. B. (1963). A patient elite: Ethnography in a hospital for the mentally retarded. *American Journal of Mental Deficiency, 68*, 372–385.

Edgerton, R. B. (1967). *The cloak of competence: Stigma in the lives of the mentally retarded.* Berkeley: University of California Press.

Edgerton, R. B. (1975). Issues relating to the quality of life among mentally retarded persons. In M. J. Begab & S. A. Richardson (Eds.), *The mentally retarded and society: A social science perspective.* Baltimore: University Park Press.

Edgerton, R. B. (1976). The cloak of competence: Years later. *American Journal of Mental Deficiency, 80*, 485–497.

Edgerton, R. B., Bollinger, M., & Herr, B. (1984). The cloak of competence: After two decades. *American Journal of Mental Deficiency, 88*, 345–351.

Edmonson, B. (1980). Sociosexual education for the handicapped. *Exceptional Education Quarterly, 1*, 67–76.

Edmonson, B., & Wish, J. (1975). Sex knowledge and attitudes of moderately retarded males. *American Journal of Mental Deficiency, 80*, 172–179.

Edmonson, B., Wish, J., & Fiechtl, K. (1977). Development of sex knowledge and attitude test for the moderately and mildly retarded. Unpublished paper, Ninonger Center, Ohio State University, Columbus.

Edwards, J. H., Harnden, D. G., Cameron, A. H., Crosse, V. M., & Wolff, O. H. (1960). New trisomic syndrome. *Lancet, 1*, 787–790.

Edwards, M., & Lilly, R. T. (1966). Operant conditioning: An application to behavioral problems in groups. *Mental Retardation, 4*, 18–20.

Efron, R. E., & Efron, H. Y. (1967). Measurement of attitudes toward the retarded and an application with educators. *American Journal of Mental Deficiency, 72*, 100–107.

Eichenwald, H. F. (1969). Toxoplasmosis. In V. C. Kelley (Ed.), *Brennemann's practice of pediatrics* (Vol. IV, Sect. 3, pp. 43–53). New York: Harper & Row.

Einhorn, A. H. (1977). Bacterial meningitis. In A. M. Rudolph (Ed.), *Pediatrics* (16th ed.) New York: Appleton-Century-Crofts.

Eisenson, J. (1965). Speech disorders. In B. B. Wolman (Ed.), *Handbook of clinical psychology.* New York: McGraw-Hill.

Elder, J. O. (1979). Coordination of service delivery system. In P. R. Magrab & J. O. Elder (Eds.), *Planning for services to handicapped persons: Community, education, health.* Baltimore: Brookes.

Elenbogen, M. L. (1957). A comparative study of some aspects of academic and social adjustment of two groups of mentally retarded children in special classes and in regular grades. *Dissertation Abstracts, 17*, 2496.

Ellis, A., & Beechley, R. (1950). A comparison of matched groups of mongoloid and non-mongoloid feeble-minded children. *American Journal of Mental Deficiency, 54*, 464–468.

Ellis, N. R. (1963a). The stimulus trace and behavioral inadequacy. In N. R. Ellis (Ed.), *Handbook on mental deficiency* (pp. 134–158). New York: McGraw-Hill.

Ellis, N. R. (1963b). Toilet training the severely defective patient: An S-R reinforcement analysis. *American Journal of Mental Deficiency, 68*, 98–103.

Ellis, N. R. (1968). Memory processes in retardates and normals: Theoretical and empirical considerations. Paper presented at the Gatlinburg Conference on Mental Retardation, Gatlinburg, TN.

Ellis, N. R. (1970). Memory processes in retardates and normals. In N. R. Ellis (Ed.), *International review of research in mental retardation* (Vol. 4). New York: Academic Press.

Ellis, N. R. (1981). On training the mentally retarded. *Analysis and Intervention in Developmental Disabilities, 1*, 99–108.

Elmer, E., Gregg, G., & Ellison, P. (1969). Late results of the failure-to-thrive syndrome. *Clinical Pediatrics, 8*, 584–588.

Elwood, M. I. (1952). Changes in Stanford-Binet IQ of retarded six-year olds. *Journal of Consulting Psychology, 16*, 217–219.

Endres, R. W. (1968). A year-round camping and outdoor education center for the mentally retarded in the northern locality of the United States. Brainerd, MN: Brainerd State Hospital.

Engel, E. (1977). One hundred years of cytogenetic studies in health and disease. *American Journal of Mental Deficiency, 82*, 109–116.

English, P. C. (1978). Failure-to-thrive without organic basis. *Pediatric Annals, 7*, 83–97.

Epple, W. A., Jacobson, J. W., & Janicki, M. P. (1985). Staffing ratios in public institutions for persons with mental retardation in the United States. *Mental Retardation, 23*, 115–124.

Epstein, S. (1973). The self-concept revisited: Or a theory of a theory. *American Psychologist, 28*, 404–416.

Erbs, R. C., & Smith, G. F. (1962). Unpublished manuscript.

Erlenmeyer-Kimling, L., & Jarvik, R. (1963). Genetics and intelligence: A review. *Science, 142*, 1477–1479.

Escalona, S. K. (1968). *The roots of individuality.* Chicago: Aldine.

Espech, J. E., & Williams, B. (1967). *Developing programmed instructional materials.* Palo Alto, CA: Fearon.

Eyman, R. K., Demaine, G. C., & Lei, T. (1979). Relationship between community environments and resident changes in adaptive behavior: A path model. *American Journal of Mental Deficiency, 83*, 330–338.

Eyman, R. K., Silverstein, A. B., & McLain, K. (1975). Effects of treatment programs on the acquisition of basic skills. *American Journal of Mental Deficiency, 79*, 573–582.

Eyman, R. K., Silverstein, A. B., McLain, R. E., & Miller, C. R. (1977). Effects of residential settings on development. In P. Mittler & J. DeJong (Eds.), *Research to practice in mental retardation: Care and intervention* (Vol. 1). Baltimore: University Park Press.

Eyman, R. K., Tarjan, G., & Cassady, M. (1970). Natural history of acquisition of basic skills by hospitalized retarded patients. *American Journal of Mental Deficiency, 75*, 120–129.

Fagan, J., Broughton, E., Allen, M., Clark, B., & Emerson, P. (1969). Comparison of the Binet and WPPSI with lower-class five-year-olds. *Journal of Consulting and Clinical Psychology, 33*, 607–609.

Falek, A., & Glanville, E. V. (1962). Investigation of genetic carriers. In F. J. Kallmann (Ed.), *Expanding goals of genetics in psychiatry.* New York: Grune & Stratton.

Fant, L. J., Jr. (1972). *Ameslan: An introduction to American Sign Language.* Silver Spring, MD: National Association for the Deaf.

Farber, B. (1959). *Prevalence of exceptional children in Illinois in 1958.* Springfield, IL: Superintendent of Public Instruction.

Farber, B. (1968). *Mental retardation: Its social context and social consequences.* Boston: Houghton Mifflin.

Farquhar, J., (1974). Offspring of PKU mothers. *Archives of Disease in Childhood, 49*, 205–208.

Favell, J. E. (1973). Reduction of stereotypes by reinforcement of toy play. *Mental Retardation, 11*, 21–23.

Favell, J. E., Azrin, N. H., Baumeister, A. A., et al. (1982). Treatment of self-injurious behavior. *Behavior Therapy, 13*, 529–554.

Favell, J. E., McGimsey, J. F., & Jones, M. (1978). The use of physical restraint in the treatment of self-injury and as positive reinforcement. *Journal of Applied Behavior Analysis, 11*, 225–241.

Favell, J. E., McGimsey, J. F., & Jones, M. L., & Cannon, P. R. (1981). Physical restraint as positive reinforcement. *American Journal of Mental Deficiency, 85*, 425–432.

Favell, J. E., McGimsey, J. F., & Schell, R. M. (1982). Treatment of self-injury by providing alternate sensory activities. *Analysis and Intervention in Developmental Disabilities, 2*, 83–104.

Favell, J. E., Risley, T. R., Wolfe, A. F., Riddle, J. I., & Rasmussen, P. R. (1981). The limits of habilitation: How can we identify them and how can we change them? *Analysis and Intervention in Developmental Disabilities, 1*, 37–43.

Fein, D., Skoff, B., & Mirsky, A. F. (1981). Clinical correlates of brainstem dysfunction in autistic children. *Journal of Autism and Developmental Disorders, 11,* 303–315.

Feldhusen, J. F., & Klausmeier, H. J. (1962). Anxiety, intelligence, and achievement in children of low, average, and high intelligence. *Child Development, 33,* 403–409.

Ferguson-Smith, M.A. (1965). Karyotype-phenotype correlations in gonadal dysgenesis and their bearing on the pathogenesis of malformations. *Journal of Medical Genetics, 2,* 142.

Fessard, C. (1968). Cerebral tumors in infancy: 66 clinicoanatomical case studies. *American Journal of Diseases of Children, 115,* 302–308.

Festinger, L. (1957). *A theory of cognitive dissonance.* New York: Harper & Row.

Feuerstein, R. (1970). A dynamic approach to the causation, prevention, and alleviation of retarded performance. In H. C. Haywood (Ed.), *Social-cultural aspects of mental retardation.* New York: Appleton-Century-Crofts.

Feuerstein, R., & Krassilowsky, D. (1967). The treatment group technique. *Israel Annals of Psychiatric and Related Disciplines, 5,* 61–90.

Feuerstein, R., Rand, Y., Hoffman, Malka, Hoffman, Mendel, & Miller, R. (1979). Cognitive modifiability in retarded adolescents: Effects of instrumental enrichment. *American Journal of Mental Deficiency, 83,* 539–550.

Field, T., Roseman, S., DeStefano, L. J., & Koweler, J. K. III. (1982). The play of handicapped preschool children with handicapped and nonhandicapped peers in integrated and nonintegrated situations. In S. G. Garwood (Ed.), Play and development. *Topics in Early Childhood Special Education, 2,* 28–38.

Field, T. (1980). Self, teacher, toy and peer-directed behaviors of handicapped preschool children. In T. Fields, S. Goldberg, D. Stern, & A. Sostek (Eds.), *High-risk infants and children: Adult and peer interactions.* New York: Academic Press.

Finberg, L. (1977). Syphilis. In A. M. Rudolph (Ed.), *Pediatrics.* New York: Appleton-Century-Crofts.

Findlay, J., Miller, P., Pegram, A., Richey, L., Sanford, A., & Semrau, B. (1974). *A planning guide to the preschool curriculum: The child, the process, the day.* Chapel Hill, NC: Chapel Hill Training Outreach Project.

Fine, M. J., 1967). Attitudes of regular and special class teachers toward the educable mentally retarded child. *Exceptional Children, 33,* 429–430.

Fine, M. J., & Caldwell, T. (1967). Self-evaluation of school related behavior of educable mentally retarded children—a preliminary report. *Exceptional Children, 34,* 324.

Fingado, M. L., Kini, J. F., Stewart, K., & Redd, W. H. (1970). A thirty-day residential training program for retarded children. *Mental Retardation, 8,* 42–45.

Finnegan, L. P. (1981). The effects of narcotics and alcohol on pregnancy and the newborn. *Annals of the New York Academy of Sciences, 362,* 136–157.

Finnie, N. R. (1975). *Handling the young cerebral palsied child at home.* New York: Dutton.

Fisch, R. O., Conley, J. A., Eysenbach, S., & Chang, Pi-Nian. (1977). Contact with phenylketonurics and their families. *Mental Retardation, 15,* 10–12.

Fischer, H. L., & Krajicek, M. J. (1974). Sexual development in the moderately retarded child: Level of information and parental attitudes. *Mental Retardation, 12,* 32–57.

Fish, B., & Shapiro, T. (1965). A typology of children's psychiatric disorders: Its application to a controlled evaluation of treatment. *Journal of the American Academy of Child Psychiatry, 4,* 35–52.

Fisher, G. M. (1962a). A note on the validity of the Wechsler Adult Intelligence Scale for mental retardates. *Journal of Consulting Psychology, 26,* 391.

Fisher, G. M. (1962b). Further evidence of the invalidity of the Wechsler Adult Intelligence Scale for the assessment of intelligence of mental retardates. *Journal of Mental Deficiency Research, 6,* 41–43.

Fisher, M. A., & Zeaman, D. (1970). Growth and decline of retardate intelligence. In N. R., Ellis (Ed.), *International review of research in mental retardation* (Vol. 4). New York: Academic Press.

Fishler, K. (1971). Psychological assessment services. In R. Koch & J. C. Dobson (Eds.), *The mentally retarded child and his family: A multidisciplinary handbook.* New York: Brunner Mazel.

Fishler, K. (1975). Mental development in mosaic Down's syndrome as compared with trisomy 21. In R. Koch & F. de la Cruz (Eds.), *Down's syndrome (mongolism) research, prevention and management.* New York: Brunner Mazel.

Fishler, K., Graliker, B. V., & Koch, R. (1965). The predictability of intelligence with Gesell Developmental Scales in mentally retarded infants and young children. *American Journal of Mental Deficiency, 69,* 515–525.

Fitzimmons, M. (1970). Bowling. In L. L. Neal (Ed.), *Recreation's role in the rehabilitation of the mentally retarded.* Eugene: University of Oregon, Rehabilitation Research and Training Center in Mental Retardation.

Flavell, J. H. (1963). The developmental psychology of Jean Piaget. Princeton, NJ: Van Nostrand.

Fleming, E. S., & Anttonen, R. G. (1971a). Teacher expectancy as related to the academic and personal growth of primary-age children. *Monographs of the Society for Research in Child Development, 36,* No. 5B. [Special issue].

Fleming, E. S., & Anttonen, R. G. (1971b). Teacher expectancy or My Fair Lady. *American Educational Research Journal, 8,* 241–252.

Fleming, J. W. (1973). *Care and management of exceptional children* (p. 45). New York: Appleton-Century-Crofts.

Floor, L., Baxter, D., Rosen, M., & Zisfein, L. (1975). A survey of marriages among previously institutionalized retardates. *Mental Retardation, 13,* 33–37.

Folstein, S., & Rutter, M. (1977). Infantile autism: A genetic study of 21 twin pairs. *Journal of Child Psychology and Psychiatry, 18,* 297–321.

Forges, N. P., Shaw, K. N. F., Kock, R., Coffelt, R. W., & Straus, R. (1966). Maternal phenylketonuria. *Nursing Outlook, 14,* 40–42.

Ford, C. E., & Hamerton, J. L. (1956). The chromosomes of man. *Nature (London), 178,* 1020–1023.

Forehand, R. (1973). Teacher recording of deviant behavior: A stimulus for behavior change. *Journal of Behavior Therapy and Experimental Psychiatry, 4,* 39–40.

Forehand, R., & Baumeister, A. A. (1970a). Effect of frustration on stereotyped body rocking: follow-up. *Perceptual and Motor Skills, 31,* 894.

Forehand, R., & Baumeister, A. A. (1970b). Body rocking and activity level as a function of prior movement restraint. *American Journal of Mental Deficiency, 74,* 608–610.

Forehand, R., & Baumeister, A. A. (1971). Stereotyped rocking as a function of situation, IQ, and time. *Journal of Clinical Psychology, 27,* 324–326.

Forsmann, H., & Akesson, H. O. (1970). Mortality of the mentally deficient: A study of 12,903 institutionalized subjects. *Journal of Mental Deficiency Research, 14,* 276–294.

Foster, R., Giddan, J. J., & Stark, J. (1973). *Assessment of Children's Language Comprehension (Manual).* Palo Alto, CA: Consulting Psychologist Press.

Fouracre, M., Connor, F. P., & Goldberg, I. (1982). The effects of a preschool program upon young educable mentally retarded children. (Cooperative Research Project No. 167). Washington, DC: U.S. Dept. of Health, Education, and Welfare, Office of Education.

Foxx, R. M. (1976). The use of overcorrection to eliminate the public disrobing (stripping) of retarded women. *Behavior Research and Therapy, 14,* 53–61.

Foxx, R. M. (1978). An overview of overcorrection. *Journal of Pediatric Psychology, 3,* 97–101.

Foxx, R. M. (1980). Harry. Behavioral treatment of self-abuse. Champaign, IL: Research Press.

Foxx, R. M., & Azrin, N. H. (1972). Restitution: A method of eliminating aggressive-disruptive behavior of retarded and brain-damaged patients. *Behavior Research and Therapy, 10,* 15–27.

Foxx, R. M., & Azrin, N. H. (1973a). *Toilet training the retarded.* Champaign, IL: Research Press.

Foxx, R. M., & Azrin, N. H. (1973b). The elimination of autistic self-stimulatory behavior. *Journal of Applied Behavior Analysis, 6,* 1–14.

Foxx, R. M., & Dufrense, D. (1984). "Harry": The use of physical restraint as a reinforcer, timeout from restraint, and fading restraint in treating a self-injuring man. *Analysis and Intervention in Developmental Disabilities, 4,* 1-13.

Foxx, R. M., & Martin, E. D. (1975). Treatment of scavenging behavior (coprophagy and pica) by overcorrection. *Behavior Research and Therapy, 13,* 153-162.

Foxx, R. M., & Shapiro, S. T. (1978). The timeout ribbon: A non-exclusionary timeout procedure. *Journal of Applied Behavioral Analysis, 11,* 125-136.

Francke, U. (1981). Gene dosage studies on Down syndrome. In F. F. de la Cruz & P. S. Gerald (Eds.), *Trisomy 21 (Down syndrome) research perspectives.* Baltimore: University Park Press.

Frankel, F., & Simmons, J. Q. III. (1976). Self-injurious behavior in schizophrenic and retarded children. *American Journal of Mental Deficiency, 80,* 512-522.

Frankenburg, W. K., Dodds, J., & Fandal, A. (1973). *Denver Developmental Screening Test Manual/ Workbook for nursing and paramedical personnel.* Denver, CO: LADOCA Project and Publishing Foundation.

Frankenburg, W. K., Downs, M., & Kazuk, E. (1973). *Denver Audiometric Screening Test Manual/ Workbook.* Denver, CO: LADOCA Project and Publishing Foundation.

Frankenburg, W. K., & Drumwright, A. (1973). *Denver Articulation Screening Exam Manual/ Workbook.* Denver, CO: LADOCA Project and Publishing Foundation.

Frankenburg, W. K., Goldstein, A. D., & Camp, B. W. The revised Denver Developmental Screening Test: Its accuracy as a screening instrument. *Journal of Pediatrics, 79,* 988-995.

Frankosky, R. J., & Sulzer-Azaroff, B. (1978). Individual and group contingencies and collateral social behaviors. *Behavior Therapy, 9,* 313-327.

Frauenheim, J. G. (1978). Characteristics of adult males who were diagnosed as dyslexic in childhood. *Journal of Learning Disabilities, 11,* 476-483.

Fredericks, H. D., Anderson, R., & Baldwin, V. (1979). Identifying competency indicators of teachers of the severely handicapped. *AAESPH Review, 4,* 81-95.

Fredericks, H. D., Baldwin, V. L., Grove, D. N., & Moore, W. G. (1975). *Toilet training the handicapped child.* Monmouth, OR: Instructional Development Corporation.

Fredericks, H. D., Baldwin, V., Grove, D., Moore, W., Riggs, C., & Lyons, L. (1978). Integrating the moderately and severely handicapped preschool child into a normal day care setting. In M. J. Guralnick (Ed.), *Early intervention and the integration of handicapped and nonhandicapped children.* Baltimore: University Park Press.

Freeman, B. J., Moss, D., Somerset, T., & Ritvo, E. R. (1977). Thumb-sucking in an autistic child overcome by overcorrection. *Journal of Behavior Therapy and Experimental Psychiatry, 8,* 211-212.

Freeman, B. J., Ritvo, E., & Miller, R. (1975). An operant procedure to teach an echolalic, autistic child to answer questions appropriately. *Journal of Autism and Childhood Schizophrenia, 5,* 169-176.

Freeman, F. N., Holzinger, K. J., & Mitchell, B. C. (1928). The influence of environment on the intelligence, school achievement, and conduct of foster children. *Twenty-seventh Yearbook of the National Society for the Study of Education, 1,* 101-217.

Freeman, R. D. (1970). Psychopharmacology and the retarded child. In F. J. Menolascino (Ed.), *Psychiatric approaches to mental retardation.* New York: Basic Books.

French, J. L. (1964). *Manual of Pictorial Test of Intelligence.* Boston: Houghton Mifflin.

Freud, A., & Burlingham, D. T. (1944). *Infants without families.* New York: International Universities Press.

Freud, S. (1949). *An outline of psychoanalysis.* New York: Norton.

Fried, P. A. (1982). Marijuana use by pregnant women and effects on offspring: An update. *Neurobehavioral Toxicology and Teratology, 4,* 415-424.

Friedlander, B. Z., Sterritt, G. M., & Kirk, G. E. (1975). *Exceptional infant: Vol. 3. Assessment and intervention.* New York: Brunner Mazel.

Friedman, P. R. (1976). *The rights of mentally retarded persons.* New York: Avon.

Fristoe, M., & Lloyd, L. L. (1979). Signs used in manual communication training with persons having severe communication impairment. *AAESPH Review, 4,* 364-373.

Fromm, E. (1953). Individual and social origins of neurosis. In C. Kluckhohn & H. A. Murray (Eds.), *Personality in nature, society, and culture.* New York: Knopf.

Fuchs, F. (1980). Genetic amniocentesis. *Scientific American, 242,* 47–52.

Fulker, D. W. (1973). A biometrical genetic approach to intelligence and schizophrenia. *Social Biology, 20,* 266–275.

Fullagar, P. K., & Glover, M. E. (1977). *Competency-based training: A manual for staff serving developmentally disabled children.* Chapel Hill, NC: Chapel Hill Training Outreach Project.

Fuller, J. L. (1954). *Nature and nurture: A modern synthesis.* New York: Doubleday.

Fulton, J. T. (1957). Closure of the human palate in the embryo. *American Journal of Obstetrics and Gynecology, 74,* 179.

Gabel, H., & Kotsch, L. S. (1981). Extended families and young handicapped children. In R. R. Fewell (Ed.), Families of handicapped children. *Topics in Early Childhood Special Education, 1,* 29–35.

Gal, P., & Sharpless, M. K. (1984). Fetal drug exposure—behavioral teratogenesis. *Drug Intelligence and Clinical Pharmacy, 18,* 186–201.

Gallagher, J. J. (1977). The sacred and profane uses of labeling. *Mental Retardation, 14,* 3–7.

Gampel, D. H., Gottlieb, J., & Harrison, R. H. (1974). A comparison of the classroom behavior of special class EMR, integrated EMR, low IQ, and non-retarded children. *American Journal of Mental Deficiency, 79,* 16–21.

Gampel, D. H., Harrison, R. H., & Budoff, M. (1972). An observational study of segregated and integrated EMR children and their non-retarded peers: Can we tell the difference by looking? Unpublished manuscript, Research Institute for Educational Problems, Cambridge, MA.

Garber, N. B., & David, L. E. (1975). Semantic considerations in the treatment of echolalia. *Mental Retardation, 13,* 8–11.

Garcia, E. E., & DeHaven, E. J. (1974). Use of operant techniques in the establishment and generalization of language: A review and analysis. *American Journal of Mental Deficiency, 79,* 169–178.

Gardner, G. E., Tarjan, G., & Richmond, J. B. (1965). *Mental retardation: A handbook for the primary physician.* Chicago: American Medical Association.

Gardner, J. M. (1969). Behavior modification research in mental retardation. *American Journal of Mental Deficiency, 73,* 844–854.

Gardner, W. I. (1958). Reactions of intellectually normal and retarded boys after experimentally induced failure. Unpublished doctoral dissertation, George Peabody College for Teachers, Nashville, TN.

Gardner, W. I. (1971). *Behavior modification in mental retardation: The education and rehabilitation of the mentally retarded adolescent and adult.* Chicago: Aldine-Atherton.

Garrett, J. J. (1966). Realistic vocational guidance. In W. M. Cruickshank (Ed.), *Cerebral palsy—its individual and community problems.* Syracuse, NY: Syracuse University Press.

Gaston, A. H. (1977). Small for gestational age (SGA) infants. In A. M. Rudolph (Ed.), *Pediatrics* (16th ed). New York: Appleton-Century-Crofts.

Gayton, W. F., & Walker, L. (1974). Down's syndrome: Informing the parents—a study of parental preferences. *American Journal of Diseases of Children, 127,* 510–512.

Gearhart, B. R. (1973). *Learning disabilities: Educational strategies.* St. Louis: Mosby.

Gebhard, P. H. (1973). Sexual behavior of the mentally retarded. In F. F. de la Cruz & G. D. LaVeck (Eds.), *Human sexuality and the mentally retarded.* New York: Brunner Mazel.

Gellner, L. (1959). *A neurophysiological concept of mental retardation and its educational implications.* Chicago: J. Levinson Research Foundation.

Gerald, P. S. (1980). X-linked mental retardation and an X-chromosome marker. *New England Journal of Medicine, 303,* 686–697.

Gerjudy, I. R., & Alvarez, J. M. (1969). Transfer of learning in associative clustering of retardates and normals. *American Journal of Mental Deficiency, 73,* 733–738.

Gerjudy, I. R., & Spitz, H. H. (1966). Associative clustering in free recall: Intellectual and developmental variations. *American Journal of Mental Deficiency, 70,* 918–927.

German, J., Kowall, A., & Ehlers, K. H. (1970). Trimethadione and human teratogenesis. *Teratology, 3,* 349–361.

Gersh, K., & Jones, R. L. (1973). Children's perceptions of the trainable mentally retarded: An experimental analysis. Unpublished manuscript, Ohio State University, Columbus.

Gershen, J. A. (1975). Galactosemia: A psycho-social perspective. *Mental Retardation, 13,* 20–23.

Geschwind, N. (1965). Disconnexion syndromes in animals and man. Part II. *Brain, 88,* 585–644.

Gesell, A. (Ed.). (1940). *The first five years of life: A guide to the study of the preschool child.* New York: Harper.

Gesell, A., & Amatruda, C. S. (1947). *Developmental diagnosis, normal and abnormal child development: Clinical methods and practical applications* (2nd ed.). New York: Paul B. Hoeber.

Gibson, D., & Gibbons, R. J. (1958). The relation of mongolism stigmata to intellectual status. *American Journal of Mental Deficiency, 63,* 345–348.

Gibson, D., & Pozsonyi, J. (1965). Morphological and behavioral consequences of chromosome subtype in mongolism. *American Journal of Mental Deficiency, 69,* 801–804.

Gibson, F. W., Jr., Lawrence, P. S., & Nelson, R. O. (1976). Comparison of three training procedures for teaching social responses to developmentally disabled adults. *American Journal of Mental Deficiency, 81,* 379–387.

Gibson, S. L. M., Lam, C. N., McCrae, W. M., et al. (1967). Blood lead levels in normal and mentally deficient children. *Archives of Diseases of Children, 42,* 573–578.

Gickling, E. E., & Theobald, J. T. (1975). Mainstreaming: Affect or effect. *Journal of Special Education, 9,* 317–328.

Gillies, S., Mittler, P., & Simon, G. B. (1963). Some characteristics of a group of psychotic children and their families. *British Psychological Society Conference Proceedings* (Reading).

Gilmer, B., Miller, J. O., & Gray, S. W. (1970). *Intervention with mothers and young children: Study of intra-family effects.* Nashville, TN: DARCEE Demonstration and Research Center for Early Education.

Ginglend, D., & Gould, K. (1962). *Day camping for the mentally retarded.* New York: National Association for Retarded Children.

Gittelman, M., & Birch, H. G. (1967). Childhood schizophrenia: Intellect, neurologic status, perinatal risk, prognosis, and family pathology. *Archives of General Psychiatry, 17,* 16–25.

Glaser, H., Heagarty, M., Bullard, D. M., Jr., & Pivchik, E. G. (1968). Physiological and psychological development of children with early failure-to-thrive. *Journal of Pediatrics, 73,* 690–698.

Glover, M. E., Preminger, J. L., & Sanford, A. R. (1978). *Early-LAP: The early learning accomplishment profile for developmentally young children: Birth to 36 months.* Winston-Salem, NC: Kaplan.

Goddard, H. H. (1912). *The Kallikak family: A study in the heredity of feeble mindedness.* New York: Macmillan.

Goffman, E. (1963). *Stigma: Notes on the management of spoiled identity.* Englewood Cliffs, NJ: Prentice-Hall.

Gola, T. J., Holmes, P. A., & Holmes, N. K. (1982). Effectiveness of a group contingency procedure for increasing prevocational behavior of profoundly mentally retarded residents. *Mental Retardation, 20,* 26–29.

Gold, A. P., Hammill, J. F., & Carter, S. (1977). Cerebrovascular diseases. In A. M. Rudolph (Ed.), *Pediatrics* (16th ed). New York: Appleton-Century-Crofts.

Gold, M. W. (1972). Stimulus factors in skill training of the retarded on a complex assembly task: Acquisition, transfer, and retention. *American Journal of Mental Deficiency, 76,* 517–526.

Gold, M. W. (1973). Research in the vocational habilitation of the retarded: The present, the future. In N. Ellis (Ed.), *International review of research in mental retardation* (Vol. VI). New York: Academic Press.

Gold, M. W. (1976). Task analysis: A statement and an example using acquisition production of a complex assembly task by the retarded blind. *Exceptional Children, 43,* 78–87.

Goldberg, M., Passow, H., & Justman, J. (1961). The effects of ability grouping. Unpublished manuscript, Teachers College, Columbia University, New York.

Goldfarb, W. (1970). Childhood psychosis. In P. H. Mussen (Ed.), *Carmichael's manual of child psychology* (Vol. 2). New York: Wiley.

Goldfarb, W., Goldfarb, N., & Pollack, R. (1966). A three year comparison of day and residential treatment of schizophrenic children. *Archives of General Psychiatry, 14,* 119–128.

Goldfarb, W. (1955). Emotional and intellectual consequences of psychologic deprivation in infancy: A reevaluation. In P. H. Hoch & J. Zubin (Eds.), *Psychopathology of childhood* (pp. 105–119). New York: Grune & Stratton.

Goldman, E. R. (1975). A state model for community services. *Mental Retardation, 13,* 33–37.

Goldman, R. D., & Hartig, L. K. (1976). The WISC may not be a valid predictor of school performance for primary-grade minority children. *American Journal of Mental Deficiency, 80,* 583–587.

Goldstein, H. (1964). Social and occupational adjustment. In H. Stevens & R. Heber (Eds.), *Mental retardation: A review of research* (pp. 214–259). Chicago: University of Chicago Press.

Goldstein, H., Moss, J. W., & Jordan, L. (1965). *The efficacy of special class training on the development of mentally retarded children.* (United States Office of Education, Cooperative Research Project Report No. 619.) Urbana: University of Illinois Press.

Goodman, H., Gottlieb, J., & Morrison, R. H. (1972). Social acceptance of EMRs integrated into a nongraded elementary school. *American Journal of Mental Deficiency, 76,* 412–417.

Goodman, L., Budner, S., & Lesh, B. (1971). The parents' role in sex education for the retarded. *Mental Retardation, 9,* 43–45.

Gordon, I. J. (1971). *A home learning center approach to early stimulation.* Gainesville, FL: Institute for Development of Human Resources.

Gordon, S. (1973). A response to Warren Johnson. In F. F. de la Cruz & G. D. LaVeck (Eds.), *Human sexuality and the mentally retarded.* New York: Brunner Mazel.

Gordon, S. (1973a). *The sexual adolescent.* Boston: Duxbury Press.

Gordon, S. (1973b). Telling it like it is. In K. Thaller & B. Thaller (Eds.), *Sexuality and the mentally retarded* (pp. 1–14). Washington: Office of Economic Opportunity.

Gorda, D. E. (1976). Occupational therapy. In R. B. Johnston & P. R. Magrab (Eds.), *Developmental disorders: Assessment, treatment, education.* Baltimore: University Park Press.

Gortmaker, S. L. (1979). The effects of prenatal care upon the health of the newborn. *American Journal of Public Health, 69,* 653–660.

Gosden, J. R., Mitchell, A. R., Gosden, C. M., Rodeck, C. H., & Morsman, J. M. (1982). Direct vision chorion biopsy and chromosome-specific DNA probes for determination of fetal sex in first trimester of prenatal diagnosis. *Lancet, 2,* 1416–1419.

Gottesman, I. I. (1963). Genetic aspects of intelligent behavior. In N. Ellis (Ed.), *Handbook of mental deficiency: Psychological theory and research.* New York: McGraw-Hill.

Gottlieb, J. (1974). Attitudes toward retarded children: Effects of labeling and academic performance. *American Journal of Mental Deficiency, 79,* 268–273.

Gottlieb, J. (1979). Education implications of mainstreaming. Papers presented at annual meeting of the American Association on Mental Deficiency, Miami Beach, FL.

Gottlieb, J. (1981). Mainstreaming: Fulfilling the promise? *American Journal of Mental Deficiency, 86,* 115–126.

Gottlieb, J., Agar, J., Kaupman, M., & Semmel, M. (1976). Retarded children mainstreamed: Practices as they affect minority group children. In R. Jones (Ed.), *Mainstreaming the minority child.* Reston, VA: Council for Exceptional Children.

Gottlieb, J., & Budoff, M. (1972). Attitudes toward school by segregated and integrated retarded children. *Proceedings of the American Psychological Association, 713–714.*

Gottlieb, J., & Budoff, M. (1973). Social acceptability of retarded children in nongraded schools differing in architecture. *American Journal of Mental Deficiency, 78,* 15–19.

Gottlieb, J., Cohen, L., & Goldstein, L. (1974). Social contact and personal adjustment as variables relating to attitudes toward EMR children. *Training School Bulletin, 71,* 9–16.

Gottlieb, J., & Davis, J. E. (1973). Social acceptance of EMRs during overt behavioral interactions. *American Journal of Mental Deficiency, 78,* 141–143.

Gottlieb, J., & Siperstein, G. N. (1976). Attitudes toward the mentally retarded: Effects of attitude referent specificity. *American Journal of Mental Deficiency, 80,* 376–381.

Gozali, J. (1972). Perception of the EMR special class by former students. *Mental Retardation, 10,* 34–35.

Graliker, B. V., Fishler, K., & Koch, R. (1962). Teenage reaction to a mentally retarded sibling. *American Journal of Mental Deficiency, 66,* 838–843.

Gray, B. B., & Ryan, B. P. (1973). *A language program for the non-language child.* Champaign, IL: Research Press.

Gray, S. W., & Klaus, R. A. (1970). The early training project: The seventh year report. *Child Development, 41,* 909–924.

Green, A. H. (1967). Self-mutilation in schizophrenic children. *Archives of General Psychiatry, 17,* 234–244.

Green, C., & Zigler, E. (1962). Social deprivation and the performance of retarded and normal children on a satiation task. *Child Development, 33,* 499–508.

Greenberg, N. H. (1971). A comparison of infant-mother interactional behavior in infants with atypical behavior and normal infants. In J. Hellmuth (Ed.), *Exceptional infant; Vol. 2. Studies in abnormalities.* New York: Brunner Mazel.

Greene, R., & Hoats, D. (1971). Aversive tickling: A simple conditioning technique. *Behavior Therapy, 2,* 389–393.

Greenspan, S., & Shoultz, B. (1981). Why mentally retarded adults lose their jobs: Social competence as a factor in work adjustment. *Applied Research in Mental Retardation, 2,* 23–38.

Greenwald, C. A., & Leonard, L. B. (1979). Communicative and sensorimotor development of Down's syndrome children. *American Journal of Mental Deficiency, 84,* 296–303.

Gregory, R. J., Lehman, R., & Mohan, P. (1976). Intelligence test results for children with and without undue lead absorption. In G. Wegner (Ed.), *Shoshone lead health project.* Boise: Idaho Department of Health and Welfare.

Gregory, R. J., & Mohan, P. J. (1977). Effect of asymptomatic lead exposure on childhood intelligence: A critical review. *Intelligence, 1,* 381–400.

Griffin, J. C., Locke, B. J., & Landers, W. (1975). Manipulation of potential punishment parameters in the treatment of self-injury. *Journal of Applied Behavior Analysis, 8,* 458–464.

Griffin, R. F., & Elsas, L. J. (1975). Classic phenylketonuria: Diagnosis through heterozygote detection. *Journal of Pediatrics, 86,* 512–517.

Griffith, B. C., Spitz, H. H., & Lipman, R. S. (1959). Verbal mediation and concept formation in retarded and normal subjects. *Journal of Experimental Psychology, 58,* 247–251.

Grinnel, M., Detamore, K., & Lipske, B. (1976). Sign it successful—manual English encourages expressive communication. *Teaching Exceptional Children, 8,* 123–124.

Grossman, F. D. (1972). *Brothers and sisters of retarded children: An exploratory study.* Syracuse, NY: Syracuse University Press.

Grossman, H. J. (1973). *Manual on terminology and classification in mental retardation* (1973 rev.). Washington: American Association on Mental Deficiency.

Grossman, H. J. (Ed.). (1977). *Manual on terminology and classification in mental retardation (1977 rev.)* Washington: American Association on Mental Deficiency.

Groves, I. D., & Carroccio, D. F. (1971). A self-feeding program for the severely and profoundly retarded. *Mental Retardation, 9,* 10–12.

Guerin, G. R., & Szatlocky, K. (1974). Integration programs for the mentally retarded. *Exceptional Children, 41,* 173–177.

Guess, D., Sailor, W., & Baer, D. M. (1974). To teach language to retarded children. In R. L. Schiefelbusch & L. L. Lloyd (Eds.), *Language perspectives—acquisition, retardation, and intervention.* Baltimore: University Park Press.

Guess, D., Sailor, W., & Baer, D. M. (1976). Children with limited language. In R. L. Schiefelbusch (Ed.), *Bases of language intervention.* Baltimore: University Park Press.

Guess, D., Sailor, W., Rutherford, G., & Baer, D. M. (1968). An experimental analysis of linguistic development: The productive use of the plural morpheme. *Journal of Applied Behavior Analysis, 1,* 297–306.

Guilford, J. P., & Hoepfner, R. (1971). *The analysis of intelligence.* New York: McGraw-Hill.

Guilford, J. P. (1967). *The nature of human intelligence.* New York: McGraw-Hill.

Gunzburg, H. C. (1958). Psychotherapy with the feeble-minded. In A. M. Clarke & A. D. B. Clarke (Eds.), *Mental deficiency: The changing outlook.* Glencoe, IL: Free Press.

Gunzburg, H. C. (1968). *Social competence and mental handicap.* Baltimore: Williams & Wilkins.

Guralnick, M. J. (1978). *Early intervention and the integration of handicapped and nonhandicapped children.* Baltimore: University Park Press.

Guskin, S. (1963). Social psychologies of mental deficiencies. In N. R. Ellis (Ed.), *Handbook of mental deficiency: Psychological theory and research.* New York: McGraw-Hill.

Hagberg, B., Hagberg, G., Lewerth, A., & Lindberg, U. (1981). Mild mental retardation in Swedish school children. *Acta Paediatrica Scandanavica, 70,* 441–444.

Hall, B. (1964). *Lund: Berlingska Bortryckeriet.*

Hall, C. S. (1970). *Theories of personality.* New York: Wiley.

Hall, J. E., & Morris, H. L. (1976). Sexual knowledge and attitudes of institutionalized and noninstitutionalized retarded adolescents. *American Journal of Mental Deficiency, 80,* 382–387.

Hall, J. E., Morris, H. L., & Barker, H. R. (1973). Sexual knowledge and attitudes of mentally retarded adolescents. *American Journal of Mental Deficiency, 77,* 706–709.

Hall, J. G., Pauli, I., & Wilson, K. M. (1980). Maternal and fetal sequelae of anticoagulation during pregnancy. *American Journal of Medicine, 68,* 122–140.

Halperin, S. L. (1945). A clinico-genetical study of mental defects. *American Journal of Mental Deficiency, 50,* 8–25.

Hamilton, J., Stephens, L., & Allen, P. (1967). Controlling aggressive and destructive behavior in severely retarded institutionalized residents. *American Journal on Mental Retardation, 71,* 852–856.

Hammill, J. F. (1977). Trauma to the nervous system. In A. M. Rudolph (Ed.), *Pediatrics* (16th ed.). New York: Appleton-Century-Crofts.

Hamre-Nietupski, S., & Williams, W. (1977). Implementation of selected sex education and social skills to severely handicapped students. *Education and Training of the Mentally Retarded, 12,* 364–372.

Hansell, N., Wodarczyk, M., & Visotsky, H. (1968). The mental health expeditor. *Archives of General Psychiatry, 18,* 392–399.

Hansen, R., Young, J., & Ulrey, G. (1982). Assessment considerations with the visually handicapped child. In G. Ulrey & S. J. Rogers (Eds.), *Psychological assessment of handicapped infants and young children.* New York: Thieme-Stratton.

Hanson, M. J. (1976). Evaluation of training procedures used in a present-implemented intervention program for Down's syndrome infants. *AAESPH Review, 1,* 36–52.

Hanshaw, J. B. (1977). In A. M. Rudolph (Ed.), *Pediatrics.* (16th ed.). New York: Appleton-Century-Crofts.

Hanson, J. W., Myrianthopoulos, N. C., Harvey, M. A. S., & Smith, D. W. (1976). Risks to the offspring of women treated with hydantoin anticonvulsants, with emphasis on the fetal hydantoin syndrome. *Journal of Pediatrics, 89,* 662–668.

Hanson, J. W., & Smith, D. W. (1975). The fetal hydantoin syndrome. *Journal of Pediatrics, 87,* 285–290.

Hanson, J. W., Streissguth, A. P., & Smith, D. W. (1978). Effects of moderate alcohol consumption during pregnancy. *Journal of Pediatrics, 92,* 457.

Hardy, J. B., & Mellits, E. D. (1972). Does maternal smoking during pregnancy have a long-term effect on the child? *Lancet, 2,* 1332–1336.

Harris, S. L., & Ersner-Hershfield, R. (1978). Behavioral suppression of seriously disruptive behavior in psychotic and retarded patients: A review of punishment and its alternatives. *Psychological Bulletin, 85,* 1352–1375.

Harris, S. L., & Romanczyk, R. G. (1976). Treating self-injurious behavior of a retarded child by overcorrection. *Behavior Therapy, 7,* 235–239.

Harris, S. L., & Wolchik, S. (1979). Suppression of self-stimulation: Three alternative strategies. *Journal of Applied Behavior Analysis, 12,* 185–198.

Harryman, S. E. (1976). Physical therapy. In R. B. Johnston & P. R. Magrab (Eds.), *Developmental disorders: Assessment, treatment, education.* Baltimore: University Park Press.

Hartup, W. W. (1970). Peer interaction and social organization. In P. H. Mussen (Ed.), *Carmichael's manual of child psychology* (3rd ed., Vol. II). New York: Wiley.

Harvey, E. R., & Schepers, J. (1977). Physical control techniques and defensive holds for use with aggressive retarded adults. *Mental Retardation, 15,* 29–31.

Harvey, J., Judge, C., & Wiener, S. (1977). Familial X-linked mental retardation with an X chromosome abnormality. *Journal of Medical Genetics, 14,* 46–50.

Hatcher, R. P. (1976). The predictability of infant intelligence scales: A critical review and evaluation. *Mental Retardation, 14,* 16–20.

Hay, W. (1951). Mental retardation problems in different age groups. *American Journal of Mental Deficiency, 55,* 191–197.

Hayden, A. H., & Haring, N. G. The acceleration and maintenance of developmental gains in Down's syndrome school-aged children. Paper presented at Fourth International Congress of the International Association for the Scientific Study of Mental Deficiency.

Hayden, A. H., & Dmitriev, V. (1975). The multidisciplinary preschool program for Down's syndrome children at the University of Washington model preschool center. In B. Z. Friedlander, G. M. Sterritt, & G. E. Kirk (Eds.), *Exceptional infants: Volume 3. Assessment and intervention.* New York: Brunner Mazel.

Hayes, S. P. (1950). Measuring the intelligence of the blind. In P. A. Zahl (Ed.), *Blindness: Modern approaches to the unseen environment.* Princeton, NJ: Princeton University Press.

Haywood, H. C., & Arbitman-Smith, R. (1979). *Modification of cognitive functions in slow-learning adolescents.* Paper presented at the 5th International Congress of the International Association for the Scientific Study of Mental Deficiency.

Heal, L. W., Colson, L. S., & Gross, J. C. (1984). A true experiment evaluating adult skill training for severely mentally retarded secondary students. *American Journal of Mental Deficiency, 89,* 146–155.

Heber, R. (1964). Personality. In H. A. Stevens & R. Heber (Eds.)., *Mental retardation: A review of research.* Chicago: University of Chicago Press.

Heber, R. F. (1957). Expectancy and expectancy changes in normal and mentally retarded boys. Unpublished doctoral dissertation, George Peabody College for Teachers, Nashville, TN.

Heber, R. F. (1959). A manual on terminology and classification in mental retardation. *American Journal on Mental Deficiency, 64* (Monograph supplement, rev. ed., 1961).

Heber, R. F. (1970). *Epidemiology of mental retardation.* Springfield, IL: Thomas.

Heber, R. F. (1976). Sociocultural mental retardation—a longitudinal study. Paper presented at Vermont Conference on the Primary Prevention of Psychopathology, June.

Heber, R. F., & Dever, R. B. (1970). Research on education and habilitation of the mentally retarded. In H. C. Haywood (Ed.), *Social-cultural aspects of mental retardation.* New York: Appleton-Century-Crofts.

Heber, R. F., Dever, R. B., & Conry, J. (1968). The influence of environmental and genetic variables on intellectual development. In H. J. Prehm, L. A. Hamerlynck, & J. E. Crosson (Eds.), *Behavioral research in mental retardation.* Eugene, OR: University of Oregon Press.

Heber, R. F., & Garber, H. (1975). The Milwaukee Project: A study of the use of family intervention to prevent cultural-familial mental retardation. In B. Z. Friedlander, G. M. Sterritt, & E. K. Girvin (Eds.), *Exceptional infant: Vol. 3. Assessment and intervention.* New York: Brunner Mazel.

Heber, R. F., Garber, H., Harrington, S., & Hoffman, C. (1972). *Rehabilitation of families at risk for mental retardation.* Madison: Rehabilitation Research and Training Center, University of Wisconsin.

Hecht, F., Bryant, J. Gauber, D., & Townes, P. L. (1964). The nonrandomness of chromosomal abnormalities. Association of trisomy 18 and Down's syndrome. *New England Journal of Medicine, 271,* 1011–1086.

Hecht, F., Hecht, B. K., & Glover, T. W. (1981). Fragile sites and X-linked retardation. *Hospital Practice, 16,* 81–84, 86–88.

Hecht, F., & Kimberling, W. J. (1971). Patterns of D chromosome involvement in human (DqSq) and (DqGq) Robertsonian rearrangements. *American Journal of Human Genetics, 23,* 361.

Hecht, F., & MacFarlane, J. P. (1969). Mosaicism in Turner's syndrome reflects the lethality of XO. *Lancet, 2,* 1197.

Heeley, A. F., & Roberts, G. E. (1965). Tryptophan metabolism in psychotic children. *Developmental Medicine and Child Neurology, 7,* 46.

Heifetz, L. J. (1977). Professional preciousness and the evolution of parent training strategies. In P. Mittler (Ed.), *Research to practice in mental retardation: Vol. I. Care and Intervention.* Baltimore: University Park Press.

Hemming, H., Lavender, T., & Pill, R. (1981). Quality of life of mentally retarded adults transferred from large institutions to new small units. *American Journal of Mental Deficiency, 86,* 157-169.

Henriksen, K., & Doughty, R. (1967). Decelerating undesired mealtime behavior in a group of profoundly retarded boys. *American Journal of Mental Deficiency, 72,* 40-44.

Henry, J. C. (1977). The effects of parent assessment and parent training of preschool mentally retarded children on Piagetian tasks of object permanence and imitation. Unpublished dissertation, Temple University, Philadelphia.

Hermelin, B., & O'Conner, N. (1967). Remembering of words by psychotic and sub-normal children. *British Journal of Psychology, 58,* 213-218.

Heron, T. E. (1978). Punishment: A review of the literature with implications for the teacher of mainstreamed children. *Journal of Special Education, 12,* 243-252.

Herr, S. (1976). The right to an appropriate free education. In M. Kindred, J. Cohen, D. Penrod, & T. Shaffer (Eds.), *The mentally retarded citizen and the law.* New York: Free Press.

Hertzig, M., Birch, H. G., Richardson, S. A., & Tizard, J. (1972). Intellectual levels of school children severely malnourished during the first two years of life. *Pediatrics, 49,* 814-820.

Herzog, E., Newcomb, C. H., & Cisin, I. H. (1972). Double deprivation: The less they have the less they learn. In S. Ryan (Ed.), *A report on longitudinal evaluations of preschool programs.* Washington: U.S. Office of Child Development.

Hess, R. D., & Shipman, V. C. (1965). Early experience and the socialization of cognitive modes in children. *Child Development, 36,* 869-886.

Hess, R. D., & Shipman, V. C. (1968). Maternal influences upon early learning. The cognitive environment of urban preschool children. In R. D. Hess & R. M. Ball (Eds.), *Early education* (pp. 91-103). Chicago: Aldine.

Hetzler, B. E., & Griffin, J. L. (1981). Infantile autism and the temporal lobe of the brain. *Journal of Autism and Developmental Disorders, 11,* 317-330.

Higenbottam, J. A., & Chow, B. (1975). Sound-induced drive, prior motion restraint, and reduced sensory stimulation effects of rocking behavior in retarded persons. *American Journal of Mental Deficiency, 80,* 231-233.

Higgs, R., Burns, G., & Meunier, G. (1980). Eliminating self-stimulatory vocalizations of a profoundly retarded girl through overcorrection. *Journal of the Association for the Severely Handicapped, 5,* 264-269.

Hill, A. L. (1974). Idiot savants: A categorization of abilities. *Mental Retardation, 12,* 12-13.

Hill, B. K., & Bruininks, R. H. (1984). Maladaptive behavior of mentally retarded individuals in residential facilities. *American Journal of Mental Deficiency, 88,* 380-387.

Hill, J. J., & Thompson, J. C. (1980). Predicting adaptive functioning of mentally retarded persons in community settings. *American Journal of Mental Deficiency, 85,* 253-261.

Hill, R. M., Vermand, W. M., Horning, M. G., McCulley, L. B., Morgan, N. F., & Houston, R. N. (1974). Infants exposed in utero to antiepileptic drugs. A prospective study. *American Journal of Diseases of Children, 127,* 645-653.

Himwich, H. E., Jenkins, R. L., Fujimore, M., Narasim-Harchari, N., & Ebersole, M. (1972). A biochemical study of early infantile autism. *Journal of Autism and Childhood Schizophrenia, 2,* 114.

Hingtgen, J. N., & Bryson, C. Q. (1972). Recent developments in the study of early childhood psychoses: Infantile autism, childhood schizophrenia, and related disorders. *Schizophrenia Bulletin, 5,* 8-53.

Hiskey, M. (1966), *Hiskey-Nebraska Test of Learning Aptitude,* Lincoln, NE: Union College Press.

Hobbs, N. (Ed.). (1975). *Issues in the classification of children* (Vols. 1, 2). San Francisco: Jossey-Bass.

Hodes, H. H. (1977). Encephalitis. In A. M. Rudolph (Ed.)., *Pediatrics.* (16th ed.). New York: Appleton-Century-Crofts.

Hodges, W. L., McCandless, B. R., & Spicker, H. H. (1967). *The development and evaluation of a diagnostically based curriculum for preschool psychosocially deprived children.* Washington: U.S. Office of Education.

Hoeltke, G. M. (1966). Effectiveness of special class placement for educable mentally retarded children. Unpublished doctoral dissertation, University of Nebraska, Lincoln.

Hoffman, E. (1971). The idiot savant: A case report and a review of explanations. *Mental Retardation, 9,* 18–21.

Holden, R. H. (1972). Prediction of mental retardation in infancy. *Mental Retardation, 10,* 28–30.

Hollis, J. H. 1967). Development of perceptual motor skills in a profoundly retarded child. Part I. Prosthesis. *American Journal of Mental Deficiency, 71,* 941–952.

Hollis, J. H. (1978). Analysis of rocking behavior. In C. E. Meyers (Ed.), *Quality of life in severely and profoundly mentally retarded people: Research foundations for improvement.* Washington: American Association on Mental Deficiency.

Holmes, L. B., Mack, C., Moser, H. W., Pant, S. S., Hall-Dorsson, S., & Matzilevich, B. (1972). *Mental retardation: An atlas of diseases with associated physical abnormalities.* New York: Macmillan.

Holsclaw, D. S., & Topham, A. L. (1978). The effects of smoking on fetal, neonatal, and childhood development. *Pediatric Annals, 7,* 201–222.

Holtzman, N. A., Welcher, D. W., & Mellits, E. D. (1975). Termination of restricted diet in children with phenylketonuria: A randomized controlled study. *New England Journal of Medicine, 293,* 1121–1124.

Honzik, M. P., MacFarlane, J. W., & Allen, L. (1948). The stability of mental test performance between two and eighteen years. *Journal of Experimental Education, 17,* 309–324.

Hook, E. W. (1973). Behavioral implications of the human XYY genotype. *Science, 179,* 139–150.

Horn, J. L. (1968). Organization of abilities and the development of intelligence. *Psychological Review, 75,* 242–259.

Horner, R. D. (1980). The effects of an environmental "enrichment" program on the behavior of institutionalized profoundly retarded children. *Journal of Applied Behavior Analysis, 13,* 473–491.

Horner, R. D., Billionis, C. S., & Lent, J. R. (1975). *Project MORE: Toothbrushing.* Bellevue, WA: Edmark.

Horner, R. D., & Keilitz, I. (1975). Training mentally retarded adolescents to brush their teeth. *Journal of Applied Behavioral Analysis, 8,* 301–310.

Horton, K. B. (1974). Infant intervention and language learning. In R. L. Schiefelbusch & L. L. Lloyd (Eds.), *Language perspectives—acquisition, retardation, and intervention.* Baltimore: University Park Press.

Horwitz, W., Kestenbaum, A., Person, C., & Jarvik, L. (1965). Identical twin idiot savant calendar calculators. *American Journal of Psychiatry, 121,* 1075–1079.

Hosking, K. E., & Ulrey, G. (1982). Overview of assessment techniques. In G. Ulrey & S. J. Rogers (Eds.), *Psychological assessment of handicapped infants and young children.* New York: Thieme-Stratton.

House, E. R., Glass, G. V., McLean, L. D., Walker, D. F., with Hutchins, E. J. (1977). No simple answer: Critique of the follow-through evaluation. Unpublished study of Center for Instructional Research and Curriculum Evaluation, University of Illinois, Urbana.

Howard-Peebles, P. N., & Markiton, R. I. (1979). A tetra-X female: Cytogenetic testing, dermatoglyphic studies, and speech impairment. *American Journal of Mental Deficiency, 84,* 252–255.

Howden, M. (1967). A nineteen year follow-up study of good, average, and poor readers in the fifth and sixth grades. Unpublished doctoral study, University of Oregon, Eugene.

Hundziak, M. Maurer, R. A., & Watson, L. S. (1965). Operant conditioning in toilet training of severely mentally retarded boys. *American Journal of Mental Deficiency, 70,* 120–124.

Hunt, E. (1976). Varieties of cognitive power. In L. B. Resnick (Ed.), *The nature of intelligence.* Hillsdale, NJ: Erlbaum.

Hunt, J. M. (1961). *Intelligence and experience.* New York: Ronald Press.

Hunter, J., & Bellamy, G. T. (1976). Cable harness construction for severely retarded adults: A demonstration of training techniques. *AAESPH Review, 1,* 2–13.

Hurley, J. R. (1965). Parental acceptance–rejection and children's intelligence. *Merrill-Palmer Quarterly, 11,* 19–31.

Hurlock, E. G. (1964). *Child development* (4th ed.). New York: McGraw-Hill.

Hutchinson, R. R. (1972). The environmental causes of aggression. In J. K. Cole & D. D. Jensen (Eds.), *Nebraska symposium on motivation.* Lincoln: University of Nebraska Press.

Hymes, J. L. (1960). Early childhood. *Children, 7,* 111–113.

Iano, R. P., Ayers, D., Heller, H. B., McGettigan, J. F., & Walker, V. S. (1974). Sociometric status of retarded children in an integrated program. *Exceptional Children, 40,* 267–271.

Illingworth, R. S. (1966). *The development of the infant and young child.* Baltimore: Williams and Wilkins.

Illingworth, R. S. (1971). *Common symptoms of disease in children.* Oxford: Blackwell Scientific Publication.

Illingworth, R. S. (1971). The predictive value of developmental assessment in infancy. *Developmental Medicine and Child Neurology, 13,* 721–725.

Ingalls, R. P. (1978). *Mental retardation: The changing outlook.* NY: Wiley.

Ingenthron, D., Ferneti, C. L., & Keilitz, I. (1975). *Project MORE: Nose Blowing.* Bellevue, WA: Edmark.

Inhelder, B. (1968). *The diagnosis of reasoning in the mentally retarded child* (2nd ed.). (W. B. Stephens and others, Trans.). New York: Chandler.

Inhorn, S. L. (1967). Chromosomal studies of spontaneous human abortion. In D. H. M. Woolam (Ed.), *Advances in teratology* (Vol. 2). New York: Logos Press Academic.

Irvin, L. (1976). General utility of easy-to-hard discrimination training procedures with the severely retarded. *Education and Training of the Mentally Retarded, 11,* 247–250.

Ispa, J., & Matz, R. D. (1978). Integrating handicapped preschool children within a cognitively oriented program. In M. J. Guralnick (Ed.), *Early intervention and the integration of handicapped and nonhandicapped children.* Baltimore: University Park Press.

Jackson, G. M., Johnson, C. R., Ackron, G. S., & Crowley, R. (1975). Food satiation as a procedure to decelerate vomiting. *American Journal of Mental Deficiency, 80,* 223–227.

Jacob, F., & Monod, J. (1961). Genetic regularity mechanisms in the synthesis of proteins. *Journal of Moleculear Biology, 3,* 318–356.

Jacobs, P. A., & Strong, J. A. (1959). A case of human intersexuality having a possible XXY sex determining mechanism. *Nature (London), 183,* 302–303.

Janicki, M. P., Mayeda, T., & Epple, W. (1983). Availability of group homes for persons with mental retardation in the United States. *Mental Retardation, 21,* 45–51.

Jarvick, L. F., Falek, A., & Pierson, W. P., (1964). Down's syndrome (mongolism): The heritable aspects. *Psychological Bulletin, 61,* 388–398.

Jarvick, L. F. (1976). Genetic modes of transmission relevant to psychopathology. In M. A. Sperber and L. F. Jarvick (Eds.), *Psychiatry and genetics.* New York: Basic Books.

Jasper, H. H., Ward, A. A., Jr., & Pope, A. (Eds.). (1969). *Basic mechanisms of the epilepsies.* Boston: Little, Brown.

Jeavons, P. M., Bower, B. D., & Dimitrihoudi, M. C., (1973). Long-term prognosis of 150 copies of West syndrome. *Epilepsia, 14,* 153–164.

Jeffree, D. M., McConkey, R., & Hewson, S. (1977). A parental involvement project. In P. Mittler (Ed.), *Research to practice in mental retardation: Vol. I. Care and intervention.* Baltimore: University Park Press.

Jensen, A. R. (1965). Rote learning in retarded adults and normal children. *American Journal of Mental Deficiency, 69,* 828–834.

Jensen, A. R. (1969). How much can we boost IQ and scholastic achievement? *Harvard Educational Review, 39* 1–123.

Jensen, A. R. (1970). A theory of primary and secondary familial mental retardation. In N. R. (Ellis (Ed.), *International review of research in mental retardation* (Vol. 4). New York: Academic Press.

Jensen, A. R. (1971). The IQs of MZ twins reared apart. *Behavior Genetics, 2,* 1–10.

Jensen, A. R. (1972). *Genetics and education.* New York: Harper and Row.

Jensen, A. R. (1973) *Educability and group differences.* London: Methuen.

Jentsch, H. (1971). Day camping with wheelchair residents at Brainerd State Hospital. *Journal of Health, Physical Education, and Recreation, 42,* 76.

Jervis, G. A. (1948). Early senile dementia in mongoloid idiocy. *American Journal of Psychiatry, 105,* 102–106.

Jervis, G. A. (1963). The clinical picture. In F. L. Lyman (Ed.), *Phenylketonuria.* Springfield, IL: Charles C Thomas.

John, V. P. (1963). The intellectual development of slum children: Some preliminary findings. *American Journal of Orthopsychiatry, 33,* 813–822.

Johnson, D. J., & Myklebust, H. R. (1967). *Learning disabilities: Educational principles and practices.* New York: Grune and Stratton.

Johnson, D. W., & Johnson, R. T. (1980). Integrating handicapped students in the mainstream. *Exceptional Children, 47,* 90–97.

Johnson, G. O. (1950). A study of the social position of mentally handicapped children in the regular grades. *American Journal of Mental Deficiency, 55,* 60–89.

Johnson, G. O. (1962). Special education for the mentally retarded—a paradox. *Exceptional Children, 29,* 62–69.

Johnson, J. C., & Mithaug, D. E. (1978). A replication survey of sheltered workshop entry requirements. *AAESPN Review, 3,* 116–122.

Johnson, R. C. (1969). Behavioral characteristics of phenylketonurics and matched controls. *American Journal of Mental Deficiency, 74,* 17–19.

Johnson, R. C., & Abelson, R. B. (1969). Intellectual, behavioral, and physical characteristics associated with trisomy, translocation, and mosaic types of Down's syndrome. *American Journal of Mental Deficiency, 73,* 852–855.

Johnson, V. M., & Werner, R. A. (1975). *A step-by-step learning guide for retarded infants and children.* Syracuse, NY: Syracuse University Press.

Johnson, W. L., & Baumeister, A. A. (1978). Self-injurious behavior. A review and analysis of methodological details of published studies. *Behavior Modification, 2,* 465–484.

Johnson, W. L., & Baumeister, A. A. (1981). Behavioral techniques for decreasing aberrant behaviors of retarded and autistic persons. In M. Hersen, R. Encor, & P. Miller (Eds.), *Progress in behavior modification* (Vol. 12). New York: Academic Press.

Johnson, W. R. (1973). Sex education of the mentally retarded. In F. F. de la Cruz and G. D. LaVeck (Eds.) *Human sexuality and the mentally retarded.* New York: Brunner Mazel.

Johnston, J. M. (1972). Punishment of human behavior. *American Psychologist, 27,* 1033–1054.

Johnston, R. B. (1976). Motor function: Normal development and cerebral palsy. In R. B. Johnston and P. R. Magrab (Eds.), *Developmental disorders: Assessment, treatment, education.* Baltimore: University Park Press.

Johnston, R. B., & Magrab, P. R. (1976). Introduction to developmental disorders and the interdisciplinary process. In R. B. Johnston & P. R. Magrab (Eds.), *Developmental disorders: Assessment, treatment, education.* Baltimore: University Park Press.

Joint Commission on Mental Health in Children. (1969). *Crisis in child mental health: Challenge for the 1970's.* New York: Harper and Row.

Jolly, D. J., Esty, A. C., Bernard, H. V., & Friedmann, T. (1982). Isolation of a genomic clone partially encoding human hypoxanthine phosphororibosyltransferase. *Proceedings of the National Academy of Sciences, 79,* 5038–5041.

Jones, F., Simmons, J., & Frankel, F., (1974). An extinction procedure for eliminating self-destructive behavior in a nine-year-old autistic girl. *Journal of Autism and Childhood Schizophrenia, 4,* 241–250.

Jones, K. L., & Smith, D. W. (1978). The fetal alcohol syndrome in early infancy. *Teratology, 12,* 1–10.

Jones, K. L., Smith, D. W., Ulleland, C. N., & Streissguth, A. P. (1973). Pattern of malformation in offspring of chronic alcoholic mothers. *Lancet, 1,* 1267–1271.

Jordan, D. R. (1972). *Dyslexia in the classroom.* Columbus, OH, Charles E. Merrill.

Jordan, L. J. (1965). Verbal readiness training for slow learning children. *Mental Retardation, 3,* 19–22.

Jordan, T. E., & DeCharms, R. (1959). The achievement motive in normal and mentally retarded children. *American Journal of Mental Deficiency, 64,* 457–466.

Kaariainen, R., & Dingman, H. F. (1961). The relation of the degree of mongolism to the degree of subnormality. *American Journal of Mental Deficiency, 66,* 438–443.

Kaback, M. M., Leisti, J. (1975). Prenatal detection of Down's syndrome: Technical and ethical considerations. In R. Koch & F. de la Cruz (Eds.) *Down's syndrome (mongolism): Research, prevention and management.* New York: Brunner Mazel.

Kagan, J. (1971). The role of evaluation in problem solving: In J. Hellmuth (Ed.)., *Cognitive studies* (Vol. 2). New York: Brunner Mazel.

Kagan, J. (1971). *Change and continuity in infancy.* New York: Wiley.

Kagan, J. (1972a). Cross-cultural perspectives on early development. Paper presented at meeting of the American Association for the Advancement of Science, Washington, December.

Kagan, J. (1972b). Do infants think? *Scientific American, 226,* 74–82.

Kagan, J., Rosman, B., Dan, D., Albert, J., & Phillips, W. (1964). Information processing in the child: Significance of analytic and reflective attitudes. *Psychological Monographs, 78,* 1.

Kagan, J., & Kogan, N., (1970). Individuality and cognitive processes. In P. H. Mussen (Ed.), *Carmichael's handbook of child psychology* (3rd ed.) Vol. 1 (pp. 1273–1365). New York: Wiley.

Kahan, E. H. (1974). *Cooking activities for the retarded child.* Nashville, TN: Abingdon Press.

Kahn, J. V. (1978). Acceleration of object permanence with severely and profoundly retarded children. *AAESPH Review, 3,* 15–22.

Kahn, J. V. (1979). Applications of the Piagetian literature to severely and profoundly mentally retarded persons. *Mental Retardation, 17,* 273–280.

Kanheman, D., Tursky, B., Shapiro, D., & Crider, A. (1969). Pupillary, heart rate and skin resistance changes during a mental task. *Journal of Experimental Psychology, 79,* 164–167.

Kalckar, H. M., Kinoshita, J. H., & Donnell, G. N. (1973). Galactosemia, biochemistry, genetics, pathophysiology and developmental aspects. *Biology of Brain Dysfunction, 1,* 33–88.

Kalisz, K., Ekvall, S., & Palmer, S. (1978). Pica and lead intoxication. In S. Palmer & S. Ekvall (Eds.), *Pediatric nutrition in developmental disorders.* Springfield, IL: Charles C Thomas.

Kamin, L. J. (1974). *The science and politics of I.Q.* New York: Halsted Press.

Kang, E. S., Sollee, N. D., & Gerald, P.S. (1970). Results of treatment and termination of the diet in phenylketonuria (PKU). *Pediatrics, 46,* 881–890.

Kanner, L. (1957). *Child psychiatry.* Springfield, IL: Charles C Thomas.

Kanner, L. (1964). *A history of the care and study of the mentally retarded.* Springfield, IL: Charles C Thomas.

Kanner, L., & Eisenberg, L. (1955). Notes on the follow-up studies of autistic children. In P. H. Hoch & J. Zubin (Eds.), *Psychopathology of childhood.* New York: Grune and Stratton.

Kaplan, F. (1969). Siblings of the retarded. In S. B. Sarason & J. Doris (Eds.), *Psychological problems in mental deficiency* (4th ed.). New York: Harper and Row.

Karan, O. (Ed.). (1979). *Habilitation practices with the severely developmentally disabled* (Vol. 2). Madison: University of Wisconsin Research and Training Center.

Karnes, M. B. (1972). *GOAL Program: Language development.* Springfield, MA: Milton Bradley.

Karnes, M. B., Hodgins, A. S., & Teska, J. A. (1969). The impact of at-home instruction by mothers on performance in the ameliorative preschool. In M. B. Karnes (Ed.), *Research and development program on preschool disadvantaged children: Final report.* Washington: U.S. Office of Education.

Kass, E. R., Sigman, M., Bromwich, R. F., & Parmlee, A. N. (1976). Educational intervention with high risk infants. In T. D. Tjossem (Ed.), *Intervention strategies for high risk infants and young children.* Baltimore: University Park Press.

Katz, I. (1970). A new approach to the study of school motivation in minority group children. In V. Allen (Ed.), *Psychological factors in poverty.* Chicago: Mackham.

Katz, P. J. (1962). Transfer of principles as a function of a course of study incorporating scientific method for the educable mentally retarded. Unpublished doctoral disseration, Teacher College, Columbia University, New York.

Kauffman, J. M., & Krouse, J. (1981). The cult of educability: Searching for the substance of things hoped for: The evidence of things not seen. *Analysis and Intervention in Developmental Disabilities, 1,* 53–60.

Kaufman, A. S. (1975). Factor analysis of the WISC-R at eleven age levels between $6\frac{1}{2}$ months and $16\frac{1}{2}$ years. *Journal of Consulting and Clinical Psychology, 43,* 135–147.

Kaufman, A. S. (1979). *Intelligent testing with the WISC-R.* New York: Wiley.

Kaufman, M. (1963). Group psychotherapy in preparation for return of mental defectives from institution to community. *Mental Retardation, 1,* 276–280.

Kaufman, M. E., & Levitt, H. (1965). A study of three stereotyped behaviors in institutionalized mental defectives. *American Journal of Mental Deficiency, 69,* 467–473.

Kaufman, M. J., Gottlieb, J., Agard, J. A., & Kukic, M. B. (1975). Mainstreaming: Toward an explication of the construct. In E. L. Meyen, G. A. Vergason, & R. J. Whelan (Eds.), *Alternatives for teaching exceptional children.* Denver: Love Publishing.

Kearsley, R. B. (1979). Iatrogenic retardation: A syndrome of learned incompetence. In R. B. Kearsley & I. E. Sigel (Eds.), *Infants at risk: Assessment of cognitive functioning.* Hillsdale, NJ: Erlbaum.

Kearsley, R. B., & Sigel, I. E. (Eds.) (1979). *Infants at risk: Assessment of cognitive functioning.* Hillsdale, NJ: Erlbaum.

Keilitz, I. Horner, R. D., & Brown, K. H. (1975). *Project MORE: Complexion care.* Bellevue, WA: Edmark.

Keller, S. (1963). The social world of the urban slum child. Some early findings. *American Journal of Orthopsychiatry, 33,* 823–831.

Kemp, B. M. (1973). The modification of meal-time spitting behavior. *Australian Journal of Mental Deficiency, 2,* 222–225.

Kempton, W. (1978). Sex education for the mentally handicapped. *Sexuality and Disability, 1,* 137–145.

Kempton, W., & Forman, R. (1976). *Guidelines for training in sexuality and the mentally handicapped.* Philadelphia: Planned Parenthood Association of Southeast Pennsylvania.

Kendall, S. R. (1977). Neonatal drug withdrawal. In A. M. Rudolph (Ed.), *Pediatrics* (16th edition). New York: Appleton-Century-Crofts.

Kennedy, R. (1966). *A Connecticut community revisited: A study of the social adjustment of a group of mentally deficient adults in 1948 and 1960.* Hartford: Connecticut State Department of health, Office of Mental Retardation.

Kennedy, W. A. (1969). A follow-up normative study of Negro intelligence and achievement. *Monographs of the Society for Research in Child Development, 34,* 126.

Kennedy, W. A. (1973). *Intelligence and economics: A confounded relationship.* Morristown, NJ: General Learning Press.

Kennedy, W. A., Van de Riet, V., & White, J. C., Jr. (1963). A normative sample of intelligence and achievement of the Negro elementary school children in the southeastern United States. *Monographs of the Society for Research in Child Development, 28,* 90.

Kent, L. R., with Klein, D., Falk, A., & Guenther, H. (1972). A language acquisition program for the retarded. In J. E. McLean, D. E. Yoder, & R. L. Schiefelbusch (Eds.), *Language intervention with the retarded.* Baltimore: University Park Press.

Keogh, B. K., & Levitt, M. L. (1976). Special education in the mainstream: A confrontation of limitations? *Focus on Exceptional Children, 8,* 1–10.

Keogh, B. K. (1973). Perceptual and cognitive styles: Implications for special education. In L. Mann & D. A. Sabatino (Eds.), *The first review of special education* (Vol. 1, pp. 83–111). Philadelphia: Journal of Special Education Press.

Kephart, N. C. (1960). *The slow learner in the classroom.* Columbus, OH: Merrill.

Kerkay, J., Zsako, S., Cotton, J. E., & Kaplan, A. (1975). Biochemical and genetic variables associated with mothers of G1-trisomy affected children. *Acta Geneticae Medicae et Gemmellologiae, 24,* 239–244.

Kerkay, J., Zsako, S., & Kaplan, A. (1971). Immunolectrophoretic serum patterns associated with mothers of children affected with the G1-trisomy syndrome. *American Journal of Mental Deficiency, 75,* 729–732.

Kessner, D. M. (1973). *Infant death: An analysis by maternal risk and health care. Contrasts in health status* (Vol. 1). Washington: Institute of Medicine, National Academy of Sciences.

Kiernan, D. W., & DuBove, R. F. (1974). Assessing the cognitive development of preschool deaf-blind children. *Education of the Visually Handicapped, 6,* 103–105.

King, R. D., Raynes, N. V., & Tizard, J. (1971). *Patterns of residential care: Sociological studies in institutions for handicapped children.* London: Routledge and Kegan Paul.

Kinney, D. K. & Kagan, J. (1976). Infant attention to auditory discrepancy. *Child development, 47,* 155–164.

Kirby, D., Alter, J., & Scales, P. (1979). *An analysis of U.S. sex education programs and evaluation methods* (Vol. 1). Bethesda, MD: Malthtech.

Kirk, S. A. (1958). *Early education of the mentally retarded: An experimental study.* Urbana: University of Illinois Press.

Kirk, S. A. (1962). *Educating exceptional children.* Boston: Houghton Mifflin.

Kirman, B. (1975). Drug therapy in mental handicapped. *British Journal of Psychiatry, 127,* 545–549.

Klapper, Z. J., & Birch, H. G. (1967). A fourteen year follow-up study of cerebral palsy: Intellectual change and stability. *American Journal of Orthopsychiatry, 37,* 540–547.

Klein, A. H., Meltzer, S., & Kenny, F. M. (1972). Improved prognosis in congenital hypothyroidism treated before age three months. *Journal of Pediatrics, 81,* 912–915.

Kleinberg, J., & Galligan, B. (1983). Effects of deinstitutionalization on adaptive behavior of mentally retarded adults. *American Journal of Mental Deficiency, 88,* 21–27.

Kliebhahn, J. (1967). Effects of goal setting and modeling on job performances of retarded adolescents. *American Journal of Mental Deficiency, 72,* 220–226.

Knights, R., Atkinson, B., & Hyman, J. (1967). Tactual discrimination and motor skills in mongoloid and non-mongoloid retardates and normal children. *American Journal of Mental Deficiency, 71,* 894–900.

Knobeloch, C. (1976). Speech and language. In R. B. Johnston & P. R. Magrab (Eds.), *Developmental disorders assessment, treatment, education.* Baltimore: University Park Press.

Koch, R. (1967). The multidisiplinary approach to mental retardation. In A. A. Baumeister (Ed.), *Mental retardation: Appraisal, education, and rehabilitation.* Chicago: Aldine.

Koch, R., Acosta, P., Fishler, K., Schaeffler, G., & Wohlers, A. (1967). Clinical observations on phenylketonuria. *American Journal of Diseases in Children, 113,* 6–15.

Koch, R., Fishler, K., & Melnyk, J. (1971). Chromosomal abnormalities in causation: Down's syndrome. In R. Koch & J. C. Dobson (Eds.), *The mentally retarded child and his family: A multidisciplinary handbook.* New York: Brunner Mazel.

Koegler, S. J. (1963). The management of the retarded child in practice. *Canadian Medical Association Journal, 89,* 1009–1014.

Kogan, K. L., & Tyler, N. (1973). Mother-child interaction in young physically handicapped children. *American Journal of Mental Deficiency, 77,* 492–497.

Kolstoe, O. P. (1975). Secondary programs. In J. M. Kaufman & J. S. Payne (Eds.), *Mental retardation: Introduction and personal perspectives.* Columbus, OH: Merrill.

Koluchova, J. (1972). Severe deprivation in twins: A case study of marked IQ change after age 7. *Journal of Child Psychology and Psychiatry, 13,* 107–114.

Koos, B. J., & Longo, L. D. (1976). Mercury toxicity in the pregnant woman, fetus, and newborn infant. *American Journal of Obstetrics and Gynecology, 126,* 390–400.

Kofchick, G., & Lloyd, L. (1976). Total communication programming for the severely language impaired: A 24-hour approach. In L. Lloyd (Ed.), *Communication assessment and intervention strategies.* Baltimore: University Park Press.

Koshlick, A., & Blunden, R. (1974). The epidemiology of mental subnormality. In A. M. Clarke & A. D. B. Clarke (Eds.), *Mental deficiency: The changing outlook* (3rd ed.) New York: Free Press.

Kostir, M. S. (1916). *The family of Sam Sixty.* Ohio Board of Administration Press Publication No. 8, Ohio State Reformatory. (Reported in L. Kanner, 1964, reference.)

Kott, M. G. (1968). Estimating the number of retarded in New Jersey. *Mental Retardation, 6,* 28–31.

Kotter, J. (1954). *Social learning and clinical psychology.* Englewood Cliffs, NJ: Prentice Hall.

Krajicek, M. J., & Roberts, P. (1976). Nursing. In R. B. Johnston & P. R. Magrab (Eds.), *Developmental disorders: Assessment, treatment, education*. Baltimore: University Park Press.

Kramm, E. R. (1963). *Families of mongoloid children*. (Children's Bureau Publication No. 401). Washington: U.S. Department of Health, Education, and Welfare.

Kravitz, H., & Boehm, S. (1971). Rhythmic habit patterns in infancy. Their sequence, age of onset, and frequency. *Child Development, 42*, 399–413.

Kravitz, H., Rosenthal, V., Teplitz, Z., Murphy, J., & Lesser, R. (1960). A study of headbanging in infants and children. *Diseases of the Nervous System, 21*, 203–208.

Kreger, K. C. (1971). Compensatory environment programming for the severely retarded behaviorally disturbed. *Mental Retardation, 9*, 29–33.

Kucera, T. (1970). Down's syndrome and infectious hepatitis. *Lancet, 1*, 569–570.

Kugel, R. B., & Reque, D. (1961). A comparison of mongoloid children. *Journal of the American Medical Association, 175*, 959–961.

Kutter, M., Lebovici, S., Eisenberg, L., Snezneviskis, A. V., Sadoun, R., Brooke, E., & Lin, T. Y. (1969). A triaxial classification of mental disorders in childhood: An international study. *Journal of Child Psychology and Psychiatry, 10*, 41–61.

Lacey, J. I. (1967). Somatic response patterning in stress: Some revision of activation theory. In M. H. Appley & R. Trumball (Eds.), *Psychological stress: Issues in research*. New York: Appleton-Century-Crofts.

LaFontaine, L. & Benjaman, G. E. (1971). Idiots savants: Another view. *Mental Retardation, 9*, 41–42.

Lagos, J. C., & Gomez, M. R. (1967). Tuberous sclerosis: Reappraisal of a clinical entity. *Mayo Clinic Proceedings, 42*, 26.

Lakin, K. C., Bradley, K. H., Harber, F. A., Bruininks, R. H., & Heal, L. W. (1983). New admissions and readmissions to a national sample of public residential facilities. *American Journal of Mental Deficiency, 88*, 13–20.

Lally, M., & Nettlebeck, T. (1977). Intelligence, reaction time and inspection time. *American Journal of Mental Deficiency, 82*, 273–281.

Lambie, D. Z., Bond, J. T., & Weikart, D. P. (1975). Framework for infant education. In B. Z. Friedlander, G. M. Sterritt, & G. E. Kirk (Eds.), *Exceptional infant: Vol. 3. Assessment and Intervention*. New York: Brunner Mazel.

Landesman-Dwyer, S., Ragozin, A. J., & Little, R. E. (1981). Behavioral correlates of parental alcohol exposure: A four-year follow-up study. *Neurobehavioral Toxicology and Teratology, 3*, 187–193.

Landesman-Dwyer, S., Sackett, G. P., & Kleinman, J. S. (1980). Relationship of size to resident and staff behavior in small community residences. *American Journal of Mental Deficiency, 85*, 6–17.

Landreth, C. (1958). *The psychology of early childhood*. New York: Knopf.

Lang, P., & Melamed, B. (1969). Case report: Avoidance conditional therapy of an infant with chronic ruminative vomiting. *Journal of Abnormal Psychology, 74*, 1–8.

Langdell, J. I. (1965). Phenylketonuria. *Archives of General Psychiatry, 12*, 363–367.

Larrabee, M. M. (1969). Involving parents in their children's day-care experiences. *Children, 16*, 149–154.

Larsen, L. A. & Bricker, W. A. (1960). *A manual for parents and teachers of severely and moderately retarded children*. Nashville, TN: Institute on Mental Retardation and Intellectual Development Papers and Reports (John F. Kennedy Center for Research on Education and Human Development, Vanderbilt University), Vol. V, No. 22.

Latimer, R. (1970). Current attitudes toward mental retardation. *Mental Retardation, 5*, 30–32.

Laurence, K. M. (1960). The natural history of hydrocephalus. *Postgraduate Medical Journal, 36*, 662.

Lee, L. L. & Canter, S. (1971). Developmental sentence scoring: A clinical procedure for estimating syntactic development in children's spontaneous speech. *Speech and Hearing Disorders, 36* 315–340.

Leff, R. B. (1974). Teaching the TMR to dial the telephone. *Mental Retardation, 12*, 12–13.

Lejeune, J., Gautier, M., & Turpin, R. (1959). Etude des chromosomes somatique de neuf enfants mongoliens. *Comptes Rendus de l'Academie des Sciences, 248,* 1721-1822.

LeJeune, J., LaForcade, J., Berger, R., Vialatte, J., Boeswillwald, M., Seringe, P., & Turpin, R. (1963). Trois cas de deletion partielle du bras court du chromosome 5. *Comptes Rendus de l'Academie des Sciences, 257,* 3098.

Leland, H., & Smith, D. E. (1965). *Play therapy with subnormal children.* New York: Grune and Stratton.

Leland, H., & Smith, D. E. (1972). Psychotherapeutic considerations with mentally retarded and developmentally diseased children. In E. Katz (Ed.), *Mental health services for the mentally retarded.* Springfield, IL: Charles C Thomas.

Lemrke, R. (1972). A theory of X-linkage of major intellectual traits. *American Journal of Mental Deficiency, 26,* 611-619.

Lenneberg, E. H. (1967). *Biological foundation of language.* New York: Wiley.

Lennox, W. G., Gibbs, E. L., & Gibbs, F. A. (1945). The brain wave pattern; a hereditary trait. *Journal of Heredity, 36,* 233.

Lensink, B. (1976). ENCOR, Nebraska. In R. B. Kugel & A. Sherer (Eds.), *Changing patterns in residential services for the mentally retarded.* Washington: President's Committee on Mental Retardation.

Leonard, M. F., Landy, G., Ruddle, F. H., & Lubs, H. A. (1974). Early development of children with abnormalities of the sex chromosomes: A prospective study. *Pediatrics, 54,* 208-212.

Lerner, I. M. (1968). *Heredity, evolution, and society.* San Francisco: Freeman.

Lerner, J. W. (1971). *Children with learning disabilities. Theories, diagnosis, and teaching strategies.* Boston: Houghton Mifflin.

Lesch, M., & Nyhan, W. L. (1964). A familial disorder of uric acid metabolism and central nervous system function. *American Journal of Medicine, 36,* 561.

Levenstein, P. (1970). Cognitive growth in preschoolers through verbal interaction with mothers. *American Journal of Orthopsychiatry, 40,* 426-432.

Levine, M. D., Carey, W. B., Crocker, A. C., & Gross, R. T. (Eds.). (1983). *Developmental-Behavioral Pediatrics.* Philadelphia: W. B. Saunders.

Levine, S., Elzey, F. F., & Fiske-Rollin, B. (1979). Developmental characteristics of severely and profoundly handicapped. *AAESPH Review, 4,* 36-51.

Levinson, A., Friedman, A., & Stamps, F. (1955). Variability of mongolism. *Pediatrics, 16,* 43.

Levinson, E. J. (1962). *Retarded children in Maine. A survey and analysis.* Orono, ME: University of Maine Press.

Levy, E., & McLeod, W. (1977). The effects of environmental design on adolescents in an institution. *Mental Retardation, 15,* 28-32.

Levy, H. L. (1974). Genetic screening. In H. Harris & K. Hirschhorn (Eds.), *Advances in human genetics* (Vol. 4). New York: Plenum.

Lewis, M., & Goldberg, S. (1969). The acquisition and violation of expectancy: An experimental paradigm: *Journal of Experimental Child Psychology, 7,* 70-80.

Lewis, P. J., Ferneti, C. L., & Keilitz, I. (1975). *Project MORE: Use of deodorant.* Bellevue, WA: Edmark.

Lilienfeld, A. (1969). *Epidemiology of mongolism.* Baltimore: Johns Hopkins University Press.

Linford, M. D., Hipsher, L. W., & Silikovitz, R. G. (1972). *Systematic instruction for retarded children: The Illinois program. Part III: Self-help instruction.* Danville, IL: Interstate.

Lipman, R. S. (1970). The use of psychopharmacological agent in residential facilities for the retarded. In F. J. Menolascino (Ed.), *Psychiatric approaches to mental retardation.* New York: Basic Books.

Lipman, R. S., & Griffith, B. C. (1960). Effects of anxiety level on concept formation: A test of drive theory. *American Journal of Mental Deficiency, 65,* 342-348.

Lippman, L. (1976). The least restrictive alternative and guardianship. In M. Kindred, J. Cohen, D. Penrod, & T. Shaffer (Eds.), *The mentally retarded citizen and the law.* New York: Free Press.

Lipsitt, L. P. (1958). A self-concept scale for children and its relation to the children's form of the Manifest Anxiety Scale. *Child Development, 29,* 463-472.

Lloyd-Still, J. D., Hurwitz, I., Wolff, P., & Shwachman, H. (1974). Intellectual development after severe malnutrition in infancy. *Pediatrics, 54,* 306–311.

Lockwood, K., & Bourland, G. (1982). Reduction of self-injurious behaviors by reinforcement and toy use. *Mental Retardation, 20,* 169–183.

Lohman, W., Eyman, R., & Lask, E. (1967). Toilet training. *American Journal of Mental Deficiency, 71,* 551–557.

Lotter, V. (1966). Services for a group of autistic children in Middlesex. In J. K. Wing (Ed.), *Early childhood autism: Clinical, educational and social aspects.* London: Pergamon.

Lotter, V. (1967). *The prevalence of the autistic syndrome in children.* Doctoral thesis, University of London.

Lovaas, O. I. Freitag, G., Gold, V. J., & Kassorla, I. C. (1965). Experimental studies in childhood schizophrenia: Analysis of self-destructive behavior. *Journal of Experimental Child Psychology, 2,* 67–84.

Lovaas, O. I. & Simmons, J. Q. (1969). Manipulation of self-destruction in three retarded children. *Journal of Applied Behavioral Analysis, 2,* 143–157.

Low, N. L. (1977). Cerebral palsy. In A. M. Rudolph (Ed.), *Pediatrics* (16th ed). New York: Appleton-Century-Crofts.

Lowenfeld, B. (1950). Psychological foundation of special methods in teaching blind children. In P. A. Zahl (Ed.), *Blindness.* Princeton, NJ: Princeton University Press.

Lowenfeld, B. (1971). Psychological problems of children with impaired vision, In W. M. Cruickshank (Ed.), *Psychology of exceptional children and youth. (3rd Ed.).* Englewood Cliffs, NJ: Prentice-Hall.

Lubchenco, L. O., Delivoria-Papadapolous, M., & Searls, S. (1972). Long-term follow-up of premature infants. II. Influence of birth weight and gestational age on sequelae. *Journal of Pediatrics, 80,* 509–512.

Lubs, H. A. (1969). A marker X chromosome. *American Journal of Human Genetics, 21,* 231–244.

Lucero, W. J., Frieman, J., Spoering, K., & Fehrenbacher, J. (1976). Comparison of three procedures in reducing self-injurious behavior. *American Journal of Mental Deficiency, 80,* 548–554.

Luckey, R. E., & Neman, R. (1976). Practices in estimating mental retardation prevalence. *Mental Retardation, 14,* 16–18.

Luckey, R. E., Watson, C. M., & Musick, J. K. (1968). Aversive conditioning as a means of inhibiting vomiting and rumination. *American Journal of Mental Deficiency, 73,* 139–142.

Ludins-Katz, F. (1972). Creative arts expression of the mentally retarded. In E. Katz (Ed.), *Mental health services for the mentally retarded.* Springfiled, IL: Charles C Thomas.

Luiselli, J. (1977). Case report: An attendant administered contingency management program for the treatment of a toilet phobia. *Journal of Mental Deficiency Research, 21,* 283–288.

Luiselli, J., Pemberton, B. W., & Helfen, C. S. (1978). Effects and side-effects of a brief overcorrection procedure in reducing multiple self-stimulatory behavior: A single case analysis. *Journal of Mental Deficiency Research, 22,* 287–293.

Luiselli, J., Reisman, J., Helfen, C. S., & Pemberton, B. W. (1979). Toilet training in the classroom: An adaptation of Azrin and Foxx's rapid toilet training procedure. *Behavioral Engineering, 5,* 89–93.

Lundeen, D. J. (1972). Speech disorders. In B. R. Gearhart (Ed.), in association with the late T. D. Vaughan, *Education of the exceptional child: History, present practices, and trends.* Scranton, PA: Intext.

Lutzker, J. R. (1978). Reducing self-injurious behavior by facial screening. *American Journal of Mental Deficiency, 82,* 510–513.

Lyle, J. (1960). Some factors affecting the speech development of imbecile children in an institution. *Journal of Child Psychology and Psychiatry, 1,* 121–129.

Lynch, E. W., Simms, B. H., Von Hippel, C. S., & Shuchat, J. (1978). *Mainstreaming preschoolers: Children with mental retardation.* Washington: DHEW Publication No. (OHDS) 79–31110.

Mabry, C. C., Denniston, J. C., & Caldwell, J. G. (1966). Mental retardation in children of phenylketonuric mothers. *New England Journal of Medicine, 275,* 1331.

MacCulloch, M. J., & Sambrooks, J. E. (1976). Concepts of autism: A review paper presented at

Burton Manor Symposium "Recent Developments in Psychiatry." Referred to in *Early childhood autism*, L. Wing (Ed.). New York: Pergamon.

MacDonald, J. D., Blott, J. P., Gordon, L., Speigel, B., & Hartmann, M. (1974). An experimental parent-assisted treatment program for preschool language delayed children. *Journal of Speech and Hearing Disorders, 39*, 395–415.

MacEachron, A. E. (1979). Mentally retarded offenders: Prevalence and characteristics. *American Journal of Mental Deficiency, 84*, 165–186.

MacEachron, A.E. (1983). Institutional reform and adaptive functioning of mentally retarded persons: A field experiment. *American Journal of Mental Deficiency, 88*, 2–12.

MacGillivroy, R. C. (1956). The larval psychosis of idiocy. *American Journal of Mental Deficiency, 60*, 570–574.

MacMillan, D. L. (1971). Special education for the mildly retarded: Servant or savant. *Focus on Exceptional Children, 2*, 1–11.

MacMillan, D. L. (1972). Paired-associate learning as a function of explicitness of mediational set by EMR and non-retarded children. *American Journal of Mental Deficiency, 76*, 686–691.

MacMillan, D. L. (1977). *Mental retardation in school and society.* Boston: Little, Brown.

MacMillan, D. L., & Borthwick, S. (1980). The new educable mentally retarded population: Can they be mainstreamed? *Mental Retardation, 18*, 155–158.

MacMillan, D. L., Jones, R. L., & Aloia, G. F. (1974). The mentally retarded label: A theoretical analysis and review of research. *American Journal of Mental Deficiency, 89*, 241–261.

MacMillan, D. L., Jones R. L., & Meyers, C. E. (1976). Mainstreaming the mildly retarded: Some questions, cautions and guidelines. *Mental Retardation, 14*, 3–10.

Madden, J. D., Chappel, J. N., Zuspan, F., Gumpel, J., Mejia, A., & Davis, R. (1977). Observation and treatment of neonatal narcotic withdrawal. *American Journal of Obstetrics and Gynecology, 127*, 199–201.

Madden, D. L., Matthew, E. B., Dietzman, D. E., Purcell, R. H., Sever, J. L., Rostafinski, M., & Mata, A. (1976). Hepatitis and Down's syndrome. *American Journal of Mental Deficiency, 80*, 401–406.

Mager, R. F. (1962). *Preparing instructional objectives.* Palo Alto, CA: Fearon Publishers.

Magaret, G. A., & Thompson, C. W. (1950). Differential test responses of normal, superior, and mentally defective subjects. *Journal of Abnormal and Social Psychology, 45*, 163–167.

Magenis, R. E., Overton, K. M., Chamberlin, J., Brady, T., & Lovrein, E. (1977). Parental origin of the extra chromosome in Down's syndrome. *Human Genetics, 37*, 8–16.

Magrab, P. R. (1976). Psychology. In R. B. Johnston & P. R. Magrab (Eds.), *Developmental disorders: Assessment, treatment, education.* Baltimore: University Park Press.

Magrab, P. R., & Elder, J. O. (1979). *Planning for services to handicapped persons. Community, education, health.* Baltimore: Paul H. Brookes.

Mahler, M. S., Furer, M., & Settlage, C. F. (1959). Severe emotional disturbances in childhood. Psychosis. In S. Arieti (Ed.), *American handbook of psychiatry* (pp. 816–839). New York: Basic Books.

Mahoney, G. J. (1975). Ethological approach to delayed language acquisition. *American Journal of Mental Deficiency, 80*, 139–148.

Mahoney, K., Van Wagenen, R., & Myerson, L. (1971). Toilet training of normal and retarded children. *Journal of Applied Behavioral Analysis, 4*, 173–181.

Malamud, N. (1964). Neuropathology. In M. A. Stevens & R. Heber (Eds.), *Mental retardation.* Chicago: University of Chicago Press.

Maloney, M. P., Ball, T. S., & Edgar, C. L. (1970). An analysis of the generalizability of sensory-motor training. *American Journal of Mental Deficiency, 74*, 458–469.

Manto, C. R., Baumeister, A. A., & Maisto, A. A. (1978). An analysis of variables related to self-injurious behavior among institutionalized retarded persons. *Journal of Mental Deficiency Research, 12*, 27–36.

Marholin, D., Lunelli, J. K., & Townsend, N. M. (1980). Overcorrection: An examination of its rationale and treatment effectiveness. In M. Hersen, R. Eisler, & P. Miller (Eds.), *Progress in behavior modification* (Vol. 9). New York: Academic Press.

Martin, B. (1975). Parent-child relations. In F. D. Horowitz (Ed.), *Review of child development research* (Vol. 4). Chicago: University of Chicago Press.

Martin, B. (1977). *Abnormal psychology: Clinical and scientific perspectives.* New York: Holt, Rinehart and Winston.

Martin, C. J. (1967). Associative learning strategies employed by deaf, blind, normal, and retarded children. *Educational Research Series, 38*, 1–158.

Martin, G. L., McDonald, S., & Omichinski, M. (1971). An operant analysis of response interactions during meals with severely retarded girls. *American Journal of Mental Deficiency, 76*, 68–75.

Martin, H. P. (1970). Microcephaly and mental retardation. *American Journal of Diseases of Children, 119*, 128–131.

Martin, L. C. (1940). Shall we segregate our handicapped? *Journal of Exceptional Children, 6*, 223–225, 237.

Martin, P. L., & Foxx, R. M. (1973). Victim control of the aggression of an institutionalized retardate. *Journal of Behavior Therapy and Experimental Psychiatry, 4*, 161–165.

Martin, R. (1981). All handicapped children are educable. *Analysis and Intervention in Developmental Disabilities, 1*, 5–11.

Martin, R. G. & Ames, B. N. (1964). Biochemical aspects of genetics. *Annual Review of Biochemistry, 33*, 235–256.

Maslow, A. H. (1954). *Motivation and personality.* New York: Harper.

Masland, R. L. (1958). The prevention of mental subnormality. In R. L. Masland, S. B. Sarason, T. Gladwin (Eds.), *Mental subnormality* (pp. 53–54). New York: Basic Books.

Mason, M. K. (1942). Learning to speak after six and one-half years of silence. *Journal of Speech Disorders, 7*, 295–304.

Matheny, A. P. (1968). Pathological echoic responses in a child: Effect of environmental mind and tact control. *Journal of Experimental Child Psychology, 6*, 624–631.

Matson, J. L., & McCartny, E. W. (1981). *Handbook of behavior modification with the mentally retarded.* New York: Plenum.

Matson, J. L., & Stephens, R. M. (1977). Overcorrection of aggressive behavior in a chronic psychiatric patient. *Behavior Modification 1*, 559–564.

Matson, J. L., Stephens, R. M., & Horne, A. M. (1976). Overcorrection and extinction—reinforcement for incompatible behavior and overcorrection. *American Journal of Mental Deficiency, 81*, 147–153.

Matson, J. L., Stephens, R. M., & Smith, C. (1978). Treatment of self-injurious behavior with overcorrection. *Journal of Mental Deficiency Research, 22*, 175–178.

Mattinson, J. (1973). Marriage and mental handicap. In F. F. de la Cruz and G. D. LaVeck (Eds.), *Human sexuality and the mentally retarded.* New York: Brunner Mazel.

Maurer, A. (1974). Corporal punishment. *American Psychologist, 29*, 614–626.

Maxfield, K. E., & Buchholz, S. (1957). *A social maturity scale for blind preschool children: A guide to its use.* New York: American Foundation for the Blind.

McAfee, R., & Cleland C. (1965). The discrepancy between self-concept and ideal self as a measure of psychological adjustment in educable mentally retarded males. *American Journal of Mental Deficiency, 80*, 63–68.

McBride, G. (1981). "Fragile" X chromosome: Major link to mental retardation. *Journal of the American Medical Association, 246*, 1631–1632.

McCall, R. B., & Melson, W. H. (1968). Attention in infants as a function of magnitude of discrepancy and habituation rate. *Psychonomic Science, 17*, 317–319.

McCandless, B. (1952). Environment and intelligence. *American Journal of Mental Deficiency, 56*, 674–691.

McCarthy, D. (1930). *The language development of the pre-school child.* (Institute of Child Welfare Monograph Series). Minneapolis: University of Minnesota Press.

McCarthy, S. (1954). Language development. In L. Carmichael (Ed.), *Manual of child psychology* (4th ed.). New York: Wiley.

McCartney, H. R., & Holden, J. C. (1981). Toilet training for the mentally retarded. In J. L. Matson &

J. R. McCartney (Eds.), *Handbook of behavior modification with the mentally retarded.* New York: Plenum.

McCarver, R., & Craig, E. (1974). Placement of the retarded in the community: Prognosis and outcome. In N. R. Ellis (Ed.), *International review of research in mental retardation* (Vol. 7). New York: Academic Press.

McClearn, G. E. (1964). Genetics and behavior development. In M. L. Hoffman and L. W. Hoffman (Eds.), *Review of child development research.* New York: Russell Sage Foundation.

McClearn, G. E. (1970). Genetic influences on behavior and development. In P. Mussen (Ed.), *Carmichael's manual of child psychology* (Vol. 1). New York: Wiley.

McClelland, D. C., Atkinson, J. W., Clark, R. A., & Lowell, E. L. (1953). *The achievement motive.* New York: Appleton-Century-Crofts.

McCormick, M., Balla, D., & Zigler, E. (1975). Resident care practices in institutions for retarded persons. *American Journal of Mental Deficiency, 80,* 1–17.

McCormick, L., Cooper, M., & Goldman, R. (1979). Training teachers to maximize instructional time provided to severely and profoundly handicapped children. *AAESPH Review, 4,* 301–310.

McCormick, L., & Goldman, R. (1979). The transdisciplinary model: Implications for service delivery and personnel preparation for the severely and profoundly handicapped *AAESPH Review, 4,* 152–161.

McCulloch, T. L. (1957). The retarded child grows up: Psychological aspects of aging. *American Journal of Mental Deficiency, 62,* 201–208.

McDevitt, S. C., Smith, D. W., & Rosen, M. (1978). Deinstitutionalized citizen: Adjustment and quality of life. *Mental Retardation, 16,* 22–24.

McFarlain, R. A., Andy, O. J., Scott, R. W., & Wheatly, M. L. (1975). Suppression of headbanging on the ward. *Psychological Reports, 36,* 315–321.

McIntire, M., Menolascino, F., & Wiley, J. (1965). Mongolism and some clinical aspects. *American Journal of Mental Deficiency, 69,* 794–800.

McIvor, W. B. (1972). Evaluation of a strategy-oriented training program on the verbal abstraction performance of EMRs. *American Journal of Mental Deficiency, 76,* 652–657.

McNemar, Q. (1942). *The revision of the Stanford-Binet scale: An analysis of the standardization data.* Boston: Houghton Mifflin.

McNemar, Q. (1964). Lost: Our intelligence? Why? *American Psychologist, 19,* 871–882.

Meeker, M. N. (1969). *The structure of intellect.* Columbus, OH: Charles E. Merrill.

Meeker, M. N. (1973). Individualized curriculum based on intelligence test patterns. In R. H. Coop & K. White (Eds.), *Psychological concepts in the classroom.* New York: Harper and Row.

Melyn, M. A., & White, D. T. (1973). Mental and developmental milestones of noninstitutionalized Down's syndrome children. *Pediatrics, 52,* 542–545.

Melnyk, J. M., & Koch, R. (1971). Genetic factors in causation. In R. Koch and J. C. Dobson (Eds.), *The mentally retarded child and his family: A multidisciplinary handbook.* New York: Brunner Mazel.

Mendels, G. E., & Flanders, J. P. (1973). Teacher expectations and pupil performance. *American Educational Research Journal, 10,* 203–212.

Menkes, J. H. (1974). *Textbook of child neurology.* Philadelphia: Lea and Febiger.

Menolascino, F. (1967). Psychiatric findings in a sample of institutionalized mongoloids. *Journal of Mental Subnormality, 13,* 67–74.

Menolascino, F. J. (1965). Emotional disturbance and mental retardation. *American Journal of Mental Deficiency, 80,* 248–256.

Menolascino, F. J. (1965). Psychiatric aspects of mongolism. *American Journal of Mental Deficiency, 69,* 653–660.

Menolascino, F. J. (1966). The facade of mental retardation: Its challenge to child psychiatry. *American Journal of Psychiatry, 122,* 1227–1235.

Merbaum, M. (1973). The modification of self-destructive behavior by a mother-therapist using aversive stimulation. *Behavior Therapy 4,* 442–447.

Mercer, J. R. (1971). The meaning of mental retardation. In R. Koch & J. C. Dobson (Eds.), *The mentally retarded child and his family. A multidisciplinary handbook* (pp. 23–48). New York: Brunner Mazel.

Mercer, J. R. (1973). *Labeling the mentally retarded.* Berkeley: University of California Press.

Mercer, J. R., & Lewis J. P. (1975). System of multicultural pluralistic assessment. Technical manual. Unpublished manuscript, University of California at Riverside.

Mesibov, G. B. (1976). Alternatives to the principle of normalization. *Mental Retardation, 14,* 30–32.

Mesibov, G. B. (1983). Current issues in autism and adolescence. In E. Schopler & G. B. Mesibov (Eds.), *Autism in adolescents and adults.* New York: Plenum.

Meyen, E. L., & Lehr, D. H. (1980). Evolving practices in assessment and intervention for mildly handicapped adolescents: The case for intensive instruction. *Exceptional Education Quarterly, 1,* 19–26.

Meyer, M. B., & Tonascia, J. A. (1977). Maternal smoking, pregnancy complications and perinatal mortality. *American Journal of Obstetrics and Gynecology, 128,* 494–502.

Meyerowitz, J. H. (1962). Self-derogation in young retardates and special class placement. *Child Development, 33,* 443–451.

Meyerowitz, J. H. (1967). Peer groups and special classes. *Mental Retardation, 5,* 23–26.

Meyers, C. E. (1971). Psychometrics. In J. Worth (Ed.), *Mental retardation and developmental disabilities* (Vol. 5). New York: Brunner Mazel.

Meyers, C. E., MacMillan, D. L., & Yoshida, R. K. (1974). Preliminary findings on the decertification of inner city EMRs. Paper presented at American Association of Mental Deficiency, Toronto.

Meyers, C. E., MacMillan, D. L., & Yoshida, R. K. (1975). *Correlation of success in transition of MR to regular class.* (Final report, grant No. 0EG-0-73-5263.) Pomona, CA: U.S. Department of Health, Education, and Welfare.

Meyers, D. G., Sinco, M. E., & Stalma, E. S. (1973). *The right-to-education child. A curriculum for the severely and profoundly mentally retarded.* Springfield, IL: Thomas.

Meyers, J. J. & Deibert, A. N. (1971). Reduction of self-abusive behavior in a blind child by using a feeding response. *Journal of Behavior Therapy and Experimental Psychiatry, 2,* 141–144.

Meyerson, L., Kere, N., & Michael, J. (1967). Behavior modification in rehabilitation. In S. W. Bijou & B. M. Baer (Eds.), *Child development: Readings in experimental analysis.* New York: Appleton-Century-Crofts.

Mickelson, P. (1947). The feebleminded parent: A study of 90 cases. *American Journal of Mental Deficiency, 51,* 644–653.

Mikkelsen, M., & Stene, J. (1970). Genetic counseling in Down's syndrome. *Human heredity, 20,* 457–464.

Milar, C. R., & Schroeder, S. R. (1983). The effects of lead on retardation of cognitive and adaptive behavior. In J. L. Matson & F. Andrasik (Eds.), *Treatment issues and innovations in mental retardation.* New York: Plenum.

Miles, R. C., Gneza, M., & Kerkay, J. (1985). A crossed immunoelectrophoretic technique for the detection of the Down's syndrome protein. *Analytical Letters, 18,* 825–835.

Milgram, N. A., & Furth, H. G. (1963). The influence of language on concept attainment in educable retarded children. *American Journal of Mental Deficiency, 67,* 733–739.

Miller, J. F., & Yoder, D. E. (1974). An ontogenetic language teaching strategy for retarded children. In R. L. Schiefelbusch & L. L. Lloyd (Eds.), *Language perspectives—acquisition, retardation, and intervention.* Baltimore: University Park Press.

Miller, J. O. (1970). Cultural deprivation and its modification: Effects of intervention. In H. C. Haywood (Ed.), *Social-cultural aspects of mental retardation.* New York: Appleton-Century-Crofts.

Miller, M. B. (1961). Locus of control, learning climate, and climate shift in serial learning with mental retardates. Unpublished doctoral dissertation, George Peabody College for Teachers, Nashville, TN.

Miller, M. H. (1967). Neuroses, psychoses, and the borderline states. In A. M. Freedman & H. I. Kaplan (Eds.), *Comprehensive textbook of psychiatry.* Baltimore: Williams and Wilkins.

Miller, R. M. (1967). Prenatal origins of mental retardation. *Journal of Pediatrics, 71,* 455.

Miller, R. V. (1956). Social status and socioempathic differences among mentally superior, mentally typical, and mentally retarded children. *Exceptional Children, 23,* 114–119.

Milunsky, A. (1975). *The prevention of genetic disease and mental retardation.* Philadelphia: Saunders.

Miniszek, N. A. (1983). Development of Alzheimer disease in Down syndrome individuals. *American Journal of Mental Deficiency, 87,* 377–385.

Minton, J., Campbell, M., Green, W. H., Jennings, S., & Samit, C. (1982). Cognitive assessment of siblings of autistic children. *Journal of the American Academy of Child Psychiatry, 21,* 256–261.

Miranda, S. B. (1976). Visual attention in defective and high-risk infants. *Merrill-Palmer Quarterly, 22,* 201–228.

Mithaug, D. E. & Hagmeier, L. D. (1978). The development of procedures to assess prevocational competencies in severely handicapped young adults. *AAESPH Review, 3,* 94–115.

Mithaug, D. E., & Haring, N. C. (1977). Community vocational and workshop placement. In N. G. Haring & L. Brown (Eds.), *Teaching the severely handicapped* (Vol. 2). New York: Grune & Stratton.

Mithaug, D. E., Mar, D. K., & Stewart, J. E. (1978). *Prevocational Assessment and Curriculum Guide.* Seattle: Exceptional Education.

Mithaug, D. E., Mar, D., Stewart, J., & McCalmon, D. (1980). Assessing prevocational competencies of profoundly, severely, and moderately retarded persons. *Journal of the Association for the Severely Handicapped. 5,* 271–284.

Mittler, P., Gillies, S., & Jukes, E. (1966). Prognosis in psychotic children: Report of a follow-up study. *Journal of Mental Deficiency Research, 10,* 73–83.

Moed, M., & Litwin, D. (1963). The employability of the cerebral palsied: A summary of two related studies. *Rehabilitation Literature, 24,* 266-271, 276.

Moerk, E. L. (1975). Paiget's research as applied to the exploration of language development. *Merrill-Palmer Quarterly, 21,* 151–170.

Molnar, G. (1974). Motor deficit of retarded infants and young children. *Archives of Physical Medicine & Rehabilitation, 55,* 393–398.

Molnar, G. E (1978). Analysis of motor disorder in retarded infants and young children. *American Journal of Mental Deficiency. 83,* 213–222.

Molnar, G. E., & Taft, L. T. (1973). Cerebral palsy. In J. Wortis (Ed.), *Mental retardation and developmental disabilities: An annual review* (Vol. 5). New York: Brunner Mazel.

Money, J. (1970). Impulse, aggression and sexuality in the XYY syndrome. *St. John's Law Review, 44,* 220–235.

Money, J. (1973). Some thoughts on sexual tension and the rights of the retarded. In F. F. de la Cruz & G. D. LaVeck (Eds.), *Human sexuality and the mentally retarded.* New York: Brunner Mazel.

Moncrieff, A. A., Koumides, O. P., Clayton, B. E., et al. (1964). Lead poisoning in children. *Archives of Diseases of Children, 39,* 1–13.

Moore, B. C., Thuline, H. C., & Capes, L. (1968). Mongoloid and nonmongoloid retardates: A behavioral comparison. *American Journal of Mental Deficiency, 73,* 433–436.

Moore, J., & Newell, A. (1974). How can Merlin understand? In L. W. Gregg (Ed.), *Knowledge and cognition.* Hillsdale, NJ: Lawrence Erlbaum.

Moore, M. G., Anderson, R. A., Fredericks, H. D., Baldwin, V. L., & Moore, W. G. (1979). *The longitudinal impact of preschool programs on trainable mentally retarded children.* Monmouth, OR: Oregon State System of Higher Education.

Morgan, C. T., & King, R. A. (1971). *Introduction to psychology* (4th ed.). New York: McGraw-Hill.

Morgan, J. B. (1979). Development and distribution of intellectual and adaptive skills in Down syndrome children: Implications for early intervention. *Mental Retardation, 17,* 247–249.

Mori, A. A., & Masters, L. F. (1980). *Teaching the severely mentally retarded adaptive skills training.* Germantown, MD: Aspen.

Morishima, A., & Brown, L. F. (1976). An idiot savant case report: A retrospective view. *Mental Retardation, 14,* 46–47.

Morishima, A., & Brown, L. F. (1977). A case report on the autistic talent of an autistic idiot savant. *Mental Retardation, 15,* 33–36.

Morris, J. L., Martin, A. J., & Nowak, M. B. (1981). Job enrichment and the mentally retarded worker. *Mental Retardation, 19,* 290–294.

Morrison, D., & Pothier, P. (1972). Two different remedial motor training programs and the development of mentally retarded preschoolers. *American Journal of Mental Deficiency, 77,* 251–285.

Moseley, A., Faust, M., & Reardon, D. M. (1970). Effects of social and non-social stimuli on the stereotyped behaviors of retarded children. *American Journal of Mental Deficiency, 74,* 809–811.

Moss, J. T., Wyatt, G., & Flora, G. (1982). Comparative teratogenicity of anticonvulsants. *Hospital Pharmacy, 17,* 230–236.

Moss, J. W. (1958). Failure-avoiding and success-striving behavior in mentally retarded and normal children. Unpublished doctoral dissertation, George Peabody College for Teachers, Nashville, TN.

Mowatt, M. H. (1970). Group therapy approach to emotional conflicts of the mentally retarded and their parents. In F. J. Menolascino (Ed.), *Psychiatric approaches to mental retardation.* New York: Basic Books.

Mulhern, T., & Baumeister, A. A. (1969). An experimental attempt to reduce stereotyping by reinforcement procedures. *American Journal of Mental Deficiency, 74,* 69–74.

Mulick, J. A., & Schroeder, S. R. (1980). Research relating to management of antisocial behavior in mentally retarded persons. *Psychological Record, 30,* 397–417.

Mulick, J. A., Schroeder, S. R., and Rojahn, J., (1980). Chronic ruminative vomiting: A comparison of four treatment procedures. *Journal of Autism and Developmental Disorders, 10,* 203–213.

Mullen, F. A., & Itkin, W. (1961). *Achievement and adjustment of educable mentally handicapped children in special classes and in regular classes.* Chicago: Chicago Board of Education.

Murphy, D. P., Shirlock, M. D. & Doll, E. A., (1942). Microcephaly following maternal pelvic irradiation for the interruption of pregnancy. *American Journal of Roentgenology, 48,* 356–359.

Murphey, R. J., Ruprecht, M. J. Baggio, P., & Nune, D. L. (1979). The use of mild punishment in combination with reinforcement of alternate behaviors to reduce to self-injurious behavior of a profoundly retarded individual. *AAESPH Review, 4,* 187–195.

Murphy, M. J., & Zahn, D. (1975). Effects of improved ward conditions and behavioral treatment on self-help skills. *Mental Retardation, 13,* 24–27.

Murray, M. A. (1959). Needs of parents of mentally retarded children. *American Journal of Mental Deficiency, 63,* 1078–1088.

Murray, S. (1972). Investigation of three teaching methods for language training. Doctoral dissertation, University of Kansas, Lawrence.

Mussen, P. H., Conger, J. J., & Kagan, J. (1963). *Child development and personality.* New York: Harper & Row.

Nadler, H. L., Inouye, T., & Hsia, D. Y. Y. (1969). Classical galactosemia. In D. Y. Y. Hsia (Ed.), *Galactosemia.* Springfield, IL: Charles C Thomas.

Naeye, R. L. (1978). Relationship of cigarette smoking to congenital anomalies and perinatal death. *American Journal of Pathology, 90,* 649–650.

Naeye, R. L. (1981). Influence of maternal cigarette smoking during pregnancy on fetal and childhood growth. *Obstetrics and Gynecology, 57,* 18–21.

Nahmias, A. J., Joesy, W. E., Naib, Z. M., Freeman, M. G., Fernandiz, R. J., & Wheeler, J. H. (1971). Perinatal risk associated with maternal genital herpes simplex virus infection. *American Journal of Obstetrics and Gynecology, 110,* 825–837.

Nahmias, A. J., & Tomeh, M. D. (1977). Herpes simplex virus infections. In A. M. Rudolph (Ed.), *Pediatrics* (16th ed.). New York: Appleton-Century-Crofts.

Nahmias, A. J., Visintine, A. M. Reimer, C. B., Buono, I. D., Shore, S. L., & Starr, S. E. (1975). Herpes simplex virus infection of the fetus and newborn. *Progress in Clinical and Biological Research, 3,* 63–77.

Nakamura, H. (1965). An inquiry into systematic differences in the abilities of institutionalized adult mongoloids. *American Journal of Mental Deficiency, 69,* 661–665.

Narot, J. R. (1973). The moral and ethical implication of human sexuality as they relate to the retarded. In F. F. de la Cruz, & G. D. LaVeck (Eds.), *Human sexuality and the mentally retarded.* New York: Brunner Mazel.

Narrol, H., & Bachor, D. G. (1975). An introduction to Feuerstein's approach to assessing and developing cognitive potential. *Interchange, 6,* 1–16.

National Institute of Child Health and Human Development. (1976). *Malnutrition, learning and behavior.* Washington: H.E.W. Publication No. 76-1036.

National Research Council, National Academy of Sciences (1972). *The effects on population of exposure to low levels of ionizing radiation.* Washington, DC: U.S. Government Printing Office.

Nawas, M. M., & Braun, S. H. (1970a). An overview of behavior modification with the severely and profoundly retarded. Part III. Maintenance of change and epilogue. *Mental Retardation, 8,* 4–11.

Nawas, M. M., & Braun, S. H. (1970b). The use of operant techniques for modifying the behavior of the severely and profoundly retarded. Part II. The techniques. *Mental Retardation, 8,* 18–24.

Nawas, M. M., & Braun, S. H. (1970c). The use of operant techniques for modifying the behavior of the severely and profoundly retarded. Part I. Introduction and initial phase. *Mental Retardation, 8,* 2–6.

Neal, L. L. (Ed.). (1970). *Recreation's role in the rehabilitation of the mentally retarded* (pp. 23–32). (Monograph No. 4.) Eugene: University of Oregon, Rehabilitation Research and Training Center in Mental Retardation.

Needleman, H. L., Gunnoe, C., Leviton, A., Reed, R., Peresie, H., Maher, C., & Barrett, B. S. (1979). Deficits in psychologic and classroom performance of children with elevated dentine lead levels. *New England Journal of Medicine, 300,* 689–695.

Neel, J. V., & Schull, W. J. (1954). *Human heredity.* Chicago: University of Chicago Press.

Neimark, E. D. (1976). The natural history of spontaneous mnemonic activity under conditions of minimal experimental constraint. In A. D. Pick (Ed.), *Minnesota symposia on child psychology* (Vol. 10). Minneapolis: University of Minnesota Press.

Neville, J. (1959). Paranoid schizophrenia in a mongoloid defective: Some theoretical considerations derived from an unusual case. *Journal of Mental Science, 105,* 444–447.

Nettelbeck, T., & Lally, M. (1976). Age, intelligence, and inspection time. *American Journal of Mental Deficiency, 83,* 398–401.

Newland, T. E. (1969). *Manual for the blind learning aptitude test: Experimental edition.* Urbana, IL: Author.

Newman, H. H., Freeman, F. N., & Holzinger, K. J. (1937). *Twins: A study of heredity and environment.* Chicago: University of Chicago Press.

Nielsen, G., Collins, S., Meisel, J., Lowry, M., Engh, H., & Johnson, D. (1975). An intervention program for atypical infants. In B. Z. Friedlander, G. M. Steritt, & G. E. Kirk (Eds.), *Exceptional infant: Vol. 3. Assessment and intervention.* New York: Brunner Mazel.

Nielsen, J. (1970). Criminality among patients with Klinefelter's syndrome and XYY syndrome. *British Journal of Psychiatry, 117,* 365–369.

Nietupski, R. (1974). Use of mouthwash. In L. Brown, W. Williams, & T. Crowner (Eds.), *A collection of papers and programs related to public school services for severely handicapped students.* Madison, WI: Madison Public Schools.

Neitupski, J., & Hamre-Nietupski, S. (1979). Teaching auxiliary communication skills to severely handicapped students. *AAESPH Review, 4,* 107–124.

Nigro, G. (1975). Sexuality in the handicapped: Some observations on human needs. *Rehabilitation Literature, 36,* 202–205.

Nihira, K. (1976). Dimensions of adaptive behavior in institutionalized mentally retarded children and adults: Developmental perspective. *American Journal of Mental Deficiency, 81,* 215–226.

Nihira, K., Foster, R., Shellhaas, M., & Leland, H., (1969). *Adaptive Behavior Scales: Manual.* Washington: American Association on Mental Deficiency.

Nirje, B. (1969). The normalization principle and its human management implications. In R. Kugel & W. Wolfensberger (Eds.), *Changing patterns in residential services for the mentally retarded.* Washington: President's Committee on Mental Retardation.

Niswander, K. R. & Gordon, M. (1972). *The women and their pregnancies.* (Vol. 1). Philadelphia: Saunders.

Nitowsky, G. M. (1975). Heterozygote detection in autosomal recessive biochemical disorders associated with mental retardation. In A. Milunsky (Ed.), *The prevention of genetic disease and mental retardation.* Philadelphia: Saunders.

Nixon, R. A. (1970). Impact of automation and technological change in employability of the mentally retarded. *American Journal of Mental Deficiency, 75,* 152–155.

Noel, B., Duport, J. P., Revil, D., Dussuyer, & Quack, B. (1974). The XYY syndrome: Reality or myth? *Clinical Genetics, J.* 387–394.

Nolley, D., Boelkins, D., Lubomira, K., Moore, M. K. Goncalves, S., & Lewis, M. (1980). Aversive conditioning within laws and guidelines in a state facility for mentally retarded individuals. *Mental Retardation, 18,* 295-298.

Nyhan, W. L. (1977). Disorders of amino acid metabolism. In A. M. Rudolph (Ed.), *Pediatrics* (16th ed.). New York: Appleton-Century-Crofts.

Nyhan, W. L. (1978). Nonketotic hyperglycinemia. In J. B. Stanbury, J. B. Wyngaarden, D. S. Frederickson (Eds.), *The metabolic basis of inherited disease* (4th ed.). New York: McGraw-Hill.

Nyhan, W. L. & Sakati, N. O. (1976). *Genetic and malformation syndromes in clinical medicine.* Chicago: Year Book Medical Publishers.

O'Brien, F. (1981). Treating self-stimulating behavior. In J. L. Matson & J. R. McCartney (Eds.), *Handbook of behavior modification with the mentally retarded.* New York and London: Plenum.

O'Brien, F., Bugle, C., & Azrin, N. H. (1972). Teaching correct eating to the mentally retarded: Reinforcement and extinction. *Journal of Applied Behavior Analysis, 5,* 67–72.

O'Connor, G. (1976). *Home is a good place: A national perspective of community residential facilities for developmentally disabled persons.* Washington: American Association on Mental Deficiency.

O'Connor, N., & Hermelin, B. (1961). Visual and stereognostic shape recognition in normal children and Mongol and non-Mongol imbeciles. *Journal of Mental Deficiency Research, 5,* 63–66.

Office of Mental Retardation Coordination. (1972). Mental retardation institutional data. *Programs for the handicapped.* Washington: U.S. Department of Health, Education, and Welfare, March 23, pp. 2–14.

Ollendick, T. H., Matson, J. L., & Martin, J. E. (1978). Effectiveness of hand overcorrection for topographically similar and dissimilar self-stimulatory behavior. *Journal of Experimental Child Psychology, 25,* 396-403.

O'Neill, C. T., & Bellamy, G. T. (1978). Evaluation of a procedure for teaching saw chain assembly to a severely retarded woman. *Mental Retardation, 16,* 37–41.

Orenstein, W. A., & Greaves, W. L. (1982). Congenital rubella syndrome: A continuing problem. *Journal of the American Medical Association, 247,* 1174–1175.

Ornitz, E. M., & Ritvo, E. R. (1968). Neurophysiologic mechanisms underlying perceptual inconstancy in autistic and schizophrenic children. *Archives of General Psychiatry, 19,* 22.

Orzack, L. H., Salloway, J., Cassell, J., Charland, B., & Halliday, H. (1969). *Residential programming and residential centers for the mentally retarded: The experience in Bridgeport.* Bridgeport, CT: Parents and Friends of Mentally Retarded Children of Bridgeport, Inc., Monograph No. 3, *On the pursuit of change* series, May 1969.

Osgood, C. E., Suci, G. J. & Tannenbaum, P. H. (1957). *The measurement of meaning.* Urbana, IL: University of Illinois Press.

Oster, J. (1953). *Mongolism.* Copenhagen: Danish Science press.

Ovellette, E. M., Rosett, H. L., Rosman, N. P., & Weiner, L. (1977). Adverse effects on offspring of maternal alcohol abuse during pregnancy. *New England Journal of Medicine, 297,* 528–530.

Owens, D., Dawson, J.C., and Losin, S. (1971). Alzheimer's disease in Down's syndrome. *American Journal of Mental Deficiency, 75,* 606–612.

Page, E. B. (1972). Miracle in Milwaukee. Raising the IQ. *Educational Research, 1,* 8–16.

Pai, A. C. (1974). *Foundations of genetics.* New York: McGraw-Hill.

Paine, R. S. (1957). Variability in manifestations of untreated patients with phenylketonuria (phenylpyruvic aciduria). *Pediatrics, 20,* 290–302.

Paine, R. S. (1964). Evolution of postural reflexes in normal infants and in the presence of chronic brain syndromes. *Neurology, 14,* 1036–1048.

Paloutzian, R. F., Hasazi, J., Streifel, J., & Edgar G. L. (1971). Promotion of positive social interaction in severely retarded young children. *American Journal of Mental Deficiency, 75,* 519–524.

Paluck, R. J., & Esser, A. H. (1971a). Controlled experimental modification of aggressive behavior in territories of severely retarded boys. *American Journal of Mental Deficiency, 76,* 23–29.

Paluck, R. J., & Esser, A. H. (1971b). Territorial behavior as an indicator of changes in clinical condition of severely retarded boys. *American Journal of Mental Deficiency, 76,* 284–290.

Palyo, W. J., Schuler, A. L., Cooke, T. P., & Apolloni, T. (1979). Modifying echolalic speech in preschool children: Training and generalization. *American Journal of Mental Deficiency, 83,* 480–489.

Pantelaskis, S. H., Chryssostomidov, D., Alexiou, D., Valaes, T., & Doxiadis, S. A. (1970). Sex chromatin and chromosome abnormalities among 10,412 liveborn babies. *Archives of Diseases of Childhood, 45,* 87–92.

Parmelee, A. H., & Michaelis, R. (1971). Neurological examination of the newborn. In J. Hellmuth (Ed.), *Exceptional infant: Vol. 2, Studies of abnormalities.* New York: Brunner Mazel.

Partington, M. W. (1962). Variations in intelligence in phenylketonuria. *Canadian Medical Association Journal, 86,* 736–743.

Pasqualini, R. Q. (1957). Psychopathology of Klinefelter's syndrome: Review of twenty-one cases. *Lancet, 2,* 164–167.

Patau, K., Smith, D. W., Therman, E., Inhorn, S. L., & Wagner, H. P. (1960). Multiple congenital anomaly caused by an extra chromosome. *Lancet, 1,* 790.

Paul, J. L., Turnbull, A. P., & Cruickshank, W. M. (1977). *Mainstreaming: A practical guide.* Syracuse, N.Y.: Syracuse University Press.

Paul, J. L. (1981). Mainstreaming: Review of research on the pros and cons of mainstreaming. Paper presented at meeting of Quebec Association for Children with Learning Disabilities, Montreal.

Paulus, A. C. (1966). A tool for the assessment of the retarded child at home. *Nursing Clinics of North America, 1,* 659.

Payne, J. S. (1971). Prevalence survey of severely mentally retarded in Wyandotte County, Kansas. *Training School Bulletin, 67,* 220–227.

Payne, J. S., & Patton, J. R. (1981). *Mental retardation.* Columbus, OH: Merrill.

Peck, J. R. & Stephens, W. B. (1965). Marriages of young male retardates. *American Journal of Mental Deficiency, 69,* 818–827.

Pei, M. (1965). *The story of language.* Philadelphia: Lippincott.

Pelosi, M. A., Frattarola, M., Apuzzio, J., Lancer, A., Cheng, T. H., Oleske, J. M., Bai, J., & Harrigan, J. T. (1975). Pregnancy complicated by heroin addiction. *Obstetrics and Gynecology, 45,* 512–515.

Pendergrass, V. E. (1972). Timeout from positive reinforcement following persistent, high-rate behavior in retardates. *Journal of Applied Behavior Analysis, 5,* 85–91.

Peniston, E. (1975). Reducing problem behaviors in the severely and profoundly retarded. *Journal of Behavior Therapy and Experimental Psychiatry, 6,* 295–299.

Penrose, L. S. (1938). *A clinical and genetic study of 1,280 cases of mental defect.* London: Medical Research Council.

Penrose, L. A. (1954). *The biology of mental defect.* London: Sidgwick and Jackson.

Perline, I. H., & Levinsky, D. (1968). Controlling maladaptive classroom behavior in the severely retarded. *American Journal of Mental Deficiency, 73,* 74–78.

Perry, T. L., Hansen, S., Tischler, B., Richards, F. M., & Sokol, M. (1973). Unrecognized adult phenylketonuria: Implications for obstetrics and psychiatry. *New England Journal of Medicine, 289,* 395–398.

Perske, R. (1979). *Mental retardation: The leading edge.* (Report of the President's Committee on Mental Retardation.) Washington: U.S. Government Printing Office, DHEW Publication No. (OHDS) 79-21018.

Peterson, D. D. (1972). Children with physical handicaps and multiple handicaps. In B. R. Gearheart (Ed.), in association with the late T. D. Vaughan, *Education of the exceptional child: History, present practices, and trends.* Scranton, PA: Intext.

Peterson, N. L., & Haralick, J. G. (1977). Integration of handicapped preschoolers: An analysis of play and social intereaction. *Education and Training of the Mentally Retarded, 12,* 235-245.

Peterson, R. F., & Peterson, L. R. (1968). The use of positive reinforcement in the control of self-destructive behavior in a retarded boy. *Journal of Experimental Child Psychology, 6,* 351-360.

Peterson, R. O., & Jones, E. M. (1964). *Guide to jobs for the mentally retarded.* Pittsburgh: American Institute for Research.

Phibbs, R. H. (1977). Hemolytic disease of the newborn (erythroblastosis fetalis). In A. M. Rudolph (Ed.), *Pediatrics* (16th ed.). New York: Appleton-Century-Crofts.

Phibbs, R. H. (1977). The newborn infant. In A. M. Rudolph (Ed.), *Pediatrics* (16th ed.). New York: Appleton-Century-Crofts.

Phillips, I. (1966). Children, mental retardation, and emotional disorder. In I. Phillips (Ed.), *Prevention and treatment of mental retardation.* New York: Basic Books.

Piaget, J. (1970). Piaget's theory. In P. H. Mussen (Ed.), *Carmichael's manual of child psychology.* (3rd ed., Vol. 1, pp. 703-732). New York: Wiley.

Picker, M., Poling, A., & Parker, A. (1979). A review of children's self-injurious behavior. *Psychological Record, 29,* 435-452.

Pickup, J., & Arsenault, P. (1976). The reduction of chronic regurgitation in a profoundly retarded individual using a multi-therapeutic paradigm. *Research and the Retarded, 3,* 82-87.

Pierce, L. (1972). Teaching time-telling. In L. Brown and E. Sontag (Eds.), *Toward the development and implementation of an empirically based public school program for trainable mentally retarded and severely emotionally disturbed students.* Madison, WI: Madison Public Schools.

Piers, E. V., & Harris, D. B. (1964). Age and other correlates of self-concept in children. *Journal of Educational Psychology, 55,* 91-95.

Pincus, J. G. & Tucker, G. (1974). *Behavioral neurology.* New York: Oxford University Press.

Pinneau, S. R. (1961). *Changes in intelligence quotient, infancy to maturity.* Boston: Houghton Mifflin.

Pitfield, M., & Oppenheim, A. N. (1964). Child rearing attitudes of mothers of psychotic children. *Journal of Child Psychology and Psychiatry, 5,* 51-57.

Poling, A., & Ryan, C. (1977). The use of brief timeout to control physical assaults: A case study. *Mental Retardation Bulletin, 5,* 136-142.

Pollack, M. (1967). Mental subnormality and childhood schizophrenia. In P. H. Hoch & J. Zubin (Eds.), *Psychopathology of mental development.* New York: Grune and Stratton.

Pollard, A., Hall, H., & Keeran, C. (1979). Community service planning. In P. R. Magrab & J. O. Elder (Eds.), *Planning for services to handicapped persons. Community, education, health.* Baltimore: Brookes.

Pollitt, E., & Eichler, A. (1976). Behavioral disturbances among failure to thrive children. *American Journal of Diseases of Children, 130,* 24-29.

Pollock, H. M. (1944). Mental disease among mental defectives. *American Journal of Psychiatry, 101,* 361-363.

Polvinale, R. A. & Lutzker, J. R. (1980). Elimination of assaultive and inappropriate sexual behavior by reinforcement and social restitution. *Mental Retardation, 18,* 27-30.

Pomeroy, J. (1964). *Recreation for the physically handicapped.* New York: Macmillan.

Porteus, S. D. (1950). *The Porteus maze test and intelligence.* Palo Alto, CA: Pacific Books.

Pototzky, C., & Grigg, A. (1942). A revision of the prognosis in mongolism. *American Journal of Orthopsychiatry, 12,* 503-510.

Pratt, M., Bumstead, D., & Raynes, N. (1976). Attendant staff speech to the institutionalized retarded: Language use as a measure of the quality of care. *Journal of Child Psychology and Psychiatry, 17,* 133-143.

Pratt, M. W. Luszcz, M. A., & Brown, M. E. (1980). Measuring dimensions of the quality of care in small community residences. *American Journal of Mental Deficiency, 85,* 188-194.

Prechtl, H., & Beintema, O. (1964). *The neurological examination of the full term newborn infant.* London: Heinemann.

Premack, D. (1971). Language in chimpanzees. *Science, 172,* 808–822.

President's Committee on Mental Retardation. (1967). *A first report on the nation's progress and remaining great needs in the campaign to combat mental retardation.* Washington: U.S. Government Printing Office.

President's Committee on Mental Retardation. (1978). *Mental retardation: The leading edge.* Washington: U.S. Govt. Printing Office, Publication No. (OHDS) 79-21018.

Prior, M. R., & Bradshaw, J. L. (1979). Hemisphere functioning in autistic children. *Cortex, 15,* 73–81.

Programs for Handicapped. (1971). Camp Hidden Valley. *Journal of Health, Physical Education and Recreation, 42,* 73–74.

Provence, S., & Lipton, R. C. (1962). *Infants in institutions: A comparison of their development with family-reared infants during the first year of life.* New York: International Universities Press.

Quay, L. C. (1963). Academic skills. In N. R. Ellis (Ed.), *Handbook of mental deficiency* (pp. 664–690). New York: McGraw-Hill.

Quaytman, W. (1953). The psychological capacities of mongoloid children in a community clinic. *Quarterly Review of Pediatrics, 8,* 255–267.

Radin, N. (1969). The impact of a kindergarten home counseling program. *Exceptional Children, 36,* 251–256.

Radin, N. (1972). Three degrees of maternal involvement in a preschool program: Impact on mothers and children. *Child Development, 43,* 1355–1364.

Raech, H. (1966). A parent discusses initial counseling. *Mental Retardation, 4,* 25–26.

Rago, W. V. (1978). Stability of territorial and aggressive behavior in profoundly mentally retarded institutionalized male adults. *American Journal of Mental Deficiency, 82,* 494–498.

Ramey, C. T. (1980). Social consequences of ecological intervention that began in infancy. In S. Harel (Ed.) The at-risk infant, *Excerpta Medica,* 440–443.

Ramey, C. T., & Campbell, F. A. (1979a). Early childhood education for psychosocially disadvantaged children: Effects on psychological processes. *American Journal of Mental Deficiency, 83,* 645–648.

Ramey, C. T., & Campbell, F. A. (1979b). *Educational intervention for children at risk for mild retardation. A longitudinal analysis.* Research report of Carolina Abecedarian Project, Frank Portor Graham Child Development Center, University of North Carolina at Chapel Hill, Chapel Hill, NC 27514.

Ramey, C. T., Campbell, F. A., & Wasik, B. H. (1982). Use of standardized tests to evaluate early childhood special education programs. *Topics in Early Childhood Special Education, 1,* 51–60.

Rarick, G. L., Dobbins, D. A., & Broadhead, G. D. (1976). *The motor domain and its correlates in educationally handicapped children.* Englewood Cliffs, NJ: Prentice-Hall.

Raynes, N. V. (1977). How big is good? The case for cross-cutting ties. *Mental Retardation, 15,* 53–54.

Reed, E. W., & Reed, S. C. (1965). *Mental retardation: A family study.* Philadelphia: Saunders.

Reed, S. C. (1955). *Counseling in medical genetics.* Philadelphia: Saunders.

Reid, A. H., & Leonard, A. (1977). Lithium treatment of cyclical vomiting in a mentally defective patient. *British Journal of Psychiatry, 130,* 316.

Reiss, I. L. (1973). Changing trends, attitudes and values on pre-marital sexual behavior in the United States. In F. F. de la Cruz and G. D. LaVeck (Eds.), *Human sexuality and the mentally retarded.* New York: Brunner Mazel.

Reiss, S., Levitan, G. W., & McNally, R. J. (1982). Emotionally disturbed mentally retarded people: An underserved population. *American Psychologist, 37,* 361–367.

Repp, A. C., & Deitz, D. E. D. (1978). On the selective use of punishment. Suggested guidelines for administrators. *Mental Retardation, 16,* 200–254.

Repp, A. C., & Deitz, S. M. (1974). Reducing aggressive and self-injurious behavior of institutionalized retarded children through reinforcement of other behaviors. *Journal of Applied Behavior Analysis, 7,* 313–325.

Repp, A. C., Deitz, S. M., & Speir, N. C. (1974). Reducing stereotypic responding of retarded persons by the differential reinforcement of other behavior. *American Journal of Mental Deficiency, 79,* 279–284.

Reschly, D. J., & Jipson, F. J. (1976). Ethnicity, geographic locale, age, sex, and urban-rural residence as variables in the prevalence of mild retardation. *American Journal of Mental Deficiency, 81,* 154–161.

Resnick, L. B., & Glaser, R. (1976). Problem solving and intelligence. In L. B. Resnick (Ed.), *The nature of intelligence.* Hillsdale, NJ: Erlbaum.

Revell, W. G., Jr., Wehman, P., & Arnold, S. (1984). Supported work model of competitive employment for persons with mental retardation. *Journal of Rehabilitation, 50,* 33–38.

Reynell, J., & Zinkin, P. (1975). New procedures for the developmental assessment of young children with severe visual handicaps. *Child Care and Health Development, 1,* 69–75.

Reynolds, W. M., & Reynolds, S. (1979). Prevalence of speech and hearing impairment of noninstitutionalized mentally retarded adults. *American Journal of Mental Deficiency, 84,* 62–66.

Rheingold, H. L. (1960). The measurement of maternal care. *Child Development, 31,* 565–575.

Rheingold, H. L. (1961). The effect of environmental stimulation upon social and exploratory behavior in the human infant. In B. M. Foss (Ed.), *Determinants of infant behavior* (pp. 143–177). New York: Wiley.

Ricci, C. S. (1970). Analysis of child-rearing attitudes of mothers of retarded, emotionally disturbed, and normal children. *American Journal of Mental Deficiency, 74,* 756–761.

Richards, B. W., & Sylvester, P. E. (1969). Mortality trends in mental deficiency institutions. *Journal of Mental Deficiency Research, 13,* 276–292.

Richardson, S. A. (1978). Careers of mentally retarded young persons: Services, jobs, and interpersonal relations. *American Journal of Mental Deficiency, 82,* 349–358.

Richardson, S. A., Koller, H., & Katz, M. (1985). Relationship of upbringing to later behavior disturbance of mildly mentally retarded young people. *American Journal of Mental Deficiency, 90,* 1–8.

Richardson, S. A., Koller, H., Katz, M., & McLaren, J. (1981). A functional classification of seizures and its distribution in a mentally retarded population. *American Journal of Mental Deficiency, 85,* 457–466.

Richmond, G., & Martin, P. (1977). Punishment as a therapeutic method with institutionalized retarded persons. In T. Thompson & J. Grabowski (Eds.), *Behavior modification of the mentally retarded* (2nd ed.). New York: Oxford University Press.

Richmond, J., & Eddy, E. (1957). Rumination: A psychosomatic syndrome. *Psychiatric Research Reports, 8,* 1–11.

Richmond, J., Eddy, E., & Green, M. (1958). Rumination: A psychosomatic syndrome in infancy. *Pediatrics, 22,* 49–55.

Ricks, D. M., & Wing, L. (1976). Language, communication and the use of symbols. In L. Wing (Ed.), *Early childhood autism* (2nd ed.). New York: Pergamon.

Rimland, B. (1971). High dosage levels of certain vitamins in the treatment of children with severe mental disorders. In D. R. Hawkins and L. Pauling (Eds.), *Orthomolecular Psychiatry.* San Francisco: Freeman.

Rincover, A. (1976). Sensory extinction: A procedure for eliminating self-stimulatory behavior in psychotic children. *Journal of Abnormal Child Psychology, 6,* 299–310.

Rincover, A., Cook, R., Peoples, A., & Packard, D. (1979). Sensory extinction and sensory reinforcement principles for programming multiple adaptive behavior change. *Journal of Applied Behavior Analysis, 12,* 221–233.

Rincover, A., & Devany, J. (1982). The application of sensory extinction procedures to self-injury. *Analysis and Intervention in Developmental Disabilities, 2,* 67–81.

Ringelheim, D. (1958). Effects of internal and external reinforcements on expectancies of mentally retarded and normal boys. Unpublished doctoral dissertation, George Peabody College for Teachers, Nashville, TN.

Ringness, T. (1961). Self-concept of children of low, average, and high intelligence. *American Journal of Mental Deficiency, 65,* 453–461.

Risley, T. R., & Wolf, M. M. (1967). Establishing functional speech in echolalic children. *Behavior Research and Therapy, 5,* 73–88.

Rivinus, T. M. (1980). Psychopharmacology and the mentally retarded patient. In L. S. Szymanski &

P. E. Tanguay (Eds.), *Emotional disorders of mentally retarded persons.* Baltimore: University Park Press.

Rivinus, T. M., & Harmatz, J. S. (1979). Diagnosis and lithium treatment of affective disorder in the retarded: Five case studies. *American Journal of Psychiatry, 136,* 551–554.

Roberts, J. A. F. (1952). The genetics of mental deficiency. *Eugenics Review, 44,* 71–83.

Roberts, P., Iwata, B. A., McSween, T. E., & Desmond, E. F., Jr. (1979). An analysis of overcorrection movements. *American Journal of Mental Deficiency, 83,* 588–594.

Robinson, C. C. (1976). Application of Piagetian sensori-motor concepts to assessment and curriculum for severely handicapped children. *AAESPH Review, 1,* 5–10.

Robinson, N. M., & Robinson, H. B. (1976). *The mentally retarded child: A psychological approach.* (2nd ed.). New York: McGraw-Hill.

Robinson-Wilson, M. A. (1976). Picture recipe cards as an approach to teaching severely retarded adults to cook. In G. T. Bellamy (Ed.), *Habilitation of the severely and profoundly retarded: Reports from the specialized training program* (pp. 99–108). Eugene, OR: University of Oregon Press.

Rodee, M. (1971). A study to evaluate the resource teacher concept when used with high level educable retardates at a primary level. Unpublished doctoral dissertation, University of Iowa, Iowa City.

Rogers, C. R. (1951). *Client-centered therapy.* New York: Houghton Mifflin.

Rogers, S. J. (1982). Assessment considerations with the motor-handicapped child. In G. Ulrey & S. J. Rogers (Eds.), *Psychological assessment of handicapped infants and young children.* New York: Thieme-Stratton.

Rogers, S. J., & Soper, E. (1982). Assessment considerations with hearing impaired preschoolers. In G. Ulrey & S. J. Rogers (Eds.), *Psychological assessment of handicapped infants and young children.* New York: Thieme-Stratton.

Rogers-Warren, A., & Baer, D. M. (1976). An analysis of two naturally covarying behaviors: Activity level and inappropriateness. Paper presented at American Psychological Association, Washington, DC. (ERIC Document Reproduction Service No. ED 136-473.)

Rohwer, W. D., Jr. (1968). Mental mnemonics in early learning. *The Record* (Teachers College), *70,* 213–216.

Rojahn, J., Mulick, J. A., McCoy, D., & Schroeder, S. R. (1978). Setting effects, adaptive clothing and the modification of head-banging and self-restraint in two profoundly retarded adults. *Behavioral Analysis and Modification, 2,* 185–196.

Rojahn, J., Mulick, J., & Schroeder, S. R. (1979). *Analysis of generalization and setting effects during overcorrection to control pica in two retarded adults.* Paper presented at the twelfth annual Gatlinburg Conference in Mental Retardation, Gulf Shores, AL.

Rojahn, J., Schroeder, S. R., & Mulick, J. A. (1980). Ecological assessment of self-protective devices in three profoundly retarded adults. *Journal of Autism and Developmental Disorders, 10,* 59–66.

Rollin, H. R. (1946). Personality in mongolism with special reference to incidence of catatonic psychosis. *American Journal of Mental Deficiency, 51,* 219–233.

Rollings, J. P., Baumeister, A. A., & Baumeister, A. A. (1977). The use of overcorrection procedures to eliminate the stereotype behaviors of retarded individuals. Analysis of collateral behaviors and generalization of suppressive effects. *Behavior Modification, 1,* 29–46.

Roos, P. (1965). Development of an intensive habit-training unit at Austin State School. *Mental Retardation, 3,* 12–15.

Roos, P. (1969). Psychological counseling with parents of retarded children. *Mental Retardation, 1,* 345–350.

Roos, P. (1973). Basic facts about mental retardation. In B. Ennis & P. Friedman (Eds.), *Legal rights of the mentally handicapped.* New York: Avon.

Rose, T. L. (1979). Reducing self-injurious behavior by differentially reinforcing other behaviors. *AAESPH Review, 4,* 179–186.

Rosecrans, C. J. (1968). The relationship of normal/21-trisomy mosaicism and intellectual development. *American Journal of Mental Deficiency, 72,* 562–566.

Rosen, M. (1972). Psychosexual adjustment of the mentally handicapped. In M. Bass (Ed.), *Sexual rights and responsibilities of the mentally retarded.* Proceedings of the American Association on Mental Deficiency, Region II, Newark, DE.

Rosen, M., Clark, G. R., & Kivitz, M. J. (1977). *Habilitation of the handicapped.* Baltimore: University Park Press.

Rosen, T. S., & Pippenger, C. E. (1976). Pharmacologic observation of the neonatal withdrawal syndrome. *Journal of Pediatrics, 88,* 1044–1048.

Rosenberg, L. E. (1977). Disorders of propronate, methylmalonate, and cabalamin metabolism. In A. M. Rudolph (Ed.), *Pediatrics* (16th ed.). New York: Appleton-Century-Crofts.

Rosenthal, R., & Jacobson, L. (1968). *Pygmalion in the classroom: Teacher expectations and pupils' intellectual development.* New York: Holt, Rinehart, and Winston.

Rosenthal, T. L., & Kellogg, J. S. (1973). Demonstration versus instructions in concept attainment by mental retardates. *Behavior Research and Therapy, 11,* 299–302.

Ross, A. O. (1964). *The exceptional child in the family: Helping parents of exceptional children.* New York: Grune & Stratton.

Ross, A. O. (1981). *Child behavior therapy.* New York: Wiley.

Ross, D. M., & Ross, S. A. (1976). *Hyperactivity: Research, theory, and action.* New York: Wiley.

Rossi, E. L. (1963). Associative clustering in normal and retarded children. *American Journal of Mental Deficiency, 67,* 691–699.

Rothman, D. J. (1979). Can de-institutionalization succeed? *New York University Quarterly, 11,* 16–22.

Rourke, R. J. (1971). A share of summer fun. (Programs for the handicapped.) *Journal of Health, Physical Education, and Recreation, 42,* 71–72.

Rowitz, L. (1980). Mental health services for the mentally retarded individual. In W. Silverman (Ed.), *A community mental health source book for professional action.* New York: Praeger.

Rubin, E. J., & Monaghan, S. (1965). Calendar calculation in a multiple-handicapped blind person. *American Journal of Mental Deficiency, 70,* 478–485.

Rubinstein, J. H., & Warkany, J. (1976). In J. Wortis (Ed.), *Mental retardation and developmental disabilities: An annual review* (Vol. VIII). New York: Brunner Mazel.

Rucker, C. N. (1968). Acceptance of mentally retarded junior high school children in academic and non-academic classes. *Dissertation Abstracts, 28,* 3038–3039.

Rucker, C. N., Howe, C. E., & Snider, B. (1969). The acceptance of retarded children in junior high academic and non-academic regular classes. *Exceptional Children, 35,* 617–623.

Ruder, K. F., & Smith, M. D. (1974). Issues in language training. In R. L. Schiefelbusch & L. L. Lloyd (Eds.), *Language perspectives—acquisition, retardation and intervention.* Baltimore: University Park Press.

Rugh, R. (1958). X-irradiation effects on the human fetus. *Journal of Pediatrics, 52,* 531–538.

Rummo, J. H., Routh, D. K., Rummo, N. J., & Brown, J. F. (1979). Behavioral and neurological effects of symptomatic and asymptomatic lead exposure in children. *Archives of Environmental Health, 34,* 120–124.

Rusch, F. R. (1979). Toward the validation of social/vocational survival skills. *Mental Retardation, 17,* 143–145.

Rusch, F., Clove, D., Hops, H., & Agosta, J. (1976). Overcorrection: Generalization and maintenance. *Journal of Applied Behavior Analysis, 9,* 498.

Rutter, M. (1966a). Prognosis: Psychotic children in adolescence and early adult life. In J. K. Wing (Ed.), *Early childhood autism.* London: Pergamon Press.

Rutter, M. (1966b). Behavioral and cognitive characteristics. In J. K. Wing (Ed.), *Early childhood autism* (1st ed.). Oxford, England: Pergamon.

Rutter, M. (1970). Autistic children: Infancy to adulthood. *Seminars in Psychiatry, 2,* 435.

Rutter, M. (1972). Psychiatric causes of language retardation. In M. Rutter and J. R. M. Martin (Eds.), *The child with delayed speech.* Philadelphia: Lippincott.

Rutter, M., Bartak, L., & Newman, S. (1971). Autism—A central disorder of cognition and language? In M. Rutter (Ed.), *Infantile autism: Concepts, characteristics and treatment.* London: Churchill.

Rutter, M., & Bax, M. (1972). Normal development of speech and language. In M. Rutter & J. A. M. Martin (Eds.), *The child with delayed speech.* Philadelphia: Lippincott.

Rutter, M., & Lockyer, L. (1967). A five to fifteen year follow-up study of infantile psychosis. I. Description of the sample. *British Journal of Psychiatry, 113,* 1169-1182.

Rutter, M., Tizard, J., & Whitmore, K. (1970). *Education, health and behavior.* London: Longman.

Ryckman, D. B., & Henderson, R. A. (1969). The meaning of a retarded child for his parents: A focus for counselors. *Mental Retardation, 3,* 4-7.

Rynders, J. E., & Horrobin, J. M. (1975). Project EDGE: The University of Minnesota's Communication Stimulation Program for Down's Syndrome Infants. In B. Z. Friedlander, G. M. Sterrit, & G. E. Kirk (Eds.), *Exceptional infant: Vol. 3. Assessment and intervention.* New York: Brunner Mazel.

Rynders, J. E., & Horrobin, J. M. (1980). Educational provisions for young children with Down's syndrome. In J. Gottlieb (Ed.), *Educating mentally retarded persons in the mainstream.* Baltimore: University Park Press.

Rynders, J. E., Spiker, D., & Horrobin, J. M. (1978). Underestimating the educability of Down's syndrome children: Examination of methodological problems in recent literature. *American Journal of Mental Deficiency, 82,* 440-448.

Sabagh, G., & Edgerton, R. B. (1962). Sterilized mental defectives look at eugenic sterilization. *Eugenics Quarterly, 9,* 213-222.

Sadler, W., & Merkert, F. (1977). Evaluating the Foxx and Azrin toilet training procedure for retarded children in a day training center. *Behavior Therapy, 8,* 499-500.

Saegert, S. (1976). Stress-inducing and reducing qualities of environments. In M. M. Proshansky, W. H. Ittelson, & L. G. Rivlin (Eds.), *Environmental psychology, people and their physical setting.* New York: Holt, Rinehart, and Winston.

Saenger, G. (1957). *The adjustment of severely retarded adults in the community.* Albany, NY: Interdepartmental Health Resources Board.

Sajwaj, T., & Hedges, D. (1971). *"Side-effects" of a punishment procedure in an oppositional retarded child.* Paper presented at Western Psychological Association, San Francisco.

Sajwaj, T., Libet, J., & Agras, S. (1974). Lemon juice therapy: The control of life-threatening rumination in a six-month-old infant. *Journal of Applied Behavior Analysis, 1,* 557-566.

Salvia, J., Clark, G. M., & Ysseldyke, J. E. (1973). Teacher retention of stereotypes of exceptionality. *Exceptional Children, 29,* 651-652.

Salvia, J., & Ysseldyke, J. E. (1978). *Assessment in special and remedial education.* Boston: Houghton Mifflin.

Sameroff, A. J., & Chandler, M. J. (1975). Reproductive risk and the continuum of caretaking casualty. In F. D. Horowitz (Ed.), *Review of child development research* (Vol. 4). Chicago: University of Chicago Press.

Sanford, A. (1973). *Learning Accomplishment Profile (LAP).* Chapel Hill, NC: Chapel Hill Training-Outreach Project.

Sanger, R. G. (1975). Facial and oral manifestations of Down's syndrome. In R. Koch and F. de la Cruz (Eds.), *Down's syndrome (mongolism): Research, prevention and management.* New York: Brunner Mazel.

Sarason, S. B. (1949). *Psychological problems in mental deficiency.* New York: Harper and Row.

Sarason, S. B. (1959). *Psychological problems in mental deficiency* (3rd ed.). New York: Harper and Brothers.

Sarason, S. B., & Doris, J. (1969). *Psychological problems in mental deficiency* (pp. 380-381). New York: Harper and Row.

Sarason, S. B., & Gladwin, T. (1958). Psychological and cultural problems in mental subnormality. In R. L. Masland, S. B. Sarason, & T. Gladwin (Eds.), *Mental subnormality.* New York: Basic Books.

Sardeman, H., Madsen, K. S., & Friis-Hansen, B. (1976). Follow-up of children of drug-addicted mothers. *Archives of Diseases in Children, 51,* 313-314.

Satter, G., & McGee, E. (1954). Retarded adults who have developed beyond expectation: I. Intellectual functions. *Training School Bulletin, 51,* 43-55.

Sattler, J. M. (1974). *Assessment of children's intelligence.* Philadelphia: Saunders.

Scally, B. G. (1968). The offspring of mental defectives. In D. H. Woolam (Ed.), *Advances in teratology* (Vol. 3). London: Logos Press.

Scally, B. G. (1973). Marriage and mental handicap: Some observations in Northern Ireland. In F. F. de la Cruz and G. D. LaVeck (Eds.), *Human sexuality and the mentally retarded*. New York: Brunner Mazel.

Scarr, S. (1985). Constructing psychology. *American Psychologist, 40,* 499–512.

Scarr, S., & McCartney, K. (1983). How people make their own environments: A theory of genotype—environmental effects. *Child Development, 44,* 424–435.

Scarr, S., & Weinberg, R. A. (1976). IQ test performance of black children adopted by white families. *American Psychologist, 31,* 726–739.

Scarr-Salapatek, S. (1975). Genetics and the development of intelligence. In F. D. Horowitz (Ed.), *Review of child development research* (Vol. 4). Chicago: University of Chicago Press.

Schaefer, E. S. (1968). *Progress report: Intellectual stimulation of culturally-deprived parents.* Washington: National Institute of Mental Health.

Schaefer, E. S. (1970). Need for early and continuing education. In V. H. Denenberg (Ed.), *Education of the infant and young child.* New York: Academic Press.

Schaefer, E. S., & Aaronson, M. (1972). Infant education research project: Implementation and implications of the home-tutoring program. In R. K. Parker (Ed.), *The preschool in action.* Boston: Allyn and Bacon.

Scheerenberger, R. C. (1976). *Deinstitutionalization and institutional reform.* Springfield, IL: Thomas.

Scheerenberger, R. C. (1982). Public residential services (1981). Status and trends. *Mental Retardation, 20,* 210–215.

Scheerenberger, R. C., & Felsenthal, D. (1977). Community settings for MR persons: Satisfaction and activities. *Mental Retardation, 15,* 3–7.

Schell, J. S. (1959). Some differences between mentally retarded children in special and in regular classes in the schools of Mercer County, Pennsylvania. *Dissertation Abstracts, 20,* 607–608.

Schiff, M., Duyme, M., Dumaret, A., Stewart, J., Tomkeiwicz, S., & Feingold, J. (1978). Intellectual status of working-class children adopted early into upper-middle-class families. *Science, 200,* 1503–1504.

Schild, S. (1971). Social work services. In R. Koch & J. C. Dobson (Eds.), *The mentally retarded child and his family: A multidisciplinary handbook.* New York: Brunner Mazel.

Schleien, S. J., Ash, T., Kiernan, J., & Wehman, P. (1981). Developing independent cooking skills in a profoundly retarded woman. *Journal of the Association for the Severely Handicapped, 6,* 23–29.

Schopler, E. (1976). Towards reducing behavior problems in autistic children. In L. Wing (Ed.), *Early childhood autism.* New York: Pergamon.

Schopler, E. (1983). Can an adolescent or adult have autism. In E. Schopler & G. B. Mesibov (Eds.), *Autism in adolescents and adults.* New York: Plenum.

Schroeder, S. R. (1972). Parametric effects of reinforcement frequency, amount of reinforcement, and required response force in sheltered workshop behavior. *Journal of Applied Behavior Analysis, 5,* 431–444.

Schroeder, S. R., Mulick, J. A., & Schroeder, C. S. (1979). Management of severe behavior problems of the retarded. In N. R. Ellis (Ed.), *Handbook of mental deficiency, psychological theory and research* (pp. 341–366). Hillsdale, NJ: Erlbaum.

Schroeder, S. R., Schroeder, C. S., Rojahn, J., & Mulick, J. A. (1981). Self-injurious behavior: An analysis of behavior management techniques. In J. L. Matson and J. R. McCartney (Eds.), *Handbook of behavior modification with the mentally retarded.* New York: Plenum.

Schroeder, S. R., Schroeder, C. S., Smith, B., & Dalldorf, J. (1978). Prevalence of self-injurious behaviors in a large state facility for the retarded: A three-year follow-up study. *Journal of Autism and Childhood Schizophrenia, 8,* 261–269.

Schurr, K. T., & Brookover, W. (1967). *The effect of special class placement in the self-concept of ability of the educable mentally retarded child.* (United States Office of Education.) East Lansing, MI: Michigan State University Press.

Schurr, K. T., Joiner, L., & Towne, R. C. (1970). Self-concept research on the mentally retarded: A review of emipircal studies. *Mental Retardation, 8,* 39–43.

Scriver, C. R. (1978). Disorders of proline and hydroxyproline metabolism. In J. B. Stanbury, J. B. Wyngarden, & D. S. Frederickson (Eds.), *The metabolic basis of inherited disease (4th ed.)*. New York: McGraw-Hill.

Segal, J. J. (1971). *Imagery: Current cognitive approaches*. New York: Academic Press.

Segal, R. (1977). Trends in services for the aged mentally retarded. *Mental Retardation, 15*, 25-27.

Sell, S. H., Merrill, R. E., Doyne, E. O., & Zimsky, E. P., Jr. (1972). Long-term of hemophilus influenzae meningitis. *Pediatrics, 49*, 206-211.

Sells, C. J., & Bennett, F. C. (1977). Prevention of mental retardation: The role of medicine. *American Journal of Mental Deficiency, 82*, 117-129.

Semmel, M. I., & Snell, M. (1979). Social acceptance and self-concept for handicapped pupils in mainstreamed environments. *Education Unlimited, 1*, 65-68.

Sever, J., & White, L. R. (1968). Intrauterine viral infections. *Annual Review of Medicine, 19*, 471.

Severy, L. J., Brighman, J. C., & Schlenker, B. R. (1976). *A contemporary introduction to social psychology*. New York: McGraw-Hill.

Shaffer, T. R., & Goehl, H. (1974). The alinguistic child. *Mental Retardation, 12*, 3-6.

Shapiro, E. J. (1979). Restitution and positive practice overcorrection in reducing aggressive-disruptive behavior: A long-term follow-up. *Journal of Behavior Therapy and Experimental Psychiatry, 10*, 131-134.

Share, J. B. (1975). Developmental progress in Down's syndrome. In R. Koch and F. de la Cruz (Eds.), *Down's syndrome (mongolism): Research, prevention and management*. New York: Brunner Mazel.

Share, J. B. (1976). Review of drug treatment for Down's syndrome persons. *American Journal of Mental Deficiency, 80*, 388-393.

Share, J. B., & French, R. W. (1974). Early motor development in Down's syndrome children. *Mental Retardation, 12*, 23.

Share, J. B., Koch, R., Webb, A., & Graliker, B. (1964). The longitudinal development of infants and young children with Down's syndrome (mongolism). *American Journal of Mental Deficiency, 68*, 685-692.

Share, J. B. & Veale, A. M. O. (1974). *Developmental landmarks for children with Down's syndrome (mongolism)*. Dunedin, New Zealand: University of Otago Press.

Shaw, C. R. (1966). *The psychiatric disorders of children*. New York: Appleton-Century-Crofts.

Shawn, B. (1964). Review of a work-experience program. *Mental Retardation, 2*, 360-364.

Shaywitz, S. E., Cohen, D. J., & Shaywitz, B. A. (1980). Behavior and learning difficulties in children of normal intelligence born to alcoholic mothers. *Journal of Pediatrics, 96*, 978-982.

Sheare, J. B. (1974). Social acceptance of EMR adolescents in integrated programs. *American Journal of Mental Deficiency, 78*, 678-682.

Shearer, D. E., & Shearer, M. S. (1976). The Portage Project: A model for early childhood intervention. In T. D. Tjossem (Ed.), *Intervention strategies for high risk infants and young children*. Baltimore: University Park Press.

Shentoub, S., & Soulairac, A. (1967). L'enfant automutilateur. Cited by A. H. Green, *Archives of General Psychiatry, 17*, 234-244.

Sherman, J. A., & Bushell, D., Jr. (1975). Behavior modification as an educational technique. In F. D. Horowitz (Ed.), *Review of child development research* (Vol. 4). Chicago: University of Chicago Press.

Sherrill, C. (1980). Posture training as a means of normalization. *Mental Retardation, 18*, 135-138.

Shia, L., Schoenbaum, S. C. Monson, R. R., Rosner, R., Stubalefield, P., & Ryan, K. J. (1983). Marijuana use with outcome of pregnancy. *American Journal of Public Health, 73*, 1161-1164.

Shih, V. E. (1978). Urea cycle disorders and other congenital hyperammonemic syndromes. In J. B. Stanbury, J. B. Wyngaarden, & D. S. Frederickson (Eds.), *The metabolic basis of inherited disease* (4th ed.). New York: McGraw-Hill.

Shih, V. E., Levy, H. L., Karolkewicz, V., Haughton, S., Efron, M. L., Isselbacher, K. J., Bentler, E., & MacCready, R. A. (1971). Galactosemia screening of newborns in Massachusetts. *New England Journal of Medicine, 284*, 753-757.

Shipe, D., Reisman, L. E., Chung, C., Darnell, A., & Kelly, S. (1968). The relationship between cytogenetic constitution, physical stigmata, and intelligence in Down's syndrome. *American Journal of Mental Deficiency, 72,* 789–797.

Shipe, D., & Shotwell, A. (1965). Effect of out-of-home care on mongoloid children. A continuation study. *American Journal of Mental Deficiency, 69,* 649–652.

Shodell, M., & Reiter, H. (1968). Self-mulitative behavior in verbal and non-verbal schizophrenic children. *Archives of General Psychiatry, 15,* 453–455.

Shotel, J. R., Iano, R. P., & McGettigan, J. F. (1972). Teacher attitudes associated with the integration of handicapped children. *Exceptional Children, 38,* 677–683.

Sidbury, J. B. (1977). Glycogenoses. In A. M. Rudolph (Ed.), *Pediatrics* (16th Ed.). New York: Appleton-Century-Crofts.

Sigel, I. E. (1963). How intelligence tests limit understanding of intelligence. *Merrill-Palmer Quarterly, 9,* 39–56.

Silver, A., & Hagin, R. A. (1964). Specific reading disability: Follow-up studies. *American Journal of Orthopsychiatry, 34,* 95–102.

Silverstein, A. B. (1964). An empirical test of the mongoloid stereotype. *American Journal of Mental Deficiency, 68,* 493–497.

Silverstein, A. B. (1966). Anxiety and the quality of human figure drawings. *American Journal of Mental Deficiency, 70,* 607–608.

Silverstein, A. B. (1968). WISC subtest patterns of retardates. *Psychological Reports, 23,* 1061–1062.

Silverstein, A. B. (1970). The measurement of intelligence. In N. R. Ellis (Ed.), *International review of research in mental retardation.* (Vol. 4). New York: Academic Press.

Silverstein, A. B., Agular, B. F., Jacobs, L. J., Levy, J., & Rubenstein, D. M. (1979). Imitative behavior by Down's syndrome persons. *American Journal of Mental Deficiency, 83,* 409–411.

Silverstein, A. B., Legutki, G., Friedman, S. L., & Takayama, D. L. (1982). Performance of Down's syndrome individuals on the Stanford-Binet intelligence scale. *American Journal of Mental Deficiency, 86,* 548–551.

Simeonsson, R. J., & Simeonsson, N. E. (1981). Medication effects in handicapped preschool children. In assessing the handicapped preschooler, *Topics in Early Childhood Special Education, 1,* 61–75.

Simpson, H. M., & Meaney, C. (1979). Effects of learning to ski on the self-concept of mentally retarded children. *American Journal of Mental Deficiency, 84,* 25–29.

Singh, N. N., & Winton, A. S. (1985). Controlling pica by components of an overcorrection procedure. *American Journal of Mental Deficiency, 90,* 40–45.

Siperstein, G. N., Bak, J. J., & Gottleib, J. (1977). Effects of group discussion on children's attitudes toward handicapped peers. *Journal of Educational Research, 70,* 131–134.

Siperstein, G. N., & Gottlieb, J. (1977). Physical stigma and academic performance as factors affecting children's first impressions of handicapped peers. *American Journal of Mental Deficiency, 81,* 455–462.

Siperstein, G. N., & Gottlieb, J. (1978). Parents' and teachers' attitudes toward mildly and severely retarded children. *Mental Retardation, 16,* 321–322.

Siva Sankar, D. V. (1969). A summary of 30 different biochemical tests in childhood schizophrenia. In D. V. Siva Sankar (Ed.), *Schizophrenia: Current concepts and research.* Hicksville, NY: P.J.D. Publications.

Skeels, H. M. (1966). Adult status of children with contrasting life experiences. *Monographs of the Society for Research in Child Development, 31,* 3.

Skeels, H. M., & Dye, H. B. (1939). A study of the effects of differential stimulation on mentally retarded children. *Proceedings and Addresses of the Sixty-third Annual Session of the American Association on Mental Deficiency, 44,* 114–130.

Skeels, H. M., & Harms, I. (1948). Children with inferior social histories: Their mental develoment in adoptive homes. *Journal of Genetic Psychology, 72,* 283–294.

Skinner, B. F. (1968). *The technology of teaching.* New York: Appleton-Century-Crofts.

Skinner, B. F. (1972). *Cumulative record: A selection of papers* (3rd ed.). New York: Appleton-Century-Crofts.

Skodak, M., & Skeels, H. M. (1949). A final follow-up study of one hundred adopted children. *Journal of Genetic Psychology, 75*, 85–125.

Slater, E., Beard, A. W., & Glithero, E. (1963). The schizophrenialike psychosis of epilepsy. *British Journal of Psychiatry, 109*, 95–105.

Slater, E., & Cowie, V. (1971). *The genetics of mental disorders.* London: Oxford University Press.

Sleith, W. (1966, January). What a mentally retarded worker can do. *Supervisory Management Magazine.*

Slitz, H. H., & DeRisi, D. T. (1978). Porteus Maze Test performance of retarded young adults and nonretarded children. *American Journal of Mental Deficiency, 83*, 40–43.

Slivkin, S. E., & Bernstein, N. R. (1970). Group approaches to treating retarded adolescents. In F. J. Menolascino (Ed.), *Psychiatric approaches to mental retardation.* New York: Basic Books.

Sloop, W. E., & Kennedy, W. A. (1973). Intstitutionalized retarded nocturnal enuretics treated by a conditioning technique. *American Journal of Mental Deficiency, 77*, 717–721.

Smeets, P. M. (1970). Withdrawal of social reinforcers as a means of controlling rumination and regurgitation in a profoundly retarded person. *Training School Bulletin, 67*, 158–163.

Smeets, P. M. (1971). Some characteristics of mental defectives displaying self-mutilative behaviors. *Training School Bulletin, 68*, 131–135.

Smith, D. (1979). Fetal drug syndromes: Effects of ethanol and hydantoins. *Pediatrics in Review, 1*, 165–172.

Smith, D. W. (1970). *Recognizable patterns of human malformation.* Philadelphia: Saunders.

Smith, D. W. (1976). *Major problems in clinical pediatrics: Recognizable patterns of human malformation* (Vol. 7, 2nd ed). Philadelphia: Saunders.

Smith, D. W., & Lyon, R. (1976). Eliminating vomiting behavior in a profoundly retarded resident. *Research and the Retarded, 3*, 24–27.

Smith, D. W., Patau, K., Therman, E., & Inhorn, S. L. (1960). A new autosomal trisomy syndrome. *Journal of Pediatrics, 57*, 338.

Smith, D. W., & Wilson, A. A. (1973). *The child with Down's syndrome (mongolism).* Philadelphia: Saunders.

Smith, G. F. (1975). Present approaches to therapy in Down's syndrome. In R. Koch, & F. de la Cruz (Eds.), *Down's syndrome (mongolism): Research, prevention and management.* New York: Brunner Mazel.

Smith, H. W., & Kennedy, W. A. (1967). Effects of three educational programs on mentally retarded children. *Perceptual and Motor Skills, 24*, 174.

Smith, K. E. (1976). Audiology. In R. B. Johnston & P. R. Magrab (Eds.), *Developmental disorders: Assessment, treatment, education.* Baltimore: University Park Press.

Smith, M. E. (1926). An investigation of the development of the sentence and the extent of vocabulary in young children. *University of Iowa Studies, 3*, [Special issue].

Smith, N. V. (1975). Universal tendencies in the child's acquisition of phonology. In N. O'Connor (Ed.), *Language, cognitive deficits and retardation.* London: Butterworths.

Smith, P. (1979). A comparison of different methods of toilet training the mentally handicapped. *Behavior Research and Therapy, 17*, 33–43.

Smith, R. S., Britton, P. G., Johnson, M., & Thomas, D. (1975). Problems involved in toilet training of institutionalized mentally retarded individuals. *Behavior Research and Therapy, 3*, 301–302.

Snell, M. E., (Ed.). (1978). *Systematic instruction of the moderately and severely handicapped.* Columbus, OH: Merrill.

Snyder, L., Apollini, T., & Cooke, T. P. (1977). Integrated settings at the early childhood level: The role of nonretarded peers. *Exceptional Children, 43*, 262–266.

Snygg, D. (1938). The relation between the intelligence of mothers and of their children living in foster homes. *Journal of Genetic Psychology, 52*, 401–406.

Solitaire, G. B., & Lamarche, J. B. (1966). Alzheimer's disease and senile dementia as seen in mongoloids: Neuropathological observations. *American Journal of Mental Deficiency, 70*, 840–848.

Sommers, D., McGregor, G., Lesh, E., & Reed, S. (1980). A rapid method for describing the efficacy of early intervention programs for developmentally disabled children. *Mental Retardation, 18,* 275–278.

Soriano, J. R. (1977). Disorders of renal tubular function. In A. M. Rudolph (Ed.), *Pediatrics* (16th ed.). New York: Appleton-Century-Crofts.

Sorotzkin, F., Fleming, E. S., & Anttonen, R. G. (1974). Teacher knowledge of standardized test information and its effect on pupil IQ and achievement. *Journal of Experimental Education, 43,* 79–85.

Sparks, H. L., & Blackman, L. S. (1965). What is special about special education revisited: The mentally retarded. *Exceptional Children, 31,* 242–247.

Spearman, C. (1923). *The nature of intelligence and the principles of cognition.* London: Macmillan.

Spearman, C. E. (1927). *The abilities of man.* New York: Macmillan.

Speer, G. S. (1940). The mental development of children of feebleminded and normal mothers. NSSE, *Thirty-ninth Yearbook,* Pt. II, 309–314.

Spellman, C., DeBriere, T., Jarboe, D., Campbell, S., & Harris, C. (1978). Pictorial instruction: Training daily living skills. In M. E. Snell (Ed.), *Systematic instruction of the moderately and severely retarded.* Columbus, OH: Merrill.

Spencer, R. L., Temerlin, M. K., & Trousdale, W. W. (1968). Some correlates of bowel control in profoundly retarded. *American Journal of Mental Deficiency, 72,* 879–882.

Spicker, H. H., & Barte, N. R. (1968). The mentally retarded. In G. O. Johnson & H. D. Bland (Eds.), *Exceptional children research review.* Washington: Council for Exceptional Children.

Spitalnick, R., & Drabman, R. (1976). A classroom time-out procedure for retarded children. *Journal of Behavior Therapy and Experimental Psychiatry, 7,* 17–21.

Spitz, H. H. (1966). The role of input organization in the learning and memory of mental retardates. In N. R. Ellis (Ed.), *International review of research in mental retardation* (Vol. II). New York: Academic Press.

Spitz, H. H., & Borys, S. V. (1977). Performance of retarded adolescents and nonretarded children on one- and two-bit logical problems. *Journal of Experimental Child Psychology, 23,* 415–429.

Spitz, H. H., & Nadler, B. T. (1974). Logical problem solving by educable retarded adolescents and normal children. *Developmental Psychology, 10,* 404–412.

Spitz, H. H., & Winters, E. H. (1977). Tic-tac-toe performance as a function of maturation level of retarded adolescents and nonretarded children. *Intelligence, 1,* 108–117.

Spitz, R. A. (1945). Hospitalism: An inquiry into the genesis of psychiatric conditions in early childhood. In A. Freud (Ed.), *Psychoanalytic study of the child* (Vol. 1, pp. 53–74). New York: International Universities Press.

Spock, B. (1961). *On being a parent of a handicapped child.* Chicago: National Society for Crippled Children and Adults.

Sroufe, L. A., & Waters, E. (1976). The ontogenesis of smiling and laughter: A perspective on the organization of development in infancy. *Psychological Review, 83,* 173–189.

Stanbury, J. B., Wyngarden, J. B., Frederickson, D. S., Goldstein, J. L., & Brown, M. S. (1983). *The metabolic basis of inherited disease* (5th ed.). New York: McGraw-Hill.

Stanfield, J. S. (1973). Graduation: What happens to the retarded child when he grows up? *Exceptional Children, 39,* 458–552.

Stanford Research Institute. (1970). *Implementation of planned variation in Head Start: Preliminary evaluation of planned variation in Head Start according to Follow-Through approaches (1969–1970).* Washington: Office of Child Development, U.S. Department of Health, Education, and Welfare.

Stanford Research Institute. (1971). *Longitudinal evaluation of selected features of the national Follow-Through program.* Washington: Office of Education, U.S. Department of Health, Education, and Welfare.

Stanovich, K. E. (1978). Information processing in mentally retarded individuals. In N. R. Ellis (Ed.), *International review of research in mental retardation* (Vol. 9, pp. 29–61). New York: Academic Press.

Stark, C. R., & Fraumeni, J. F. (1966). Viral hepatitis and Down's syndrome. *Lancet, 1,* 1036.

Stebbins, L. B., St. Pierre, R. G., Proper, E. C., Anderson, R. B., & Cerva, T. R. (1977). *Education as experimentation: A planned variation model.* Cambridge, MA: ABT Associates Report for U.S. Office of Education.

Stedman, D. J. (1963). Associative clustering of semantic categories in normal and retarded subjects. *American Journal of Mental Deficiency, 67,* 700–704.

Stedman, D. J. (1970). The hypothetical community, a template for planning mental retardation programs. *North Carolina Journal of Mental Health, 4,* 26–29.

Stedman, D. J., & Eichorn, D. H. (1964). A comparison of the growth and development of institutionalized and home-reared mongoloids during infancy and early childhood. *American Journal of Mental Deficiency, 69,* 391–401.

Steed, F. R. (1974). *A special picture cook book.* Lawrence, KA: H and H Enterprises.

Stein, J. U. (1962). Adapted physical education for the educable mentally handicapped. *Journal of Health, Physical Education, and Recreation, 33,* 30–31, 50–51.

Stephen, E., & Hawks, G. (1974). Cerebral palsy and mental subnormality. In A. M. Clarke and A. D. B. Clarke (Eds.), *Mental deficiency: The changing outlook,* (3rd ed.). New York: Free Press.

Sternlicht, M. (1966). Psychotherapeutic procedures with the retarded. In N. R. Ellis (Ed.), *International review of research in mental retardation* (Vol. 2). New York: Academic Press.

Sternberg, R. J. (1981). The nature of intelligence. *New York University Education Quarterly, 12,* 10–17.

Sternberg, R. J., & Powell, J. S. (1983). Comprehending verbal comprehension. *American Psychologist, 38,* 878–893.

Stillman, R. D. (1975). *Assessment of deaf-blind children: The Callier-Azusa scale.* Dallas: Callier Center for Communication Disorders, University of Texas/Dallas.

Stippich, M. E. (1940). The mental development of children of feebleminded mothers: A preliminary report. NSSE, *Thirty-ninth Yearbook,* Pt. II, 337–350.

Stoker, B. (1977). The postural characteristics of the severely mentally retarded. Unpublished thesis, Texas Woman's University.

Stoller, A. (1968). Virus-chromosome interactions as a possible cause of cases of Down's syndrome (mongolism) and other congenital anomalies. *Advances in Teratology, 3,* 7–126.

Stoller, A., & Collmann, R. D. (1965). Incidence of infective hepatitis followed by Down's syndrome nine months later. *Lancet, 2,* 1221–1223.

Stone, L. J., & Church, J. (1957). *Childhood and adolescence.* New York: Random House.

Stone, N. W. (1975). A plea for early intervention. *Mental Retardation, 13,* 16–18.

Stott, D. H. (1960). Observations on retest discrepancy in mentally sub-normal children. *British Journal of Educational Psychology, 30,* 211–219.

Stott, D. H. (1973). Follow-up study from birth effects of prenatal stresses. *Developmental Medicine and Child Neurology, 15,* 770–787.

Strain, P. S. (1975). Increasing social play of severely retarded preschoolers with socio-dramatic activities. *Mental Retardation, 13,* 7–9.

Strauss, A., & Lehtinen, L. (1947). *Psychopathology and education of the brain-injured child.* New York: Grune and Stratton.

Streissguth, A. P., Herman, C. J., & Smith, D. W. (1970). Intelligence, behavior, and dysmorphogenesis in the fetal alcohol syndrome. *Journal of Pediatrics, 92,* 363.

Strichart, S. S. (1974). Effects of competence and nurturance on imitation of non-retarded peers by retarded adolescents. *American Journal of Mental Deficiency, 78,* 665–674.

Strichart, S. S., & Gottlieb, J. (1975). Imitation of retarded children by their nonretarded peers. *American Journal of Mental Deficiency, 79,* 506–512.

Strickland, O., & Arrell, V. (1967). Employment of the mentally retarded. *Exceptional Children, 33,* 21–29.

Strupp, H. H. & Hadley, S. W. (1977). A tripartite model of mental health and therapeutic outcomes: With special reference to negative effects in psychotherapy. *American Psychologist, 32,* 187–196.

Sutherland, B. S., Umbarger, B., & Berry, H. K. (1966). The treatment of phenylketonuria: A decade of results. *American Journal of Diseases of Children, 3,* 505-523.

Sulzbacher, S., & Houser, J. E. (1968). A tactic to eliminate disruptive behaviors in the classroom: Group contingent consequences. *American Journal of Mental Deficiency, 73,* 88-90.

Syden, M. (1963). Guidelines for a cooperatively conducted work-study program for educable mentally retarded youth. *Mental Retardation, 2,* 91-94, 120-123.

Szmuness, W., & Prince, A. M. (1971). The epidemiology of serum hepatitis (SH) infections: A controlled study in two closed institutions. *American Journal of Epidemiology, 94,* 585-595.

Szmuness, W., Prince, A. M., Etling, G. F., & Pick, R. (1972). Development and distribution of hemagglutinating antibody against hepatitis B antigen in institutionalized populations. *Journal of Infectious Diseases, 126,* 498-506.

Taft, L. T., & Cohen, H. J. (1977). Mental retardation. In A. M. Rudolph (Ed.), *Pediatrics* (16th ed.). New York: Appleton-Century-Crofts.

Talkington, L. W., Hall, S., & Altman, R. (1971). Communication deficits and aggression in the mentally retarded. *American Journal of Mental Deficiency, 76,* 235-237.

Tanner, B. A. & Leiler, M. D. (1975). Punishment of self-injurious behavior using aromatic ammonia as the aversive stimulus. *Journal of Applied Behavior Analysis, 8,* 53-57.

Tansley, A. E., & Gulliford, R. (1960). *The education of slow learning children* (2nd ed.). London: Routledge and Kegan Paul.

Tarjan, G., Dingman, H., Eyman, R., & Brown, S. (1960). Effectiveness of hospital release programs. *American Journal of Mental Deficiency, 64,* 609-617.

Tarjan, G., Wright, S. W., Eyman, R. K., & Keeran, C. J. (1973). Natural history of mental retardation: Some aspects of epidemiology. *American Journal of Mental Deficiency, 77,* 369-378.

Tarpley, H. D., & Schroeder, S. R. (1979). Comparison of DRO and DRI on rate of suppression of self-injurious behavior. *American Journal of Mental Deficiency, 84,* 188-194.

Tate, B. G. (1972). Case study: Control of chronic self-injurious behavior by conditioning procedures. *Behavior Therapy, 3,* 72-83.

Tate, B. G., & Baroff, G. S. (1966). Aversive control self-injurious behavior in a psychotic boy. *Behavior Research and Therapy, 4,* 281-287.

Taylor, E. M. (1959). *Psychological appraisal of children with cerebral defect.* Cambridge, MA: Harvard University Press.

Telford, C. W., & Sawrey, J. M. (1967). *The exceptional individual.* Englewood Cliffs, NJ: Prentice-Hall.

Terman, L. M. (1916). *The measurement of intelligence.* Boston: Houghton Mifflin.

Terman, L. M., & Merrill, M. A. (1960). *Stanford-Binet intelligence scale.* Boston: Houghton Mifflin.

Terman, L. M., & Merrill, M. A. (1973). *The Stanford-Binet intelligence scale—Third Revision* (with 1972 by R. L. Thorndike). Boston: Houghton Mifflin.

Thiessen, D. D. (1972). *Gene organization and behavior.* New York: Random House.

Thomas, A., Chess, S., & Birch, H. G. (1968). *Temperament and behavior disorders in children.* New York: New York University Press.

Thompson, C. W., & Magaret, G. A. (1947). Differential test responses of normals and mental defectives. *Journal of Abnormal and Social Psychology, 42,* 255-293.

Thompson, M. M. (1963). Psychological characteristics relevant to the education of the mongoloid child. *Mental Retardation, 1,* 148-151, 185-186.

Thompson, T., & Carey, A. (1980). Structured normalization: Intellectual and adaptive changes in a residential setting. *Mental Retardation, 18,* 193-197.

Thompson, T., & Grabowski, J. (Eds.). (1977a). *Behavior modification of the mentally retarded* (2nd ed.). New York: Oxford University Press.

Thompson, T., & Grabowski, J. (1977b). Ethical and legal guidelines for behavior modification. In T. Thompson & J. Grabowski (Eds.), *Behavior modification of the mentally retarded* (2nd ed.). New York: Oxford University Press.

Thompson, T., & Manson, R. (1983). Overhydration: Precautions when treating urinary incontinence. *Mental Retardation, 21,* 139-143.

Thompson, W. R. (1960). Early environmental influences on behavioral development. *American Journal of Orthopsychiatry, 30,* 306-314.

Thompson, W. R., & Grusec, J. E. (1970). Studies of early experience. In P. H. Mussen (Ed.), *Carmichael's manual of child psychology* (p. 606). New York: Wiley.

Thorndike, E. L. (1927). *The measurement of intelligence.* New York: Teachers College, Columbia University.

Thorndike, R. L. (1973). *Stanford-Binet intelligence scale—Third revision.* Form L-M 1972 norms tables. Boston: Houghton Mifflin.

Thorne, F. C. (1948). Counseling and psychotherapy with mental defectives. *American Journal of Mental Deficiency, 52,* 263–271.

Thurstone, L. L. (1938). Primary mental abilities. *Psychometric Monographs,* No. 1. [Special issue].

Thurstone, L. L., & Thurstone, T. G. (1941). *Factorial studies of intelligence.* Chicago: University of Chicago Press.

Thurstone, T. G. (1959). *An evaluation of educating mentally handicapped children in special classes and regular grades.* Chapel Hill: University of North Carolina Press.

Tillman, M. H., & Osborne, R. T. (1969). The performance of blind and sighted children on the Wechesler Intelligence Scale for Children: Interaction effects. *Education of the Visually Handicapped, 1,* 1–4.

Tizard, B. (1968). Observations of over-active imbecile children in controlled and uncontrolled environments. I: Classroom studies. *American Journal of Mental Deficiency, 72,* 540–547.

Tizard, J. (1974). Longitudinal studies: Problems and findings. In A. M. Clarke & A. D. B. Clarke (Eds.), *Mental deficiency: The changing outlook* (3rd ed.). Glencoe, IL: Free Press.

Tizard, J., & Grad, J. (1961). *The mentally handicapped and their families: A social survey.* London: Oxford University Press.

Tjo, J. H., & Levan, A. (1956). The chromosome number of man. *Hereditas, 42,* 1–6.

Tjossem, T. D. (Ed.). (1976). *Intervention strategies for high risk infants and young children.* Baltimore: University Park Press.

Topper, S. T. (1975). Gesture language for a non-verbal severely retarded male. *Mental Retardation, 13,* 30–31.

Town, C. H. (1939). *Familial feeblemindedness.* Buffalo: Foster and Stewart.

Towne, R. C., & Joiner, L. M. (1966). *The effects of special class placement on the self-concept of ability of the educable mentally retarded child.* East Lansing, MI: Office of Educational Publications.

Tredgold, A. F. (1937). *A textbook of mental deficiency* (6th ed.). Baltimore: Wood.

Treffry, D., Martin, G., Samuels, J., & Watson, C. (1970). Operant conditioning of grooming behavior of severely retarded girls. *Mental Retardation, 8,* 30–34.

Tronick, E., & Brazelton, T. B. (1975). Clinical uses of the Brazleton Neonatal Behavioral Assessment. In B. Z. Friedlander, G. M. Steritt, & G. E. Kirk (Eds.), *Exceptional infant: Volume 3: Assessment and intervention.* New York: Brunner Mazel.

Trott, M. (1977). Application of Foxx and Azrin's toilet training method for the retarded in a school programme. *Education and Training of the Mentally Retarded, 12,* 336–338.

Turkel, H. (1963). Medical treatment of mongolism. *Proceedings of the 2nd International Congress on Mental Retardation,* Vienna.

Turner, G., Daniel, A., & Frost, M. (1980). X-linked mental retardation, macro-orchidism, and the X 27 fragile site. *Journal of Pediatrics, 96,* 837–841.

Turner, G., & Opitz, J. M. (1980). Editorial comment: X-linked mental retardation. *American Journal of Medical Genetics, 7,* 407–415.

Turner, G., & Turner, B. (1974). X-linked mental retardation. *Journal of Medical Genetics, 11,* 109–113.

Turner, M. W. (1958). *A comparison of social status of mentally retarded children enrolled in special classes.* Unpublished doctoral dissertation, Indiana University, Bloomington.

Turnure, J. E. (1970a). Distractibility in the mentally retarded: Negative evidence for an orienting inadequacy. *Exceptional Children, 37,* 181–186.

Turnure, J. E. (1970b). Children's reactions to distractors in a learning situation. *Developmental Psychology, 2,* 115–122.

Twardosz, S., & Sajwaj, T. (1972). Multiple effects of a procedure to increase sitting in a hyperactive retarded boy. *Journal of Applied Behavioral Analysis, 5*, 73-78.

Tymchuk, A. (1979). The mentally retarded in later life. In O. J. Kaplan (Ed.), *Psychopathology of aging.* New York: Academic Press.

Ulleland, C. H. (1972). The offspring of alcoholic mothers. *Annals of the New York Academy of Sciences, 197,* 167-169.

Ulrey, G. (1982). Assessment of cognitive development during infancy. In G. Ulrey & S. J. Rogers (Eds.), *Psychological assessment of handicapped infants and young children.* New York: Thieme-Stratton.

Upchurch, T. T., Ham, L., Daniels, R., McGhee, M. R., & Burnett, M. (1980). *A better way: An illustrated guide to protective intervention techniques.* Butner, NC: Murdoch Center.

U.S. Department of Health, Education, and Welfare. (1968). *Syphilis: A synopsis.* Washington: Public Health Service, publication No. 1660.

U.S. Department of Health, Education, and Welfare. (1973). *Feeding the child with a handicap.* Washington: U.S. Government Printing Office, stock No. 1729-00025.

Uzgiris, I. C., & Hunt, J. McV. (1975). *Assessment in infancy.* Urbana: University of Illinois Press.

Valencia, J. I., DeLuzzio, C. B., & De Coriat, L. F. (1963). Heterosomic mosaicism in a mongoloid child. *Lancet, 2,* 488.

Valentine, G. H. (1966). *The chromosome disorders.* London: Hineman.

Vanderheiden, D. H. (1975). Blissymbols and the mentally retarded. In G. Vanderheiden and K. Grilley (Eds.), *Nonvocal communication techniques and aids for the severely physically handicapped.* Baltimore: University Park Press.

Vanderheiden, D. H., Brown, W. P., MacKenzie, P., Reinen, S. & Scheibel, C. (1975). Symbol communication for the mentally handicapped. *Mental Retardation, 13,* 34-37.

Vanderveer, B., & Schweid, E. (1974). Infant assessment: Stability of mental functioning in young retarded children. *American Journal of Mental Deficiency, 79,* 1-4.

Van Osdol, B. M. (1972). Art education for the MR. *Mental Retardation, 10,* 51-53.

Van Osdol, B. M. & Carlson, L. (1972). A study of developmental hyperactivity. *Mental Retardation, 10,* 18-23.

Van Wagenen, R. K., Meyerson, L., Kerr, N. J., & Mahoney, K. (1969). Field trials of a new procedure for toilet training. *Journal of Experimental Child Psychology, 8,* 147-159.

Veall, R. M. (1974). The prevalence of epilepsy among mongols related to age. *Journal of Mental Deficiency Research, 18,* 99.

Vellutino, F. R., Steger, B. M., Moyer, S. C., Harding, C. J., & Niles, J. A. (1975). Has the perceptual deficit hypothesis led us astray? An examination of current conceptualizations in the assessment and treatment of exceptional children. In W. Pryzwansky, S. Rosenthal, J. Stikeleather, & T. Taylor (Eds.), *Proceedings of the fourth Annual Conference of the North Carolina Association for Children with Learning Disabilities.* Chapel Hill, NC: NCACLD, Route 2, Box 114.

Vernon, P. E. (1950). *The structure of human abilities.* New York: Wiley.

Villee, D. B. (1975). *Human endocrinology. A developmental approach.* Philadelphia: Saunders.

Vukelich, R., & Hake, D. F. (1971). Reduction of dangerously aggressive behavior in a severely retarded resident through a combination of positive reinforcement procedures. *Journal of Applied Behavior Analysis, 4,* 215-225.

Vulpé, S. G. (1977). *Assessment battery.* Toronto: National Institute of Mental Retardation.

Vygotsky, L. J. (1962). *Thought and language.* Cambridge: Massachusetts Institute of Technology Press.

Wabash Center for the Mentally Retarded, Inc. (1977). *Guide to early developmental training.* Boston: Allyn and Bacon.

Wald, P. M. (1976). Basic personal and civil rights. In M. Kindred, J. Cohen, D. Penrod, & T. Shaffer (Eds.), *The mentally retarded citizen and the law.* New York: Free Press.

Walker, K. P., & Gross, F. L. (1970). IQ stability among educable retarded children. *Training School Bulletin, 66,* 181-187.

Walker, V. (1972). The efficacy of the resource room for educating mentally retarded children. Unpublished doctoral dissertation. Temple University, Philadelphia.

Wallace, J., Burger, D., Neal, H. C., Van Brero, M., & Davis, D. E. (1976). Aversive conditioning use in public facilities for the mentally retarded. *Mental Retardation, 14*, 17-19.

Wallach, L., Wallach, M. A., Dozier, M. G., & Kaplan, N. E. (1977). Poor children learning to read do not have trouble with auditory discrimination but do have trouble with phoneme recognition. *Journal of Educational Psychology, 69*, 36-39.

Warburg, M. (1960). Anophthalmos complicated by mental retardation and cleft palate. *Acta Ophthalmologica, 38*, 394-409.

Warkany, J. (1968). The role of sensitive or critical periods in teratogenesis. In G. M. McKhann, S. J. Yaffe, & G. S. Sharon (Eds.)., *Drugs and poisons in relation to the developing nervous system*. Washington: U.S. Public Health Service.

Warkany, J. (1971). *Congenital malformations: Notes and comments*. Chicago: Year Book Medical Publishers.

Warkany, J. (1975). Etiology of Down's syndrome. In R. Koch and F. de la Cruz (Eds.), *Down's syndrome (mongolism): Research, prevention, and management*. New York: Brunner Mazel.

Warren, K. (1962). An investigation of the effectiveness of educational placement of mentally retarded children in a special class. *Dissertation Abstracts, 23*, 2211.

Warren, S. A., & Burns, N. R. (1970). Crib confinement as a factor in repetitive and stereotyped behavior in retardates. *Mental Retardation, 8*, 25-29.

Watson, L. S., Jr., and Bassinger, J. F. (1974). Parent training technology: A potential service delivery system. *Mental Retardation, 12*, 3-10.

Watson, L. S., Jr., and Uzzell, R. (1981). Teaching self-help skills to the mentally retarded. In J. L. Matson & J. R. McCartney (Eds.), *Handbook of behavior modification with the mentally retarded*. New York: Plenum.

Wayne, M., & Melnyr, W. (1973). Toilet training of a blind retarded boy by operant conditioning. *Journal of Behavior Therapy and Experimental Psychiatry, 4*, 267-268.

Weber, W. W. (1967). Survival and sex ratio in trisomy 17-18. *American Journal of Human Genetics, 19*, 369.

Webster, D. R., & Azrin, N. H. (1973). Required relaxation: A method of inhibiting agitative-disruptive behavior of retardation. *Behavior Research and Therapy, 11*, 67-68.

Webster, T. G. (1970). Unique aspects of emotional development in mentally retarded children. In F. J. Menolascino (Ed.), *Psychiatric approaches to mental retardation*. New York: Basic Books.

Wechsler, D. (1949). *Wechsler Intelligence Scale for Children*. New York: Psychological Corp.

Wechsler, D. (1955). *Wechsler Adult Intelligence Scale, Manual*. New York: Psychological Corp.

Wechsler, D. (1967). *Manual for the Wechsler Preschool and Primary Scale of Intelligence*. New York: Psychological Corp.

Wechsler, D. (1974). *Wechsler Intelligence Scale for Children—Revised*. New York: Psychological Corp.

Wechsler, D. (1981). *WAIS-R Manual. Wechsler Adult Intelligence Scale—Revised*. New York: Harcourt Brace Jovanovich.

Weeks, M., & Gaylord-Ross, R. (1981). Task difficulty and aberrant behavior in severely handicapped students. *Journal of Applied Behavior Analysis, 14*, 449-462.

Wehman, P. (1977). *Helping the mentally retarded acquire play skills*. Springfield, IL: Thomas.

Wehman, P. (1979). *Curriculum design for the severely and profoundly handicapped*. New York: Human Sciences Press.

Wehman, P. (1981). *Competitive employment: New horizons for severely disabled individuals*. Baltimore: Brookes.

Wehman, P., Hill, J. W., & Koehler, F. (1979). Helping severely handicapped persons enter competitive employment. *AAESPH Review, 4*, 274-290.

Wehman, P., Hill, M., Goodall, P., Cleveland, P., Brooke, V., & Pentecost, J. H., Jr. (1982). Job placement and follow-up of moderately and severely handicapped individuals after three years. *Journal of the Association for the Severely Handicapped, 7*, 5-16.

Wehman, P., Renzaglia, A., Schutz, R., Karan, O. (1976). Stimulating productivity in two profoundly retarded workers through mixed reinforcement contingencies. In O. Karan, P. Wehman, A. Renzaglia, & R. Schutz (Eds.), *Habilitation practices with the severely developmentally disabled.* Madison: University of Wisconsin Rehabilitation Research and Training Center.

Wehman, P., Schleien, S., & Kiernan, J. (1980). Age appropriate recreation programs for severely handicapped youth and adults. *Journal of the Association for the Severely Handicapped, 5,* 395–407.

Wehman, P., Schutz, R., Renzaglia, A., & Karan, O. C. (1977). The use of positive practice training in work adjustment with two profoundly retarded adolescents. *Vocational Evaluation and Work Adjustment Bulletin, 14,* 14–22.

Weikart, D. P., et al. (1970). *Longitudinal results of the Ypsilanti Perry preschool project.* Ypsilanti, MI: High/Scope Educational Research Foundation.

Weisberg, H. F. (1982). *Water, electrolyte, and acid-base balance.* Baltimore: Williams and Wilkins.

Weise, P., Koch, R., Shaw, R. N. F., & Rosenfeld, M. J. (1975). The use of S-hydroxytryptophan in the treatment of Down's syndrome. In R. Koch & F. de la Cruz (Eds.), *Down's syndrome (mongolism): Research, prevention and management.* New York: Brunner Mazel.

Welch, E.A. (1966). The effects of segregated and partially integrated school programs on self-concept and academic achievement of educable mental retardates. *Dissertation Abstracts, 26,* 5533–5534.

Wells, K. C., Forehand, R. L., Hickey, K., & Green, K. D. (1977). Effects of a procedure derived from the overcorrection principle on manipulated and nonmanipulated behaviors. *Journal of Applied Behavior Analysis, 10,* 679–687.

Wenar, C. (1971). *Personality development from infancy to adulthood.* Boston: Houghton Mifflin.

Werry, J. S. (1970). Some clinical and laboratory studies of psychotropic drugs in children: An overview. In W. L. Smith (Ed.), *Drugs and cerebral function.* Springfield, IL: Thomas.

Wertelcki, W., Schindler, A. M., & Gerald, P. S. (1966). Partial deletion of chromosome 18. *Lancet, 2,* 641.

Wheeler, A. J., Miller, R. A., Duke, J., Salisbury, E. W., Merritt, V., & Horton, B. (1977). *Murdoch Center C and Y program library. A collection of step-by-step programs for the developmentally disabled.* Butner, NC: Murdoch Center.

White, D., & Kaplitz, S. E. (1964) Treatment of Down's syndrome with a vitamin-mineral-hormonal preparation. *Proceedings of the International Copenhagen Congress on the Scientific Study of Mental Retardation, 1,* 224.

White, J., & Taylor, D. J. (1967). Noxious conditioning as a treatment for rumination. *Mental Retardation, 5,* 30–33.

White, R. W. (1959). Motivation reconsidered: The concept of competence. *Psychological Review, 66,* 297–333.

Whitman, T. L., & Scibak, J. W. (1979). Behavior modification research with the severely and profoundly retarded. In N. R. Ellis (Ed.), *Handbook of mental deficiency, psychological theory and research* (pp. 289–340). Hillsdale, NJ: Erlbaum.

Whitman, T. L., Scibak, J. W., & Reid, D. H. (1983). *Behavior modification with the severely and profoundly retarded: Research and applications.* New York: Academic Press.

Weiner, G., Rider, R. V., Oppel, W. C., Fischer, L. K., & Harper, P. A. (1965). Correlates of low birth weight: Psychological status at six to seven years of age. *Pediatrics, 35,* 434–444.

Wiest, G. (1955) Psychotherapy with the mentally retarded. *American Journal of Mental Deficiency, 59,* 640–644.

Willer, B., & Intagliata, J. (1982). Comparison of family-care and group homes as alternatives to institutions. *American Journal of Mental Deficiency, 86,* 588–595.

Willerman, L. (1979). Effects of families on intellectual development. *American Psychologist, 34,* 923–929.

Willerman, L., & Stafford, R. E. (1972). Maternal effects on intellectual functioning. *Behavior Genetics, 2,* 321–325.

Williams, C. E. (1971). A study of the patients in a group of mental subnormality hospitals. *British Journal of Mental Subnormality, 17,* (Part I, No. 32), 29–41.

Williams, R. L. (1970). Black pride, academic relevance, and individual achievement. *Counseling Psychologist, 2,* 18–20.

Wilson, G. W., Desmond, M. M., & Verniaud, W. M. (1973). Early development of infants of heroin-addicted mothers. *American Journal of Diseases of Children, 126,* 457-462.

Wilson, G. W., McCreary, R., Kean J., & Baxter, J. C. (1979). The development of preschool children of heroin-addicted mothers: A controlled study. *Pediatrics, 63,* 135-141.

Wilson, W. (1970). Social psychology and mental retardation. In N. R. Ellis (Ed.), *International review of research in mental retardation* (Vol. 4). New York: Academic Press.

Windle, C. (1962). Prognosis of mental subnormals. *American Journal of Mental Deficiency, 66* [Monograph supplement].

Winett, R. A., & Winkler, R. C. (1972). Current behavior modification in the classroom: Be still, be quiet, be docile. *Journal of Applied Behavior Analysis, 5,* 499-504.

Wing, L. (1972). *Autistic children: A guide for parents and professionals.* New York: Brunner Mazel.

Wing, L. (1976). Diagnosis, clinical description and prognosis. In L. Wing (Ed.), *Early childhood autism* (2nd ed.). New York: Pergamon Press.

Winton, P. J., & Turnbull, A. P. (1981). Parent involvement as viewed by parents of preschool handicapped children. In R. R. Fewell (Ed.), Families of handicapped children. *Topics in Early Childhood Special Education, 1,* 11-20.

Wisniewski, K., Howe, J., Williams, D. G., & Wisniewski, H. M. (1978). Precocious aging and dementia in patient's with Down's syndrome. *Biological Psychiatry, 13,* 619-627.

Witkin, H. A., Faterson, H. F., Goodenough, D. R., & Birnbaum, J. (1966). Cognitive patterning in mildly retarded boys. *Child Development, 37,* 301-316.

Witt, S. (1981). Increase in adaptive behavior level after residence in an intermediate care facility for mentally retarded persons. *Mental Retardation, 19,* 75-79.

Wittner, M. (1977). Toxoplasmosis. In A. M. Rudolph (Ed.), *Pediatrics.* New York: Appleton-Century-Crofts.

Wolf, J. M., & Anderson, R. M. (1969). *The multiply handicapped child.* Springfield, IL: Thomas.

Wolf, M. M., Birnbrauer, J., Lawler, J., & Williams, T. (1970). The operant, extinction, re-instatement, and re-extinction of vomiting behavior in a retarded child. In R. Ulrich, T. Stachik, & J. Mabry (Eds.), *Control of human behavior: From cure to prevention* (Vol. 2). Glenview, IL: Scott, Foresman.

Wolf, M. M., Risley, T., Johnson, M., Harris, F., & Allen, E. (1967). Application of operant conditioning procedures to the behavior problems of an autistic child. A follow-up and extension. *Behavior Research and Therapy, 5,* 103-111.

Wolfensberger, W. (1967). Counseling the parents of the retarded. In A. A. Baumeister (Ed.), *Mental retardation: Appraisal, education and rehabilitation.* Chicago: Aldine.

Wolfensberger, W. (1972a). *The principle of normalization in human services.* Toronto: National Institute on Mental Retardation.

Wolfensberger, W. (1972b). *Citizen advocacy for the handicapped, impaired, and disadvantaged: An overview.* Washington: Department of Health, Education, and Welfare, publication No. (OS) 72-42.

Wolfensberger, W. (1976). Reaction comment to advocacy. In M. Kindred, J. Cohen, D. Penrod, & T. Shaffer (Eds.), *The mentally retarded citizen and the law.* New York: Free Press.

Wolfensberger, W., & Glenn, L. (1975). *PASS 3: A method for the quantitative evaluation of human services.* Toronto: National Institute on Mental Retardation.

Wolfensberger, W., & Kurtz, R. A. (Eds.). (1969). *Management of the family of the mentally retarded.* Chicago: Follett.

Wolfesnberger, W., & Menolascino, F. J. (1970). A theoretical framework for the management of parents of the mentally retarded. In F. J. Menolascino (Ed.), *Psychiatric approaches to mental retardation.* New York: Basic Books.

Wood, J. W., Johnson, K. G., & Yoshiaki, O. (1967). In utero exposure to the Hiroshima atomic bomb. An evaluation of head size and mental retardation: Twenty years later. *Pediatrics, 39,* 385-392.

Woodward, M. (1963). The application of Piaget's theory to research in mental deficiency. In N. R. Ellis (Ed.), *Handbook of mental deficiency.* New York: McGraw-Hill.

Wright, H. T. (1971). Prenatal factors in causation. In R. Koch & J. Dobson (Eds.), *The mentally retarded child and his family: A multidisciplinary handbook* (pp. 70-72). New York: Brunner Mazel.

Wright, M. M., & Menolascino, F. J. (1966). Nurturant nursing of mentally retarded ruminators. *American Journal of Mental Deficiency, 71,* 451–459.

Wright, S. W., & Tarjan, G. (1957). Phenylketonuria. *American Journal of Diseases of Children, 93,* 405–419.

Wrightsman, L., Jr., (1962). The effects of anxiety, achievement motivation, and importance upon performance on an intelligence test. *Journal of Educational Psychology, 52,* 150–156.

Yando, R. M., & Zigler, E. (1971). Outerdirectedness in the problem-solving of institutionalized normal and retarded children. *Developmental Psychology, 4,* 277–288.

Yawkey, T. D. (1982). Effects of parents' play routines on imaginatve play in their developmentally delayed preschoolers. In S. G. Garwood (Ed.), Play and development, *Topics in Early Childhood Special Education, 2,* 66–75.

Yoder, D. E., & MIller, J. F. (1972). What we may know and what we can do: Input toward a system. In J. E. McLean, D. E. Yoder, & R. L. Schiefelbusch (Eds.), *Language intervention with the retarded: Developing strategies.* Baltimore: University Park Press.

Yoshida, R., MacMillan, D., & Meyers, C. (1976). The decertification of minority group EMR students in California: Its historical background and an assessment of student achievement and adjustment. In R. Jones (Ed.), *Mainstreaming the minority child.* Reston, VA: Council for Exceptional Children.

Yoshida, R. K., & Meyers, C. E. (1975). Effects of labeling as EMR on teachers' expectancies for change in a student's performance. *Journal of Educational Psychology, 67,* 521–527.

Young, P. T. (1961). *Motivation and emotion.* New York: Wiley.

Zackai, E., Mellman, M. J., Neiderer, B., & Hanson, J. W. (1975). The fetal trimethadione syndrome. *Journal of Pediatrics, 87,* 280–284.

Zaleski, W. A., Houston, C. S., Pozsonyi, J., & Ying, K. K. (1966). The XXXXY chromosome anomaly: Report of three new cases and review of 30 cases from the literature. *Canadian Medical Association Journal, 94,* 1143.

Zehr, M. D., & Theobald, D. E. (1978). Manual guidance used in a punishment procedure: The active ingredient in overcorrection. *Journal of Mental Deficiency Research, 22,* 263–272.

Zeigob, L., Alford, G., & House, A. (1978). Response suppressive and generalization effects of facial screening on multiple self-injurious behavior in a retarded boy. *Behavior Therapy, 9,* 688.

Zeigob, L., Becker, J., Jenkins, J., & Bristow, A. (1976). Facial screening: An analysis of clinical applicability. *Journal of Behavior Therapy and Experimental Psychiatry, 7,* 355–357.

Zelazo, P. R. (1972). Smiling and vocalizing: A cognitive emphasis. *Merrill-Palmer Quarterly, 18,* 349–365.

Zelazo, P. R. (1979). Reactivity to perceptual-cognitive events: Application for infant assessment. In R. B. Kearsley & I. E. Sigel (Eds.), *Infants at risk: Assessment of cognitive functioning.* Hillsdale, NJ: Erlbaum.

Zelazo, P. R., Hopkins, J. R., Jacobson, S. M., & Kagan, J. (1974). Psychological reactivity to discrepant events: Support for the curvilinear hypothesis. *Cognition, 2,* 385–393.

Zelazo, P. R., Kagan, J., & Hartmann, R. (1975). Excitement and boredom as determinants of vocalization of infants. *Journal of Genetic Psychology, 126,* 107–117.

Zellweger, H., & Abb, G. N. (1963). Chromosomal mosaicism and mongolism. *Lancet, 1,* 827.

Zigler, E. (1966). Research on personality structure in the retardate. In N. R. Ellis (Ed.), *International review of research in mental retardation* (Vol. 1). New York: Academic Press.

Zigler, E. (1967). Familial mental retardation: A continuing dilemma. *Science, 155,* 292–298.

Zigler, E., & Balla, D. (1971). Luria's verbal deficiency theory of mental retardation and performance on sameness, symmetry, and opposition tasks: A critique. *American Journal of Mental Deficiency, 75,* 400–413.

Zigler, E., & Balla, D. (1977). Impact of institutional experience on the behavior and development of retarded persons. *American Journal of Mental Deficiency, 82,* 1–12.

Zigler, E., & Butterfield, E. C. (1968). Motivational aspects of changes in IQ test performance of culturally deprived nursery school children. *Child Development, 39,* 1–14.

Zigler, E., & Muenchow, S. (1979). Mainstreaming: The proof is in the implementation. *American Psychologist, 34,* 993–996.

Zimmerman, B. J., & Rosenthal, T. L. (1974). Observational learning of rule-governed behavior by children. *Psychological Bulletin, 81,* 29–42.

Index